Abdominal and General Ultrasound

VOLUME 1

This volume is part of a self-contained two volume work entitled
Abdominal and General Ultrasound. Additionally, it forms an integral part of
CLINICAL ULTRASOUND a comprehensive text together with its companion
titles, *Ultrasound in Obstetrics and Gynaecology* and *Cardiac Ultrasound*, each of
which may also be purchased separately.

For Churchill Livingstone

Publisher: Simon Fathers
Project Editor: Clare Wood-Allum
Indexer: Michele Clarke
Production Control: Neil Dickson
Sales Promotion Executive: Caroline Boyd

For Longman Malaysia

Production Co-ordination: Shirley Kerk

CLINICAL ULTRASOUND a comprehensive text

Abdominal and General Ultrasound

VOLUME 1

Edited by

David Cosgrove MA MSc FRCR FRCP
Consultant in Nuclear Medicine and Ultrasound, Royal
Marsden Hospital, London, UK

Hylton Meire FRCR
Consultant Radiologist, King's College Hospital, London, UK

Keith Dewbury BSc MB BS FRCR
Consultant Radiologist and Honorary Senior Lecturer,
Southampton University Hospitals, Southampton, UK

Associate Editor: Pat Farrant DCRR DMU
Superintendent Research Sonographer, King's College
Hospital, London, UK

Foreword by

Barry B. Goldberg MD
Professor of Radiology, Director, Division of Diagnostic
Ultrasound, Thomas Jefferson University Hospital,
Philadelphia, Pennsylvania, USA

CHURCHILL LIVINGSTONE
EDINBURGH LONDON MADRID MELBOURNE NEW YORK AND TOKYO 1993

CHURCHILL LIVINGSTONE
Medical Division of Longman Group UK Limited

Distributed in the United States of America by Churchill
Livingstone Inc., 650 Avenue of the Americas, New York,
N.Y. 10011, and by associated companies, branches and
representatives throughout the world.

First published 1993

ISBN 0-443-04277-2

British Library Cataloguing in Publication Data
A catalogue record for this book is available from the
British Library.

Library of Congress Cataloging in Publication Data
A catalog record for this book is available from the Library
of Congress.

The
publisher's
policy is to use
**paper manufactured
from sustainable forests**

Printed and bound in Great Britain by
William Clowes Limited, Beccles and London

Foreword

There has been rapid progress in the development of ultrasound almost since its beginnings in the late 1940s. However, it was not until the mid 1970s with the development of gray scale and real time ultrasound that it became an accepted clinical procedure. In the 1980s, with the development of color Doppler as well as the miniaturization of transducers allowing for the development of a variety of endoluminal transducers, its worldwide acceptance expanded exponentially.

In the past few years, the revenue generated from ultrasound equipment sales has exceeded that of all other imaging modalities, including magnetic resonance imaging. With this rapid expansion of ultrasound in a variety of areas throughout the world, the need for education has also expanded. No matter how good the equipment purchased and the number of transducers employed, the key for the success of ultrasound diagnosis and improved patient care depends on the abilities of the individual physicians and sonographers who use this technique. This series of books covering all of ultrasound, not only the major areas such as the abdomen, echocardiography, and obstetrics and gynecology, but also newly developed and more novel uses, makes an important contribution to raising the standards of knowledge in this field.

Chapters from a diverse group of contributors, recognized for their expertise, have been coordinated by the editors into a comprehensive text that meets the needs of those individuals wishing to have a complete knowledge of the current usefulness of ultrasound in medicine. Used as a complete compendium or as individual books on specific areas of interest, this work should become a standard in every ultrasound library throughout the world. It should prove of value not only to those experienced in ultrasound, both physicians and non-physicians, but also to students wishing to obtain an in-depth knowledge of the multiple uses of ultrasound. I extend my congratulations on this unique accomplishment to the editors as well as to the many contributors to this well illustrated and referenced text.

B.B.G.

Preface

Most textbooks, at least in the field of diagnostic imaging, stem from the wish of the authors or editors to make their special expertise more widely available. The origin of *Clinical Ultrasound* is rather unusual in that it is a response to a proposal by the publishers, Churchill Livingstone, that the time was right for a comprehensive ultrasound textbook with a strong clinical content.

At first approach, we have to confess to having been sceptical of the need for such a textbook and we were most reluctant to embark on such a monumental task but, as we began to review the field, it was possible to envisage it being broken down into more manageable components. It was also clear that there really was no comprehensive textbook on the market, all of the available books concentrating on a particular application or body region.

An initial hurdle was to secure the editorship of Dr Peter Wilde to oversee the cardiology section; initially Peter was as reluctant as the rest of us, having heavy commitments on his hands but, fired by the prospect of a comprehensive and strongly clinical reference work, he was persuaded. The Cardiology section has been completely under his editorship, though it adheres to the general format and goals of the entire book.

For the remaining large sections, a decisive influence in our agreeing to proceed was the fact that Pat Farrant was enthusiastic, something she may have come to regret as time went by! Pat agreed to take control of the massive task of handling all of the editing and advising that underlay the organising of the extensive text and innumerable figures together with their orientation diagrams,[1] keeping track of where alterations had to be entered, checking that tables referred to in the text were, in fact, contained in the chapter or appendix and generally managing the entire process of creation and collation which extended to double the 18 months that we had originally anticipated. However, that was not all for, as we got further into the project, Pat was also called upon to contribute large portions of chap-

ters that had somehow fallen by the wayside and her input into almost every section has been absolutely invaluable. It was in the knowledge that she would give this kind of support that we entered the 'battle'. None of us foresaw just how protracted a battle it would become nor how large Pat's contribution would turn out to be – 'siege' would have been a more apposite term!

We would also like to thank our families and friends who have borne with us during the past three stressful years. Special thanks are due to Christine Dewbury and Gill Meire for their continuing support and encouragement, and for hosting so many editorial meetings.

From this explanation, our intentions should be clear. We have aimed to provide an up-to-date textbook on clinical diagnostic ultrasound that would cover the entire gamut of its applications, both imaging and Doppler. Because of its clinical basis, the physics of ultrasound does not feature as a formal topic, though its important practical consequences and implications, especially in newer, less familiar areas such as Doppler, are covered.

Diagnostic ultrasound has become so extensive that, inevitably, this had to be a large book and a small team of specialists could not hope to cover the entire field. Therefore, we commissioned a large number of contributing authors from Europe and the Americas, most well known experts in their own areas. We stand to lose friends however, because we have exercised strong editing rights in the interests of maintaining a uniform style – we hope our loyal contributors will feel that our sometimes heavy alterations have contributed to the overall quality of the book and will not take offence that we have freely altered their prose and even sometimes substituted scans that seemed clearer or that made the intended point better.

With respect to the division of material through the book, the separation of Cardiology from the other applications already referred to, made it obvious that this should form a separate volume that is available on its own. Obstetrics and Gynaecology formed a second distinct section and so we have arranged that this also be a separate volume with its own page numbering and index. The other

---

[1] Actually there are approximately 3000 figures and 500 tables!

two volumes, which contain the remaining applications (abdominal, small parts, vascular, miscellaneous), are offered together as two sections of a single book: the pages are numbered through and they are indexed together in the expectation that few users will need only one of the pair.

We hope that *Clinical Ultrasound* will become a reference work for all who use ultrasound in their clinical practice and that users will find in it comprehensive answers to their everyday needs. It should provide critical information in a form that is easy to look up, as well as form the basis for specialist training.

1992

H.M.
D.C.
K.D.

Terminology and scan position indicators

The aim of this book is to serve both as a reference text and as an aid to education and teaching. During the editorial process it was clear to us that the terminology used to describe ultrasound appearances is extremely diverse, confusing and occasionally inaccurate. We have therefore unified the terminology in *Clinical Ultrasound*. In doing this we have considered the two main interactions between the ultrasound beam and the tissue; namely reflection and attenuation.

Meaningless terms such as 'sonolucent' and 'echo dense' have been eradicated. We also considered the use of the prefixes 'hyper-' and 'hypo-' a source of confusion and found several instances where the secretaries typing the manuscripts had confused the two.

Where backscattered amplitude is being discussed the ultrasound appearances are described as of reduced, normal or increased reflectivity (by inference compared with that which would normally be expected).

The above features of *Clinical Ultrasound* have been incorporated in an attempt to make these volumes more valuable and easier to understand, and it is hoped that the terminology we have used will encourage readers to consider more carefully the terminology they use to describe their own ultrasound findings.

The relatively small field of view of modern ultrasound scanners, and the infinitely variable planes of imaging, sometimes lead to difficulties in interpreting the anatomy and orientation of an ultrasound image. Rather than using extensive free narrative to describe the positions from which images have been obtained we have used a system of body markers on which the position of the scans has been indicated. When referring to these the reader should be aware that the scans indicating a lateral area of contact do not necessarily imply that the patient was moved into an oblique or decubitus position but simply that the transducer was located on the lateral aspect of the patient.

The orientation of the conventional extracavitory images included in this book has generally been adjusted such that longitudinal scans are viewed as if from the patient's right side and transverse scans as if from the patient's feet. Unfortunately there is no standardisation for the orientation of intracavitory images and, in general, these have been displayed with the orientation unaltered from that supplied by the individual authors. We have not attempted to identify the position of the transducer or the orientation of the image for intracavitory scans as these should be clear from the accompanying text in each case.

1992

H.M.
D.C.
K.D.

Contributors to Abdominal and General Ultrasound

Paul L. Allan BSc MB BS DMRD FRCPE FRCR
Senior Lecturer, Department of Medical Radiology,
University of Edinburgh; Honorary Consultant
Radiologist, Royal Infirmary, Edinburgh, UK

Mary Y. Anthony MB BS DCH MRCP
Lecturer in Paediatrics, Academic Unit of Paediatrics,
Leeds General Infirmary, UK

Jeffrey C. Bamber MSc PhD
Lecturer in Physics as Applied to Medicine, Institute of
Cancer Research, Royal Marsden Hospital, Sutton,
Surrey, UK

Luigi Barbara MD
Professor of Medicine and Head of Department of
Internal Medicine and Gastroenterology, University of
Bologna, Italy

Jane Bates DCR DMU
Superintendent Sonographer, St James's University
Hospital, Leeds, UK

Roland Blackwell BSc MSc FIEE FInstP FIPSM
Chief Physicist, The Middlesex Hospital, London, UK

Luigi Bolondi MD
Associate Professor, University of Bologna, Italy

Maria Chiara Bossi MD
Senior Registrar, Radiology Department, Ospedale San
Paolo, Milan, Italy

David O. Cosgrove MA MSc FRCR FRCP
Consultant in Nuclear Medicine and Ultrasound, Royal
Marsden Hospital, London, UK

Fausto Croce MD
Department of Radiology, Civil Hospital, Busto Arsizio
(VA) Italy

A. N. Dardenne MD
Associate Professor, Université Catholique de Louvain;
Chief, Uroradiology and Ultrasound Section,
Department of Radiology and Diagnostic Imaging,
Saint-Luc University Hospital, Brussels, Belgium

Michel M. J. Dauzat MD
Maitre de Conférences des Universités, Faculté de
Médecin de Montpellier; Praticien des Hopitaux, Unité
d'Exploration Vasculaire, Centre Hospitalier
Universitaire, Nîmes, France

Jean-Michel de Bray MD
Neurologist and Physiologist, Vascular Investigations
Department, Centre Hospitalier Universitaire, Angers,
France

Rose de Bruyn MB BCh DMRD FRCR
Consultant Paediatric Radiologist, The Hospitals for
Sick Children, London, UK

Ghislaine Deklunder MD
Maître de Conférences de Physiologie; Praticien
Hospitalier du Service Explorations Fonctionnelles
Cardiovasculaires, Centre Hospitalier Régional
Universitaire de Lille, France

Lorenzo E. Derchi MD
Radiologist, Instituto di Radiologia Dell Universita,
Ospedale S. Martino, Genova, Italy

Keith C. Dewbury BSc MB BS FRCR
Consultant Radiologist and Honorary Senior Lecturer,
Southampton University Hospitals, Southampton, UK

Claire Dicks-Mireaux BA MB BS MRCP FRCR
Consultant Radiologist, The Hospitals for Sick Children,
London, UK

Paul A. Dubbins MB BS BSc FRCR
Consultant Radiologist, Plymouth General Hospital,
Plymouth, UK

Pat Farrant DCRR DMU
Superintendent Research Sonographer, X-Ray
Department, King's College Hospital, London, UK

John A. Fielding MB ChB FRCR DMRD
Consultant Radiologist, Department of Radiology, Royal
Shrewsbury Hospital, Shrewsbury, UK

Christopher D. R. Flower MA FRCP(C) FRCR
Consultant Radiologist, Addenbrookes Hospital,
Cambridge, UK

Bruno Fornage MD
Professor of Radiology and Chief, Section of
Ultrasound, The University of Texas, M.D. Anderson
Cancer Center, Houston, USA

Richard Fowler MB BS MRCP DMRD FRCR
Consultant Radiologist, The General Infirmary, Leeds;
Senior Clinical Tutor, University of Leeds, UK

Stefano Gaiani MD
Registrar, Department of Internal Medicine, University
of Bologna, Italy

Steven Garber BSc MB BS MRCP FRCR
Senior Registrar in Radiology, The Middlesex Hospital,
London, UK

Anders Glenthøj MD
Chief Pathologist, Centralsygehuset Hillerød, Hillerød,
Denmark

Peter B. Guyer DM MS FRCP FRCR DMRD
Consultant Radiologist and Honorary Senior Lecturer,
Southampton University Hospitals, Southampton, UK

Christopher R. Hill BA PhD DSc FIEE FInstP HonFRCR
Professor of Physics as Applied to Medicine, Institute of
Cancer Research and Royal Marsden Hospital
(University of London), Sutton, UK

Hans Henrik Holm MD PhD
Professor and Head, Department of Ultrasound, and
Chief Surgeon, Department of Urology, Herlev
Hospital, University of Copenhagen, Denmark

Henry C. Irving MB BS DMRD FRCR
Consultant Radiologist, St James's University Hospital,
Leeds, UK

Charles Janbon MD
Professeur des Universités, Service de Médicine Interne
B. et Angiologie, Hôpital St Eloi, Montpellier, France

Tim Jaspan MB ChB BSc MRCP FRCR
Consultant Neuroradiologist, University Hospital,
Nottingham, UK

Anton E. Joseph MSc FRCR
Consultant Radiologist, Head of Ultrasound and Nuclear
Medicine, St George's Hospital, London, UK

Steen Karstrup MD
Department of Diagnostic Radiology, Herlev Hospital,
University of Copenhagen, Denmark

Ian J. Kenney BSc MB ChB DMRD FRCR
Consultant Paediatric Radiologist, Royal Alexandra
Hospital for Sick Children, Brighton, UK

Jean-Pierre Laroche MD
Consultant Angiologist to University Hospital
Montpellier, Nîmes, France

William R. Lees FRCR
Consultant Radiologist, The Middlesex Hospital,
London, UK

Malcolm I. Levene MD FRCP
Professor of Paediatrics and Head of Academic Unit of
Paediatrics and Child Health, Leeds General Infirmary,
Leeds, UK

Caroline Lewis MRCP FRCR
Senior Registrar, Department of Radiology, St George's
Hospital, London, UK

David J. Lomas MA MRCP FRCR
Honorary Senior Registrar, Department of Radiology,
Addenbrookes Hospital, Cambridge; Clinical Lecturer,
University of Cambridge, UK

François-Michel Lopez MD
Professeur de Radiologie, Faculté de Montpellier-Nîmes;
Chef de Service du Département d'Imagerie Médicale,
CHU Nîmes, France

Lesley M. MacDonald MB BS DMRD FRCR
Consultant Radiologist, St Thomas' Hospital, London,
UK

Hylton B. Meire FRCR
Consultant Radiologist, King's College Hospital,
London, UK

Paula Murphy MB BCh MRCPI FFR(RCSi) FRCR
Consultant Cardiovascular Radiologist, Bristol Royal
Infirmary, Bristol, UK

Renato Nessi MD
Associate Professor of Radiology, University of Milan,
Italy

Christian Nolsøe MD
Associate Professor, Department of Ultrasound, Herlev
Hospital, University of Copenhagen, Denmark

Jan Fog Pedersen MD PhD
Head of Ultrasound Laboratory, Department of
Radiology, Glostrup Hospital, University of
Copenhagen, Denmark

Graham R. Plant MB BS FRCR
Consultant Radiologist, Basingstoke Hospital,
Basingstoke, UK

J. B. C. M. Puylaert MD PhD
Radiologist, Westeinde Hospital, The Hague,
Netherlands

David Rickards FRCR FFRDSA
Consultant Radiologist, The Middlesex Hospital and the
St Peter's Institute of Urology, London, UK

Andrew J. S. Saunders FRCR FRCP
Consultant Radiologist, Guy's Hospital, London, UK

Sally T. Scott MB BS(Hons) DMRD FRCR
Consultant Radiologist, West Dorset General Hospitals
NHS Trust, West Dorset Hospital, Dorchester, UK

Philip J. Shorvon MA(Cantab) MB BS MRCP FRCR
Director of Radiology, Central Middlesex Hospital,
London, UK

Luigi Solbiati MD
Department of Radiology, Civil Hospital, Busto Arsizio
(VA), Italy

Gail ter Haar MA(Oxon) MSc PhD
Team Leader, Therapeutic Ultrasound, Physics
Department, Royal Marsden Hospital, Sutton, UK

Søren Tobias Torp-Pedersen MD
Head, Department of Ultrasound, Herlev Hospital,
University of Copenhagen, Denmark

Judith A. W. Webb BSc MD FRCP FRCR
Consultant Radiologist, St Bartholomew's Hospital,
London, UK

David J. Wilson MB BS BSc MRCP FRCR
Consultant Radiologist, Nuffield Orthopaedic Centre,
Oxford; Clinical Lecturer, University of Oxford, UK

John P. Woodcock PhD FInstP
Director of Medical Physics Services, South Glamorgan
Health Authority; Professor of Bioengineering,
University of Wales College of Medicine, Cardiff, Wales

Contents

VOLUME 2

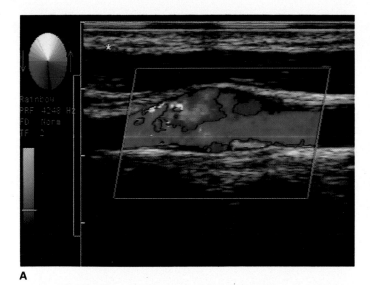

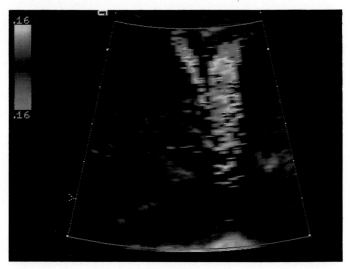

Plate 2   Pixels in the colour image. The pixels within CDI images are much larger than those in grey scale imaging and therefore give rise to jagged vessel margins and usually lead to inappropriately wide display of narrow vessels. This image has been magnified to demonstrate this.

A

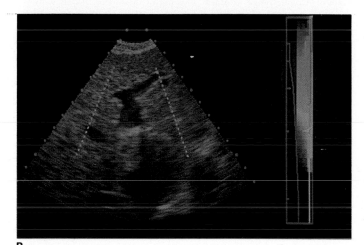

B

Plate 1   Physiological vortices. A: Longitudinal scan of the carotid bulb. Complex vortices (red) are present due to boundary layer separation. This is a normal flow characteristic. **B:** Transverse scan of the left portal vein. The CDI sensitivity has been reduced to show only the highest velocity flow which can be seen to follow a spiral course through this vessel (compare with Fig. 7B).

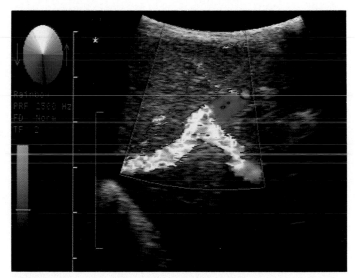

Plate 3   Mosaic artefact due to aliasing. The flow velocity in this patent ductus venosus exceeds the aliasing limit giving rise to the mosaic artefact. Normal velocity flow within the left branch of the portal vein gives rise to a correctly coded blue signal.

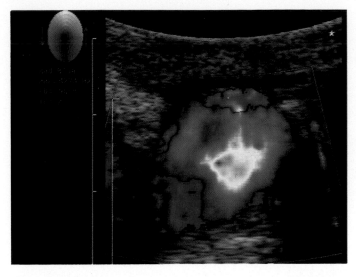

Vol. 1, Ch. 5

Plate 4 Apparent flow reversal due to aliasing. In this transverse scan of a large vein in which there is parabolic flow the flow velocity in the centre of the vessel exceeds the aliasing limit. The coding passes from blue through white to red without a break indicating that this is true aliasing.

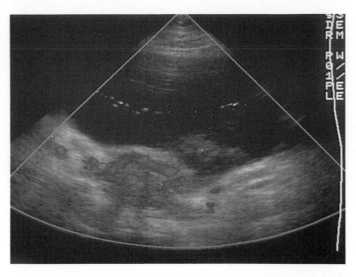

Vol. 1, Ch. 5

Plate 6 Colour range artefact. Imaging of these deep vessels within the pelvis required a low PRF. In order to overcome aliasing the PRF has been increased and has resulted in range ambiguities giving rise to artefactual colour signals within the bladder.

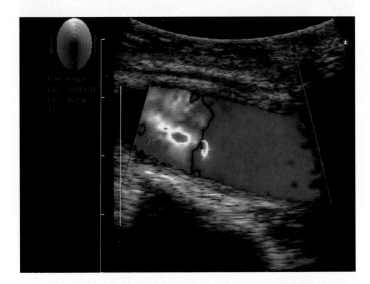

Vol. 1, Ch. 5

Plate 5 True flow reversal. Same case as Plate 4, longitudinal scan. There is a small area of aliasing within the red flow segment. The radial orientation of the imaging pulses arising from this curvilinear array gives rise to flow effectively towards the transducer in the red segment of the vessel and away from the transducer in the blue segment. At the point where the flow is at right angles to the beams there is a small black gap between the red and blue segments confirming true flow reversal at this point.

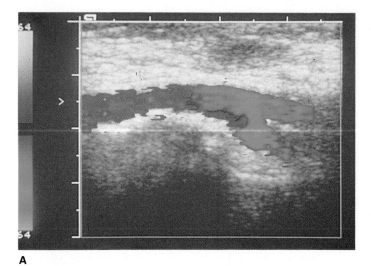

A

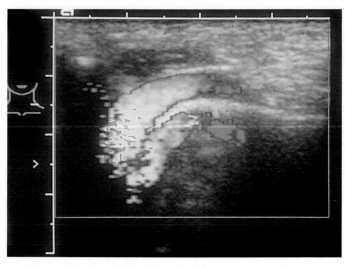

Vol. 1, Ch. 5
Plate 8 Mirror artefact. The subclavian artery has been imaged as it curves over the apex of the lung. The lung surface acts as a specular reflector and gives rise to a mirror image artefact with an apparent duplicate vessel lying beneath the lung surface.

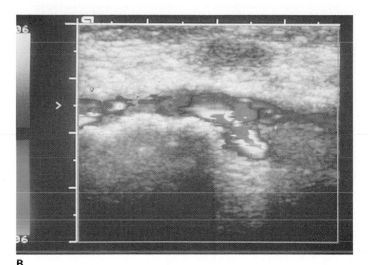

B

Vol. 1, Ch. 5
Plate 7 Aliasing and its correction. A: The axillary artery has been examined with an inappropriate velocity range and consequent low PRF. The colour flow image is corrupted by aliasing. **B:** The velocity range, and therefore PRF, have been markedly increased to overcome the aliasing. Note the apparent change in flow direction similar to that seen in Plate 5, in this case due to a curved vessel imaged with a straight linear array.

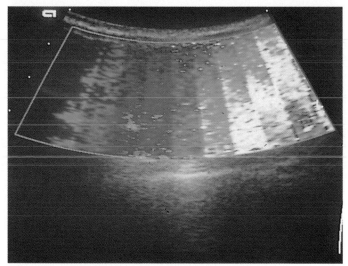

Vol. 1, Ch. 5
Plate 9 Frame rate artefact. Scan obtained during rapid backwards and forwards longitudinal movement of the transducer. The separate blocks of colour demonstrate the way in which the colour information is obtained during time blocks, each of which may be relatively long if a low frame rate is in use.

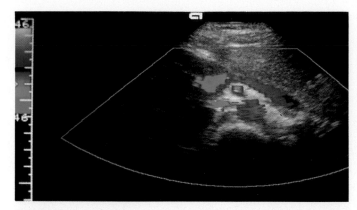

Vol. 1, Ch. 8
Plate 1   Normal peripancreatic vessels. The aorta, SMA and IVC are seen in transverse section with the splenic vein and proximal portal vein crossing transversely anterior to the SMA.

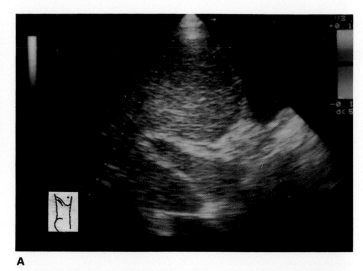

A

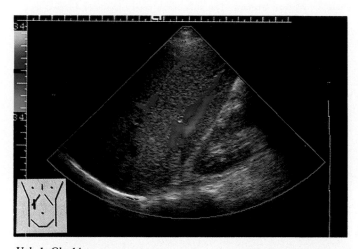

Vol. 1, Ch. 14
Plate 1   Colour Doppler of the right lobe of the liver. The flow in the main portal vein is shown as a red colour because it runs towards the transducer; whereas the flow in the hepatic vein is coded as blue because it is away from the transducer.

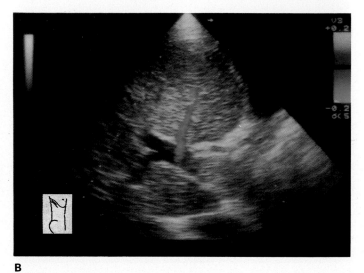

B

Vol. 1, Ch. 17
Plate 1   Tumour involvement of the portal vein. A: Though solid tissue completely fills the vessel's lumen, colour flow mapping displays a little hepatopetal flow. **B:** A portal vein branch shows reversed flow.

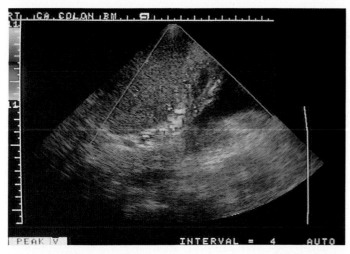

Vol. 1, Ch. 19
Plate 1 Colour Doppler scan showing portal collaterals in the gallbladder wall.

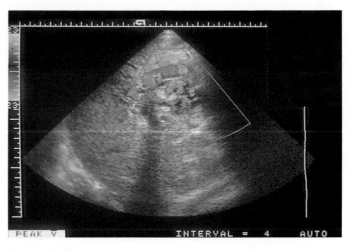

Vol. 1, Ch. 19
Plate 3 Cavernous transformation of the portal vein. Colour Doppler demonstrates blood flowing in small collaterals.

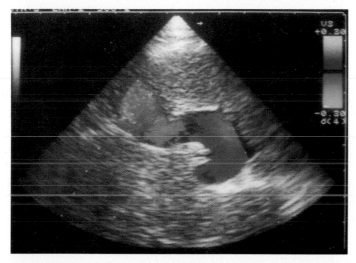

Vol. 1, Ch. 19
Plate 2 Colour flow mapping of a dilated and tortuous intrahepatic portal branch in a patient with portal hypertension. Flow is represented in red (towards the probe) or blue (away from the probe) depending on the vessel direction with respect to the ultrasound beam.

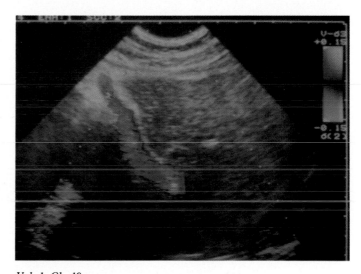

Vol. 1, Ch. 19
Plate 4 Colour Doppler of the umbilical vein. The red colour indicates flow towards the transducer (hepatofugal).

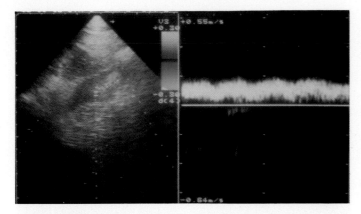

Vol. 1, Ch. 19
Plate 5 Budd-Chiari syndrome. Colour Doppler ultrasound of the inferior vena cava shows reversed (red) and continuous flow (arrow).

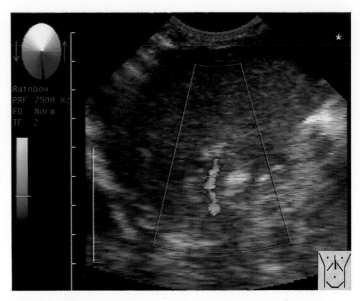

Vol. 1, Ch. 20
Plate 1 Arterial signal in portal vein occlusion. There is a strong forward flow signal in the region of the porta hepatis. This is due to continuous high velocity flow in the hepatic artery in the absence of portal vein flow.

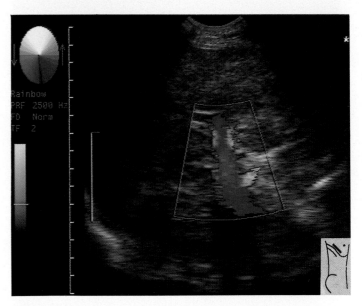

Vol. 1, Ch. 20
Plate 2 Colour Doppler detection of the hepatic artery. The colour map velocity coding has been adjusted to highlight the higher systolic velocities in the artery as orange against the slower red portal vein flow.

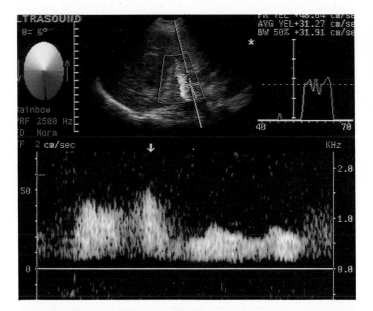

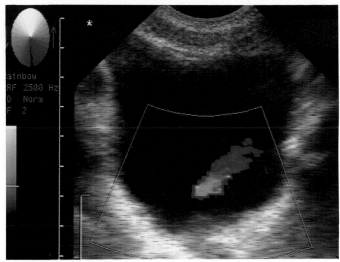

Plate 3 Low velocity arterial flow. The high velocity flow within the portal vein prevented identification of the artery on the colour flow image. Spectral Doppler studies reveal the presence of a low velocity arterial signal adjacent to the high velocity venous signal.

Plate 1 Colour flow imaging of ureteral jets. Sagittal colour Doppler scan of the full bladder. Urine is seen jetting into the bladder.

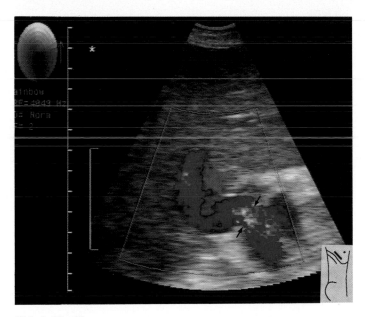

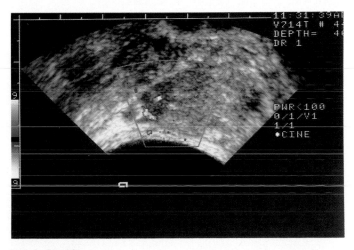

Plate 2 Transverse axial prostate ultrasound showing an echo-poor area in the right peripheral zone associated with increased blood flow on colour Doppler. The two features together make the diagnosis of carcinoma very much more probable.

Plate 4 Post-transplant portal vein study. There is a mild narrowing at the anastomosis (arrows) with a moderately high velocity jet through the anastomosis (coded yellow). Within the intrahepatic portal vein there is a coarse vortex, the reverse flow component is coded purple.

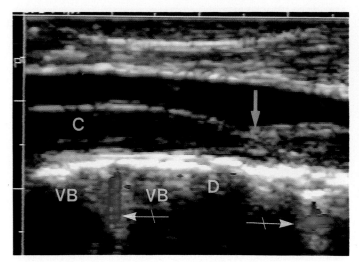

Plate 1 Sagittal IOSU in a 36-year-old woman with a 2 year history of mild spastic paraparesis. The spinal cord (arrow) is tethered to a focal defect of the dura. Note the normal basivertebral veins (hatched arrows) within the vertebral bodies (VB). Further images demonstrated their continuity with the anterior longitudinal spinal veins. C – spinal cord, D – intervertebral disc.

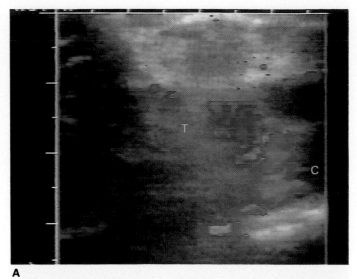

A

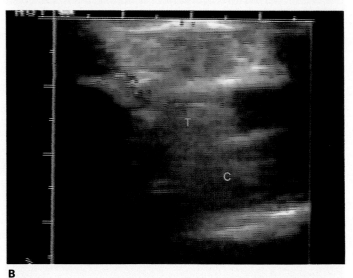

B

Plate 3 CSF flow. Same patient as in Figure 10. Sagittal plane colour Doppler imaging demonstrates pulsed CSF flow in a caudad direction **A:** during systole (encoded red, with some of the flow directed ventrocephalad accounting for part of the jet transforming to blue) and **B:** cephalad flow (blue) during diastole. T – cerebellar tonsil, C – spinal cord.

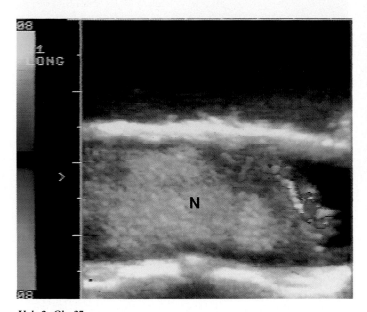

Plate 2 Neurofibroma. Same case as Figures 4 and 6. Colour Doppler imaging demonstrates surface vessels at the caudal extremity of the intradural neurofibroma (N).

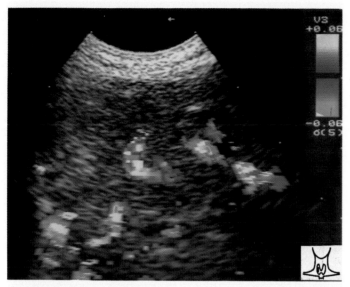

Plate 1 Large toxic adenoma,
isoreflective and hypervascular.

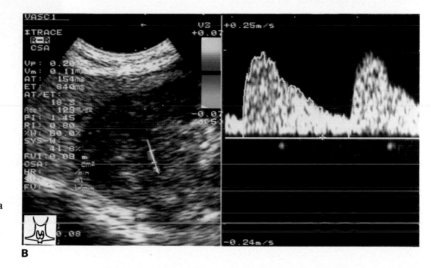

A

B

Plate 2 Benign and malignant thyroid masses. Same
patients as Figure 13B and D. **A:** With colour Doppler
flow is confined to the halo. This was a follicular adenoma
at pathological examination. **B:** There is flow within the
lesion and there are arterial signals with high systolic
peaks. This was a papillary cancer.

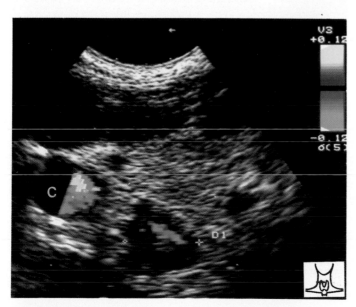

Plate 3 A small parathyroid carcinoma with internal vascular
signals. Ultrasound differentiation from a benign mass is impossible.
C – carotid artery.

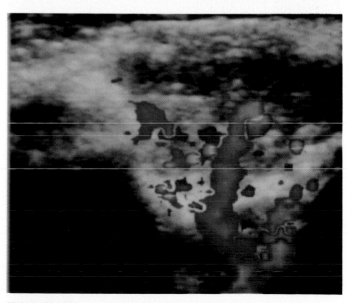

Plate 4 Neck haemangioma with significant colour flow signals.
(Figure courtesy of Dr D. O. Cosgrove.)

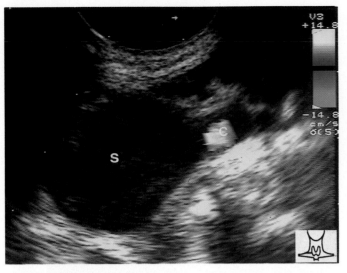

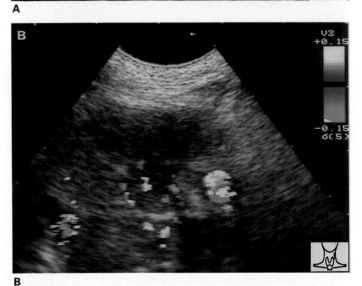

Vol. 2, Ch. 39
Plate 5 25 mm Schwannoma (S) of the neck, close to the carotid artery (C). No flow signals are detected.

Vol. 2, Ch. 39
Plate 6 35 mm chemodectoma of the carotid body. The carotid artery is seen crossing the tumour (**A**) which shows intense flow signals (**B**).

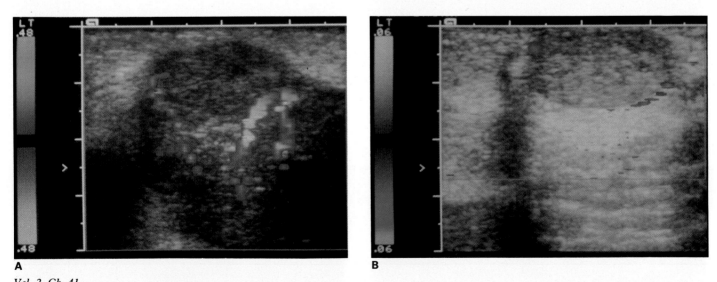

Vol. 2, Ch. 41
Plate 1 Colour Doppler in breast lesions. The neovascularity typical of breast carcinomas can usually be demonstrated on colour Doppler as tortuous vessels in and around the lesion (**A**) whereas no vessels can be demonstrated in fibroadenomas (**B**) unless they are large or of the juvenile type. Regions of benign mammary change, even when focal (**C**), are also devoid of signals.

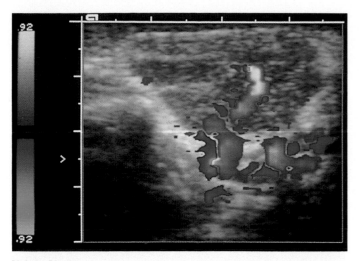

Vol. 2, Ch. 47
Plate 1   Haemangioma of the neck. Several tortuous vessels are seen supplying this apparently solid tumour. Note the relative lack of vessels within the lesion, many haemangiomas show surprisingly little intrinsic flow. The size of the vessels is exaggerated in this image due to 'colour capture' over a period of 4 seconds.

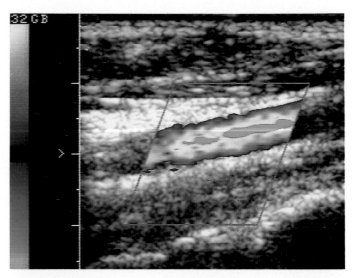

Vol. 2, Ch. 48
Plate 1   Colour Doppler image of a normal common carotid artery. This image has been captured during peak systole. There is high velocity flow in the centre of the vessel (aliased to green) with decreasing velocities towards the vessel wall indicating a parabolic velocity profile.

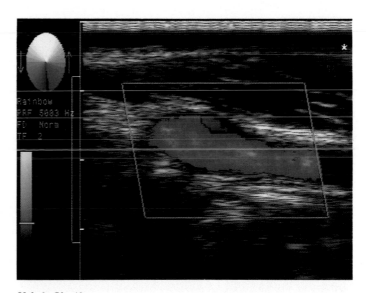

Vol. 2, Ch. 48
Plate 2   Colour Doppler image of a normal carotid bulb. Boundary layer separation has given rise to a small area of flow reversal (blue) within the bulb.

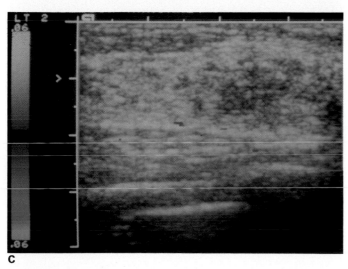

C

Vol. 2, Ch. 41
Plate 1 (see opposite for caption)

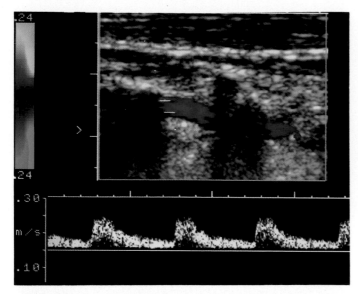

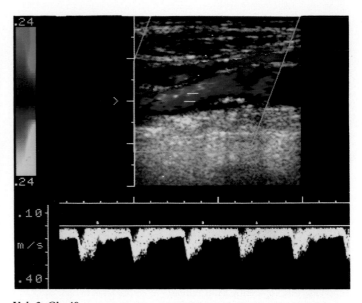

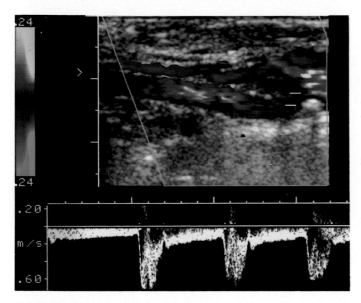

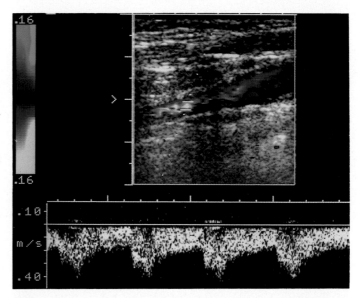

Vol. 2, Ch. 48
Plate 3 Colour coded Doppler imaging of the second (V2) part of the vertebral artery, between the transverse processes, in a normal subject.

Vol. 2, Ch. 48
Plate 5 Colour coded Doppler imaging of the internal carotid artery. There is no significant blood flow disturbance around and downstream from this partly calcified plaque with a smooth surface.

Vol. 2, Ch. 48
Plate 4 Colour coded Doppler imaging of a stenosis of the origin of the vertebral artery. A branch artery and the vertebral vein are also seen.

Vol. 2, Ch. 48
Plate 6 Colour coded Doppler imaging of a moderate carotid artery stenosis.

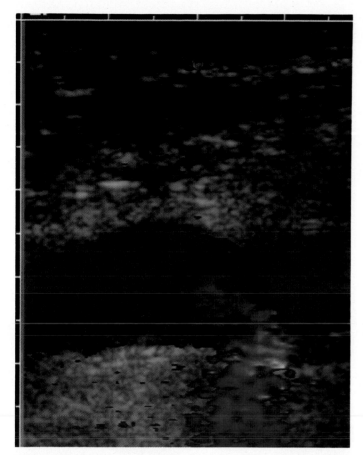

Vol. 2, Ch. 49
Plate 1   Colour flow image of the normal common, superficial and deep femoral veins (see Fig. 20).

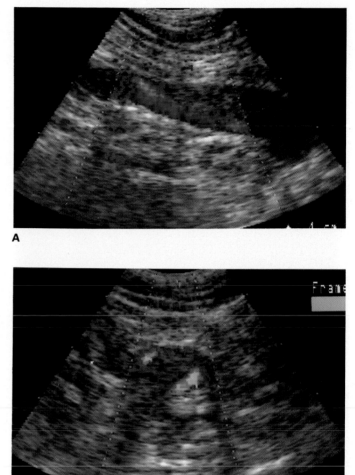

A

B

Vol. 2, Ch. 49
Plate 2   Colour coded Doppler image of a moderately reflective thrombus incompletely obstructing the lumen of the superficial femoral vein in **A:** longitudinal and **B:** transverse sections.

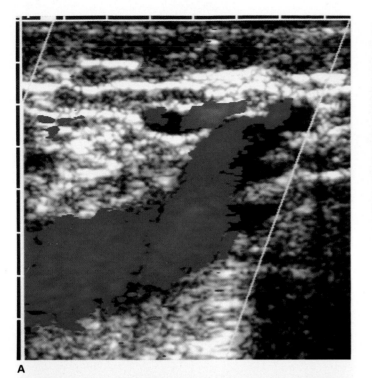

A

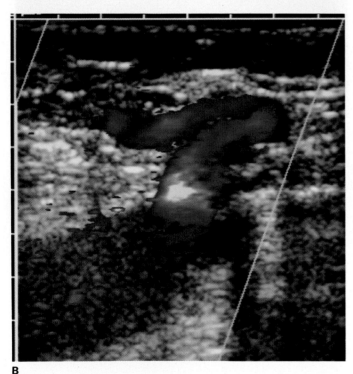

B

Plate 3 Internal saphenous vein. A: Normal blood flow during quiet respiration and **B:** venous reflux in the internal saphenous vein during the Valsalva manoeuvre.

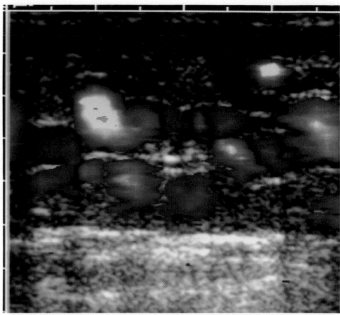

Plate 4 Varicose veins in the calf. Colour Doppler image of a large varicose network in the calf.

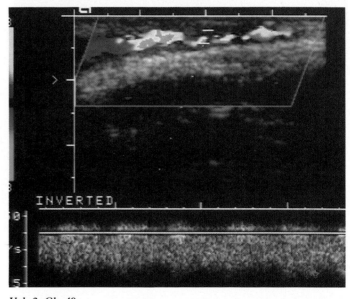

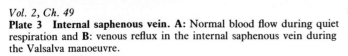

Plate 5 Arteriovenous fistula. Colour Doppler image and Doppler spectrum of the efferent vein of an arteriovenous fistula for haemodialysis (longitudinal section).

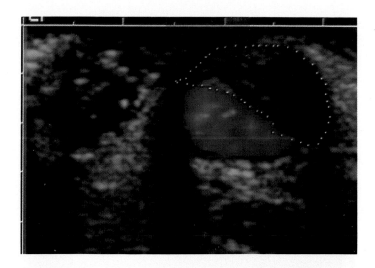

Vol. 2, Ch. 49
Plate 6   Colour Doppler image of a partial thrombosis in the efferent vein of an arteriovenous fistula for haemodialysis (transverse section).

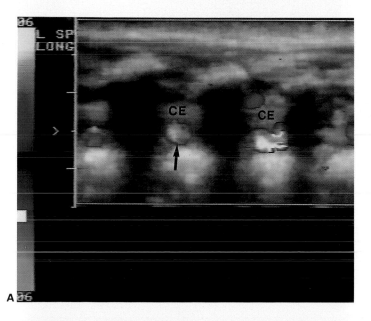

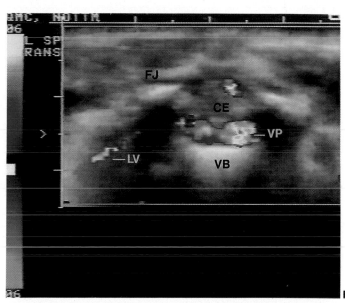

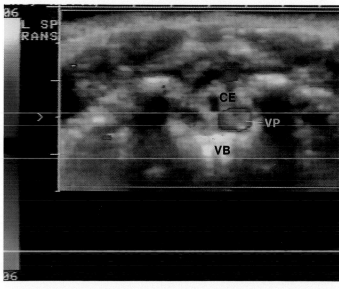

Vol. 2, Ch. 53
Plate 1   Vascular anomaly. Colour Doppler images of the lumbar spine. **A:** Sagittal scan. Large veins are identified in the anterior epidural space (arrow) and within the thecal sac (arrowhead). CE – cauda equina. **B:** Transverse scan at L3/4. VP – venous plexus, FJ – facet joint, LV – lumbar vein, VB – vertebral body. **C:** Transverse scan at L2.

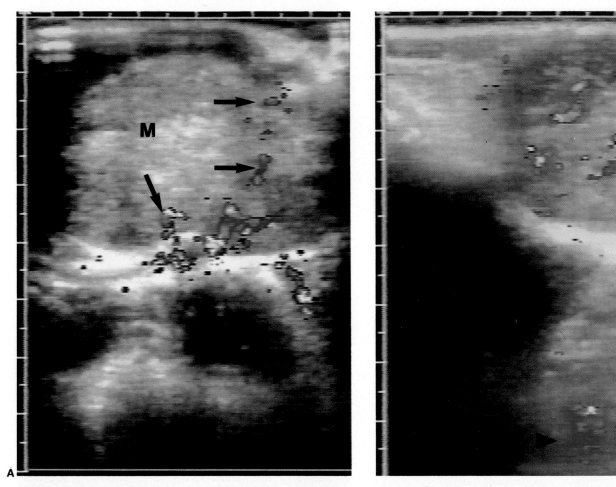

Vol. 2, Ch. 53
Plate 2 Vascular sacrococcygeal tumour. A: Transverse and **B**: sagittal colour Doppler images demonstrate prominent tumour vessels (arrows) within the mass (M) suggestive of an aggressive lesion. A very vascular tumour was macroscopically totally excised, histology confirming a highly malignant embryonic tumour. Widespread metastatic disease developed 2 months after resection of the mass. An iliac vessel is intersected on the sagittal scan (arrowhead).

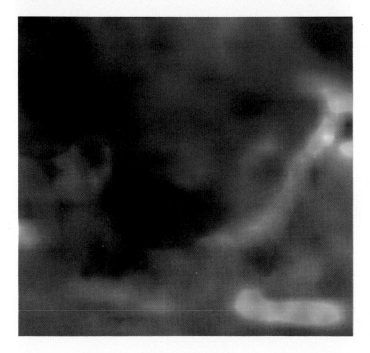

Vol. 2, Ch. 57
Plate 1 Colour coded tissue segmentation. Using an in vitro measuring scanner, quantitative images of ultrasound velocity, attenuation and reflectivity of a 3 cm × 3 cm block of liver tissue were obtained. The liver was fatty and contained a metastatic deposit from a soft tissue sarcoma. The three measurements were coded in red, green and blue respectively and combined to form a 'parametric image' in which the metastasis is displayed as purple (top left) and the fatty liver as brownish yellow. The margin between the tumour and the liver is seen as a bright line, as are vessels. This type of composite image, which is akin to colour Doppler, codes complex information in a readily assimilated form and may be the most useful way to display the large amounts of data that tissue characterisation systems can offer. (Refs 54 and 55.)

History – now and then

Christopher R. Hill

'History is bunk' – but we can learn from it

Although Henry Ford's famous dictum may be unpopular with professional historians, it finds some justification in the field of investigative ultrasound, whose history includes a considerable mixture of unrecognised achievements and ill-founded ideas. The story is none the less a fascinating one for its own sake and has been recorded by several authors in more detail than present space allows,[1-4] as well as in a useful bibliography of the early literature.[5]

In this chapter we shall look particularly at the development of ideas in the field. The present 'received wisdom' has arisen, on the one hand from some remarkable pioneering work, often carried out in the teeth of professional scepticism, and sometimes even derision, but also from a number of misjudgements and failures of scientific understanding, some of which may still influence current practice and inhibit its effective advance. To learn useful lessons from history one needs, like Henry Ford, to be on the look-out for 'bunk' dressed up for purposes of self justification.

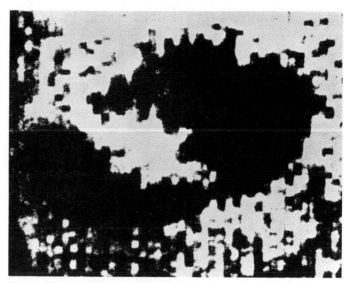

Fig. 1 Ultrasound transmission scan ('radiograph') of the human head published by the Dussik brothers[7] in 1942. Hindsight would indicate however that the image owes more to artefact than to anatomy (see text).

Origins of the concepts and technology behind investigative ultrasound

Concepts

The dream of being able to explore the living anatomy of the human body must go back at least to the days of the great anatomists, exemplified by the work of Vesalius in the 16th Century. The practical means for achieving this non-invasively were of course lacking until recently but the general concept may have arisen, if only subconsciously, as witness the words of Thomas Hardy (in 'The Return of the Native', published in 1878 and thus contemporary with Rayleigh, the great theoretician of acoustics): 'Compound utterances address themselves to their senses, and it was possible to view by ear the features of the 'neighbourhood'. Acoustic pictures were returned from the darkened scenery; although still not seen as having application to anatomy, this appears to have been first focused on to practical application by a British physicist, Richardson in 1912, for detection of icebergs.[6]

The great step that had made an instant reality of medical imaging was however Röntgen's discovery of X-rays in 1895, and the concept that this had brought with it, that of the shadowgraph or 'radiograph', dominated people's thinking for the next 50 years or more. Indeed, the first steps towards making an anatomical image with ultrasound were taken by the Austrian brothers Dussik in 1937, using essentially that principle.[7] They scanned over a human head, immersed in water, using a transmitter-receiver pair of quartz crystal transducers; the result that they published in 1942 is illustrated in Figure 1. However, they gave no grounds for believing that the image portrayed real anatomy and, with the benefit of hindsight, current assessment must be that the data are essentially artefactual.

Technological foundations

The essential technological foundations for modern investigative ultrasound can be described under the following headings: acoustical theory, practical means for electro-acoustic conversion ('transduction'), fast electronic pulse technology, and video display and recording. All of these became available in practically usable form in the 75 year period culminating in 1945, with the further important component of contemporary technology – digital processing – following soon afterwards.

Prior to 1870 there seems to have been little coherent intellectual basis for the science of acoustics. Writing in 1873 to the then J. W. Strutt (later, and more generally known as, Lord Rayleigh) Clerk Maxwell remarked 'I am glad you are writing a book on Acoustics . . . . You speak modestly about a want of sound books in English. In what language are there such, except Helmholtz, who is sound not because he is German but because he is Helmholtz?'. Rayleigh had in fact started work on his book in December 1872, at the outset of a 3 month honeymoon trip on a Nile sailing boat.[8] The result, his 'Theory of Sound'[9] immediately became, and has remained, one of the great classic texts in physics and provided the intellectual foundation for the subject of Acoustics and, thus, of Ultrasonics.

It is a remarkable and double coincidence, first that only three years after the publication of Theory of Sound came the discovery, quite independently, of the physical phenomenon that makes possible the investigative use of ultrasound, that of the piezo-electric effect[10] and, second, that the two brothers who were its discoverers were those whose surname was shortly to become, for quite other reasons, widely famous in medical science: Jean and Pierre Curie. Their observations were made in single crystals of tourmaline, although the phenomenon was soon recognised as being more general in occurrence and specifically to occur in quartz, which became widely used in practice. It was not until the 1950's that the phenomenon was effectively exploited in the more versatile composite ceramic materials (e.g. lead zirconate titanate – PZT) and, later still, plastics, that are now in almost universal use in medical applications.

In a further manifestation of the apparently small world of turn-of-the-century science it was a graduate student of Pierre Curie, Paul Langevin who was to go on to develop Richardson's idea and become the practical pioneer of acoustic pulse-echo techniques, in their 1914 to 1918 wartime application to underwater detection of submarines. This work was secret and unpublished at the time. In a sense it was technologically premature since it pre-dated the thermionic triode valve and thus lacked straightforward means for either generation or amplification of electrical pulses. It, and related work elsewhere, laid the foundations for subsequent developments, first in marine SONAR (Sound Navigation and Ranging) and subsequently in RADAR (Radio Detection and Ranging), non-destructive materials testing and medical imaging.

Interestingly, Langevin's work also was the first to arouse interest in the possible biological consequences, whether harmful or otherwise, of ultrasound exposure, since he noticed damage to the fish in Cherbourg harbour when they strayed into his high power beam. A remarkable early follow up of this observation, together with an account of some of the technological problems coped with by Langevin, was reported by Wood and Loomis in 1927.[11]

An important link between Langevin's work in acoustics and its application to medicine was forged by the Russian engineer, S. Y. Sokolov, who pioneered the use of ultrasound echo methods for flaw detection in metals,[12] foresaw the extension of such methods to the gigahertz frequency (and corresponding micron resolution) microscopy applications which have only quite recently been realised, and invented the ultrasonic analogue of the television camera (the 'Sokolov Camera') which enables direct transformation of ultrasonic image data into electrical signals.[13] During the 1939 to 1945 war these concepts led naturally into work on ultrasonic non-destructive testing and radar, both of which, in turn, relied on the recently developed cathode-ray display tube and the associated technology of television, that had been built up by Baird and others during the 1930's.

The 'post-War' period (1948 to 1960)

With the above background, and following the intensive technological development work stimulated by the needs of the war, particularly that directed towards radar, the essential ingredients had become available for the implementation of investigative ultrasound. In what happened next, although enormous credit is due to the very small number of far-sighted pioneers, the real cause for surprise should not be that the development occurred, but rather how blind was the conventional wisdom to its significance and thus how slowly its potential benefits came to be exploited. Although a relative latecomer, the present author must be numbered amongst the blind in this context. The reasons behind such blindness can only be speculative. It is none the less important to be aware of the influences that can divert otherwise logical and potentially valuable advances.

The Second World War concluded with the nuclear bombing of Hiroshima and Nagasaki, events that led to widespread and deep feelings of awe and guilt. One of the consequences was the creation of the International Atomic Energy Agency, one of whose principal functions was, as some kind of communal reparation, to act as a wealthy patron of a particular Phoenix, nuclear medicine. It is ironical that the relatively benign role played by ultrasound in wartime led to its neglect by the post-War, guilt-ridden public imagination.

Also, by this time, diagnostic radiology seemed to have reached a state of relative equilibrium and most radiologists were unreceptive to the prospect of a radically new imaging technology (which nuclear medicine had not become at this stage), that might complement X-ray examination even for problems in which this was known to be unsatisfactory.

During the war ultrasonic echo methods had been developed, principally by Firestone in the USA and Sproule in Britain, for detecting cracks in metal structures, and by 1949 three separate groups in the USA had become interested in their medical potential: Ludwig and Struthers at the US Naval establishment at Maryland, Wild, a British trained surgeon in Minneapolis who recruited help from a local US naval air station, and Howry, a radiologist at Denver. All three groups initially worked with A-scan techniques and whilst the former, who were interested in locating gallstones and foreign bodies, never apparently progressed beyond that, the two others both developed B-scan imaging methods, but with differences that may have had considerable influence on subsequent development.

Together with his electronic engineering colleague, Reid, Wild, whose interest was in elucidating histopathology, and particularly that of cancer, developed a B-scanner working at 15 MHz and designed to be sensitive even to low level tissue echoes, at the calculated cost of producing images with a good range of grey scale but of somewhat fuzzy

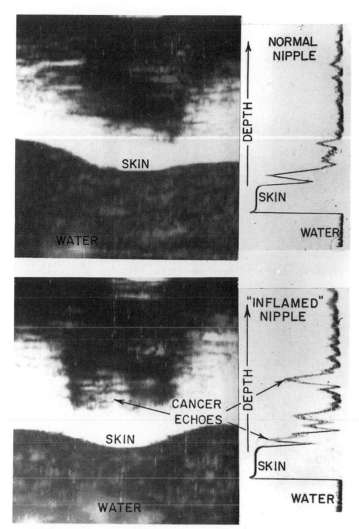

Fig. 2   **Early B-scan of the breast**, published by Wild & Reid in 1953 and reported as showing the presence of a tumour in the region of the nipple.[3]

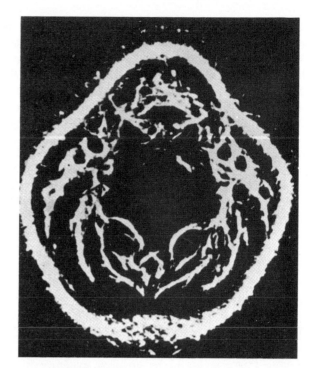

Fig. 3   **Cross-sectional image of the neck** obtained by Howry, in about 1954, using a water-immersion compound scanner.[14]

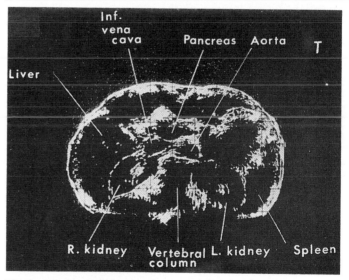

Fig. 4   **An outstanding example from the Bistable Image School**: a transverse cross-section of the abdomen, 16 cm above the umbilicus, obtained by Holm[15] in 1970.

appearance (Fig. 2). In retrospect this work can be seen to be the true forerunner of modern imaging procedures, but, perhaps because of failure to solve the technical problem of image display with adequate dynamic range compression, and in spite of an extensive, vigorous and imaginative programme of work,[3] the potential value of the images was not generally perceived in the early days.

Howry's approach was somewhat different, being in essence a prototype of the reconstruction tomography that came into its own with the development of X-ray CT, and had the practical outcome of images that emphasised the location of organ boundaries (Fig. 3).[14] In his original 'Somatom' apparatus (although this was shown later not to be essential) the anatomy of interest was immersed in a waterbath and echo data were received from all possible orientations and superimposed in their correct relative locations in order to form the final image. This approach, which became known as 'compound scanning', had the

apparent strength, particularly at the height of its development, of providing images reminiscent of anatomical line drawings (Fig. 4). It became a standard procedure until the development of high sensitivity, high resolution techniques showed both the diagnostic importance of low level echoes[16] and the serious impact of movement artefact that occurs in compound scanning.[17]

The vogue for compound scanning was in fact lent strength at one stage through developments in display device technology. In the 1950's the only available means, apart from photography, for even temporarily storing complete images was to use display CRT's with 'long persistence' phosphors – an unsatisfactory procedure because their low luminance levels called for scanning in virtually total darkness, and consequent long observer accommodation times. Subsequent developments of 'storage' display tubes initially provided only a bistable (black or white) display, which emphasised the appearances of simple anatomy but provided no half tones with which to display tissue echoes (Fig. 5). However, human conservativeness is such that later developments allowing a return to good half tone ('grey scale') display were initially greeted by some diagnosticians with appreciable disapproval.

A curious aspect of the compound scanning era was the myth that grew up (propagated in many standard text books and may even persist still, to explain the success of the technique) that the echoes recorded were only those received from 'specularly reflecting' (i.e. essentially flat) interfaces. There seems to be no clear evidence for this model and indeed even simple consideration of the three-dimensional nature of the geometry concerned would indicate that most specular reflectors would not be expected to return echoes in the plane of scan. The more tenable physical explanation of the effect would now seem to lie in the signal-to-noise enhancement that results from multiple sampling of diffusely backscattered echoes, the strongest of which arise from connective tissue around organ boundaries.

A number of other principal items in the technical armoury of present day diagnostic ultrasound date from this period. For his work on bowel, Wild developed, and used clinically, the first ultrasonic endoscope (Fig. 6),[18] whilst, at about the same time, Edler and Hertz in Sweden opened up applications to cardiology by introduction of M-mode recording.[19] Again at this time it was Wild who took the first steps towards deriving quantitative information about tissue type from features of the ultrasonic echo: in modern parlance 'tissue characterisation'.[20] What is in a sense a special case of tissue characterisation, although it has come to be seen almost as a technology in its own right – Doppler flow detection and measurement – was developed and published by Satomura[21,22] in Japan in 1956. Finally, these early users of ultrasound were conscious of using an essentially novel form of diagnostic radiation which might have unforeseen consequences for their patients, or even for themselves, and it was once again Wild who seems to have been the first to investigate, in however preliminary a fashion, this possibility,[23] as early as 1951.

Clinically, Wild was interested in cancer, particularly of the breast and large bowel, and time, even with the advent of CT, has vindicated his far-sightedness in these and many other sites of the disease. Equally clearly however he

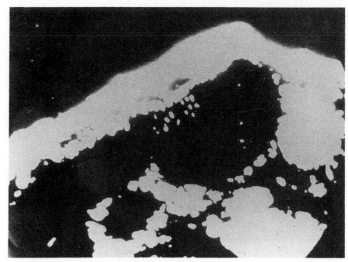

A

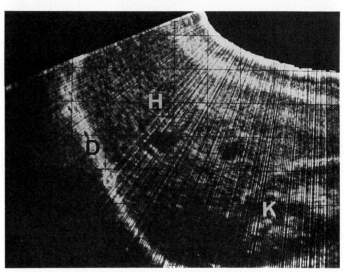

B

Fig. 5 Two liver scans published in the same journal issue in 1973 and illustrating the diversity of image appearances at that time. **A:** Scan apparently obtained with an unfocused transducer and recorded through a bistable display device.[32] The author's caption reads: 'Supine transverse scan of a liver showing two transonic nodules bordered by an echogenic band (metastasis of a gastric cancer)'. **B:** Scan obtained on the equipment illustrated in Figure 8, with a 3 MHz focused transducer, logarithmic signal compression and 'open shutter' recording directly on to film,[16,33] ('scratchy potentiometer artefact' is painfully visible!). The authors' caption reads: 'longitudinal section of liver, 6 cm to right of midline, showing diaphragm (D), normal liver (H), normal right kidney (K) and two small areas of replacement of normal architecture by small discrete areas of Hodgkin's disease'.

was taking on in the breast one of the more difficult areas of diagnostic imaging and it is thus hardly surprising that the clear demonstration of the worth of his results here was slow to come.

Howry's initial interest (as indeed had been the Dussiks', one of whom was a psychiatrist) was, by contrast, in the brain, which was perhaps a natural site for a

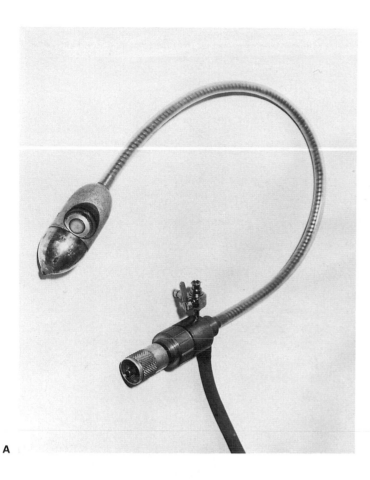

A

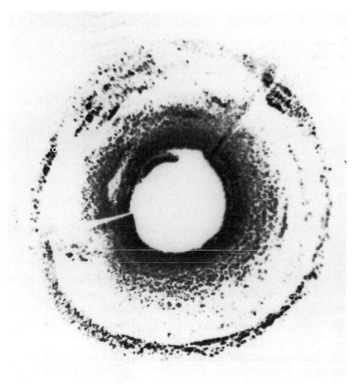

B

Fig. 6 A: Prototype of an ultrasonic endoscope, designed and built by Wild,[18] in about 1957. **B:** Example of a rectal scan obtained with it.

radiologist to attack at that time, knowing as he did that it presented a substantial set of clinical problems that could not be solved satisfactorily by conventional techniques. Even more than Wild, Howry soon discovered that the adult brain is a very difficult organ to study with ultrasound because of overlying bone and subsequent authors have confirmed this to present almost insuperable problems.[24] None the less, again in ironic contrast to Wild, Howry's interest in the brain attracted a considerable number of followers, to the extent that a substantial proportion of the 'second generation' of ultrasound pioneers were recruited through an interest in neurology: names such as White in Canada, de Vlieger in Holland, Alvisi in Italy, Mayneord in Britain and Kikuchi, Tanaka and Wagai in Japan.

As already mentioned, another organ that received relatively early attention was the heart, largely because it was found that useful kinetic information could be derived by relatively simple M-mode techniques. For similar reasons interest arose at an early stage in studies of the eye, where useful optometric and other information (again with early attempts at 'tissue characterisation') could be derived from straightforward A-scan methods. In this connection it is interesting to note that, as White has pointed out,[5,25] approximately 60% of all papers on echography published prior to the year 1970 were related to applications in either neurology or ophthalmology, a figure that had dropped below 5% by 1982.[26]

The abdomen seems to have proved a difficult region in the early days, probably for the reasons suggested above in relation to cancer investigation and, of the relatively few early published papers in this area, the great majority were concerned with location of stones.

Obstetric applications similarly attracted little interest until, from the publication of the early work of Donald and co-workers, commencing in 1958[27] (although with its origins traceable to the work of Mayneord's group[28,29] commencing in 1951), it became apparent that, even with the then somewhat primitive state of the technology, it was quite possible to derive several types of data having vital bearing on obstetric management: e.g. fetal skull size, placental position and differential diagnosis of hydatidiform mole. Arguably this was the key advance that led to the eventual acceptance of ultrasound as a generally respected clinical imaging tool, as indeed it also led to the production of the first commercial B-scanner – the 'Diasonograph' – designed on Clydeside to shipbuilders mechanical specifications and driven by a multitude of wartime electronic valves (Fig. 7).

This is to anticipate. Perhaps the event that was to mark the close of the 'classical period' of diagnostic ultrasound was the withdrawal of Wild's US Public Health Service research grant. At $0.5 million this was, at the time of the award in 1962, the largest single medical grant ever given to an individual. The decision to stop payments and confiscate his equipment[30] led to the following entry in the

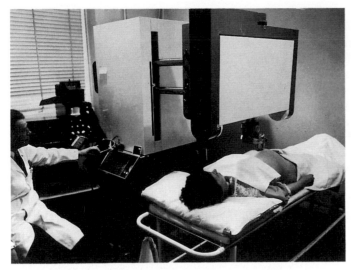

Fig. 7 Professor Ian Donald, at the Queen Mother's Hospital, Glasgow, working with an early model Diasonograph, manufactured in 1964 by Smiths Industries in Glasgow: the first B-scanner to have been produced commercially. In the background (above Donald's hand) is the Smiths 'Mark 7 supersonic Flaw Detector' that was used by Dr Stuart Campbell in his early work on biparietal cephalometry. Photograph by courtesy of Mr J. E. E. Fleming and with permission of the British Medical Ultrasound Society Historical Collection.

Guinness Book of Records: 'A sum of $16,800,000 was awarded to Dr. John J. Wild, at the Hennepin District Court, Minnesota, USA on 30th November 1972 against the Minnesota Foundation and others for defamation, bad faith, termination of a contract, interference with professional business relationship and $10.8 million in punitive damages'.[4] The award was subsequently much reduced by the Minnesota Supreme Court, but not before its members had resigned en bloc over the issue, an event that was itself unique in American legal history.

Modern times

Thus, by about 1963, virtually all the essential concepts underlying modern diagnostic ultrasound had been demonstrated – even something approaching real time scan acquisition had been achieved by the indomitable Wild.[3] None the less, much remained to be done: the technique was essentially unrecognised outside a very small band of enthusiasts and the only equipment being produced commercially were industrial flaw detectors.

Donald and Brown's Diasonograph went into commercial production in the mid-1960's with an initial run of six units. In this the transducer was mounted so as to move within a rectangular measuring frame (Fig. 7), which proved to be good, if somewhat cumbersome engineering design. Some other manufacturers soon followed however with what proved to be a more ergonomically satisfactory arrangement of 'compound B-scanner' in which the transducer was mounted on the end of articulated measuring arm (Fig. 8). Thus, by the time of the First World Con-

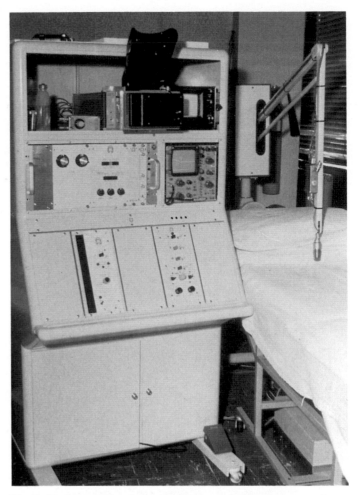

Fig. 8 Early example of an articulated-arm design of compound B-scanner (scanning arm originally manufactured by Kretz, with electronics developed at the Royal Marsden Hospital[16]).

gress of Ultrasound in Medicine held in Vienna in October 1969,[31] there was already an interesting variety of commercial scanners on offer. However, display devices were still either of the long persistence or bistable types and this, taken with the remarkable fact that most, if not all, transducers were unfocused and (in abdominal and obstetric scanners) operated at between 1 and 2 MHz, resulted in indifferent image quality (Fig. 5).

In relation to the shortcomings in display devices at that time it is noteworthy that the best available technique for recording images of good quality was direct recording from a non-storage display monitor onto photographic film, with the camera shutter held open during the scanning procedure. It was to a large extent careful optimisation of this procedure that enabled Kossoff's group in Sydney to achieve such outstanding results at this time.

Transducer design was however being worked on by a number of groups. The present author for example in 1971, incorporated a 3 MHz, 10 cm focus transducer in an articulated arm abdominal scanner and this, working together with the well-conceived developments in electronics and display that were due to the Sydney group, led to dramatic improvements in image quality[34] and corresponding extensions of clinical usefulness.

Perhaps more significant in the long-term were developments that had commenced in the late 1960's of transducer arrays – a technology that derived, albeit in miniaturised form, from underwater acoustics. Here Somer[35] and Bom,[36] both working in Holland, pioneered the phased and simple linear array techniques respectively that are in widespread use today. A major practical outcome of array technology was, of course, the facility of real time imaging, but the alternative of fast automatic mechanical scanning devices – rockers and rollers, or 'whizzers' – was also becoming available,[37] with some substantial advantages for certain applications, once the problems of mechanical reliability had been solved.

The majority of scanners of this period were far from 'user friendly' – a situation that posed a considerable barrier in terms of training and also of integration into conventional clinical or radiological practice. The Australian 'Octoson', with its derivatives, was a remarkable and imaginative attempt to solve this problem: an automated scanner (not unlike CT, with whose development it was contemporary but conceptually independent) in which the patient lies on a membrane-covered waterbed containing a set of scanning transducers.[38] This device might have seemed ideally suited to the pattern of work of radiology departments and it was certainly capable of producing spectacular and informative images (Fig. 9). Eventually, however it failed to gain general acceptance, and the reason for this failure may have been that it took away from ultrasound the very feature that distinguishes it from the bulk of radiological examinations – its clinical interactiveness.

A strand of thought that has occupied the attention of a number of workers in the field relates to the problems of conveying to the diagnostician, through an essentially two-dimensional image acquisition procedure, information about a three-dimensional object. Developments in this direction are proceeding to this day in spite of partial solution to the problem offered by effective 'real time' or 'cine-echographic' procedures but an interesting early approach was that of T. G. Brown, based on the use of a modified articulated arm scanner.[39]

The advances that have occurred over the past 15 years will be familiar to many readers. On the technical side these have often come about through general advances in technology: for example, developments in miniaturisation and in high frequency transducers have led to much improved equipment for interventional and 'small parts' examination whilst fast and affordable digital technology has made possible innovations such as colour flow Doppler imaging.

It will have to be for future historians, with the benefit of longer perspectives, to define the factors that have de-

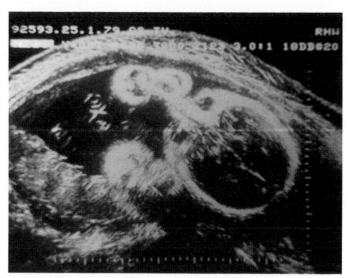

Fig. 9 Image of a pregnant abdomen, showing a cross-sectional view of a fetal skull, taken at the Royal Hospital for Women, Sydney, in 1979, with the 'CAL Octoson' (courtesy Drs G. Kossoff and W. Garrett).

termined the particular patterns of clinical use of ultrasound that we see today. One set of such factors derives of course from the nature of the technology: its successes and failures. Here one can cite for example its flexibility and real time characteristics that contribute to its value for early and rapid extensions of clinical examination, and its apparent safety and patient-friendliness that suit it to both obstetrics and paediatrics. Another factor however has been its relationship to complementary imaging methods, particularly CT and MRI, which also underwent a phase of rapid development during this period. The interactions of these different but related developing technologies have been complex, particularly as they have involved the attitudes and activities both of diagnosticians and of technologists. To the future historian it may well appear that ultrasound in the 1980's was experiencing a period of relatively undeserved neglect, whilst the attractions, both real and apparent, first of CT and then of MRI, gripped the attention of both radiologists and manufacturers.

The scientific background

Although it could be argued that it has so far had rather limited impact on commercial technology and clinical practice, part of the recent history of medical ultrasound has been in the area of basic physical science, particularly that to do with the propagation and scattering of ultrasound in human tissues. It is difficult to put exact dates to the outset of such work: measurements of tissue absorption coefficient, for example, were being made in the 1950's in connection with experiments on ultrasonic surgery.[40] To the extent, however, that pulse-echo methods essentially rely on the physical process of acoustic backscattering it is indicative that a review of that subject by Chivers in 1973 was only able to find two references to observations of the phenomenon in human or animal tissues (and one of those related to frozen fish).[41,42] The subject is thus quite recently established.

The question of safety

We have already seen that curiosity as to the possible ill effects of the novel form of biophysical stress represented by pulse-echo ultrasound goes back to Wild's work in the 1950's. Even prior to that however there was a considerable body of evidence, albeit often of dubious quality, on the biology underlying attempts to use ultrasound for treatment of conditions ranging from cancer to 'Violinspieler-Krampf'.[43]

In connection with their early work in obstetrics, Donald and colleagues,[44] no doubt correctly concluding that 'the proper study of mankind is man', carried out what was to be the first (but retrospective, and not rigorously controlled) epidemiological study of the consequences of ultrasound exposure for obstetric examination, with generally negative and thus reassuring findings. Somewhat earlier the present author had been invited to write what was to be the first systematic review of the subject[45] and identified, in addition to epidemiology, the two other and complementary lines of evidence on the subject as being, first, the elucidation of fundamental mechanisms of biological action and, second, the more empirical toxicological type of studies, on both of which there was then an emerging literature.

Subsequently the field has expanded greatly and has survived a number of superficially alarming publications claiming evidence of significant hazard. These claims have been found to be unsustainable. A minor industry has emerged in the writing of reviews on the question of the existence of hazards, with accompanying recommendations for minimising their possible impact.[46,47]

An unfortunate impediment that affected much of the early work on so-called 'ultrasound bioeffects' was the absence of an appropriate experimental and theoretical framework of metrology – the science and practice of measuring and recording – for ultrasonic fields. Until quite recently the conventional wisdom was to report values of acoustic intensity, based on measurements with a radiation force balance. This was not for any clearly defined scientific reason but because the measurement seemed reasonably easy to perform and had become conventional and thus incorporated into a number of national guidelines

and regulations. A focus for international collaboration and discussion on this topic was the 'Medical Ultrasonics' Working Group of International Electrotechnical Commission (IEC), whose various members presented the first major symposium on the subject in 1971.[48] From such work has emerged the modern consensus that measurements should be carried out on fundamental acoustic field quantities and that the most appropriate and practical measurement to be carried out is that of acoustic pressure, for which purpose a range of miniature hydrophones have been developed over the past few years.

Is this something of an abstruse technicality that has little to do with the real world of patients and their problems? Indeed not! An important factor in the recent history of diagnostic ultrasound has been the substantial public apprehension, as to both the validity of the evidence on safety and the possible problems that may arise from overdiagnosis.[49]

Conclusion

Arthur Koestler in 'The Sleepwalkers' gives a penetrating commentary on the often blind and stumbling manner in which – contrary to the conventional wisdom – many of the major historical advances in scientific perception have actually come about. This theme has resonances in the history of diagnostic ultrasound, where advance, or lack of it, can now, with the benefit of hindsight, be seen often to have been the result of whim, quirks of personality and tides of fashion both in the medico-scientific professions and also in industry.

To derive lessons for the future is always a hazardous task but a good general one would be to avoid the attitude of the middle-aged conservative professional that 'this is all I know on earth, and all I need to know': many radiologists and others in this category were taken unawares by the advent of diagnostic ultrasound and could be so again.

The current state of the art has come about through empirical and at times random processes, with little benefit from systematic insight into the underlying physics of the data-gathering procedure. A lesson from this interim historical review is that one could reasonably anticipate further advances in image quality as and when such insight is eventually achieved. Put another way, if it is indeed true that ultrasound has been relatively neglected as a field of physical science with applications in medical investigation, we should not be surprised if eventually its technical quality, and thus its clinical efficacy, turn out to have potential for advance relatively greater than those of some of the other, complementary imaging methods.

REFERENCES

1 Hill C R. Medical ultrasonics: an historical review. Brit J Radiol 1973; 46: 899–905

2 White D N. Ultrasound in Medical Diagnosis. Kingston, Ontario: Ultramedison. 1976

3 Wild J J. The use of pulse-echo ultrasound for early tumour detection: history and prospects. In: Hill C R, McCready V R, Cosgrove D O. eds. Ultrasound in Tumour Diagnosis. Tunbridge Wells: Pitman Medical. 1978: p 1–16

4 Wells P N T. History. In: de Vlieger M, Holmes J H, Kazner E, et al. eds. Handbook of Clinical Ultrasound. New York: Wiley. 1978: p 3–13

5 White D, Clark G, Carson J, White E. Ultrasound in Biomedicine: cumulative bibliography of the world literature to 1978: Oxford: Pergamon. 1982

6 Richardson M L F. Apparatus for warning a ship at sea of its nearness to large objects wholly or partly under water: UK Patent No. 1125: 1912

7 Dussik K T, Dussik F, Wyt L. Auf dem Wege zur Hyperphonographie des Gehirnes. Wien Med Ochenschr 1947; 97: 425–429

8 Rayleigh, 4th Baron (Lord). Life of Lord Rayleigh. London: Edward Arnold. 1924

9 Rayleigh, 3rd Baron (Lord). Theory of Sound. London: Macmillan. 1877

10 Curie J, Curie P. Sur l'electricite polaire dans cristaux hemiedres a face inclinees. Compt Rend Seances Acad Sci 1880; 91: 383–389

11 Wood R W, Loomis A L. The physical and biological effects of sound-waves of great intensity. Phil Mag S.7. 1927; 4: 417–436

12 Sokolov S Y. Improvements in and relating to the detection of faults in solid, liquid or gaseous bodies. UK Patent No.477; 139: 1937

13 Hill C R. Ultrasonic imaging: review article. J Phys E 1976; 9: 153–162

14 Howry D H, Bliss W R. Ultrasonic visualization of soft tissue structures of the body. J Lab Clin Med 1952; 40: 579–592

15 Holm H H. Ultrasonic scanning in the diagnosis of space-occupying lesions of the upper abdomen. Br J Radiol 1971; 44: 24–36

16 Hill C R, Carpenter D A. Ultrasonic echo imaging of tissues: instrumentation. Br J Radiol 1976; 49: 238–243

17 Taylor K J W, Hill C R. Scanning techniques in grey scale ultrasonography. Br J Radiol 1975; 48: 918–920

18 Wild J J, Reid J M. Current developments in ultrasonic equipment for medical diagnosis. IRE Trans Ultrasonic Eng 1957; 5: 44–58

19 Edler I, Herz C H. The use of ultrasonic reflectoscope for the continuous recording of movements of heart walls. K Fysiogr Sallsk Lund Forh 1954; 24: 1–19

20 Wild J J, Neal D. Use of high-frequency ultrasonic waves for detecting changes of texture in living tissues. Lancet 1951; 1: 655–657

21 Satomura S. A study on examining the heart with ultrasonics: I. Principle; II. Instrument. Jpn Circ J 1956; 20: 227

22 Satomura S. Ultrasonic Doppler method for the inspection of cardiac functions. J Acoust Soc Am 1957; 29: 1181–1185

23 French L A, Wild J J, Neal D. Attempts to determine harmful effects of pulsed ultrasonic vibrations. Cancer 1951; 4: 342–344

24 White D N. The effects of the skull upon the spatial and temporal distribution of a generated and reflected ultrasonic beam. Kingston, Ontario: Ultramedison. 1976

25 White D N. Personal communication. 1989

26 White D N, Carson J, White E. Cumulative bibliography of the world literature 1979–82. Ultrasound Med Biol 1987; 13: 1987

27 Donald I, MacVicar J, Brown T G. Investigation of abdominal masses by pulsed ultrasound. Lancet 1958; 1: 1188–1195

28 Mayneord W V. Report for the Physics Department of the Royal Cancer Hospital. In: BECC Annual Report for 1951. London: British Empire Cancer Campaign. 1951

29 Donald I. Sonar – the story of an experiment. Ultrasound Med Biol 1974; 1: 109–117

30 Wild J J. The origin of soft tissue ultrasonic echoing and early instrumental application to clinical medicine. In press

31 Bock J, Ossoinig K. Ultrasonographia Medica (3 volumes) Vienna: Verlag der Wiener Medizinischen Akadamie. 1971

32 Melki G. Ultrasonic patterns of tumours of the liver. JCU 1973; 1: 306–314

33 Taylor K J W, Carpenter D A, McCready V R. Grey scale echography in the diagnosis of intrahepatic disease. JCU 1973; 1: 284–287

34 Kossoff G. Improved techniques in ultrasonic cross-sectional echography. Ultrasonics 1972; 10: 221–227

35 Somer J C. Electronic sector scanning for ultrasonic diagnosis. Ultrasonics 1968; 6: 153–159

36 Bom N, Lancee C T, Honkoop J, Hugenholtz P G. Ultrasonic viewer for cross-sectional analyses of moving cardiac structures. Biomed Eng 1971; 6: 500–503 and 508

37 McDicken W N, Bruff K, Paton J. An ultrasonic instrument for rapid B-scanning of the heart. Ultrasonics 1974; 12: 269–272

38 Kossoff G, Carpenter D A, Robinson D E, Radovanovich G, Garrett W J. Octoson – a new rapid, general purpose echoscope. In: White D, Barnes R. eds. New York: Plenum. Ultrasound in Medicine 1976; 2: 333–339

39 Brown T G. Visualization of soft tissues in two and three dimensions – limitations and development. Ultrasonics 1967; 5: 118–124

40 Dunn F, Edmonds P D, Fry W J. Absorption and dispersion of ultrasound in biological media. In: Schwan H P. ed. Biological engineering. New York: McGraw-Hill. 1969

41 Chivers R C. The scattering of ultrasound by human tissues. PhD Thesis: University of London. 1973

42 Hill C R, Chivers R C, Huggins R W, Nicholas D. Scattering of ultrasound by human tissue. In: Fry F J. ed. Ultrasound: its applications in medicine and biology. Amsterdam: Elsevier. p 441–493

43 Bergmann L. Der Ultraschall. Stuttgart: Hirzel. 1954

44 Hellman L M, Duffus G M, Donald I, Sunden B. Safety of diagnostic ultrasound in obstetrics. Lancet 1970; 1: 1133–1135

45 Hill C R. The possibility of hazard in medical and industrial applications of ultrasound (review). Br J Radiol 1968; 41: 561–569

46 Anonymous. Biological effects of ultrasound: mechanisms and clinical implications. NCRP Report No.74. Bethesda: National Council on Radiation Protection and Measurements. 1983

47 Hill C R, ter Haar G R. Ultrasound. In: Suess M J, Benwell-Morison D A. eds. Non-Ionizing Radiation Protection. WHO Regional Publications, European Series, No.25. Copenhagen: World Health Organisation. 1989

48 Hill C R. Ultrasound dosimetry: session summary. In: Reid J M, Sikov M R. eds. Interaction of ultrasound and biological tissues. DHEW Publication (FDA) 73-8008. Rockville: US Dept. of HEW. 1972: p 153–158 and 159–214 for related papers

49 Anonymous. Future use of new imaging technologies in developing countries. WHO Publication, Technical Report Series No. 723. Copenhagen: World Health Organisation. 1985

2

Ultrasound equipment

Roland Blackwell

INTRODUCTION

There are some ultrasound images which make the interpretation not only believable, but obvious. Others leave us feeling far less confident. What is it about an image that assists our critical faculties in this way? Those who also have to spend hundreds of hours scanning know that some machines require little attention to adjustments whilst others, even amongst the most modern, seem fussy and time wasting.

The question, 'which is the best machine and probe selection for my purposes?' seems appropriate; regrettably, because of the progress in ultrasound technology, a specific answer is inevitably transient. It is more important for the user to understand the basis of equipment quality and efficiency to enable the best use to be made of the equipment currently owned and the most appropriate tool for the job to be selected without being misled by the manufacturers advertising and packaging.

There is little doubt that, over recent years, digital control of the scanner has been fundamental to the dramatic improvements in image quality which have been achieved. For many years, computer control has been available to assist in 'housekeeping' functions. This has allowed on-screen measurements, image annotation, look-up tables and the presetting of control settings for different applications. However, the important contribution of digital control to scanning has been through the manipulation of beams and echoes and in image processing. To the user, the most obvious development in scanning equipment has been the range of probes available. However, without digital control the new probe technologies, by themselves, would not have been particularly effective.

In this chapter digitisation is described and the way it is used in conjunction with probes and displays to overcome some of the earlier limitations in the quality of image production explained.

Components of a diagnostic image

Images which make diagnosis straightforward always have high spatial resolution. Spatial resolution may be loosely taken to mean the ability to see small structures, both along the beam (axial resolution) and across it (lateral resolution). This is desirable, not only in the centre of the image but also at the edges. High contrast resolution, the ability to distinguish between different types of tissue, is also crucial. For good contrast resolution small echoes must be capable of being displayed at the same time as large ones without 'noise' and artefacts cluttering up the image. Good contrast resolution at depth depends upon sensitivity sufficient for small echoes to be displayed to beyond the maximum depth of diagnostic importance.

These features depend upon image forming techniques such as dynamic focusing, aperture control, apodisation, image smoothing and edge enhancement which can best be achieved by digital control. Digitisation, in the context of image processing, will be reviewed before the slightly more complex issue of digital beam control.

Digital imaging

After each ultrasound pulse has been launched into the body, a string of echoes arrive back at the probe where they are turned into a voltage by the transducer. The voltage pattern produced by the echoes from the pulse contains the information required to fill in the greys along one line of the image. This voltage pattern could be drawn out as a graph. Just like any other graph, the shape could be recorded as a series of co-ordinates with the Y axis representing voltage (echo intensity) and the X axis representing time (depth in the body). The original can be reconstructed, given the series of co-ordinates: digitisation is simply the technique of changing the voltage pattern from the echoes into a series of voltage/time co-ordinates (Fig. 1). For image processing, these values are stored in a computer memory where they are used as the raw data from which the image is modified and later reconstructed, line by line, as the display.

Each computer memory element is essentially a group of switches which can be individually turned on or off under electronic control. The on/off state of each switch is used to represent the binary digits 0 and 1. The computer can write a number into any memory element by setting the switches or it can read a number from the memory by testing the position of the switches. Thus, a stored binary number can be read as often as desired or changed to a new value.

Measurement of the go-and-return time of the reflected sound pulse requires an extremely accurate timing device. Computers all contain an accurate 'clock' which, like a stop watch, allows the exact measurement of very small time intervals to be made. It consists of an electronic oscillator which switches a small voltage on and off tens of millions of times each second. These voltage pulses are generated with a constancy which may be likened to a watch which, even after years without adjustment, will never be inaccurate by more than 1 or 2 seconds (a fluctuation of less than one part in 50 000). The go-and-return time interval, along with the beam direction information, determines the computer address of the pixels to be filled with echo information.

Each memory element must be filled with a number representing the appropriate echo amplitude. The clock is used to control an analogue to digital converter (ADC) which continually reads the echo voltages to be stored. The ADC is a very fast voltmeter which reads out each voltage sample as a number. It can obtain a voltage reading in less than 40 nanoseconds (i.e. up to 25 million readings per second) which will enable the radio frequency (rf) voltage

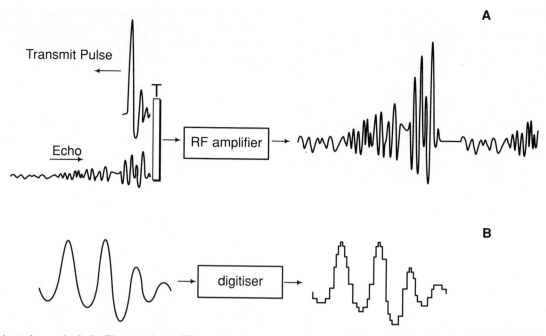

Fig. 1 The pulse-echo method. A: The transducer (T) launches a pulse into the body. The returning train of echoes is turned into a voltage pattern corresponding to the sound pressure fluctuations in the echo. The voltage pattern is amplified by a radio frequency amplifier. **B:** The single echo voltage pattern shown is digitised and appears at the output of the analogue to digital converter as a series of voltage steps. The voltage value of each step is stored in digital memory to give a series of co-ordinates, one being time, the other the voltage. These co-ordinates are used later to reconstruct the image.

signal to be sampled and stored. More usually, some smoothing of the signal is first performed to obtain the outline of the radio frequency pulses (Fig. 2). This outline is called the 'video' signal and need only be sampled at about four million readings per second. This relatively slow digitisation rate is less expensive, but also less flexible.

To turn the stored echo intensity values back into a voltage pattern for display the scan converter requires the use of a device called a 'digital to analogue converter' (DAC). This device 'reads' each stored number and immediately generates a voltage corresponding to it. By presenting the stored values in rapid succession to the DAC, a waveform which mimics the original voltage pattern is produced.

Digitisation at very high rates is difficult to do accurately. Fortunately, a relatively low precision can be tolerated because echoes of substantially different amplitude are all displayed with the same shade of grey. This is inevitable because the strongest echo produces a voltage which may be up to a million times stronger than the smallest echo (the dynamic range). Even after correction by the time-gain compensation (TGC) control for attenuation, the range is as much as 350 to one; this range of brightness levels cannot be displayed on a video screen.

The precision to which a voltage reading is recorded is given by the number of significant figures used. However, recording, say, 1.3561 is no more useful than the less precise 1.4 volts if the shade of grey is the same at both of these voltages anyway. Computers handle numbers using the binary system. For recording echo voltages, up to eight binary digits or bits (*BI*nary digi*TS*) are used. The use of more bits than this is expensive and gives a greater precision than is necessary. Eight bits allows the display of 256 shades of grey. Experiments on perception suggest that observers get better at interpreting images in a noisy background until 256 shades of grey are used, but then there seems to be no further improvement.[1]

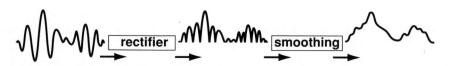

Fig. 2 Rectification. The echo voltage signal is usually turned into a 'video' signal before digitisation. The negative voltage portions of the waveform are inverted by a rectifier and the envelope of the fluctuations is produced by smoothing to form the video waveform.

The number of bits used to record a voltage is called the word length or depth. The more bits used the more closely the original intensity fluctuations can be followed (Fig. 3). Some scanners use only a four bit word, but many record the echo using eight bits and then use six bits for display. If effective image processing is to be undertaken, then the greater word depth is required to record the echo pattern if significant errors are to be avoided when arithmetical procedures are undertaken. The display of an image using a small word depth gives an image which has contours around it, a rather 'oily' appearance, which is called quantisation error (Fig. 4).

Scan conversion

In clinical practice, the only satisfactory way of handling images is in video format. Video monitors, tape recorders, discs and imagers all have remarkably high quality and are inexpensive; they are the obvious choice for display and storage.

To display the image from a linear array scanner in video format, a video camera could be pointed at an oscilloscope

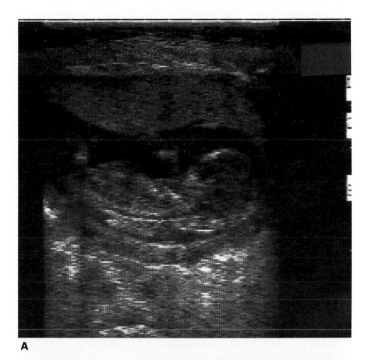

A

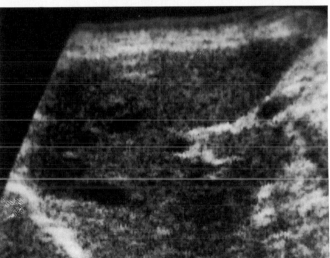

B

Fig. 4 Contouring. A: This image of a fetus is taken with scanning equipment in which the number of bits in the video signal has been restricted. The picture has rather obvious blotches of different greys. **B:** The same appearance seen in a liver image digitised to 4 bits.

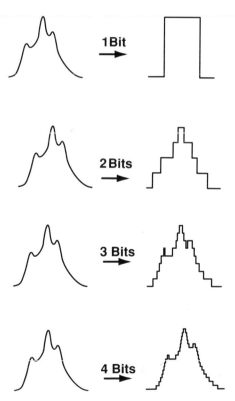

Fig. 3 Digitisation. A small portion of video signal is shown alongside the output which is produced after digitisation using different word depths. When only one bit is used, all voltage samples below a certain value are recorded as zero (displayed as black) and those above this value are recorded as the digit one (displayed as white), producing a bistable image. The shape of the video waveform is recorded more faithfully as the number of bits used increases.

screen on which the real time image is displayed. Indeed, in early machines this is exactly what was done, but the results were degraded by the complex electro-optical signal path. A direct link, bypassing the camera, is preferable but carries its own problem: ultrasound images are built up from a number of vertical or radial lines generated at a rate that depends on the speed of sound in the body. The video image, however, is built up from horizontal lines generated at a rate suitable for TV transmission. A device is required which will enable a scan to be stored in the ultrasound scan format and displayed in the video format. The commonly used device to perform this conversion is called a 'digital scan converter'.

The scan converter is made up of a large number of computer memory elements which store the entire echo information derived from the scan. This information enables a digital image comprising a mosaic of tiny rectangular picture elements, called pixels, to be produced. Each memory element has an 'address' which relates it to a single pixel in the image. The address where the value of the echo amplitude is to be stored is determined by the exact direction from which the echo originates and the time taken for the go-return passage of the ultrasound pulse. The stored information enables the appropriate shade of grey to be displayed in each pixel after the stored number is converted back to a voltage by a digital to analogue converter.

The scan converter contains enough memory elements to match one to each pixel in the image (Fig. 5). There are typically 512 pixels across the image and 512 down making 262 144 in all. This arrangement is referred to as a 512×512 memory matrix or memory plane. Each memory element has an address which identifies the pixel related to it. The addresses are arranged to identify pixels in columns down and rows across the image.

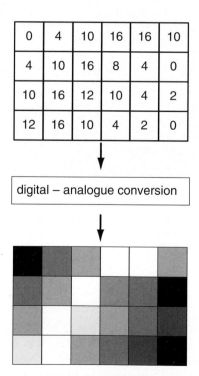

Fig. 5 Digital memory. The memory is like a set of addressed 'pigeon holes' each containing the voltage value corresponding to part of the image. A small section of memory elements is shown with the corresponding image pixels, each of which displays a grey level determined by the number in the memory cell. The number in the memory element is translated by the digital-to-analogue converter to a voltage to produce the display.

Consider the formation of a linear array image. As the voltage values from the first pulse arrive they are stored, one to a memory element, in the column of addresses relating to the first image line. The values from the second ultrasound pulse are stored in the second column of addresses and so on until the memory addresses for the entire image frame are full up. When the memory is full the video system reads out and displays the first video line. This is formed from the values stored in the top row of addresses. The next row is fed out for the next video line and so on until the video image frame is complete.

A real time ultrasound scanner presents new image frames one after another to produce the real time effect. Having produced the first frame, the second and subsequent frames must be stored using the same memory elements. The values required for the first column of the second frame are obtained and these overwrite the values which are already stored in the memory matrix. The overwriting process continues line by line to produce sequential frames. It is not essential to wait until the frame is completely overwritten before rows of values for the video are read out – both read and write processes can proceed together.

Frame freeze

Frame freeze enables a single frame to be examined or a structure measured using the on-screen calipers. The freeze mechanism is simply a mechanical switch which stops new echo values overwriting those already stored. The same stored values are read out time and time again onto the video display. Unfreezing the image restores the overwrite process.

It should be noted that some scanners continue to transmit ultrasound pulses even though the frame freeze is on. Such unnecessary insonation of the patient is a poor design feature.

Smoothing the image

The video lines, scan lines and other visible features caused by the scanning process are called 'structured noise', and should be reduced to a minimum by image processing.

A typical linear array is about 10 cm in length and produces about 125 ultrasound lines. However, there may be 512 pixels in each row across the image to be filled up with echo information. Thus, there is only one echo value available for every four pixels across the screen. If the empty pixels are not filled in, an image with obvious gaps between the vertical lines is displayed. The three empty pixels between those receiving data can be filled with calculated values. Using the recorded values in the pixels either side of the empty pixels, calculated values can be graded to give a smooth transition from one measured

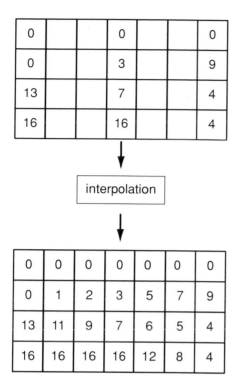

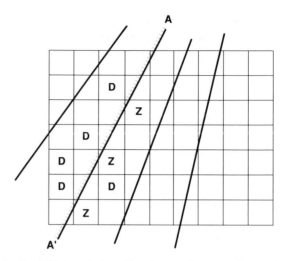

Fig. 6 Spatial smoothing. A small section of memory is shown in the upper part of the diagram. The linear array produces only enough echo information to fill every third column. The computer calculates values so that the empty columns are filled with interpolated echo amplitudes.

Fig. 7 Spatial interpolation. The diagram illustrates the way in which the axes of several consecutive ultrasound beams cross the pixels in the image. One vector (line A – A′) has time intervals marked on it indicating the instants at which digitisation takes place. As the beam crosses the corners of the pixels marked Z, it remains within the pixel for too short a time for the voltage to be measured. Similarly, the pixels marked D are not entered at all by the ultrasound beam. Conversely, many pixels have the ultrasound beams cross them in such a way that there are a substantial number of voltage readings and a policy has to be derived for indicating which reading will be stored for these memory locations.

value to the next (Fig. 6). This process is called 'line interpolation'.

When recording a sector scan a more difficult problem is encountered. The direction of the ultrasound vectors crosses the grid of pixels at an angle so that some pixels never receive a value, others have the vector clip the corner of the pixel leaving little time for a voltage value to be obtained. Still others have the ultrasound vector cross the pixel diagonal so that many values of echo voltage are generated for that pixel (Fig. 7). A design strategy has to be adopted on how to use the digitised data. The voltage value actually recorded for the pixel may be the largest, smallest or some sort of weighted average of the digitised voltages.

If nothing is done about the empty pixels a series of black spots appear over the image as if pepper had been sprinkled on it. These spots are called 'drop out'. The strategy for smoothing drop out gives a distinctive appearance to the scan. One solution is to adapt the size of the pixels so that some are square and others are oblong, the shape being chosen to ensure that the ultrasound vector always passes through the middle of the cell. The vertical spacing of the pixels may also be chosen so that they always fall on video lines. This technique makes good use of all available information but, unless further processing is undertaken, produces a slightly 'smeared' appearance to the

image in the distal part of the scan where the scan lines are diverging significantly.

There are various other strategies which can be used. One is the 'moving nine point average' smoothing technique. In this process a complete frame is stored and then smoothed by replacing the value in each pixel by the average of that value and its eight surrounding neighbours. This smoothing strategy, and variants of it, can produce visually pleasing results.

Smoothing out coherent radiation speckle (frame averaging)

The limit of axial resolution for a scanner is about half the pulse length and for lateral resolution it is approximately equal to the beam width (Fig. 8). In practice, the resolution of parenchymal echoes appears to be better than the theoretical limit of resolution (Fig. 9). The reason is that parenchymal tissue gives rise to small echoes which are so close together that they interfere with each other and generate a random pattern (Fig. 10). There is a loss of the one to one correspondence between the image and the tissues. This 'tissue texture' pattern is called 'coherent radiation speckle'. It must be remembered that the texture does not relate to the real texture of the tissue.

In some diagnostic situations the ability to determine small changes in the reflectivity of tissues is essential. In these cases the speckle pattern can be obtrusive. The speckle pattern may be smoothed out to leave an im-

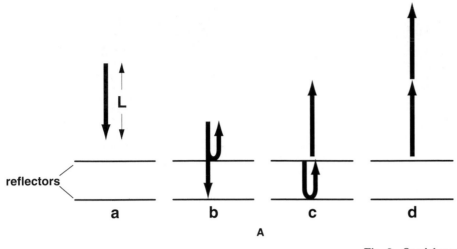

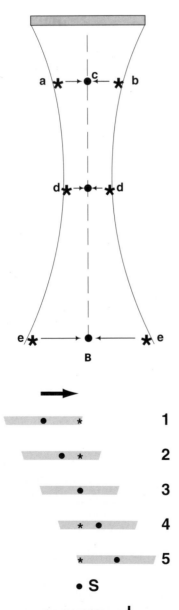

Fig. 8 Spatial resolution. A: Axial resolution. Two reflecting surfaces are separated by half of the pulse length. The diagram suggests that the limit of axial resolution occurs when the distance between them is half the pulse length. The broad arrows represent the physical length of an ultrasound pulse which, in (a), is travelling towards the two reflecting surfaces. In (b) the pulse is crossing the first surface and has just reached the second. An echo, half a pulse length in extent, has already been reflected from the first surface. In (c) an echo of the entire pulse length has been reflected from the first surface and the transmitted energy has now been reflected from the second surface and follows the first echo. In (d) both echoes are travelling back towards the transducer and the head of the second echo just touches the tail of the first echo. This is the condition required for the two surfaces to be resolved. **B:** Lateral (azimuthal) resolution. A reflector anywhere within the beam is displayed as if it was on the axis of the beam. Thus, reflectors a and b (*) are displayed as if they were situated at c and only show as a single echo (i.e. they will not be resolved as separate structures). Lateral resolution is equal to the effective beam width and is best at the focus (d–d) and worst where the beam is widest (e–e). **C:** As a beam is swept in the direction of the arrow across a small reflector (*) a line (L) is displayed instead of the ideal spot (S). Sections 1 to 5 illustrate the beam at the point where the reflector is situated. In 1 the beam has just reached the reflector, which is displayed on the axis of the beam (a). In 2 the reflector is nearer to the position where it is actually displayed, while in 3 the reflector is on the axis and is displayed in its correct position. As the beam moves still further across the reflector (4 and 5) the error increases in the opposite direction. The result is that a point reflector is displayed as a line (L) which has the same length as the beam width.

pression of the overall reflectivity of the tissue. Smoothing relies on small movements of the speckle pattern as the tissue is moved by cardiac or muscular action or as the probe is moved. (The way the speckle pattern moves has itself been used as an indication of pathology.) Although the speckle pattern moves, the general brightness of the region does not change so that, if the frames are super-imposed, the movement averages out the speckle but leaves the average brightness of an area on the display.

For this technique a number, typically nine, of identical computer memories have to be provided. The first frame is stored in the first memory in the usual way. The second frame does not overwrite the first, but is stored separately in the second memory, the third in the third and so on

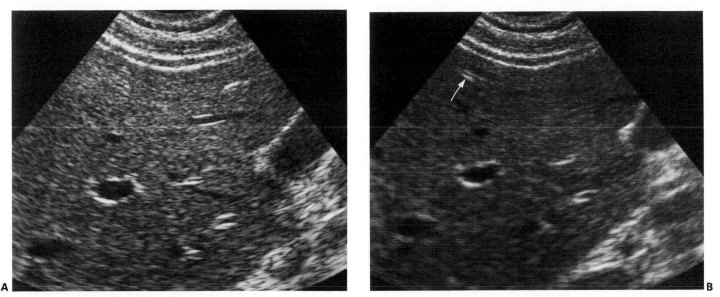

Fig. 9 Image speckle and its reduction. A: An image of the liver with a mechanical annular array sector scanner. There is apparent fine detailed structure, especially in the near field of the transducer. This is virtually all artefact due to random speckle. **B**: An image of the same area with frame averaging applied. The random speckle has mostly cancelled out whilst the real information – in this case a small portal vein branch (arrow) – is reinforced.

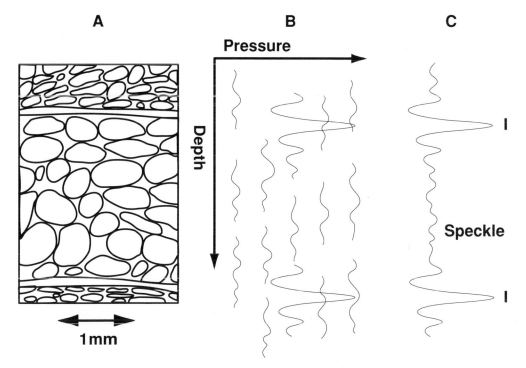

Fig. 10 Production of speckle. A: Three tissue types are depicted. The interfaces give rise to scattered echoes each of which occurs before the previous echo has completely died away. **B**: These pressure waves are drawn staggered across the page to show their time relationship. As the pressure waves overlap interference occurs. At some positions the echoes cancel out and sometimes they reinforce each other and **C**: a random pressure pattern, called coherent speckle, is produced. The large echoes (I) from the boundaries to the central region are correctly identified, but the correspondence between 'an echo' displayed on the image and the presence of a reflecting structure in the tissue is lost in the regions where significant interference occurs.

until the eighth frame has been stored. The value of the echo in the first pixel in each frame store is now averaged and the result stored in the ninth memory as the value to be displayed. Similarly, the series of echoes in the second pixel addresses are averaged and stored in the second pixel of the ninth memory and so on until all of the elements in the ninth memory are full. This memory matrix is then read out to give the video information for display. Subsequent frames now overwrite the eight originally stored, the values for the displayed ninth store being recalculated as each new frame is stored. Variants are used in which a smaller number of frames are selected for averaging, or by weighting the calculated average value for each pixel so that the most recent frame has a greater influence on the image.

The initial phase of any clinical ultrasound examination requires rapid survey of the tissues. Frame averaging is only meaningful when the slice to be averaged is identical in each frame. If the probe or tissues are moving rapidly (e.g. when imaging the heart) different sections are averaged together and result in a smeared image. If detailed study of small changes in tissue reflectivity is not required, the frame averaging should be turned off. It is essential that this function can be controlled by the user.

Volume scanning

The reduction in the cost of computer memories has made it realistic to use many memory planes. This has opened up the possibility of scanning through a large number of anatomical planes sequentially and storing them all. The scan can then be reconstructed in any desired plane (Fig. 11). Even more recent is the combination of high level echoes from many planes to produce a three-dimensional representation of anatomical structures such as the prostate or the intraluminal architecture of blood vessels. The clinical value of these new techniques is not yet established.

Zoom

An area of the scan can be magnified on the display by the use of zoom. There are two types of zoom (Fig. 12). 'Read zoom' is used to enlarge a frozen image and 'write zoom' is used to enlarge the display while scanning is taking place.

In read zoom grey level values are read from only a small part of the computer memory and the pixels are displayed larger. The effect is rather like taking a magnifying glass to the image. If magnification scale factor is too large the image matrix becomes rather obvious and the grainy effect becomes obtrusive.

In write zoom use is made of the fact that digital samples are usually received fast enough for several samples to occur in each pixel. When this is the case, the image scale may be enlarged to the point when only one sample occurs in each pixel. The amount of tissue represented by each pixel is decreased but the displayed size of the pixel is unchanged. In this case there is true magnification without loss of definition. Any further enlargement requires an increase in digitisation rate.

As the scale factors are increased there is a larger space between the scan lines so that further smoothing is required to maintain an acceptable image. It is possible, using sophisticated signal processing, to introduce more real scan lines so that definition is improved (see below).

Recording the image (gamma correction)

If we view a film or recording of a scan, it should look just like the image which was seen on the screen. This situation

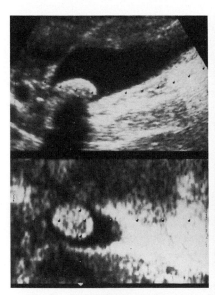
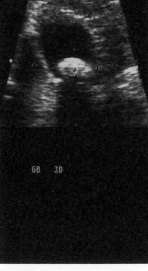

Fig. 11 Three-dimensional reconstruction. These three images of a gallstone are in orthogonal planes (i.e. at right angles to each other). These images were generated by computer controlled selections of data obtained during a single scan of the entire volume. Scans in any desired plane can be obtained from the same data. (Picture by courtesy of Kretz UK Ltd.)

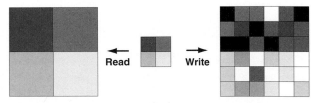

Fig. 12 Zoom. The four pixels in the centre of the diagram represent part of the image which is to be enlarged by the zoom control. 'Zoom on read' is achieved by displaying each pixel larger than it was originally. There is no new information presented. In 'zoom on write' the pixels are the same size as originally but far more of them are used to display the section of the original image. There is a consequent increase in displayed information.

is difficult to achieve because the eye can respond to a huge range of brightness levels, but film has a far more limited range (Fig. 13). Film density swings from black to white over a small range of subject brightness so that a direct photograph of the display screen results in a film with a loss of grey levels. To achieve an acceptable recording, it is necessary to photograph an image in which the change in greys is limited by compression of the contrast so that a rather 'muddy' looking image is photographed.

The digital to analogue scan converter performs a process rather like 'painting by numbers', each stored voltage value representing a shade of grey. A child who drops the painting-by-numbers box and gets the colours muddled up can still paint a consistent, if somewhat strange, picture. The stored values of voltage can similarly be changed by an electronic 'look up' table before they are fed to the DAC. In this way the stored values can be used to generate simultaneously one image for viewing and another for display on the camera tube. This process is called 'gamma correction', the gamma characteristic being the name given to the plot of the film response to different light levels.

Post-processing

The facility to change the displayed grey shade assigned to each echo amplitude, used in gamma correction, also enables the contrast and brightness of the viewed image to be altered after storage in the memory. This is only useful if the image was originally stored with an adequate word

depth. Post-processing implies that the image is modified after storing it in the memory.

The range of echo intensities coming from the tissues is extremely large, typically 100 dB (i.e. the amplitude of the strongest echo voltage is 100 000 times that of the weakest). Half of this range is due to attenuation and may be compensated for by the TGC, but the other half is due to the change in tissue reflectivity which is the feature used to generate the ultrasound image. Even assuming that the TGC was set correctly, the strongest reflection from a soft tissue interface gives a stored voltage about 300 times bigger than the smallest; this range of reflectivities cannot be displayed on a video screen without loss of information. In some way the echo information must be compressed before it is displayed. A compression characteristic must be chosen, using a front panel control, to emphasise the diagnostic feature of interest.

If linear compression is chosen, the echo amplitude is allowed to change substantially before a change in grey

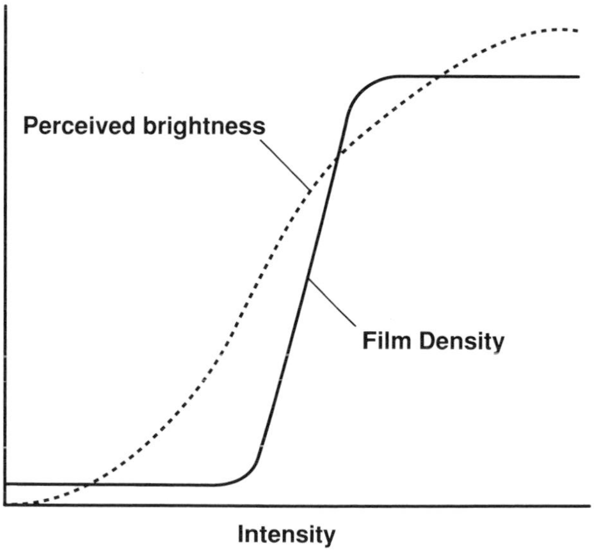

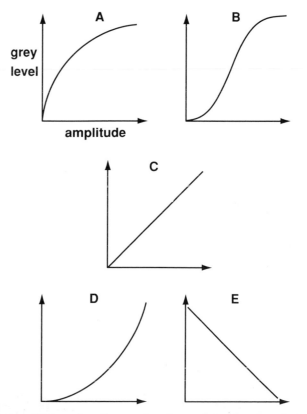

Fig. 14 Compression. Compression characteristics show how the grey tone of an echo displayed on the image varies with the echo amplitude. Characteristics are usually a variant of one of five types. **A:** is a logarithmic curve which emphasises changes in small echoes. **B:** is a sigmoid curve which suppresses the smallest echoes but emphasises changes in mid-range echoes. **C:** is a linear characteristic where the input amplitudes are evenly distributed across the available grey tones **D:** is an exponential characteristic which gives heavy emphasis to outlines. **E:** Characteristics with a negative slope reverse black and white on the image (this may be necessary for photographic recording).

Fig. 13 Gamma correction. The eye can perceive a range of brightness of over 100 000 000 to 1 (dashed line). Conversely, exposed film changes from clear to maximum density over a relatively small range of brightness (solid line). The contrast of the image must be reduced to match the film characteristic if the film image is to look like the display seen directly on the screen.

shade is registered on the display (Fig. 14). This is particularly appropriate if outlines, showing the shape and size of organs, are to be measured. If, however, it is the small changes in reflectivity of tissues which are diagnostically important, then small changes in echo intensity need to produce a detectable change in grey on the display. In this case it is usual to display all large echoes, perhaps half the total range, as white. The remaining echoes are graded so that small changes in the reflectivity region of interest give noticeable changes in grey. The reflectivity changes which are important may be amongst the smallest echoes in which case a logarithmic characteristic is used. However, for mid-range echoes a sigmoid characteristic ('S' curve) is appropriate.

Selection of the best characteristic to use has a strong subjective element because individual perception of detail changes from one person to another. If you like a particular characteristic and you get satisfactory results, use it, even though a colleague is sure a different one is correct.

Pre-processing

Before a series of echoes is stored some signal processing usually takes place. This is termed pre-processing. The exact functions performed before storage and after storage vary slightly from machine to machine. TGC and edge enhancement are almost always performed as pre-storage functions, and radio frequency digitisation obviously must be performed before storage.

Radio frequency digitisation

When the echo returns to the transducer it produces a voltage pulse at the same frequency as the ultrasound wave which is within the frequency band used in radio. The voltage waveform is immediately processed by a radio frequency (rf) amplifier which is tuned to the frequency of the pulse. A different radio frequency amplifier has to be used for each probe of a different frequency. It is conventional to rectify and smooth the waveform as soon as possible to produce a video signal because the design of

electronic circuits to handle video frequencies is far less demanding than for rf. The smoothing circuit produces a voltage tail on the video signal of an echo so that, instead of a dot being displayed, it appears as a 'comma' (Fig. 15). If the digitisation is fast enough, the rf signal, modified only by some TGC, can itself be stored in memory. This makes the possibilities of subsequent signal processing much more flexible and also enables the echo to be displayed without the tail. The image is consequently cleaner.

Automatic time-gain control (TGC)

The TGC compensates for the attenuation of sound as it passes into the tissues in such a way that deep echoes from identical structures appear equally reflective to superficial echoes. Accurate adjustment of the TGC characteristics has always been a major source of difficulty to operators. To obtain an automatically compensated scan is very desirable. There are many successful designs of automatic TGC while others are poor in that they introduce artefacts in the region of large fluid spaces, such as liquor amnii, the bladder or gallbladder. The low attenuation of these structures confuses the system and produces incorrect compensation beyond the low attenuation region. It is therefore important that an automatic TGC can be overridden by the operator.

In essence, automatic TGC is based upon detection of the fall of echo intensity along each ultrasound line by smoothing out the rapid fluctuations due to the changes in reflectivity. This approximates to the shape of the attenuation profile which, when inverted, gives the ideal shape for the TGC characteristic (Fig. 16). The averaging may take place over just one line, by using one line to correct the next, or by strategies which use the information contained in an entire frame.

Edge enhancement

To achieve good axial resolution well-defined echoes must be displayed. Echo definition may be enhanced by processing the echo voltages so that the upswing of each echo is

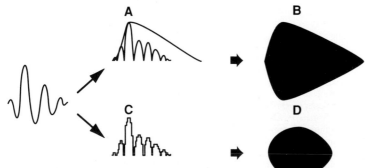

Fig. 15 Digitisation of the rf. When a rectified pulse (**A**) is smoothed the envelope of the trailing edge does not follow the original voltage waveform but rather decays at a constant rate from the peak voltage. This effect produces a display spot with a tail (**B**). If the rectified wave itself is digitised (**C**) and used to drive the display, the tail is not present and so a more circular spot is displayed (**D**). This results in a crisper image.

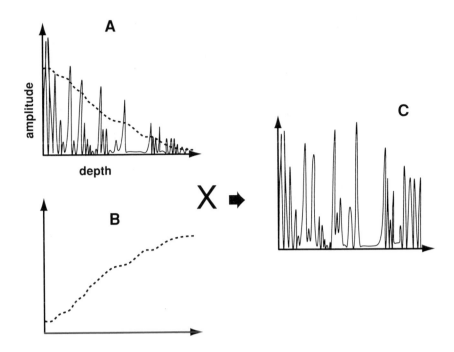

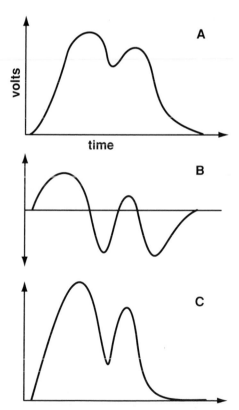

Fig. 16 Automatic TGC. A: Attenuation results in deep echoes having progressively less intensity. The average rate of decrease (dotted line) of the voltage produced by the echoes is measured at every instant to produce a decay characteristic. **B:** The decay characteristic is inverted, (i.e. the reciprocal of each voltage value is derived) to give the 'ideal' TGC characteristic. **C:** The original echo amplitudes are multiplied by the TGC values to give automatically corrected amplitudes.

emphasised. This is called 'edge enhancement'. One edge enhancement technique is termed 'differentiate and add' (Fig. 17). A voltage proportional to the slope of the leading edge of an echo is generated and added back into the original echo voltage. The boundaries of structures usually give rise to strong reflections which, even when the reflectors are closely spaced, will make outlines better defined and improve resolution. The amplitude of the added voltage can be adjusted to give different degrees of enhancement. A drawback is that the differentiation process also enhances noise and must therefore be used sparingly.

Measurement

'On screen measurement' facilities are based on a standard piece of digital electronics. However, the design of the user controls often makes a substantial difference to the acceptability of a particular scanner. The design must enable the system to be rapid and convenient to use. If the measurement process is cumbersome, requiring a number of key strokes, a measurement may easily take a few seconds longer on one system than on another. In many investigations perhaps 10 measurements are made on a typical patient. A poor system can easily waste an additional 1 minute measurement time per patient. Over a day this amounts to sufficient time to see another patient.

Systems which require the operator to depress a control and wait while a caliper moves slowly across the screen are time wasters, as are systems which move the caliper spots back to the middle of the screen and destroy the previous reading as soon as the frame freeze is released. Calipers

Fig. 17 Edge enhancement. The video voltage waveform, shown in (**A**), comes from two echoes but the change in brightness of the display is not sufficient for this to be noticed. The voltage waveform in (**B**) is the differential of A, i.e. the voltage is proportional to the rate at which the original waveform changes. In (**C**), the differentiated voltage pattern has been added to the video voltage waveform to give a resultant signal in which the voltage from the leading edges of the echoes rises more steeply and the trough between them is much deeper. This 'edge enhance' process makes the echoes on the display more easily distinguished.

which remain on screen and are controlled by tracker ball or joystick are generally quicker to use.

Measurement precision

On screen measurements are made by positioning the calipers on the image of the structure to be measured. The boundary of the structure will be at least one pixel wide. Measurements are recorded from the centre of one chosen pixel to the centre of the other (Fig. 18): there is no way of knowing if the true reading was from the outside corners of the pixels, the inside corners, or somewhere in between – in all cases the displayed distance is the same. The precision of the reading is thus equal to plus or minus the diagonal of the pixel which, at low magnifications, can be half a millimetre. Most scanners, therefore, give readings to the nearest millimetre; others appear to give high accuracy by reading in 0.1 mm steps, but the reading actually increments by 0.3 mm steps. Higher accuracy readings are possible if high frequencies are used (e.g. small parts scanning) or in write zoom.

Digital beam control

The major problem in generating an image is to know from exactly where each echo originates. The range of an echo is determined from the time delay from launching a pulse and its subsequent arrival back at the transducer. The round trip distance is derived from the product of the time delay and the speed of sound. There is a variation of some 4% in the speed of sound in soft tissues so that there is a small uncertainty in determining the depth from which an

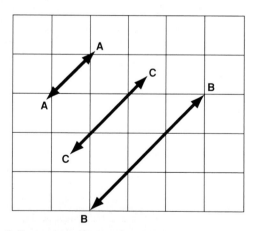

Fig. 18 Caliper errors. On screen measurement calipers are designed to display the distance between the centre points of the pixels where the calipers are placed. Calipers placed on the inside corners of the pixels (A – A) will give an identical reading to calipers placed on the outer corners of the pixels (B – B). Regardless of where the exact echo positions are, the reading will be that relating to (C – C). The uncertainty in the reading is equal to ± the diagonal of one pixel. Measurements on a full sized image on the best equipment currently available are subject to an error of ± 0.25 mm. Uncertainties of 1 mm are not uncommon.

echo originated. The resulting image distortion is usually imperceptible and cannot usually be corrected for.

Of much greater significance is the uncertainty in the direction from which an echo originates. The direction is always taken to be along the axis of the beam as it leaves the probe, but echoes, in fact, occur from anywhere across the beam which is disturbingly wide over much of its path. An echo from one side of the beam will be displayed at exactly the same point as a similar echo from the other side (Fig. 8C). This makes for inherently poor lateral resolution. The fact that the beam is most intense along its axis helps to give reasonable results, but positive improvements are necessary. One solution is to focus the beam electronically, both on send and receive, under computer control.

An equally significant problem is caused by grating lobes, low intensity beams generated at an angle to the main beam from all array probes. Although of low intensity, strong reflectors situated in the grating lobe give echoes which are easily detected and are displayed erroneously as if they came from the axis of the main beam (Fig. 19). Grating lobe artefacts limit the maximum amplification factor, which needs to be as high as possible to boost small echoes, because the resulting artefact swamps the image. The artefact can be significantly reduced by a digital technique called 'apodisation'. If apodisation is used, a much wider range of echo amplitudes can be displayed.

Synthetic aperture techniques

Array transducers, whether linear, steered (phased) or annular, can be made to behave as though they had a completely flexible shape, focusing and directing the beam in unexpected ways. Thus, an aperture is synthesised.

Wave interference Fundamental to the technique is the way sound waves interact with each other. Sound is a longitudinal compression wave. Any volume of tissue in the beam contains an excess of molecules during the high pressure phase of the wave and a reduction during the low pressure phase. Two ultrasound transducers, spaced by a small distance and operating at the same frequency and amplitude, give rise to waves which cross each other. A small volume of tissue, situated where the pressure peaks coincide, receives an excess of molecules from one wave and a further excess from the other. Consequently, the amplitude of the pressure wave in this volume is doubled. Conversely, a volume of tissue, situated where a pressure peak and trough coincide, experiences an increase in molecules from one source and a reduction from the other, leaving the net number of molecules in the volume unchanged. Thus, the pressure waves cancel out.

If there is a row of small sound sources, then a wave front, where all of the molecules move together in the same direction, is formed in a direction tangential to the waves from each transducer at the points where reinforcement

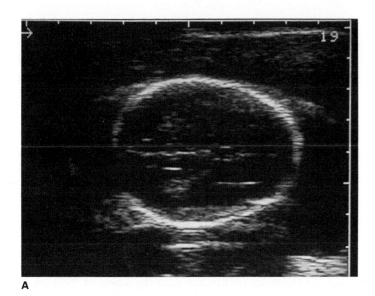

A

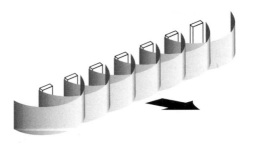

Fig. 20 Wavefront from an array. Each element in the array produces a sound wave at the same moment. The wavelet from each element spreads out and crosses the wavelets from the other elements. At the crossing points constructive interference occurs and reinforces the wave. The waves combine as shown to produce a wavefront which propagates as a beam in the direction of the arrow. In other directions there is cancellation due to destructive interference.

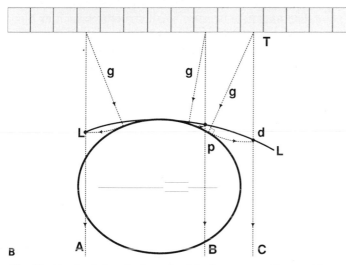

B

Fig. 19 Grating lobe. A: A grating lobe is seen extending to either side of the fetal head. **B:** The paths of just three beams, A, B and C are shown, but the argument applies to all beams. Each beam has a number of grating lobes (g), one of which, such as T-p, strikes the fetal head at a right angle. Although the energy in the lobe is small, the specular reflection has sufficient energy to be registered at the probe. The echo is displayed on the main beam at d, which has the same path length, T-d, as the grating lobe path T-p. A similar process is shown for beams A and B and occurs for all beams between A and C. The artefact is the locus of all such echoes.

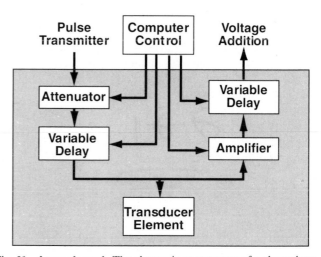

Fig. 21 Array channel. The electronic components of a channel are shown in the shaded area of the diagram. For dynamic focusing and apodisation, and for beam steering, each element in the group is connected to a channel. Each element in the channel can be adjusted by computer control.

occurs (Fig. 20). A beam always propagates in a direction at right angles to the wavefront.

Channels Array transducers are made from a sheet of piezo-electric material which has been cut into small elements. For array transducers to achieve their full potential each element must be accessed by its own electronic circuit. A wire contacts the element and then branches, one side connecting to a trigger pulse generator, an attenuator and a delay, and the other side connecting to a delay and an amplifier. The whole system of electronics connecting to each element is called a 'channel' (Fig. 21). Every com-

ponent in a channel may be adjusted instantaneously by computer control. To economise, many scanners use fewer channels than there are elements, and may not have the full complement of components to each channel.

On the pulse generation side, the pulser generates the trigger voltage which shocks each element into vibration. The voltage may be as high as 500 volts and is applied to the element for about one tenth of a microsecond. The attenuator reduces the voltage which reaches the transducer element. Delays are devices which pass a voltage pattern, unchanged in shape, from the input to the output, with a small, controllable time delay between the signal entering and emerging.

On the receive side the delay performs the same function as on the send side. The amplifier is a radio frequency amplifier whose gain (amplification factor) can be varied.

Phased array scanners

Phased array scanners produce a sector scan by steering the beam electronically. This has the advantage over mechanical sector scanners that there are no moving parts to wear out and, more significantly, that the beam can be switched instantly to any direction without passing through the intermediate scan line directions. This facility makes it possible to produce time-position traces, or duplex Doppler spectral displays, simultaneously with an image. The pulses producing the spectral display, time-position scan or A-scan can be interleaved with image lines. This happens sufficiently fast for the movement indication and image to be displayed together.

A phased array probe contains a large number, perhaps as many as 128, thin transducer elements. A small time delay is imposed between the application of the trigger pulse to each element (Fig. 22). The wave front from each element is circular because the elements are small compared to the wavelength. The wave from the first element to be triggered has time to propagate further than the wave from the adjacent element which is triggered fractionally later. The wave from the second element, in turn, propagates further than its neighbour and so on.

Earlier, it was stated that the wave front will be tangential to the wavelets. The result here is that the ultrasound pulse propagates at an angle to the probe face. The angle of propagation is dependent only upon the time delay between trigger pulses. This time delay is altered after each ultrasound pulse has been generated so that the beam angle changes to give the required 'windscreen wiper' sector scanning action.

When the beam is steered to large angles (greater than about 30°) to the probe axis, the first cycle of the pressure wave from one of the last elements to be triggered can readily interfere with the second cycle from one of the first elements to be triggered. This particular interference results in a relatively intense grating lobe, the direction of which is at a large angle to the primary beam and so may cause significant artefacts.

Focusing

Weakly focused lenses on single element transducers in mechanical sector scanners are used to narrow the beam over the central part of the image at the focal depth. Mechanical lenses are fixed focus. They improve the image significantly in the focal region but degrade it distally.

It is less obvious how the beams from linear and phased array transducers could be focused. Lenses can only be used to focus the beam at right angles to the scanning plane. Such lenses reduce the slice thickness of the scan in the focal region (Fig. 23). Scans are relatively tolerant of poor slice thickness because small structures such as blood vessels run parallel to the surface and seem well-resolved in cross-section. Less obvious structures, however, may be poorly resolved. Scans improve in contrast and spatial resolution if the slice thickness is narrow.

Electronic focus 'on send' An electronic focusing technique is required to bring the beams from array scanners to a focus – once again the wave interference principle is used. The beam is produced by a selected group of elements in the array, the channels being used so that the

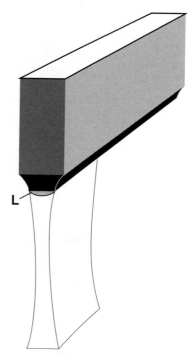

Fig. 23 Orthogonal focusing. A cylindrical lens along the face of a linear array focuses the beam in a direction at right angles to the scan plane. The consequent reduction in the beam width reduces the slice thickness thus improving the partial volume effect.

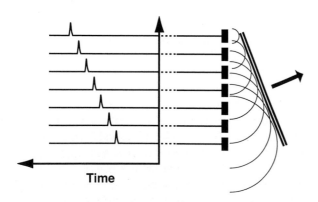

Time

Fig. 22 Electronic beam steering. A few transducer elements from a phased array transducer are portrayed along with a timing diagram showing the time delays between the trigger pulses applied to each element. The waves propagating from the lower elements have time to travel further than those from the upper elements. The interference between the waves causes the wavefront to be at an angle to the probe face. The pulse travels in a direction determined by the delays.

trigger pulses to the inner elements are progressively delayed with respect to the pulses applied to the outer elements. The circular wave fronts from the outer elements have time to propagate further than the waves from the inner elements: by constructive interference the resulting wave front will be curved (Fig. 24).

The beam propagates at right angles to the wave front so that the curved wave front brings the beam to a focus. Adjustment of the values of the delays applied to the trigger pulses changes the curvature of the wave front and alters the focal depth. The focal depth can be selected from the control panel of the scanner.

It is often desirable to focus at more than one depth in each image. This is achieved by building up the scan in strips, or zones, with the focus centred on each strip. The delays are adjusted under computer control so that first the focus is set close to the probe. All echoes occurring beyond the focal zone are rejected by an electronic 'range gate' and are not stored in memory. Having collected the echoes for the first strip, the delays are reset to give a deeper focus. The next zone starts at the depth at which the first zone cuts off and ends beyond the new focal point. The process is repeated to collect successively deeper strips until the

image is complete. The disadvantage of this technique is that the image frame rate is slowed down, making it more difficult to follow moving structures. (The display frame rate is maintained so that image flicker is minimised.) In addition the total sound energy deposited in the patient is increased, although the improved resolution may significantly reduce the total scanning time required to reach a diagnosis.

'Focus on receive' It would be convenient if the scanner could be continuously refocused, like a pair of binoculars, to track the position from which echoes are being received. This would avoid the problem of having to rescan with the focus set to different depths and would make it possible, in principle, to make the focus equally good at all depths. This can be done by computer control of the channels as the echoes are received.

Echoes radiate back toward the probe along spherical wave fronts. All elements on the array receive some of the sound energy in the echo, but at slightly different times. A small reflector will produce an echo which is detected first by the nearest element in the array and at later times by elements at a greater distance (Fig. 25). If the echo voltages from all of the elements are added together as they arrive, the time differences between them produces an elongated or smeared echo which, in turn, results in loss of resolution.

A correction for the time delays can be made if it is assumed that the echoes came from the axis of the beam. The distance from the reflector to each element in the array can be calculated for reflectors at any depth. Because the speed of sound in tissues is fairly constant, the expected time delays between the reception of the echoes can be derived. The echo voltages at each of the elements can then be synchronised by a computer which adjusts the delays in the channels. After synchronisation of the echoes, the summed voltages result in a large signal. If the echo did not originate on the beam axis, the delays in each of the channels, which have been calculated for an on-axis echo, will not synchronise the signals: summing produces only a small fluctuating voltage. Thus, on-axis echoes will be preferentially amplified, the same result as achieved by conventional focusing.

As the ultrasound pulse moves into the body, the focal point needs to be moved to coincide with the depth echoes are currently coming from. This gives real time focal tracking, achieved by continuously adjusting the delay values under computer control. In general, the more channels there are in the array the more accurately the beam can be focused. The complexity and cost of equipment rises with the number of channels, but the additional image quality is impressive.

Annular arrays

Techniques of focus on send and receive apply also to an-

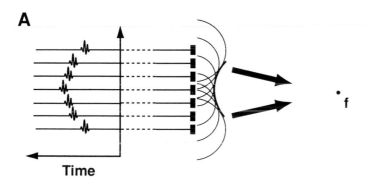

A

Time

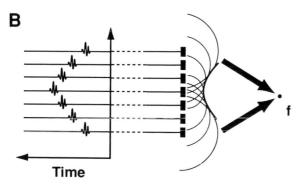

B

Time

Fig. 24 Electronic focusing. A small group of transducer elements is shown with a timing diagram of the trigger pulses applied to each element. The outer elements are triggered first so that the wave has time to propagate further than the waves from the inner elements. Interference effects cause the wavefront to be curved and the pulse propagates toward a focal area, f. In **A**: the time delays between the trigger pulses are smaller than in **B**: so the focus is further from the probe.

A

B

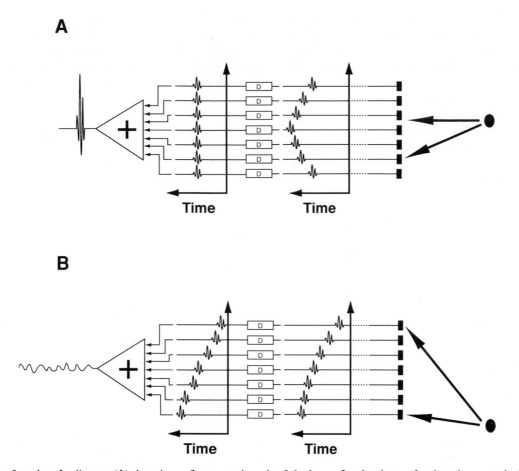

Fig. 25 Receive focusing. In diagram (**A**) there is a reflector on the axis of the beam. It takes longer for the echo to reach the outer elements than the central element. The timing diagram of the arrival of the echo at each element is shown. The voltages are passed through delays which bring the waves back into phase. When the waves are summed a large echo voltage is produced. In diagram (**B**) the reflector is off-axis. The relative arrival times at the elements is now different. The same delays are applied as in (A) but this moves the echo voltages further out of phase so that no voltage summation occurs and low level noise results.

nular array transducers. The significant advantage of annular arrays is that focusing is achieved both in the image plane and also across it (i.e. in both scanned and orthogonal planes). The shape of the beam is conical rather than the wedge shape produced by linear and phased arrays. For annular array transducers to be effective they need a large diameter. The mechanical problems of scanning the beam by oscillating a large array are considerable. Some instruments keep the array stationary and reflect the beam into the patient from an oscillating acoustic mirror. Annular arrays have weaker grating lobes and have potential for producing better spatial resolution.

Some experimental attempts to develop basic dynamic focus for linear arrays in the plane at right angles to the image plane have been attempted. The transducer elements are divided into three strips along the probe. The trigger pulses to the inner strip are delayed with respect to the outer resulting in a coarse, but variable, focus.

Dynamic aperture and f number

Photographers are familiar with the fact that a large lens aperture enables a photograph to be strongly focused on a subject in the middle foreground. The same considerations apply to ultrasound scanning. The width of the beam at the focus determines the lateral resolving power of the system and is calculated as the product of the wavelength and the focal length divided by the aperture. In optics, the focal length divided by the aperture is the familiar unit known as the 'f number'. The same term is used in ultrasound.

The resolving power in the focal zone improves as the f number decreases and also as the frequency increases. From other physical considerations it is known that it is impossible to obtain a focal spot smaller than a wavelength. An ideal f number where the beam width is twice the wavelength (i.e. 1 mm at 3 MHz) is f2. To obtain high resolution at f2 focused at 20 cm, the aperture would need to be 10 cm implying that the entire length of the linear array was used. At first sight it would seem that this would result in the disastrous situation of only a single ultrasound line being available to produce the scan!

A solution is found in the same principle that lay behind 'focus on receive'. If all of the elements in the array are used, the sound field floods the target area. Now, instead of emphasising echoes from the axis of the beam, the delays can be suitably changed so that echoes from any selected off-axis point are synchronised (Fig. 26). This possibility frees the designer from being constrained by where the axis of the ultrasound beams lies – the lines are created on receive rather than send. This technique is also valuable for the zoom function since the spacing between the lines created can be adjusted to the required value, and permit Regional Expansion Selection. Focus on send is used in conjunction with this technique with the image created one line to a pulse and the beam steered and focused to the region of the body where the echo line is to be generated. Clearly, an aperture of f2 can be achieved with a small number of elements when echoes originating near to the probe are being focused. To accommodate this fact, more and more elements are switched into circuit as echoes are received from deeper into the tissues. This is termed 'dynamic aperture'.

Apodisation

Grating lobes give rise to serious artefacts. They can be attenuated by 'apodisation' in which elements at the outer edges of the transducer are energised less strongly than the central elements. Similarly, if the echo is amplified less in the channels connected to the outer elements then, again, the echoes received from the grating lobes are attenuated (Fig. 27). The process is also referred to as 'spatial filtering' and enables the display dynamic range to be increased facilitating the ability to display small changes in tissue reflectivity. The consequent improvement in contrast resolution has considerable diagnostic advantage.

Probe construction

The digital techniques described would be of little value without high quality probes. Probe manufacture has steadily improved but there are inevitable design compromises. For instance, damping improves resolution but degrades sensitivity; more channels improve performance but make the cable stiff and bulky, and so on. A decision must always be reached on the balance between options, and the optimum probe design usually has to be found by experience gained in a particular clinical situation.

Resolution and frequency

The frequency of a transducer is determined by the thickness of its piezo-electric sheet. Usually the entire probe must be changed to alter the frequency though multi-element mechanical sector probes are available where each

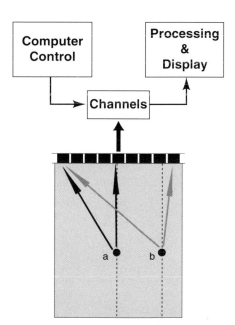

Fig. 26 Receive 'steering'. Figure 25 illustrated how an on-axis reflector is brought into focus electronically by delaying the echoes at the inner elements to bring them into phase with echoes arriving at the outer elements slightly later. By selecting different delays it is equally possible to bring the echoes from an off-axis reflector into phase. Thus, by suitable computer control of the channels the reflector at (b) can be emphasised while the on-axis echo (a) is rejected. The process depends upon a calculation of the distances from the reflector to each element in the array.

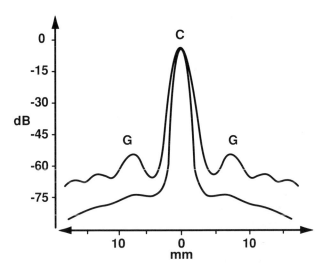

Fig. 27 Apodisation. The figure shows how the relative intensity of two beams varies from one side of the beam to the other. The large peak is the main lobe with the central axis at C. The upper trace has prominent grating lobes (G). When apodisation is applied (lower trace) the grating lobes are almost completely suppressed.

element produces a different frequency, and it is possible to drive a transducer at a slightly different frequency than its resonance. If the probe has to be changed, it saves a great deal of time and effort if it can be switched in and out of circuit without having to pull out a large multiway plug and insert another.

The use of high frequency probes allows both lateral and axial resolution to be improved. Narrower beams can be produced as the wavelength decreases (frequency increases) and lateral resolution improves as the beam width decreases. Similarly, as was shown earlier, the axial resolution is about half of the pulse length. As there are usually the same number of cycles in a pulse, regardless of frequency the pulse length will also decrease and the resolution will be improved.

A compromise must be made between resolution and sensitivity. Attenuation of sound at diagnostic frequencies is approximately proportional to frequency. Thus, higher frequencies are absorbed more strongly by the tissues so that deeper tissues cannot be imaged without using inordinately high power levels. This consideration usually restricts the diagnostic frequency range to between 1 and 20 MHz with the most used frequencies being between 2 and 7 MHz.

Sensitivity

The depth of penetration depends on the sensitivity of the probe which, in turn, depends upon many factors including frequency, damping, quarter wave matching, material and aperture.

At lower frequencies the attenuation of the sound pulse is less, making visualisation of deep tissues easier, but with the penalty of reduced resolution.

Shock excited transducers resonate with their natural frequency though in fact the pulse encompasses a spectrum of frequencies. The frequency quoted for a probe is actually that at which the spectral power is maximum (Fig. 28). Because the attenuation of a sound wave is proportional to its frequency, the higher frequencies in the spectrum are preferentially removed causing the centre frequency of echoes to drop as they originate from deeper in the patient. Some scanners use a radio frequency amplifier which is retuned to lower frequencies to keep track of the expected centre frequency of deeper echoes. Retuning allows a higher amplification factor to be used and makes the equipment more sensitive.

One form of tissue characterisation, which has been offered on commercial scanners, is based on the change in frequency content of echoes from different tissues. At present, the results are heavily dependent upon the equipment used so that, clinically, the technique has been disappointing.

Damping   To achieve high axial resolution the ultrasound pulse must contain as few cycles as possible. Efficient damping is required to stop the transducer ringing. This is achieved by moulding a backing block, possessing optimum mechanical properties, onto the back of the transducer. Sometimes, an electronic resonant circuit applied across the transducer is used to give further damping. Pulses as short as two cycles are achieved. Regrettably, efficient damping also makes the transducer insensitive.

Sensitivity and reverberation   Reverberation is an annoying artefact in which a cloud of echoes extends deep from the proximal edge of an area known to be echo-free. It is mainly caused by the poor absorption of echo energy by the transducer material. The energy which is not absorbed (typically 80%) is reflected back into the tissues producing a 'ghost' image. To minimise reverberation, the sound energy in the echo must be transmitted into the transducer more efficiently.

The technique which is commonly used to improve sen-

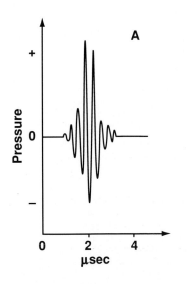
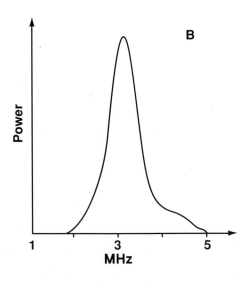

Fig. 28   Spectrum of a pulse. A: The pressure fluctuations in a pulse from a commercial probe, marked 3 MHz by the manufacturer, are displayed. **B:** A Fourier power spectrum of the pulse in (A) shows that a wide range of frequencies is present in the pulse. The plot shows that maximum power (i.e. the predominant frequency) is at 3 MHz but there is a significant amount of power at other frequencies.

sitivity is 'quarter wave plate' matching. The transducer is coated with a layer of a material with an impedance which is the geometric mean of the impedance of the tissues and the transducer material. The thickness is made equal to one quarter of the wavelength used. For long pulses the energy in the pulse is transferred to the transducer with very high efficiency but, since the short pulses used in imaging encompass a range of frequencies, matching is imperfect.

A further problem is the production of a single material with the correct impedance. It is simpler to manufacture a series of materials of graded acoustic impedance, which produces identical results and achieves high efficiencies. These are described as 'multiple matching layer transducers', and give good results reducing reverberation and allowing higher frequencies to be used with improved resolution.

Another technique, which has been used for high frequency probes, involves the use of a transducer material with a specific acoustic impedance much closer to that of soft tissue than the traditional ceramic materials. Transducers have been made from plastics such as polyvinylidene diflouride (PVDF). They have the additional advantage of being acoustically rather 'dead' so that the need for backing material is reduced. Although these transducers are good at receiving ultrasound, they are inefficient at producing it. Their major use is as hydrophone transducers. There is some interest in fabricating array transducers from the material, but this will probably necessitate mounting amplifiers directly onto the transducer elements themselves because the electrical impedance of plastics is very high.

Aperture and sensitivity Large aperture probes not only enhance focusing but also improve sensitivity. The transducer is rather like a sail on a ship – extensive canvas collects significant force even when the breeze is light. Similarly, a large transducer collects more ultrasound energy and makes the transducer more sensitive. The large apertures used for imaging at depth also enhance the sensitivity available for detecting deep echoes.

Transducer ageing Hundreds of millions of pulses are produced by a probe in its lifetime. It is not unusual for the transducer material to start to loose its piezo-electric properties as the crystal structure becomes disordered. The probe slowly becomes less sensitive. Probes must be regarded, rather like X-ray tubes, as consumable items with a typical life of 3 or 4 years of intensive use.

Sub-dicing

Each transducer element in a linear array probe may be sliced into a number of thinner elements that are connected together electrically. This process is designed to eliminate 'stationary noise' which appears as a cloud of echoes immediately beyond the transducer.

A transducer vibrates at its resonant frequency which is determined by its thickness. However, it also vibrates along and across at frequencies determined by its width and length (Fig. 29). In single element probes the width and length of the transducer are much greater than the thickness, hence sideways vibrations are of much lower frequency than the frequency from the wanted thickness-mode vibration and are eliminated by the tuned amplifiers. In a linear array transducer the width of each element is much the same as the thickness so that the sideways pulse has the same frequency as the interrogating pulse and is not tuned out. These thickness-mode vibrations travel along the array and generate echoes from the interfaces between the elements. These echoes are interpreted as originating within the tissues. By sub-dicing the elements, the frequency of the sideways pulse is made much higher than that of the wanted pulse and can again be eliminated by tuning the amplifier.

Probe ergonomics

The majority of what has been explained is profoundly important to image quality, but is not immediately obvious to the user except in manufacturers' literature. Of far more

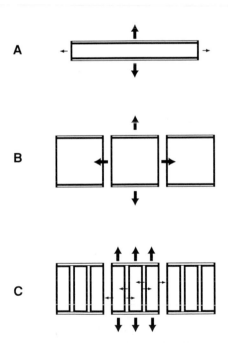

Fig. 29 Sub-dicing. When a transducer vibrates a sound wave is generated from the sides of the elements in addition to their faces. The resonant frequency of the sideways vibration depends upon the width of the element. **A:** In the case of a single element transducer the frequency of the unwanted part is much lower than the main beam and is tuned out by the radio frequency amplifier. **B:** However, in a linear array, the elements have square cross-sections and the pulse from the transducer sides has an identical frequency to the main pulse and cannot be eliminated by tuning. **C:** By dividing the elements further, but connecting them electrically, the pulse from the sides has a much higher frequency and again can be tuned out.

direct interest is the selection of probes. The range of available probes is huge. In general, probes should be lightweight, robust, convenient to hold, easy to change and perform well in practice.

General considerations Mechanical probes have the advantage that they are simple and seem to produce clearer Doppler signals. However, a typical scanner produces about 100 000 000 frames per year. It is clear that even a well-engineered mechanical probe will wear after a few years of use.

The lenses used on phased and linear array scanners are often made of silicon rubber to form a convex shape: silicon rubber is hygroscopic and lenses can be damaged if left in coupling gel for long periods of time. Similarly, cleaning spirits can cause damage.

Footprint For many applications the access area of the patient through which a satisfactory scan can be obtained, is small. In such cases the region of the probe in contact with the patient, the 'footprint', must be appropriate. An obvious example is cardiac scanning where a sector scanner is essential because of the small footprint which will fit into the window afforded by the intercostal spaces.

If good visualisation of superficial tissues is important a larger footprint is essential. A linear or curvilinear array is required. Sometimes angling of a probe into an anatomical area involves pressing one end of a linear array hard against the skin, causing discomfort. A curvilinear array is then preferable and produces good results. An instance is a longitudinal scan into the pelvis. Linear array probes are available from which the beam can be steered into the pelvis by phasing the last group of elements in the array.

Intra-corporeal probes It is desirable to place the transducer close to the target organ; this may often be achieved by intra-corporeal scanning. There is a number of reasons for this. The near complete reflection of sound at gas or air/tissue interfaces make an external approach to some organs effectively impossible. Similarly, the scattering and absorption of sound by tissues make the use of high frequencies, with their potential for markedly improved resolution, unusable for structures at depth if an external approach is used. Finally, although the speed of sound changes only slightly in soft tissues, angulated fat/muscle interfaces refract the sound beam by several degrees and may produce significant artefacts (see Ch. 4). Avoidance of superficial musculature is similarly helpful.

There is a wide range of intra-corporeal probes operating in most of the traditional modes of scanning, including linear and curvilinear arrays, mechanical sectors, and radial (plan position indication) probes. These are used as endoscopic, transoesophageal, trans-rectal, trans-vaginal, transurethral and even intravascular probes.

In all cases, taking the transducer inside the patient makes additional demands on the design. The electrical integrity of the probe and cable must be an order of magnitude better than for external scanning. The contours of the entire device must be smooth and able to be satisfactorily disinfected. The size and shape must be acceptable to the patient.

Because of the restricted nature of access to the probe contact area, needle guides are often useful to constrain the passage of the needle to the plane of the scan and along a marked vector on the image.

Intra-operative probes Intra-operative probes, like other intracorporeal probes, are capable of high resolution. There is a wide range of application because there are few parts of the anatomy which cannot be scanned. Once the skull or abdomen is opened ultrasound access, without interference from bone or gas, is usually assured. These probes are particularly useful for guiding the surgeon to a particular structure or foreign body.

The features of intra-operative probes are a small footprint and a probe casing and cable which do not get in the way of the operative field. In addition, the microbiological integrity of the device must be of a higher order than for any other probes.

Safety

Improvements in resolution and sensitivity, particularly in some Doppler and colour flow mapping techniques, and the use of annular array transducers have led manufacturers to raise the acoustic power output of equipment. Machines are available that produce beams 1000 times more intense than some of those used a decade ago. Spatial peak pulse average intensities of 10 Wcm^{-2} and peak negative pressures of -4 MPa (-40 atmospheres) have been measured from commercially available scanners. At these levels there is no question that mechanisms for cellular modification exist. It is important that all users make a risk–benefit judgement and know the output of their equipment.

Duplex scanners ensure that pulsed Doppler signals are obtained from the desired vessel. If the same elements are used to generate the image and to derive the Doppler signal there is no uncertainty about the co-planar nature of the image and the Doppler vector thus ensuring that the Doppler signal comes from the desired vessel. These systems must be set up to optimise the image, rather than the Doppler signal. The low sensitivity of the system and the broad bandwidth of the pulse make it very difficult to detect the minute echoes from blood corpuscles. The only solution is to use exceedingly high power pulses with the attendant uncertainties about hazard. This is of particular concern with trans-vaginal probes.

The alternative of using separate imaging and Doppler paths has attractions. The Doppler and the imaging processors can be optimised independently so that less power is required in the Doppler interrogating pulse. A problem with using a single probe is that, because most blood vessels run parallel to the surface of the body, the beam intersects the vessel at an angle close to 90°. Because the Doppler shift is proportional to the cosine of this angle the shift amplitude is small. With a separate probe system there can be a significant off-set between the two probes, making the angle between the Doppler beam and the blood vessels more acute and improving the Doppler signal. The same angling of the Doppler beam relative to the imaging beam can be achieved by steering in a linear array.

Several types of duplex scanners with separate imaging and Doppler probes are available. Some have Doppler probes which clip onto a linear array at a fixed angle and others house a steerable Doppler probe in the same housing as a mechanical sector probe. Although these probes may be less convenient the importance of safety must always be taken into account.

Use of controls

When performing real time scanning the effect of adjusting controls is immediately evident on the image. Thus, optimum adjustment is a matter of repeated corrections until the desired result is obtained. However, there is a logic to adjustments which will achieve the best results with the maximum efficiency.

Adequate preparation of the patient, although not a control, is essential if good images are to be obtained. If insufficient coupling medium (gel) is used, both initially and throughout the scanning process, no amount of adjustment of controls will produce the desired result. Similarly, care must be taken to avoid bubbles in the acoustic path. This is relevant when using coupling medium in a sheath over the probe. Obvious bubbles should be eliminated.

At the start of the day, the contrast, brightness and focusing of the display screens and hard copy devices must be checked. If these are poorly adjusted some of the already limited dynamic range will be lost. Adjustments are the same as on a domestic TV. The use of a grey scale bar or test card generated by the scanner facilitates adjustment.

The settings of other scanner controls must be optimised for the particular anatomical section being scanned. The required frequency of probe and its focal depth (for mechanical sector and other fixed focus probes) can be predicted from the application: high frequency, short focus probes are selected for scanning superficial structures and vice versa. Before scanning, TGC and compression characteristics are set to some reasonable value determined by experience or by a control which presets suitable values for typical examinations.

A quick scan to survey the area is undertaken in order to position the probe over the specific area of interest before making further adjustments. The first adjustment required is to the TGC aiming to use the minimum power consistent with a diagnostic image, and to achieve an even balance of echoes between near and far structures.

The distal part of the image determines the minimum acceptable acoustic power level. According to the type of TGC the 'far' or 'overall' gain, or the sliding adjusters for the deepest part of the required image, are set to a high level and the output power is reduced until this part of the image has the required displayed brightness. If sliders are used, the image is now 'evened up' zone by zone starting at the deepest and moving towards the most superficial. If, alternatively, a four control system is used, the near gain is next set, then any delay (to account for the absence of attenuation as the sound passes through any large echo-free spaces such as the bladder), and finally the slope. If the slope is too steep there will be a bright band across the middle of the image.

For cardiac scanning in M-mode the adjustment of the TGC slope is designed to emphasise a particular group of echoes such as the valves. Consequently the slope is steep and set across the valves whose movement is to be measured.

Having set the TGC on a low magnification image, the appropriate zoom or scroll is applied so that the region of interest occupies a significant proportion of the display screen. Now dynamic focus and edge enhance are used to optimise spatial resolution. On some mechanical sector scanners the line density can be changed. Slow sweeps giving high density may also improve spatial resolution. High frame rate small angle sectors are used when rapidly moving structures, such as cardiac valves, are to be followed.

Finally the compression control is adjusted to obtain the desired contrast resolution or to enhance outlines for measurement. For examinations where the differentiation of tissue types is critical, frame averaging may be used to smooth out speckle and improve contrast.

As the examination progresses there will usually be need for repeated small adjustments to the controls for the best images.

REFERENCES

1 Geiger M L, Ohara K, Doi K. Investigation of basic imaging properties in digital radiography. 9. Effect of displayed grey levels on signal detection. Medical Physics 1986; p 312–318

FURTHER READING

Fish P. Physics and instrumentation of diagnostic medical ultrasound. Chichester: John Wiley. 1990
Powis R, Powis W. A thinkers guide to ultrasonic imaging. Baltimore-Munich: Urban and Schwarzenberg. 1984
McDicken N. Diagnostic ultrasonics. Third edition. Chichester: John Wiley. 1990

Patient preparation and scanning techniques (general)

Paul A. Dubbins

INTRODUCTION

Ultrasound has long been described as an operator dependent technique, the quality of image and therefore the accuracy of diagnosis depending upon the familiarity of the operator with the equipment, with the use of multiple acoustic windows and with imaging artefacts. To some degree the advent of high resolution real time ultrasound has made this dependence less marked. The awkwardness of the static scanner of 10 years ago was sufficient disincentive to all but the most committed of sonographers. With real time ultrasound even an untrained person can produce an image but the technique still relies for its accuracy on the expertise of the operator and interpreter. Careful attention to the practice of scanning remains vital for good diagnosis.

Preparation

Preparation for an ultrasound examination is simple. For ultrasound scans of the upper abdomen a 6 hour fast is generally recommended, although this is not absolutely essential. Some would suggest that fasting the patient does little to improve visualisation of the upper abdominal organs and may even increase the amount of intestinal gas as a result of aerophagy. Indeed it is occasionally unavoidable to scan a patient unprepared, for example when the clinical condition demands urgent evaluation. In diabetic patients it is recommended that the 'portions' are taken as fluid rather than solid food. Although fasting does not reduce the amount of intestinal gas this is not the only reason for the preparation. Perhaps most important is the distension of the gallbladder that is afforded by a 6 hour fast. Non-visualisation of the gallbladder is generally taken as evidence of gallbladder disease as are contraction of the gallbladder lumen and thickening of the gallbladder wall. Because these features are normal findings following the functional contraction after a meal, they may be confusing.

Fasting also ensures that the stomach is empty and that the small bowel is not distended with food and fluid. Although real time has allowed the appreciation of peristalsis, occasionally a food and fluid filled bowel loop may masquerade as an intra-abdominal mass and the stomach full of food may obscure the pancreas. Attempts to reduce bowel gas by the use of such agents as activated charcoal or dimethyl siloxane have been disappointing.

In the newborn and infant it is often useful to scan during a feed to ensure a contented and relatively immobile patient.

Pelvic examination[1]

Traditionally the ultrasound examination of the pelvis has required a full urinary bladder. The variable amount of fluid and time required to fill the bladder has long been a source of frustration to both patient and operator. Typical instructions are to drink five or six glasses of fluid approximately 1 hour before the examination. The amount of fluid required varies not only with the patient but also with the time of day. More fluid is required in the morning as a result of the relative dehydration of an overnight sleep than for bookings in the afternoon. However, even the most careful planning will inevitably result in patients arriving for appointments with empty bladders, but an hour later all will be painfully full at exactly the same time! Although trans-vaginal scanning for gynaecological problems and trans-rectal scanning for disease of the prostate and seminal vesicles (and also of the rectum and pelvic peritoneal 'pouches') may replace much transabdominal scanning, the field of view remains limited and for the foreseeable future the full bladder technique will remain in use.

Filling the bladder has several functions; it displaces bowel out of the pelvis and acts as an acoustic window to structures within the pelvic peritoneal cavity (Fig. 1). In the female it straightens the axis of the uterus and demonstrates more clearly the relationship of the uterine fundus to the ovaries. However, an overfull bladder may distort anatomy,[2] e.g. by making a normal gestation sac appear irregular and flattened, producing a falsely enlongated cervix and consequently an apparent 'low lying placenta' or by displacing structures beyond the optimum focus of the transducer. Partial emptying of the bladder is required in these situations. Even with optimum bladder filling, partial and then complete emptying of the urinary bladder may be useful for a number of reasons:

a) to document bladder emptying;
b) to remove back pressure on the kidneys;

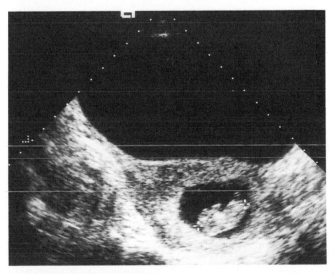

Fig. 1 Transverse scan of the pelvis, through a filled urinary bladder. The bladder provides a window to the pregnant uterus containing an embryo (measurement cursors).

c) to demonstrate any pelvic mass displaced into the abdomen by the full bladder;

d) to avoid confusion between a large pelvic cyst and the urinary bladder;

e) to examine the side walls of the false pelvis (the iliac fossae) for evidence of iliac lymphadenopathy, muscle asymmetry etc. (Fig. 2). It is frequently possible to perform a limited pelvic examination when a patient presents with an empty bladder (Fig. 3).

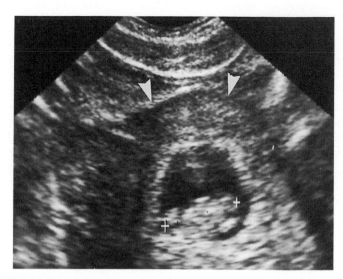

Fig. 3 Obstetric scan – empty bladder. Scan through the pelvis in a patient with an empty bladder. Compression with the transducer allows the demonstration of the fundus of the uterus (arrowheads). The pregnancy can be identified in this case without recourse to a full bladder or to the trans-vaginal approach.

The use of fluid infused into the rectum has been advocated as a method of differentiation of bowel from masses and for the determination of their relative position in the pouch of Douglas or recto-vesical pouch. With real time this is rarely necessary since usually the demonstration of natural peristalsis and mass movement can allow this differentiation. The technique is occasionally used in the evaluation of large bowel pathology and water or saline enemata with ultrasound monitoring has been advocated to reduce intussusceptions though the traditional barium reduction is a better technique.

Upper abdominal ultrasound

Anatomy Knowledge of the position occupied by the various organs within the abdomen and pelvis and their relationship with surface markings is required for the proper performance of ultrasound. The relationship for example of the liver with the right costal margin must be understood not only for the adequate demonstration of the liver itself, but also the use of the liver as an acoustic window to other intra-abdominal organs. The normal axes of organs such as the kidneys must be remembered if a scan plane demonstrating the long axis of the structure is to be achieved.[3]

Although a knowledge of sectional anatomy is a self-evident requirement both in the performance and in the interpretation of ultrasound scans; knowledge of the anatomical relationships for example of the liver to the kidney, gallbladder to portal vein branches etc. is essential if intra-abdominal structures are to be correctly identified and adequately demonstrated.

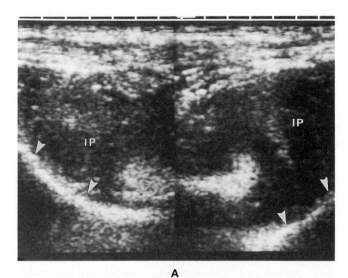

A

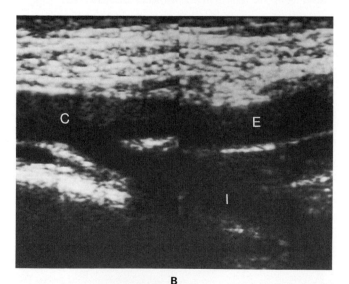

B

Fig. 2 Pelvic scans – empty bladder. A: Transverse scan of the pelvis with an empty bladder. This is a split screen, linear array scan using compression to demonstrate the muscles of the greater pelvis. The iliac bones are demonstrated bilaterally (arrowheads) with the ilio-psoas muscles overlying them (IP). The muscle on the left is enlarged and relatively echo-poor in this patient with a left ilio-psoas haematoma. **B:** Oblique scan of the iliac fossa following the course of the common (C) and external (E) iliac arteries. The postero-medial origin of the internal iliac artery (I) is also shown.

Transducer selection The choice of transducer type is partly personal preference, although the advantages of a small faced sector scanner are significant in abdominal and pelvic scanning. The small footprint, yet wide field of view, allows the transducer to be placed where acoustic windows are limited: in the intercostal spaces, the sub-xyphoid region and low in the pelvis when the bladder cannot be completely filled. Linear arrays are more cumbersome and the larger footprint makes them less suitable for intercostal scanning, for example. However, the field of view in the near zone is much more extensive than the sector scanner; therefore for superficial structures, such as the muscles of the anterior abdominal wall (Fig. 4), small parts scanning and superficial intra-abdominal organs such as the gallbladder and aorta in slim patients, the linear array provides optimum imaging. Curved arrays are more flexible than linear arrays. Tightly curved (microconvex) arrays suffer from the same limitations of field of view in the near zone as do sector scanners.

Frequency and focus Electronic focusing for phased and linear arrays and for annular mechanical sector transducers has made the selection of transducer for a particular working depth less critical although setting the optimum focus remains important. Fixed focus transducers are still in wide use and with these it remains important to select the optimum transducer not only for frequency of sound transmission but also for focal zone at the depth of the area of interest. The selection of transducer frequency follows a simple rule: the highest frequency possible should be selected that allows adequate penetration to the area of interest at low to medium power levels. Generally this implies the use of high frequency transducers for superficial structures while lower frequencies must be used for more deeply placed organs.

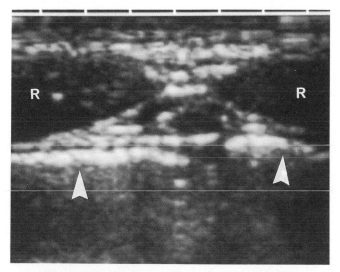

Fig. 4 High frequency linear array scan demonstrating the structures of the anterior abdominal wall. R – rectus abdominis, Arrowheads identify the transversalis fascia and peritoneum.

Occasionally the use of a stand-off is useful. To some degree this achieves the same effect as using a transducer with a shorter focus, since the stand-off displaces the face of the probe from the skin surface and from the structures under examination. With the variety of frequencies now available this is not often necessary, although it can be of value in the assessment of superficial structures, particularly when using a sector scanner since it widens the field of view in the near zone. Occasionally the use of a stand-off allows the visualisation of a superficial structure when the ideal transducer is not available.

Patient position The supine position is standard for an abdominal ultrasound examination. This position owes as much to history as to patient comfort: with the original static scanners it was difficult to examine the patient in any other position. With real time equipment the patient may be scanned supine, standing or even sitting if this is appropriate. Indeed a flexible approach to patient position is necessary to achieve optimum images in all patients and any images at all in patients in whom position is dictated by other factors such as age, infirmity, intensive care paraphernalia, drainage tubes etc.

Supine: the starting point for most examinations. It allows muscle relaxation, and flattens the abdomen (Fig. 5A).

Decubitus[4-6] (right and left) (Fig. 5B): raising alternately the right and left sides causes descent of the liver and the spleen further into the abdomen and allows axial scanning of the kidneys and retroperitoneum (Fig. 6). This and the oblique position encourage free fluid into the most dependent position and displace gas from the mid-abdomen. The left posterior oblique position is ideal for scanning the gallbladder and proximal biliary tract (Fig. 5C). In the right posterior oblique position the distal bile duct may be visualised through the fluid filled antrum and pylorus. Use of these different positions after ingestion of fluid may allow better visualisation of many of the retroperitoneal structures.

Upright:[7] this causes the liver and gallbladder to descend into the abdomen, changes the position of biliary calculi and distends the intra-abdominal veins, many of which act as landmarks for intra-abdominal organs. The pancreas for example is more frequently visualised in the erect position than any other.

Prone: the prone position is used rather less than hitherto but may be useful for visualisation of the kidneys, particularly during interventional procedures (Fig. 5D). The patient may crouch on all fours, scanning from a ventral position to detect small amounts of ascitic fluid and to demonstrate stone movement in difficult cases of gallbladder calculi (Fig. 5E).

Sitting: this is the optimal position for the evaluation of pleural fluid since it is in this position that most pleural aspirations are performed. Furthermore it may be necessary to examine dyspnoeic patients in this position and in

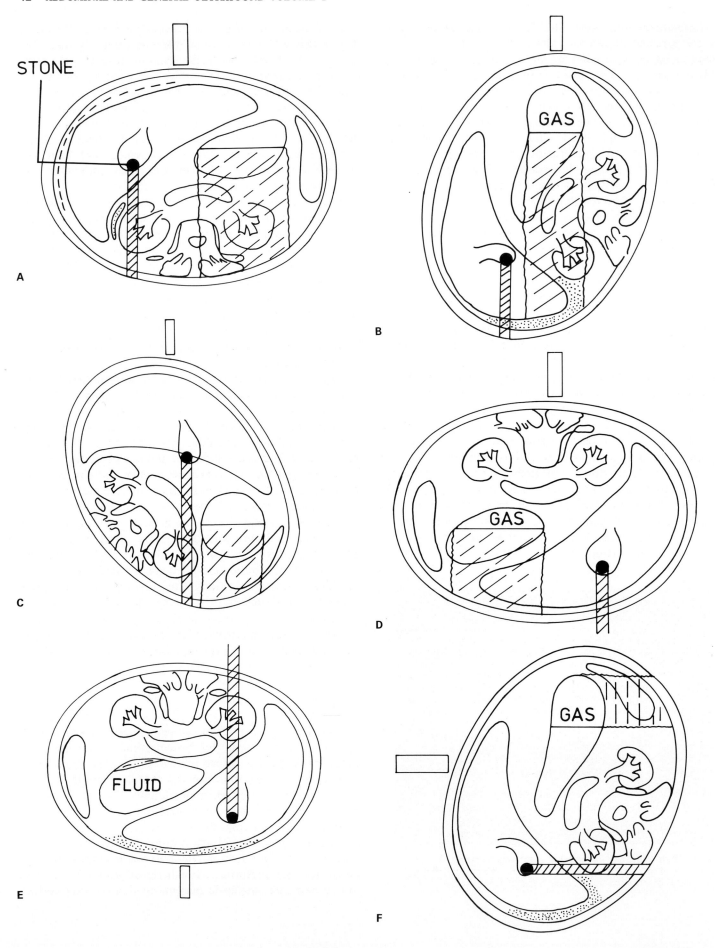

extreme cases, when only limited diagnostic information is required (for example the documentation of hepatic metastases), it is possible to examine patients without their having to be manhandled from the comfort of their wheelchair!

In infants and young children the sonographer may have to use all of these positions in rapid succession. Often very young children are best examined in the mother's arms when their position may be unorthodox and variable.

Changes in patient position often improve the demonstration of intra-abdominal anatomy and pathology. However, it is important to be aware of the differences in anatomical appearances and of imaging artefacts that such changes produce. Knowledge of the expected shift of bowel gas, of free fluid and acoustic shadowing will allow a more complete evaluation (Fig. 5).

Scan technique and planes of scan Although static scanning was cumbersome, it demanded a scan technique of obsessional discipline. It is no longer necessary or even possible to perform scan plans at half or one centimetre intervals over the entire abdomen, but instead real time ultrasound can provide multiple images at millimetre intervals. To realise the full potential of this capability, a careful methodical approach to scan technique is still required.

Orthodox scan planes remain the starting point for most ultrasound examinations. Sagittal planes of scan can be achieved by sweeping the transducer in the sagittal plane slowly from midline to right and to left starting at the xiphisternum and ending in both flanks. The probe should be alternately angled up and then down to visualise the dome of the diaphragm and more inferiorly placed struc-

Fig. 5 Effect of posture on anatomy. A: Supine scanning position. Section of the upper abdomen showing the contribution to image quality and image artefacts by various abdominal structures. The left upper quadrant is obscured by gas in the stomach. A stone in the gallbladder produces acoustic shadowing which may obscure structures deep to this. Fluid will collect in Morrison's pouch or may track over the surface of the liver. **B:** Right posterior steep oblique. Shadowing from the gas in the stomach now obscures midline structures and some of the structures in the right upper quadrant including some of the fluid that has collected in Morrison's pouch. The spleen and left kidney however, are well-demonstrated in this plane. **C:** Left posterior steep oblique position. This plane of scan demonstrates the right upper quadrant structures well but gas in the stomach obscures the left upper quadrant. **D:** The prone position. Less commonly used than hitherto, access to the kidneys is occasionally facilitated. This approach is used during interventional procedures of the renal tract, for example percutaneous nephrostomy. **E:** Prone position. It is occasionally valuable to place the transducer on the dependent portion of the abdomen in oblique, decubitus or prone positions. This allows the detection of small volumes of fluid in the peritoneal cavity, may improve images of the stomach and occasionally allow the identification of mobile calculi indistinguishable from bowel gas on other views. **F:** Scanning in the right posterior steep oblique position. Ascites and fluid in the bowel collects in the more dependent portion. This allows the detection of small amounts of fluid in Morrison's pouch and may also allow visualisation of the head and body of the pancreas through fluid in the body and antrum of the stomach.

tures such as the inferior margin of the liver, gallbladder, pancreas etc. In the transverse plane the transducer may be placed beneath the xiphisternum and moved slowly down the abdomen angling to right and to left to complete the survey. Modified scan planes from the axial approach are often necessary, angling the transducer cephalad for example, to visualise the hepatic veins and caudad, using the left lobe of the liver as an acoustic window, to image a pancreas otherwise obscured by bowel gas. Other modifications of scan planes are necessitated by surface anatomy, organ anatomy and patient well-being. Demonstration of the common bile duct is best performed with the patient in the left posterior oblique position and the scan plane angled from the right shoulder to the left pelvic brim, a line which follows the usual lie of the hepatic pedicle.[8] The long axis of the kidneys is best seen in a scan plane at an angle to the sagittal, recognising the more lateral position of the lower poles. Similarly in the coronal plane the axis of scan must take into account the fact that the lower poles are more anteriorly placed than the upper poles. The scan of the pancreas also follows an oblique plane with the tail displaced cephalad.

Intercostal views of the liver and spleen require that the scan plane follow the intercostal spaces to allow maximum visualisation of organ parenchyma. While these unusual scan planes allow accurate assessment of parenchymal texture, they often cause difficulties with the assessment of gross anatomy and of anatomical relationships. Indeed unfamiliar scan planes may be confusing while the production of unusual artefacts makes diagnosis more difficult.

The coronal scan plane used for evaluation of the kidneys, major vessels and retroperitoneum can be achieved by placing the probe in the patient's flank with the patient in the lateral decubitus position (Fig. 6). This is ideal for demonstration of the lateral branches of the major vessels, particularly the renal arteries and moving the probe more posteriorly and angling slightly anteriorly towards the lumbar spine produces a true coronal scan through the axis of the kidney, thereby demonstrating the continuity between the collecting system and renal pelvis.

Pelvic ultrasound

The scan planes used for evaluation of pelvic organs are similar to those for the upper abdomen. Sagittal and transverse scans form the basis for most examinations. However, to make full use of the filled urinary bladder as an acoustic window, it is important to place the ultrasound probe on the contralateral side of the pelvis to the area of interest, angling across the bladder. Similarly, in the transverse plane, angulation both superiorly and inferiorly may demonstrate the pelvic anatomy more clearly. The angulation of the probe in pelvic examination is particularly important: the ultrasound beam must be orientated normal to the axis of the uterus for optimum demonstration of the

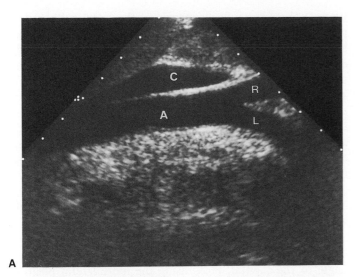

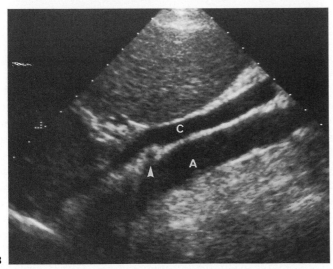

Fig. 6   Coronal scans showing the retroperitoneum. A: Long axis coronal scan from the right flank demonstrating the inferior vena cava (C), the aorta (A) and bifurcation into right and left iliac arteries (R, L). **B:** Coronal scan through the right upper quadrant demonstrating the liver, inferior vena cava (C) and the aorta (A). The origin of the right renal artery (arrowhead), a lateral branch of the aorta, is well-shown in this plane which is ideal for Doppler assessment.

endometrial canal and the different appearances of the endometrium during the menstrual cycle. Similarly an off-axis plane of scan may be necessary to demonstrate the uterus which deviates to right or left of midline. Following bladder emptying, the pelvic organs may be re-examined: occasionally it is possible to image the fundus of the uterus in an anteverted position together with laterally placed ovaries related to the internal iliac vessels (Fig. 3). With the bladder empty, the scan plane should follow the course

of the iliac vessels along the line between the umbilicus and the palpable pulsation of the femoral artery in the groin. This allows demonstration of the common and external iliac arteries and any associated lymphadenopathy. Transverse scans along the same course complete the examination.

For the most part, with liberal use of acoustic gel, gentle pressure of the transducer is all that is required to achieve adequate imaging of the intra-abdominal organs. Occasionally rather firmer pressure is required, for example, when angling the probe underneath the costal margin to visualise the liver close to the dome of the diaphragm. Deliberate compression of the abdomen with the probe is, however, often extremely valuable. By displacing bowel gas from the pelvis it often allows the demonstration of previously obscured iliac vessels, uterus, ovaries etc. after bladder emptying (Fig. 3). Similarly probe compression is often necessary to demonstrate the abdominal aorta, although care must be taken if an aortic aneurysm is suspected. An important example is the use of graded compression in the assessment of suspected appendicitis when the displacement of bowel gas from the right iliac fossa allows acoustic access to the thickened appendix and associated peri-appendiceal fluid.[9] Compression, however, has a wider role in the evaluation of the bowel itself: occasionally fluid filled bowel can mimic bowel thickening or other intra-abdominal pathology – careful but firm compression with the ultrasound probe will allow the differentiation of real from apparent bowel pathology.

Doppler

Although Doppler ultrasound is considered elsewhere in this text (see Ch. 5) it is worthwhile to reiterate the differences in technique that Doppler ultrasound requires. Doppler evaluation of all vessels requires that there is a vector of flow towards or away from the transducer. Imaging is best when the ultrasound beam is at right angles to the structure under investigation (Fig. 6): at this angle no Doppler signal is produced. The combination of ultrasound imaging and Doppler examination is therefore a compromise between the requirements of the two techniques, particularly in the abdomen.

Summary

Adequate, accurate diagnosis by ultrasound requires an extensive knowledge of anatomy, both surface and sectional, of pathology and of the sonographic appearances that may result from pathology. If any information is to be derived from an ultrasound examination, then this must be performed with strict attention to examination technique.

REFERENCES

1 Sample W F, Lippe B M, Gyepes M T. Gray scale ultrasonography of the normal female pelvis. Radiology 1977; 125: 477
2 Baker M E, Mahony B S, Bowie J D. Adverse effect of an overdistended bladder on first trimester sonography. AJR 1985; 145: 597
3 Whalen J P. Caldwell Lecture: Radiology of the abdomen impact of new imaging methods. AJR 1979; 133: 585
4 Athey P A, Tamez L. Lateral decubitus position for demonstration of the aortic birfurcation. JCU 1979; 7: 154
5 Isikoff M B, Hill M C. Sonography of the renal arteries: left lateral decubitus position. AJR 1980; 134: 1177
6 Pardes J G, Auh Y H, Kneeland J B, et al. The oblique coronal view in sonography of the retroperitoneum. AJR 1985; 144: 1241
7 McMahon H, Bowie J D, Beezhold C. Erect scanning of pancreas using a gastric window. AJR 1979; 132: 587
8 Behan M, Kazam E. Sonography of the common bile duct: value of the right anterior oblique view. AJR 1978; 130: 701
9 Puylaert J B. Acute appendicitis: US evaluation using graded compression. Radiology 1986; 158: 355

Artefacts

David O. Cosgrove

INTRODUCTION

Strictly an artefact is any man-made object; in imaging the term is used in a looser sense to describe unwanted information generated in the process of image formation.[1-3] Almost always artefacts interfere with interpretation though there are occasional instances where they contain diagnostically useful clues (e.g. acoustic shadowing). Ultrasound is particularly prone to artefacts: their recognition and avoidance form a major part of the skill and art of sonography.[4,5]

Noise

Two types of noise beset all imaging systems, random and structured. All electrical components produce random voltage changes at low level; when these are amplified they appear as a fluctuating, moving pattern of fine grey spots resembling a snow storm. Since the scanner's electronic components are designed to keep such noise at low levels, it is only seen when high degrees of amplification are applied and so is usually most obvious in the deeper parts of the image where the TGC amplifier adds most to the overall receiver gain (Fig. 1). Because this type of noise is random in time its effects can be reduced by temporal smoothing (the scanner controls for this are labelled 'frame averaging' or 'persistence' on some machines). With this technique the information in two or more images is added together. The 'real' information is reinforced whilst the random noise tends to cancel out. Random noise can also be produced as an acoustic artefact by chaotic vibrations in the body or in the transducer at ultrasonic frequencies; in practice these are too low in amplitude to produce detectable signals.

Random noise may also be produced by electrical interference, but in this case it usually forms patterned signals such as flashes or bars in the image; structured noise such as this is known as clutter (Fig. 2). It is caused by pick-up of extraneous signals in the radio-frequency band by the transducer acting as an antenna or by electrical pulses breaking through into the mains cable or interconnecting cables to attachments such as recorders. The noise they produce is usually easily recognised as artefact, the interference appearing randomly or intermittently, sometimes coinciding with the switching of a nearby motor or diathermy unit. Transient pulses can also wreak havoc with the digital circuitry of the scanner computer causing it to lock-up or otherwise misbehave. Mains filters or even shielding of the scanning room may be required in severe cases.

There are numerous other sources of noise such as interference from the scan-head motor and faulty connections and soldered joints which may affect ultrasound scanners, but they are uncommon and generally not diagnostically confusing, though rectification requires specialist

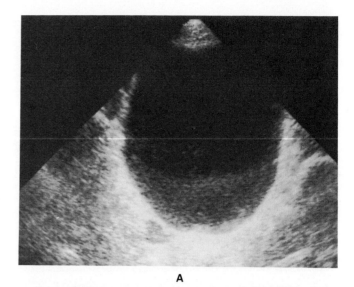

A

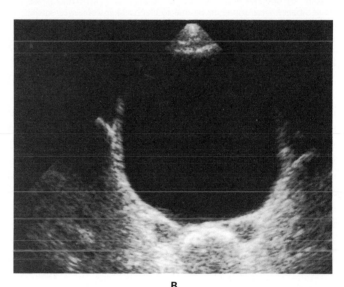

B

Fig. 1 Gain related noise. A: The combination of high overall gain and the high TGC amplification at depth may produce random noise in the image. Though this is present throughout the deeper parts of the image, because it is masked by the echoes from tissue structure, the noise is most obtrusive in echo-free regions such as within the urinary bladder. **B:** In this case, correction of the excessive gains removed the noise but this cannot always be achieved without also darkening structure whose display is required.

service engineers. Structured noise due to multiple reflections is discussed on page 54.

Scattering and specular interfaces

Two distinct types of ultrasound echo formation can be recognised and each produces important artefacts. Echoes arising from small regions[6] (around the ultrasound wavelength, say 0.1 to 1 mm) where there is a change in

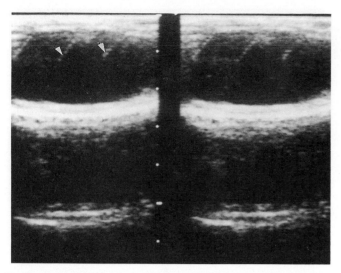

Fig. 2 Structured noise. Persistent oblique bars (arrowheads) on these images were found to be due to electrical interference to the scanner by a nearby diathermy apparatus. Similar effects can be produced by radio transmitters and by stray fields from poorly shielded TV monitors and video recorders. CB radio transmitters are particularly troublesome offenders.

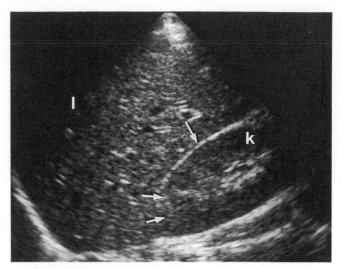

Fig. 3 Specular and scattered echoes. Scattered signals account for the low intensity parenchymal echoes from the liver (l) and kidney (k). Their appearance is independent of the direction of the ultrasound beam. Specular echoes arise from the flatter structures of the peritoneal and fascial layers separating the liver from the kidney. These echoes are strongly dependent on the angle between the beam and the surface, being intense when the surface is aligned at 90° (arrow) but weak or even completely absent when the beam runs along the interface (short arrows).

impedance are known as scattered echoes because they are sent out more or less uniformly in all directions.[7] It follows that the amount of ultrasound energy returning to the transducer from each scattering structure is extremely low (e.g. if the scattering is truly omnidirectional, then only some 0.25% is received by the transducer, depending on its diameter and on the depth of the scatterer); generally this signal will be too weak to be detected. However, when an array of such weak scatterers lies in the beam (this is the usual situation when for example they are the surfaces related to liver lobules or renal tubules), their individual echoes combine to form an interference pattern, summing in some directions and subtracting in others (Fig. 3). Signals strong enough to be detected are produced. The near random pattern that results is known as speckle; it is the acoustic equivalent of the speckled texture seen under laser light, for example in a hologram. The ultrasound pattern, though isotropic (i.e. uniform regardless of scanning direction), is only remotely related to the real tissue structure: the displayed texture is actually a convolution of the real structure by the ultrasound beam characteristics. Thus a pixel on the ultrasound image of the parenchyma of say, the liver, cannot be expected to correspond to a real interface in the organ. Because the speckle pattern is as much produced by the transducer as by the tissue, the same organ will produce a different texture with different transducers so that organs with different histological structures may have indistinguishable appearances on ultrasound – an example is the near-identical texture of liver and spleen.

When the reflecting surface is flat (relative to the ultrasound wavelength), it behaves as a mirror so that the direction of reflection equals the angle of incidence. Since the focused beam of ultrasound is not dispersed, all of the reflected energy can be picked up by the transducer so that the signals are much stronger than for scatterers. However they are intensely directional and can only be detected when the transducer is correctly situated i.e. when the surface is at right angles to the beam for the standard pulse-echo imaging. As the surface is tilted away from the right angle, the signal intensity falls off rapidly; in fact, were it not for the tolerance afforded by the beam width and the fact that real biological surfaces are rarely mirror-smooth, any tilting of the surface from 90° would cause the echo to be lost and this constraint would apply in both the scanned and orthogonal planes. In practice most interfaces are detectable up to angles of more than 60°, albeit with diminished intensity, depending on the particular structures involved (Fig. 3).

However, beyond some limiting angle, flat surfaces are not imaged and this can be most confusing (Fig. 4). It accounts for the apparent communication sometimes seen between the IVC and the aorta when these lie close together, for the failure to image the sides of the globe of the eye and for the invisibility of the superior surface of the urinary bladder in ascites scanned from certain angles. Such 'missing' surfaces can always be demonstrated by scanning from other angles: the sonographer needs to be aware of the problem to avoid serious diagnostic errors.

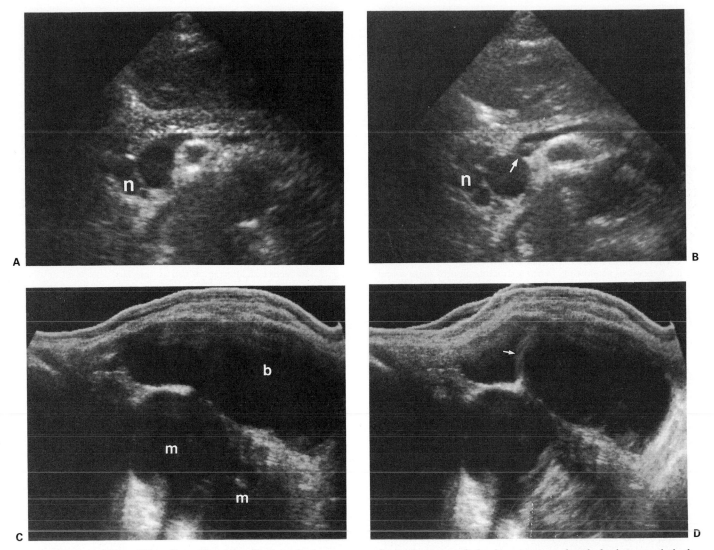

Fig. 4 Missing surfaces. When flat surfaces that lie along the beam are not depicted, very confusing images are produced. **A:** An example is the wall between a dilated lower common bile duct and the adjacent portal vein in the head of the pancreas. The duct seems to form part of the vein and may be missed altogether. **B:** The interface is readily detected when the transducer is appropriately angled (arrow). (The obstruction was caused by enlarged lymph nodes (n) in the head of the pancreas.) **C:** A similar situation applies in the pelvis when a cystic mass lies above the bladder (b). **D:** If the interface (arrow) is not detected, the cystic mass may be missed completely, being interpreted as part of the bladder itself. Figures C and D are from a patient with cystadenocarcinoma of the ovary with peritoneal metastases (m).

Shadowing and enhancement

The commonest form of shadowing (and its counterpart, enhancement) are perhaps not true artefacts and their presence provides important diagnostic information about the attenuation of the tissues responsible for them (Table 1).[8,9] Shadowing occurs when a region of the tissue has a higher attenuation coefficient than the majority of the tissue in the scan; since the TGC (which corrects for the attenuation with depth) can only be set for an average value, an inadequate correction will be applied to this region so that both it and the tissues deep to it are depicted as less reflective than they actually are (Fig. 5). The dark band is referred to as an acoustical or distal shadow. Conversely, if a region of tissue attenuates less than its surroundings, echoes from it and the deeper tissue are

Table 1 Types of shadowing

Type	Source
attenuation	attenuation higher than TGC compensation
reflective	near-total reflection
edge	from curved surfaces

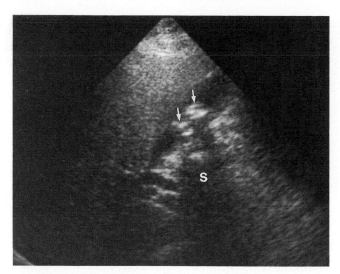

Fig. 5 Acoustical shadowing. When a structure absorbs more sound energy than its surroundings, the TGC correction is inadequate for that region and the deeper structures appear darker – this is known as acoustical or distal shadowing, here produced by gallstones in the gallbladder (arrows). s – shadowing.

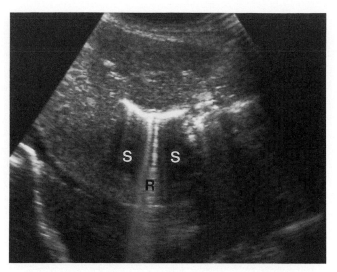

Fig. 7 Reflective shadowing. When an interface reflects all or almost all of the incident sound energy, a situation that is typical of gas (here, gas in the common bile duct) so little penetrates that a band of distal shadowing (S) results. Though the effect is the same as with absorptive shadowing (compare with Fig. 5) the mechanism is different. The intense flat reflector that the gas forms often leads to reverberation artefacts (R) that partially fill the shadow (compare with Fig. 14).

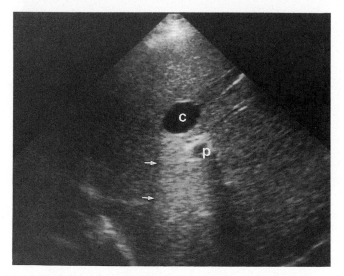

Fig. 6 Enhancement. The fluid in a cyst absorbs very little of the sound energy passing through it so that the TGC, which has been adjusted to correct for attenuation in the surrounding tissues (here, the liver) is locally excessive. The deeper tissues are depicted as being more reflective giving a lighter band (arrows) known as distal or acoustic enhancement. c – cyst, p – portal vein.

Thus these effects provide clues to the attenuation of the tissue regions responsible.

Since shadowing is simply loss of acoustical signal for a tissue region, it can also be produced by an extremely efficient reflector (Fig. 7).[10] A gas bubble or region of calcification for example, where 99% and 80% of the incident sound beam is reflected back respectively, will cast an acoustic shadow because very little of the energy penetrates to insonate the deeper tissues (in addition, any echoes from them would probably not cross the reflective layer on the return journey since they would be re-reflected distally). However, it should be noted that, for most soft tissues, only a small proportion of the loss of energy from the beam (i.e. the attenuation) is due to reflection (in fact only between 1% and 20%) so that echogenicity does not correlate well with attenuation. Echogenic fluids (e.g. crystalline bile or a pyonephrosis) are examples where strong echoes are associated with enhancement (Fig. 8).

An interesting and confusing form of shadowing is seen deep to the edges of strongly curved surfaces such as vessels, cyst walls and the fetal skull (Fig. 9). Fine, dark lines are seen extending distal to such edges; in the case of a cyst they are striking by contrast with the enhancement from the cyst itself. Two explanations have been offered (Fig. 10). In the refractive model the ultrasound beam is dispersed as it is reflected from the curved edge because the leading edge of the ultrasound beam strikes it at a different angle than the trailing edge. Thus the ultrasound energy is spread through a larger tissue region and so the returning echoes are weaker resulting in a 'shadow', at the

over-corrected and appear as a bright band known as 'enhancement' (Fig. 6). This enhancement has no relation to the increase in tissue contrast produced by the injection of 'contrast' agents e.g. gas bubbles in echocardiography or iodinated compounds in X-radiology. The degree of shadowing and enhancement are determined by the difference in attenuation from the surrounding structures as well as the path length through the anomalous region.

same time the velocity differences may focus the beam in the region immediately deep to the structure, increasing the enhancement.[11] Simple geometrical reflection, as from a flat surface, would not have the same effect, for a mirror image of the tissues it strikes will be superimposed on the band immediately behind the edge; this is the mirror image artefact, see below. The other explanation presumes that the tissue forming the wall of the curved structure has a higher attenuation than the surrounding tissue; the ultrasound beam passing along the edge must pass through three to four times as much of this tissue than that crossing at the diameter and therefore will be attenuated more. The

effect is familiar to those who have used a hacksaw in plumbing: cutting a pipe is difficult at first, becoming easier towards the centre of the pipe before becoming more difficult again as the full thickness of the other side is cut. In this model the edge shadows are a form of attenuation, but only of the wall material, not of the contents. The two mechanisms could coexist in different situations.

Whichever explanation is accepted, the importance is that edge or refractive shadows do not have the same diagnostic significance as bulk shadowing. They are commonly seen in situations where shadowing alerts to the presence of calcification (e.g. from vessel walls in the renal sinus) or

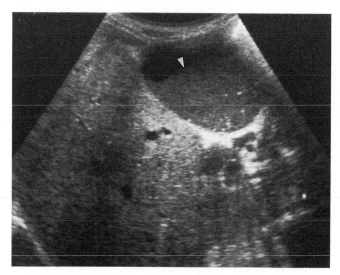

Fig. 8 Echogenic fluid. Since in many real situations only a small amount of energy is removed from the beam by reflection, it is quite possible to encounter debris-containing fluids that are accompanied by enhancement. In this example echogenic bile (arrowhead) partly fills the gallbladder.

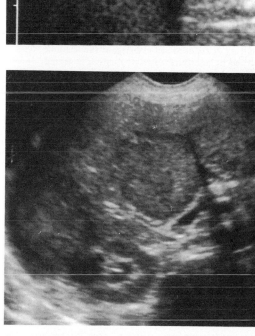

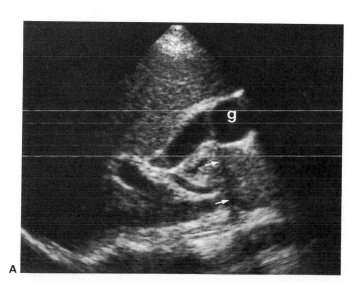

Fig. 9 Edge shadows. Edge or refractive shadows are commonly produced by smooth curved surfaces. In **A**: such a shadow (arrows) is seen beyond a fold within the gallbladder (g), while in **B**: an epididymal cyst (c) has had the same effect. However the curved surfaces of solid structures can also produce edge shadows (arrows), seen in this case also from the upper pole of the testis (t) itself and from the edge of the head of the epididymis (e). Masses can have the same effects: in **C**: a metastasis at the porta hepatis has caused edge shadows.

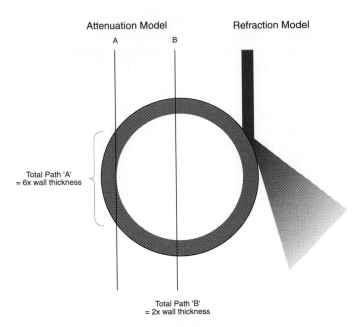

Fig. 10 Mechanisms of edge shadows. Edge shadows are fine echo-poor lines extending deep to the edges of strongly curved structures. Two possible mechanisms are illustrated. On the left is the attenuation model which proposes that the wall is more attenuating than the surrounding tissue; since the beam traversing the edge of the wall 'B' must traverse three times the thickness of the wall as the beam 'A' passing through the diameter of the curved structure, it is more heavily attenuated. On the right is the refractive model which proposes that the beam is dispersed as it reflects from the curved edge which is struck at more than the critical angle; the returning echoes from the spreading beam have less energy than echoes from a confined beam, so that, even though they are reflected from the interfaces they encounter, their intensity is reduced. In either case the shadows should not be construed as signifying high attenuation as would ordinarily be the case.

of sinister lesions (e.g. from Cooper's ligaments in the breast); they must be recognised for what they are and dismissed.

Multiple echoes

A basic and critical assumption in pulse-echo ultrasound is that the ultrasound beam returns directly to the transducer after a single reflection.[12] Where the geometry allows multiple reflections to occur, multiple images are formed; sometimes these are very confusing. Repeat echoes are more likely to occur where the reflections are strong and this implies flat surfaces giving specular echoes. Since the path lengths for multiples are longer, the corresponding images are depicted as lying deeper in the body and they are weakened as the ultrasound is attenuated. Therefore multiple echoes are more likely to be observed when the surfaces are close together and when the intervening tissue is of low attenuation, especially when it is fluid.

An example of a single repeat echo is the mirror image artefact where a repeat image of a structure is depicted on the 'other side' of a specular reflector and equidistant from it.[13,14] This effect is readily demonstrated for the diaphragm: imaged from below through the liver, echoes commonly appear above the diaphragm and sometimes discrete structures in the normal liver or focal lesions can be recognised there (Fig. 11). This is not the appearance of lung (which is seen as an intensely reflective band when imaged intercostally) and is attributable to the beam reflecting back into the liver from the diaphragm.[15] The reflecting surface is probably the air/pleura interface since the muscle of the diaphragm itself would be expected to act as a scatterer rather than a specular reflector.

Generally this artefact is not a diagnostic problem and on rare occasions it may actually be useful, for example when it reveals enhancement from a peripheral liver cyst which would otherwise be invisible as it falls onto the diaphragm; since this is already shown as a full white on the screen no further increase in intensity can be depicted. In other situations the mirror artefact is confusing; in the pelvis for example, a repeat echo of the bladder or of echogenic structures immediately posterior to it (the rectum or sigmoid) may appear as a deeper line marking the back of an echo-poor mass (Figs 12 and 13). In fact the echo-poor region is the mirror image of the bladder. The typical position should arouse suspicion that it is artefactual and the back wall of the 'mass' often lies beyond the position of the sacrum and so is anatomical nonsense. A further clue is the weak superior and inferior walls compared to the strong anterior and posterior walls.

Multiple repeat echoes are known as reverberations. They are produced when two strong reflectors lie parallel to each other. By far the commonest example of this is when a flat surface such as a gas bubble or a stone is parallel to the skin surface where the skin/transducer interface forms the second reflector (Fig. 14). Ultrasound reflected off the gas bubble travels back to the transducer in the usual way to generate a correctly placed image, but a proportion of the echo is re-reflected back into the tissue, retracing its path. On its second reflection from the gas surface it produces a second image at twice the depth of the real image. Sequential repeat echoes are depicted deeper behind the first ('real') echo. A striped pattern results with the deeper multiple echoes becoming weaker because of loss of sound energy due to incomplete reflection at the surfaces and to attenuation by the intervening tissues. Since weaker echoes appear to be narrower than stronger ones, the reverberating bands become shorter as well as less intense with depth. The spacing between the bands depends on the distance between the reflectors; if they are very close together the echoes may merge to form a reflective band in which the individual components cannot be discerned (Fig. 15). A bright streak appears on the display, forming a tail distal to the image of the causal structure, itself usually strongly reflective. The whole complex looks rather like a comet with its tail.[16] This is

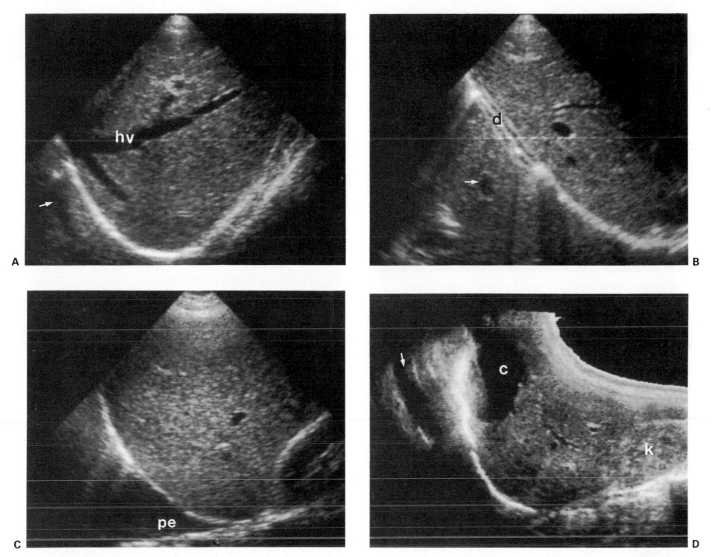

Fig. 11 Mirror image artefacts. The apparent tissue normally visualised above the diaphragm in the right lower zone of the chest is actually artefactual, being produced by the air/pleura interface acting as an acoustic mirror. Sometimes recognisable structures feature in the artefact, forming 'ghost images'. An example is a branch of the right hepatic vein (arrow in **A**) while in **B**: a blood vessel (arrow) is cut in cross-section. In this image the diaphragm appears as a triple layered structure: probably this is a mirror image of thickening of the diaphragmatic peritoneum. **C**: Since the artefact depends on reflection from the air surface, where this is replaced, such as by consolidation or a pleural effusion (pe) the artefact no longer occurs. **D**: Pathological changes may appear as 'ghost lesions'; an example is the cystic lesion (c) in the upper part of the right lobe of the liver. It has its mirrored counterpart (arrow), seemingly within the chest. This was a cystic metastasis. d – diaphragm, hv – hepatic vein, k – kidney.

commonly seen with foreign bodies such as surgical clips, implants (including IUCDs) and catheters. Bullets and shrapnel may also cause the comet-tail effect, as may small fluid cavities such as the Aschoff-Rokitansky sinuses in the wall of the gall bladder in adenomyosis. Presumably here the sound reverberates within each fluid space, echoing repeatedly from the walls of the 'cysts'. The same phenomenon probably accounts for the comet-tail commonly seen distal to frothy or foamy collections of gas bubbles, the sound reflecting repeatedly from the outer surfaces of the gas bubbles in all directions in the inter-

vening fluid so that a continuous stream of sound escapes, some of which returns to the receiving transducer. The effect is often observed from gas within the duodenal cap and is transient as a peristaltic wave moves the gas on.

Velocity errors

An important assumption of scanners is that the velocity of ultrasound in soft tissues is constant. In fact this is not quite valid, fat, for example, conducting ultrasound some

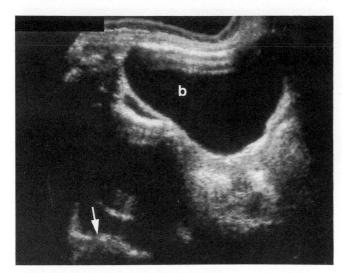

Fig. 12 False pelvic mass. Ultrasound reflecting from the gas surfaces in pelvic bowel loops may be re-reflected into the tissues and produce a second-time-around echo depicted at twice the depth of the gas surface (arrow). Here it may simulate a deep interface forming the back wall of a pseudomass which is nothing more than a mirror artefact. The typical geometry, the anatomical impossibility of a mass lying so far posteriorly and the lack of superior and inferior walls are clues to its artefactual nature. b – bladder.

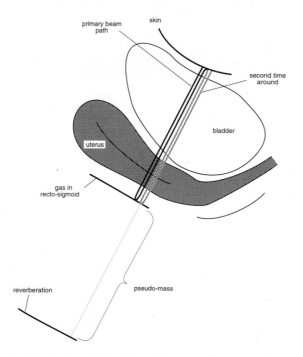

Fig. 13 Mechanism of the false pelvic mass. The strong interface of bowel gas immediately posterior to the bladder acts as a mirror, reflecting the sound beam back to the transducer from which a proportion is re-reflected into the tissues to give a repeat or second-time-around image that simulates the back wall of a large pelvic mass.

10% to 15% more slowly than most other soft tissues (Table 2).[17-20] Prosthetic materials show more marked deviation, silicone used for breast augmentation and testicular implants, for example, having a very much lower velocity.

The average velocity of 1540 m/s used to calibrate scanners is the delay-to-depth conversion constant, set so that every 13 μs delay in the echoes after the transmit pulse corresponds to 1 cm depth on the final image. Where a tissue conducts more slowly, the echoes from deeper structures will be further delayed and therefore be depicted as originating from deeper in the body (Fig. 16A).[20-22] This distortion does not affect the lateral dimension, since this is set by the scanning action of the transducer rather than by the speed of sound. For the most part velocity errors are too small to be clinically important, though, especially for silicone implants, the effects may be surprisingly marked. However in ophthalmic measurements, where great precision is required, the distortion caused by the significantly higher velocity in the lens can be important. The speed of sound in the lens is 1620 m/s; regions of the retina imaged through it appear closer than the parts imaged through the sclera so that a shelf-like anterior distortion is produced (known as Baum's bumps after the sonologist who first described them) (Fig. 16B).[23]

Changes in velocity also produce refractive artefacts; the ultrasound beam deviates from its straight line path when it crosses obliquely between two tissues of different velocity. (Fig. 17). The beam is bent towards the 90° degree line when entering a 'slower tissue' and vice versa. The scanner, of course, continues to operate on the assumption that the beam follows a straight line so that reflectors distant to the surface are incorrectly plotted to the side of their true position. The degree of displacement depends both on the speed of sound difference and on the distance of the object from the surface. A particular situation where this lateral distortion is important clinically is in pelvic scans by the transabdominal route. The beam crossing the wedge shaped fat space around the rectus muscle is refracted so that deep pelvic structures (e.g. the uterus or prostate) can appear stretched laterally (Figs 18 and 19).[24,25] An obstetrical measurement made under these circumstances will be in serious error. In extreme cases the object, e.g. a gestational sac, may seem to be duplicated giving rise to the appearance of twins – this is one reason for the phenomenon of the 'vanishing twin' noted when ultrasound was introduced for early pregnancy. The distortional displacement disappears when the transducer is moved so as to image the pelvis through the centre of the muscle; the appearance is thus easily recognised as artefactual. It is also less common in longitudinal scans because the alignment of the fat/muscle interface is changed, and this effect is less common in the epigastrium, presumably because there is less fat here.

The mechanism by which the ultrasound beam is

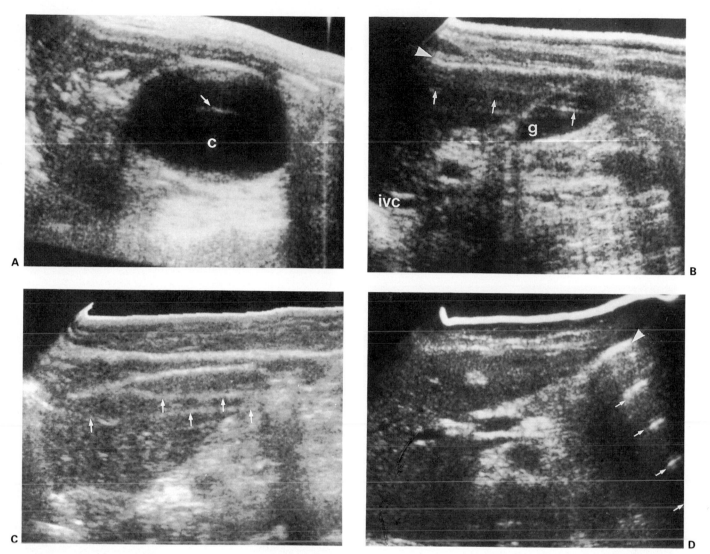

Fig. 14 Reverberation artefacts. A: A second-time-around signal occurs when a strong reflector, in this example the anterior surface of a pancreatic pseudocyst (c), lies parallel to the skin-transducer surface so that some of the received signal is re-reflected into the tissue to be received as a false surface (arrow) at twice the depth of the real surface. The mechanism is the same as for the false pelvic mass (see Fig. 13). **B:** When the surface is longer, for example the fat-fascial interface of the anterior abdominal wall (arrowhead), the reverberation artefact is more extensive (small arrows) though it is more obvious where it falls over an echo-free region, such as the gallbladder (g). There are actually several parallel reverberation artefacts, corresponding to the various layers of the abdominal wall. ivc – inferior vena cava. **C:** Where there is no fluid space to reveal them, reverberations may be more difficult to detect (arrows). This type of artefact is much less troublesome with matched layer transducers because less of the received signal is re-reflected from their surface. **D:** If the reflective layer responsible for the reverberation artefact is superficial (in this case the stomach, arrowhead) multiple reverberations may appear in the image to produce a zebra stripe pattern (arrows).

focused depends on the compression and rarefaction waves of which it is composed coinciding in their proper phase at the focal zone and, symmetrically, at the transducer surface during receive mode focusing. If the velocity in the intervening tissue is different from the calibrated value, the focal zone will be shifted; more importantly, when the intervening tissue has heterogeneous velocities, the focusing effect will be disturbed because the waves will not coincide precisely, some arriving early when the propagation path includes tissues of a high velocity, others arriving late when the path includes fat, for example. The beam is thus defocused, degrading the lateral resolution. This effect probably accounts for the marked variation in ultrasound image quality from patient to patient, despite which the quality of images from obese subjects is sometimes surprisingly good. The larger the transducer aperture used, the worse the effect; this is probably why sophisticated systems such as high resolution linear arrays in which 100 or more elements are used to form each ultrasound line and give such exquisite images in 'easy' subjects, perform badly with 'difficult' subjects, in whom images from smaller, simple transducers are less degraded.

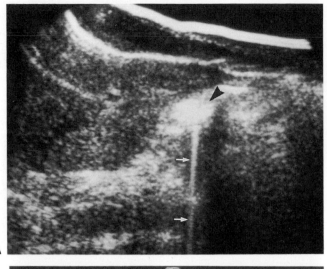

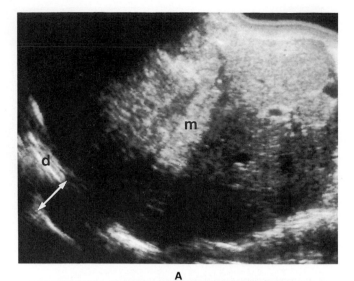

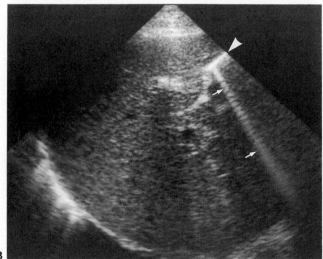

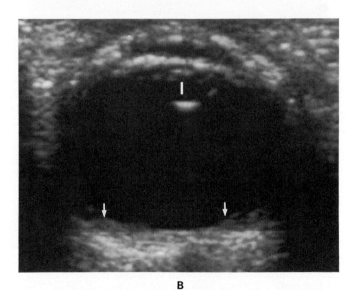

Fig. 15   A and B: Comet tail artefact. When a pocket of gas forms a foam, there is the possibility for multiple, almost random reflection paths between the bubbles to produce trains of echoes. They are seen as intensely reflective lines (arrows) extending deep to the gas. This is seen most commonly in the duodenum (arrowheads).

Fig. 16   Velocity errors. When traversing a region where it is conducted slowly, the sound beam takes longer to complete the go-and-return pathway, so that echoes from beyond it are depicted deeper in the image than their real positions. **A:** In this example, a fatty metastasis (m) in the liver has slowed the sound beam so that the diaphragm (d) appears to have a shelf (arrow). **B:** The reverse situation, where a high velocity region is traversed, as is the case for the lens (l) of the eye, moves the portion imaged through it closer. The resulting distortion, known as 'Baum's Bumps' (arrows), can cause serious errors in eye diameter measurements.

Table 2   Velocity of ultrasound in biologically important materials (From Wells 1969, Goss 1978 and Bamber 1986)

Tissue type	Velocity (m/s)
Air	330
Fat	1450
Water (20°C)	1480
Amniotic fluid	1510
Brain	1565
Blood	1570
Kidney	1560
Muscle	1580
Liver	1600
Uterus	1630
Skin	1700
Lens of eye	1650
Fascia	1750
Perspex	2680
Bone	3500
Soft tissue average	1540

Beam width

Unfortunately the real ultrasound beam shape falls far short of the desired uniformly thin laser beam configuration that would be optimal.[26] A typical actual focused beam (Fig. 20) consists of a disturbed region immediately in front of the transducer surface, then a near zone that progressively narrows to the focus, after which it spreads in the far zone. In addition to this main beam there are

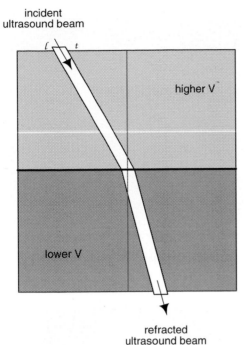

incident
ultrasound beam

higher V

lower V

refracted
ultrasound beam

Fig. 17 Refraction of ultrasound. When the ultrasound beam crosses obliquely between two tissues of differing velocities, the beam is refracted to emerge in a new direction. The situation is exactly the same as the refraction of a light beam. The diagram illustrates the effect of crossing into a material that conducts the ultrasound more slowly: the sound in the leading edge of the beam (l) is slowed first, while sound towards the trailing edge (t) is affected later. This results in the entire beam being refracted towards the 90° direction. The converse occurs when the deeper medium conducts faster.

side lobes, low energy beams directed at angles away from the centre line.

Axial resolution depends on the pulse length which is mainly determined by the wavelength; typically this might be 0.3 mm for a 5 MHz transducer and does not change significantly with depth. In contrast the width of the main beam defines the lateral resolution of the ultrasound image because adjacent objects can only be separately resolved if the beam is narrower than the distance between them.[27] If the beam is wider they are depicted as one larger object on the screen. Because of the complex trumpet-shape of the typical practical ultrasound beam, lateral resolution varies

Fig. 18 Refractive artefacts. A: Refraction of the ultrasound beam by the fatty tissues in the anterior abdominal wall can produce split or double images such as this apparent double IUCD in the uterus (arrows). **B:** Its artefactual nature is clear when the duplication disappears on moving the transducer slightly to one side. (The left ovarian cyst was functional). **C:** The 'split image' artefact is less common in the upper abdomen, perhaps because there is usually less fat and less muscle here, but occasionally apparent duplication of the coeliac axis is seen (arrows). The aortic wall also appears to be stretched laterally. a – aorta, s – stomach.

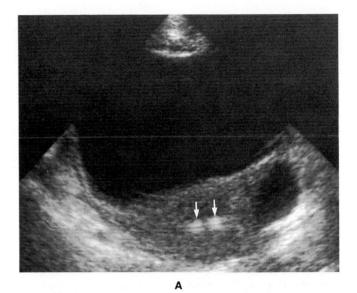

A

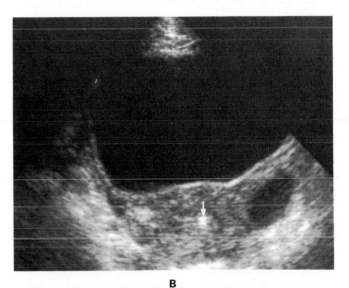

B

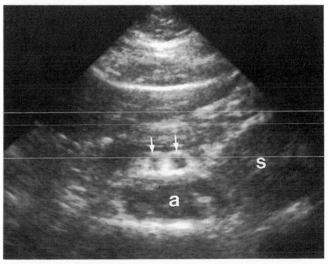

C

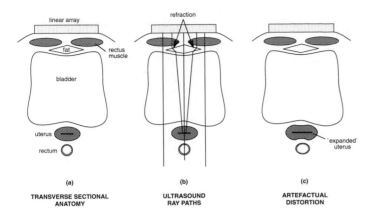

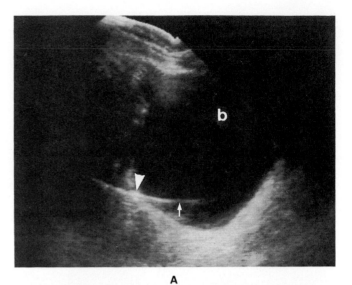

A

Fig. 19 Double images in the pelvis. When the ultrasound beam strikes the slower-conducting layer of fat, it is bent towards the midline so that medial structures are displayed lateral to their true position (**B**). They therefore appear laterally stretched (**C**) or even duplicated leading to confusing or even serious diagnostic errors.

with depth, being best at the focal zone and deteriorating rapidly beyond it.

The edges of the beam are not sharply defined; the ultrasound energy is concentrated on the centre line of the beam and falls off progressively from the centre line with a Gaussian distribution. This means that a strong reflector will continue to give detectable echoes further from the central axis than a weak reflector. In clinical terms this means that the resolution of ultrasound is better for weak reflectors. Strong reflectors tend to blur laterally and are therefore seen as cigar-shaped smears or streaks so that their width is exaggerated. This is the beam width artefact (Fig. 21), and is most obvious when the smearing overlaps an echo-free structure, often encountered when a gassy or bony structure lies adjacent to a fluid space. However, it also leads to the general tendency to infill echo-free regions such as ducts and in part for the discrepancy between the

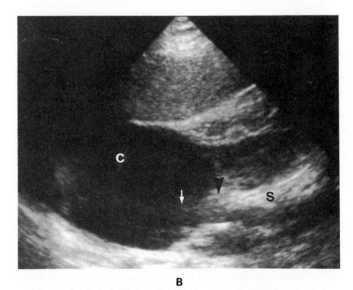

B

Fig. 21 Beam width artefact. Echoes arising from structures at the edge of the ultrasound beam, which has a finite width, are depicted as lying in the centre-line of the beam. The more intense the reflection, the further off-axis its echoes will be received. **A:** In this example the strong echoes from a pocket of gas in a pelvic gut loop (arrowhead) smear across the bladder (arrow). **B:** A weaker beam spread artefact misplaces echoes from the more reflective sinus tissues (arrowhead) into a renal cyst (arrow). As is often the case with artefacts, they are more obvious when the false signal overlies an echo-free region but, in fact, are present everywhere to a greater or lesser extent, depending on the beam shape (mainly determined by focusing) and the reflectivity of the off-axis interfaces. b – bladder, c – cyst, s – renal sinus.

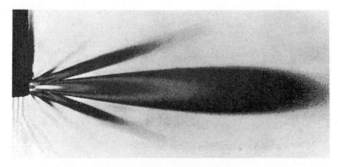

Fig. 20 Ultrasound beam shape. In this Schlieren tank photograph of the ultrasound field from an unfocused disc transducer, the main beam is accompanied by several side lobes emitted at angles from the central axis. The width of the main beam limits resolution in the transverse direction. The side lobes cause falsely positioned images. (From: Bergmann L. Der ultraschall und sein unwendung in wissenschaft und technik. Stuttgart: S. Heizel Verlage. 1954).

ultrasound and X-ray measurements of the calibre of the bile and pancreatic ducts (the remaining discrepancy being attributable to the magnification on X-ray and to duct dilatation caused by contrast agents).

Beam width artefacts also occur in the orthogonal plane, i.e. across the slice thickness. With circular transducers (either the simple disc type or annular arrays) the beam is

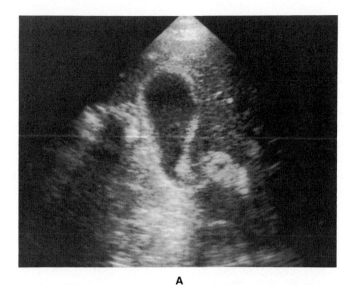

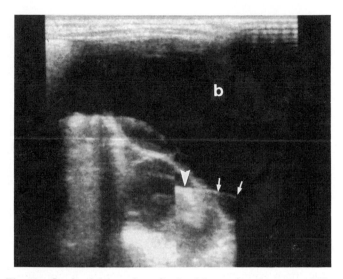

A

Fig. 23 **Grating lobe artefact.** Grating lobe artefacts have essentially the same effects as simple beam spread artefacts but are more severe and only occur with array transducers. They often have a convex shape (arrows). This example arose from a gas-containing pelvic gut loop (arrowhead). b – bladder.

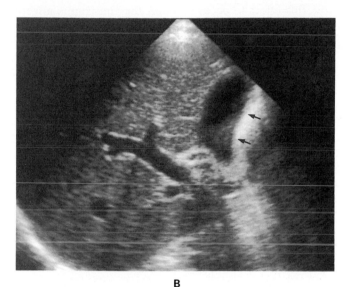

B

Fig. 22 **Orthogonal beam width artefact.** The low level echoes within this gallbladder (**A**) are not due to debris or echogenic bile but are a beam width artefact arising from gas in the adjacent duodenum (arrows in (**B**)); because the artefact arises out of the plane of the tomogram, this variant of the beam width artefact is more difficult to recognise.

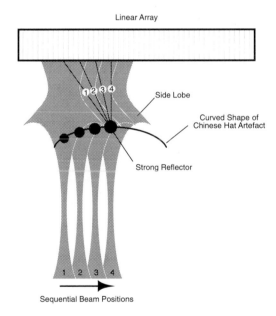

Fig. 24 **Mechanism of the Chinese hat artefact.** When a side or grating lobe strikes a strongly reflective target (1), a weak signal will be received and registered as originating slightly deeper than the real target depth because the oblique line-of-sight takes longer for the beam to traverse than the direct line that results when the beam is correctly centred on the target (4). The result is a cigar-shaped artefact whose ends are depicted as lying deeper than the centre, recalling the shape of a Chinese hat.

symmetrical in all planes, but for linear and phased arrays the beam is wider in the orthogonal plane. Orthogonal beam spread artefacts are exactly the same as the slice thickness artefact in the CT except that the ultrasound beam is non-uniform; low level information derived from signals in adjacent planes is spuriously depicted in the image plane.[28,29] Typically echo-poor bands or lines are noted within echo-free spaces (Fig. 22). They may mislead the operator into thinking that the fluid contains debris. Because the 'offending' reflector is not visualised within the image the orthogonal beam width artefact is more dif-

ficult to recognise than the same artefact occurring within the scanned plane.

Unfortunately this description of the shape of the ultrasound beam is incomplete because the profile is even further complicated by the inevitable presence of side lobes and, for array transducers, of grating lobes also.[30,31] Both these are misdirected, aberrant lines of ultrasound energy transmitted alongside the main beam and have their counterpart in off-axis regions of sensitivity when the transducer is in the receive mode. Side lobes are generated as part of the beam focusing mechanism, whether by applied lenses or by curving of the transducer face, and consist of ill-defined beams, the first some 20° away from the main beam and much weaker than it (by about 40 dB). For a disc transducer they form a series of rings, while in the case of linear arrays they are asymmetrical, being differently positioned in the two planes.

Grating lobes are similar but are produced in array transducers of all types; however, they tend to be more discrete and powerful. Grating lobes are less marked when the array elements are small and numerous because the array then approximates more closely to a continuous transducer. Because they are much weaker than the main beam, only strong reflectors cause serious side and grating lobe artefacts in clinical practice but, if a gas bubble or bone surface happens to lie at the position of a side lobe then its grating lobe echo will be depicted in the line of the main beam (Fig. 23). The result is a convex-shape streak that has been dubbed the 'Chinese hat artefact' (Fig. 24). Because these artefacts may be consistent on rescanning the region, they may be rather confusing. Often the cause can be visualised within the image, but side lobes can extend beyond the imaged area and do also occur in the orthogonal plane.

Time sampling problems

Some interesting and important artefacts arise from the fact that there is an upper limit for the rate at which ultrasound pulses can be repeated. This is set by the speed of sound in tissue and the depth penetration required. If the next pulse is sent before the deepest echoes from the first have faded away, then these late echoes will be received immediately after the second pulse transmission. The scanner has no means of identifying which transmit pulse is responsible and plots these deep echoes as nearby reflectors from the second pulse. The process is repeated for subsequent pulses. Thus a distant structure is imaged as though it lies close to the transducer. Flickering 'objects' are seen in the near field and their depth can be altered by changing the pulse repetition frequency (PRF).[32] Since the PRF is usually linked to the depth of field, they move with a change in scale. Properly adjusted scanners should not allow this effect to occur, though the constraints affecting duplex Doppler (both pulsed and colour) may force a compromise in this respect.

The limited frame rate can also obscure the motion of fast-moving structures such as heart valves, because their position is not being sampled sufficiently frequently for a true rendition of their movement to be displayed. Generally this results in a jerky, cartoon-like rendition of the movement, but in some cases the movement can seem to be slowed or even reversed in direction.[33] This phenomenon, known as aliasing, is rare in real-time imaging but is extremely important in Doppler (see Ch. 5).

REFERENCES

1 Robinson D E, Kossoff G, Garrett W J. Artefacts in ultrasonic echoscopic visualization. Ultrasonics 1966; 4: 186–194
2 Laing F C. Commonly encountered artifacts in clinical ultrasound. Semin Ultrasound 1983; 4: 1–25
3 Kremkau F W, Taylor K J W. Artifacts in ultrasound imaging. J Ultrasound Med 1986; 5: 227–237
4 Sanders R C. Atlas of ultrasonographic artifacts and variants. Chicago: Year Book. 1986
5 Oliva L. Gli artefatti in echotomographia. Milano: Masson. 1989
6 Wells P N T, Halliwell M. Speckle in ultrasonographic imaging. Ultrasonics 1981; 19: 225–232
7 Burchard C B. Speckle in ultrasound B-scan. IEEE Transactions on Sonics and Ultrasonics 1978; SU-25: 1–6
8 Suramo I, Paivanslo M, Vuoria P. Shadowing and reverberation artifacts in abdominal ultrasonography. Eur J Radiol 1985; 5: 147–151
9 Robinson D E, Wilson L S, Kossoff G. Shadowing and enhancement in ultrasonic echograms by reflection and refraction. JCU 1981; 9: 181–188
10 Sommer F G, Taylor K J. Differentiation of acoustic shadowing due to calculi and gas collections. Radiology 1980; 135: 399–403
11 Ziskin M C, LaFollette P S, Blathras K, Abraham V. Effect of scan format on refraction artefacts. Ultrasound Med Biol 1990; 16: 183–191
12 Bly S H, Foster F S, Patterson U S, Foster D R, Hunt D W. Artefactual echoes in B-Mode images due to multiple scattering. Ultrasound Med Biol 1985; 11: 99–111
13 Cosgrove D O, Garbutt P, Hill C R. Echoes across the diaphragm. Ultrasound Med Biol 1978; 3: 388–392
14 Gardner F J, Clark R N, Kozlowski R. A model of a hepatic mirror image artifact. Medical Ultrasound 1980; 4: 18–21
15 Fried A M, Cosgrove D O, Nassiri D K, McCready V R. The diaphragmatic echo complex: an in vitro study. Invest Radiol 1985; 20: 62–67
16 Thickman D I, Ziskin M C, Goldemburg N J, Linder B E. Clinical manifestations of the comet tail artifact. J Ultrasound Med 1983; 2: 225–230
17 Wells PNT. Physical principles of ultrasonic diagnosis. London: Academic Press
18 Goss S A, Johnstone R A, Dunn F. Comprehensive compilation of principle properties of mammalian tissues. Ultrasound Med Biol 1978; 3: 373–379
19 Bamber J C. Attenuation and absorption. In: Hill C R. ed. Physical principles of medical ultrasonics. Chichester: Ellis Horwood. 1986: Ch 5
20 Pierce G, Golding R H, Cooperberg P L. The effects of tissue velocity changes on acoustical interfaces. J Ultrasound Med 1982; 1: 85–187
21 Richman T S, Taylor K J W, Kremkau F W. Propagation speed artefact in a fatty tumour (myelolipoma). J Ultrasound Med 1983; 2: 45–47
22 Mayo J, Cooperberg P L. Displacement of the diaphragmatic echo by hepatic cysts: a new explanation with computer simulation. J Ultrasound Med 1984; 3: 337–340

23 Baum G. Ultrasonography in clinical ophthalmology. Trans Pa Acad Ophthalmol Otolaryngol 1964; 68: 265–270

24 Müller N, Cooperberg P L, Rowley V A, Mayo J, Ho B, Li D B. Ultrasonic refraction by the rectus abdominis muscles: the double image artefact. J Ultrasound Med 1984; 3: 515–520

25 Sauerbrei E E. The split image artefact in pelvic ultrasonography: anatomy and physics. J Ultrasound Med 1985; 4: 29–34

26 Goldstein A, Parks J A, Osborne B. Visualization of B-scan transducer transverse cross-sectional beam patterns. J Ultrasound Med 1982; 1: 23–35

27 Jaffe C C, Taylor K J. The clinical impact of ultrasonic beam focusing patterns. Radiology 1979; 131: 469–472

28 Fiske C E, Filly R A. Pseudo-sludge. Radiology 1982; 144: 631–632

29 Goldstein A, Madrazo B L. Slice-thickness artifacts in gray-scale ultrasound. JCU 1981; 9: 365–375

30 Laing F C, Kurtz A B. The importance of ultrasonic side-lobe artifacts. Radiology 1982; 145: 763–768

31 McKeighen R E. The influence of grating lobes on image quality using real-time linear arrays. J Ultrasound Med 1982; 1, 7 (suppl): 83

32 Goldstein A. Range ambiguities in real-time ultrasound. JCU 1981; 9: 83–90

33 Morrison D C, McDicken W N, Smith D S A. A motion artefact in real time ultrasound scanners. Ultrasound Med Biol 1983; 9: 201–203

5

Doppler

Hylton B. Meire

INTRODUCTION

The basic principles of ultrasound pulse-echo imaging have been covered repeatedly in numerous previous texts and are not therefore included in this book. However, the application of the Doppler principle to detect moving blood has only relatively recently gained clinical acceptance and is a rapidly expanding field.[1-5] Correct interpretation of the information obtained from Doppler ultrasound presupposes a knowledge of the principles of both blood flow and Doppler ultrasonics and for this reason both are discussed in some detail in this chapter.

The characteristics of blood flow

Blood is a viscous medium and as it moves throughout the vascular tree there is a drag effect between the moving blood and the vessel walls.[6,7] As a result of these two factors the speed of the blood near the vessel wall is generally less than that toward the centre of the vessel. There is thus a 'velocity profile' across the vessel (Fig. 1).[8] If the vessel is straight the profile is symmetrical and, in steady venous flow, is generally parabolic in shape (Fig. 1). In this situation the blood can be considered to be flowing in a number of concentric laminae (streamlines), the velocity within each lamina increasing towards the centre of the vessel. This form of flow is frequently referred to simply as 'laminar flow' but the use of this term does not imply any particular velocity profile or gradient across the vessel.

Normal venous flow

Normal flow in peripheral veins at rest is slow, continuous and unmodulated with a velocity of typically only 2 or 3 cm per second (Figs 2A and 2B). As limb perfusion increases as a result of exercise the venous velocities increase dramatically, but flow usually remains unmodulated.

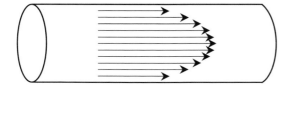

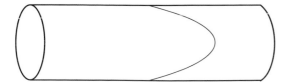

Fig. 1 Normal blood flow. The vessel walls exhibit a drag effect upon the adjacent blood giving rise to a parabolic flow profile across the vessel.

Flow within more central veins, typically jugular, iliac, intra-abdominal and intrathoracic veins, is normally modulated to a variable extent by the cardiac pulsations. The atrial (a) and ventricular (v) waves are conducted from the right atrium into the superior and inferior venae cavae and cause transitory reductions in flow velocity or even flow reversal (Figs 2C and 2D). In addition there is usually also some modulation of venous flow induced by normal breathing movements. The degree by which flow is modulated by both cardiac pulsations and respiration is very variable from patient to patient but in general the modulation is greatest in those vessels closest to the heart.

It is generally assumed that the flow profile in major veins is approximately parabolic in shape (see below) and this assumption is probably valid for most medium sized veins. In larger veins the drag has little or no effect in the peripheral streamlines and most of the central blood moves at the same velocity, thus approximating to plug flow (Fig. 3).

On the occasions when volume flow calculations are attempted the vessel is often assumed to be circular in cross-section. Whilst this is almost always true for arteries it is seldom true for veins: most are normally somewhat elliptical and those that lie superficially are particularly prone to distortion by pressure from the overlying transducer.

Normal arterial flow

The characteristics of blood flow within arteries is extremely complex. The arterial wall is elastic and dilates significantly as the systolic pressure wave passes.[9-11] This radial expansion causes a transitory increase in cross-sectional area of 20% to 25% in medium sized healthy arteries and, during the expansion phase, there is necessarily some radial movement of blood to fill the increased lumen size. The pulsatile changes in vessel dimensions and the radial component of flow are almost invariably ignored in current Doppler studies and calculations.

During systole there is rapid acceleration of the moving blood column with a subsequent rapid deceleration in early diastole. Flow throughout diastole is determined by a wide range of factors including cardiac dynamics, the state of the local vascular tree and the nature of the circulation supplied by the artery under examination. These factors, commonly referred to as upstream, local and downstream, are discussed in more detail later in this chapter.

The flow velocity in diastole is invariably lower than that in systole (Fig. 4A) and, when there is little distal perfusion (for example in the vascular bed of a muscle at rest), diastolic flow is very low; in addition the elastic recoil of the distal arterial tree may cause transitory reversal of flow during early diastole (Fig. 4B). The waveform shown in Figure 4A characterises flow in vessels supplying capillary beds with low flow resistance, typically the brain, liver,

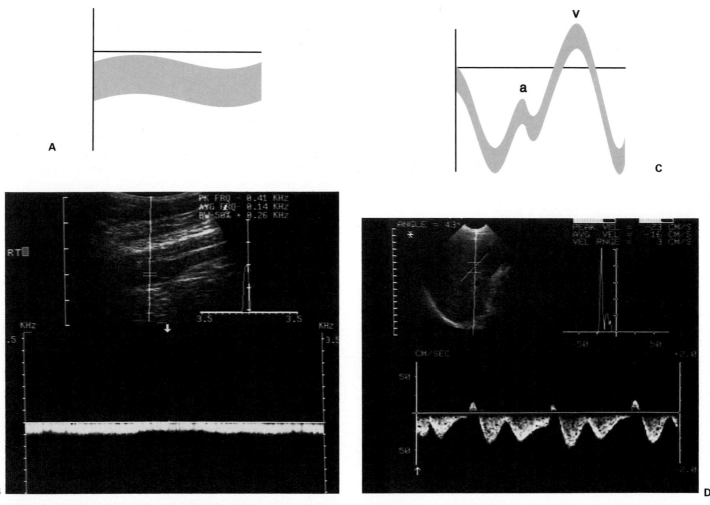

Fig. 2   Normal venous flow. A: Diagrammatic representation of venous flow in a peripheral vein showing gentle respiratory modulation. **B:** Spontaneous low velocity flow in a femoral vein showing minimal respiratory modulation. **C:** Schematic representation of blood flow in a central vein. Forward flow is reduced by the atrial 'a' wave and is temporarily reversed by the ventricular 'v' wave transmitted from the right ventricle. **D:** Normal pulsatile flow in an hepatic vein. Note that in all the above examples flow is away from the probe and forward flow is therefore below the baseline.

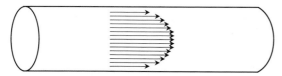

Fig. 3   Normal flow in a large vein. In large veins the drag effect does not reach the centre of the vessel thus giving rise to central flattening of the velocity profile.

kidneys, placenta and pregnant uterus, and this waveform is commonly described as a 'low resistance' waveform. The waveform in Figure 4B is termed 'high resistance' and, in addition to normal muscles at rest, may be seen in a range of pathological conditions elsewhere in the body.

Simultaneous with the changes in velocity throughout the cardiac cycle the velocity profile across an artery also changes (Fig. 5). As a general rule, flow during diastole approximates to parabolic flow but, in systole, the power of the left ventricular ejection forces almost all of the blood to move with the same velocity, giving rise to a profile approximating to plug flow. The temporal changes in velocity profile in arteries supplying a higher vascular resistance bed may be extremely complex with the different flow laminae showing simultaneous flow in opposite directions during certain phases of the cardiac cycle (Fig. 6).

Flow axis

For the purpose of making measurements from Doppler signals it is always assumed that all the flow streamlines

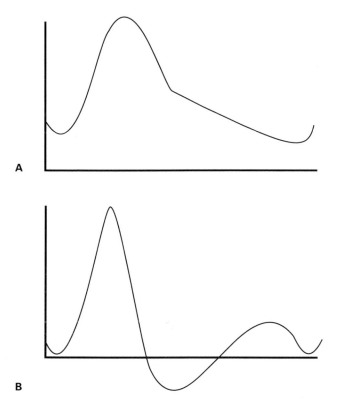

Fig. 4 **Normal arterial flow. A:** In vessels supplying low resistance vascular beds there is continuous forward flow throughout the cardiac cycle. **B:** Arterial flow to high resistance vascular beds shows varying degrees of diastolic flow reduction with early diastolic flow reversal if the resistance is high.

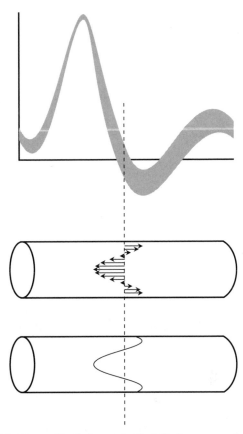

Fig. 6 **Velocity profile during early diastolic flow reversal.** When flow reverses in early diastole the reversal occurs first in the centre of the column of moving blood whilst the blood nearer the vessel wall is still moving in a forward direction. This gives rise to a biphasic velocity profile and simultaneous forward and reverse flows in the spectral analysis.

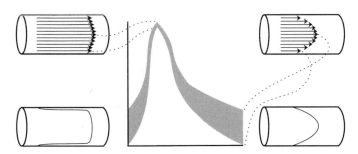

Fig. 5 **Changes in arterial velocity profile throughout the cardiac cycle.** During peak systole most of the blood is moving at one velocity giving rise to a flat flow profile and a narrow range of frequencies in the Doppler spectrum. During diastole the velocities are lower and the range of velocities wider giving rise to a parabolic flow profile and a wide range of frequencies in the spectrum.

within a vessel are moving in a direction parallel to the vessel wall. This is only true in parallel walled straight vessels; the direction and parallelism of the flow streamlines may be very different in the region of junctions, bends and branches (Fig. 7)[12] which may give rise to areas of physiological vortex formation or flow reversal (Plate 1).

Flow in abnormal arteries

Narrowing, for example due to atheromatous plaques, disturbs the normal flow streamlines[13] and the nature and degree of this disturbance varies according to the size and characteristics of the plaque.

It is generally assumed that smooth plaques which reduce the lumen by less than 50% do not reduce the volume of blood flowing through a vessel segment. However, if the volume flow is maintained despite a reduction in the vessel cross-sectional area, there must necessarily be an increase in flow velocity at the site of the narrowing (Fig. 8). The flow velocity and velocity profile is normal both proximal and distal to the lesion.

If the surface of the plaque is rough or ulcerated, even if the plaque itself is quite small, local flow disturbance occurs over the surface of the plaque, usually with small vortices developing within the craters on the plaque surface (Fig. 9). The flow characteristics above and below the lesion remain normal, the vortices usually only propagating for a few millimetres downstream.

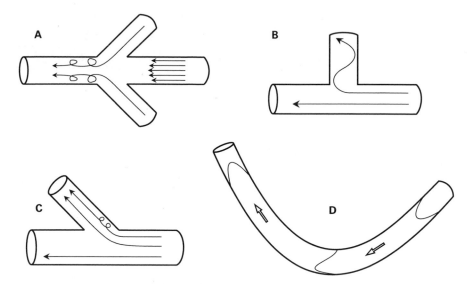

Fig. 7 Normal flow at junctions, branches and bends. A: Normal venous laminar flow is disturbed at major junctions, for example between the renal veins and IVC, giving rise to vortex formation at and just beyond the junction. **B:** A coarse vortex may arise at an acutely angled branch, for example at the bifurcation of the portal vein within the liver (see Plate 1B). **C:** As blood enters the origin of an obtusely angled branch flow near the wall may become disturbed due to 'boundary layer separation' and give rise to small localised vortices (see Plate 1A). **D:** In curved vessels the normal symmetry of the velocity profile is distorted in the region of the curve.

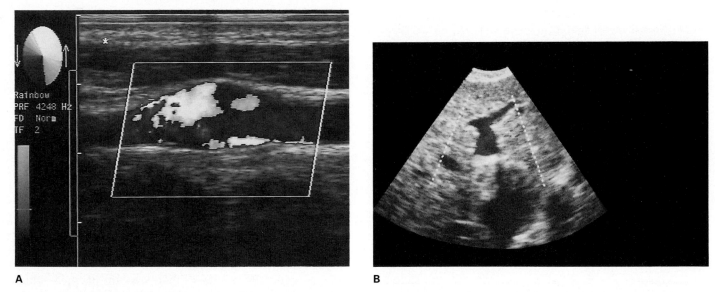

Plate 1 Physiological vortices. A: Longitudinal scan of the carotid bulb. Complex vortices (red) are present due to boundary layer separation. This is a normal flow characteristic. **B:** Transverse scan of the left portal vein. The CDI sensitivity has been reduced to show only the highest velocity flow which can be seen to follow a spiral course through this vessel (compare with Fig. 7B). This figure is reproduced in colour in the colour plate section at the front of this volume.

Stenoses of greater than 50% are associated with a more marked increase in flow velocity through the stenosis with flow disturbance (Fig. 10). The increase in peak velocity is approximately proportional to the severity of the stenosis[14] and the high velocity jet may propagate for 2 to 3 cm distal to the lesion. Proximal to the lesion there is a reduction in flow velocity below that which would normally be expected at that anatomical site.

Stenoses of greater than 90% produce a drastic reduction in volume flow with a high velocity and extremely disturbed flow through and beyond the stenosis (Fig. 11).

The basis of Doppler ultrasound

The detection of blood flow with ultrasound depends on the Doppler principle (Fig. 12) which determines that,

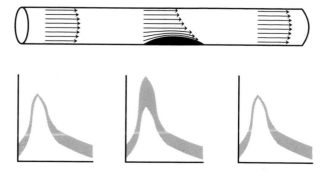

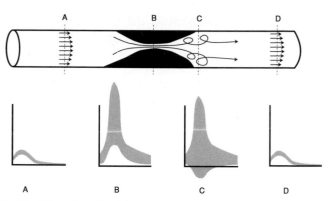

Fig. 8 Flow over a low grade stenosis. Proximal and distal flow remains normal but there is a slight acceleration at the site of the stenosis resulting in an increased range of velocities in the Doppler spectrum during systole.

Fig. 11 Flow through a high grade stenosis. Proximal and distal flow is drastically reduced (A and D). The flow velocity through the stenosis is greatly increased (B) and there is severe vortex formation beyond the stenosis (C).

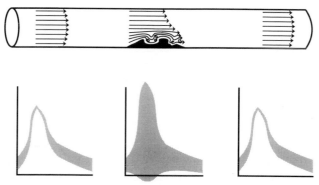

Fig. 9 Flow over an ulcerated atheromatous plaque. If the stenosis is less than 50%, flow above and below the plaque is normal. As the flow streamlines enter the craters in the plaque, small vortices are generated and propagate for short distances downstream. These give rise to widening of the spectral breadth with true simultaneous forward and reverse flow that is usually only apparent during systole since they are most likely to be produced when the flow velocity is fast.

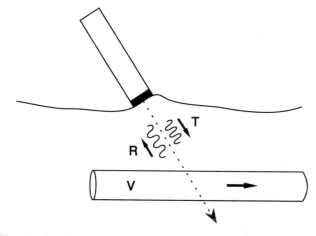

Fig. 12 The Doppler principle. The frequency of the transmitted ultrasound pulse (T) is altered when it is reflected from a moving structure, in this case blood flowing within the vessel (V). When the direction of blood flow is away from the transducer the frequency of the returning wave (R) is reduced.

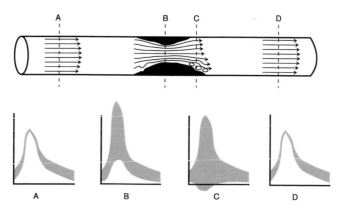

Fig. 10 Flow through a 50% to 90% stenosis. Though the proximal and distal profiles are normal, there is an overall velocity reduction roughly in proportion to the severity of the stenosis. At the site of the stenosis there is an increase in peak velocity and gross spectral broadening with true flow reversal. The flow disturbance may be propagated for 2 to 3 cm downstream.

when ultrasound is reflected from a moving structure, the frequency of the reflected waves is different from that of the incident waves. The degree to which the frequency is altered is determined both by the speed and direction of movement of the blood cells, movement towards the transducer increasing the frequency and vice versa. Analysis of the Doppler shifted frequency permits assessment of the speed and relative direction of the blood flow. The equation which determines the value of the Doppler shift frequency is:

$$f_d = \frac{2V\ (\text{Cos }\theta)\ f}{c}$$

where f_d is the Doppler shifted frequency

V is the speed of the moving blood

θ is the angle between the ultrasound beam and the direction of movement of the blood

f is the transmitted ultrasound frequency

c is the speed of ultrasound (1540 m/s).

In any Doppler examination the ultrasound frequency and speed are fixed and the Doppler shifted frequency therefore depends on the speed of the blood and the beam/vessel angle. The beam/vessel angle (θ) is of great importance in clinical Doppler examinations[15] since when θ is 90° its cosine is 0 (Fig. 13) and therefore no Doppler signal is obtained. Conversely if the ultrasound beam can be aligned along the direction of the long axis of the vessel θ is 0, the cosine of θ 1 and the maximum possible Doppler shift frequency is obtained. In practice this alignment is seldom achievable and a compromise has to be accepted. In general, however, it is advisable to try to position the ultrasound transducer in such a way that the beam/vessel angle is no greater than 60°.

In clinical examinations, there is never a single Doppler shift frequency and the returning ultrasound signal contains a spectrum of frequencies determined by the distributions of different blood velocities across the vessel.

The interpretation of the Doppler signal, and any calculations made from information derived from the Doppler signal, assume that the whole width of the vessel under interrogation is exposed to a uniform ultrasound field. This is termed 'uniform insonation' and the degree to which this is achieved in practice is determined by the size, depth and orientation of the blood vessel together with the characteristics of the ultrasound beam (Fig. 14).[16] If the beam is significantly narrower than the blood vessel, little or no signal is obtained from the slow moving blood at the periphery of the vessel. This may lead to an overestimation of the mean flow velocity in the vessel or to failure to detect areas of flow disturbance near the vessel wall.

The simplest of medical ultrasound Doppler equipment utilises two separate transducers, one transmitting a con-

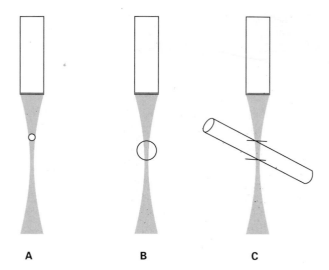

A   **B**   **C**

Fig. 14   Uniform insonation. A: If the vessel is no larger than the effective width of the ultrasound beam the whole vessel lumen can be assumed to be uniformly insonated. **B:** If the vessel is significantly wider than the beam a high proportion of the slow moving peripheral blood may not be sampled giving rise to a falsely high assessment of the overall flow velocity. **C:** The sample volume is also determined by the size of the range gate which should match the vessel diameter (see Figure 15).

tinuous ultrasound tone whilst the second receives the returning echoes.[2] These devices still have wide clinical application in such areas as fetal heart detection and for the assessment of patency of peripheral arteries. These 'continuous wave' (CW) machines can be small, simple and inexpensive but suffer from the major disadvantage that there is no information concerning the depth from which any Doppler shifted signals originate. Any vessel or other moving structure anywhere along the length of the ultrasound beam gives rise to a signal and all such signals are mixed together in the resulting Doppler output.

In those clinical situations where it is necessary to identify signals from within individual closely adjacent vessels, or from limited areas within a single vessel, it is necessary to employ pulse-echo ultrasound similar to that used for conventional imaging. In imaging ultrasound, the depth from which each individual echo originates is calculated from knowledge of the speed of transmission of ultrasound in the tissues and the time taken between transmission of the ultrasound pulse and reception of a specific echo. Provided the duration of the transmitted pulse is of sufficient length for its frequency to be measured accurately, the frequency of the returning echoes can also be measured, in addition to determining the depth from which they arose. This 'pulsed Doppler' has been combined with conventional imaging to produce 'duplex Doppler'[17,18] and has been fundamentally responsible for the recent rapid increase in clinical applications of Doppler ultrasound. Modern duplex Doppler systems permit the operator to identify the depth or range of depths from which Doppler signals are to be acquired, whilst suppressing any signals

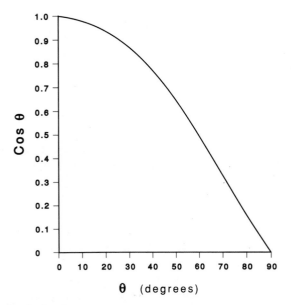

Fig. 13   Cosine θ.

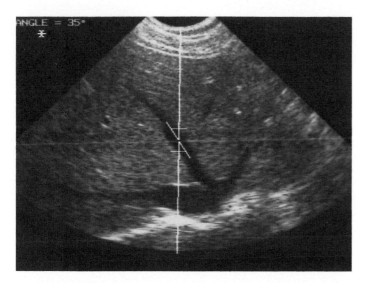

Fig. 15 Sample volume and range gate size. The portion of the ultrasound beam from which Doppler signals are received is marked by the operator using 'range gates' which appear in this figure as short lines at right angles to the ultrasound path. The separation of these range gates determines the sample volume and this should be adjusted to ensure that the whole vessel cross-section is being sampled.

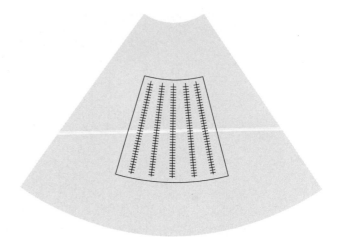

Fig. 16 Colour flow imaging. Within the colour flow region of interest there are large numbers of sequential range gates along each line of site. The number and spacing of the range gates and lines of site vary with make of equipment and control settings.

arising from outside the defined sample volume. The depth and dimensions of the sample volume are determined by a combination of the ultrasound beam width and the position of the 'range gate' markers which are set by the operator (Fig. 15).

Colour Doppler/colour flow imaging

Colour flow imaging (CFI) is a relatively recent technical development whereby the Doppler shifted information is used to generate a colour overlay on the conventional 2D grey scale image.[19–21] In order to achieve this, it is necessary to detect the Doppler flow information at a large number of sites within the image in rapid succession. This necessitates the use of a great deal of additional electronic hardware and sophisticated software and significant compromises are generally employed by equipment manufacturers in order to limit both the complexity and cost of the equipment.

The principle is similar to that of conventional single range gate Doppler but, instead of detecting flow in a single large sample volume, numerous small adjacent sample volumes are created along the lines of site of several consecutive pulses (Fig. 16). The number of adjacent range gates along each line of sight varies from equipment to equipment and with different control settings and may be from 32 to 128 samples. Similarly the number of consecutive pulses from which Doppler information is acquired also varies in the range of 32 to 128 and the colour display therefore contains from 1024 to 16 384 colour elements. Calculating the Doppler frequency content for each in-

dividual range gate takes a significant time and computational power and there is thus a limit on the number of picture elements which can be interrogated in a given time interval. If the user requires a large number of picture elements to produce finer detail in the colour image, a significant time penalty is suffered with the frame rate falling to as low as two per second. Conversely if a high frame rate is required, for example in cardiological imaging, it is only possible to display a small number of relatively large picture elements giving rise to poor spatial and frequency resolution. These compromises dictate that manufacturers generally optimise their equipment either for cardiac or abdominal purposes and machines optimised for one of these clinical applications are usually inappropriate for use in the other.

The Doppler information obtained from each range gate is analysed to determine the direction of movement and a relatively crude assessment of the mean velocity. This information is then turned into a colour signal which is added to the appropriate pixel in the 2D display (Plate 2). Flow towards the transducer is customarily coded red and flow away, blue. However, the user is able to change this or to substitute a wide range of other colour maps to the velocity information.

In the majority of clinical applications it is not necessary to interrogate the entire field of view for Doppler information; when a smaller region of interest is selected, all the available colour picture elements can be allocated to this region, thereby reducing pixel size and significantly improving the resolution of the colour image as well as the frame rate.

A great many technological refinements have been developed in modern colour Doppler imaging systems to improve flow detection, suppress confusing signals from moving soft tissues and to improve both spatial and tem-

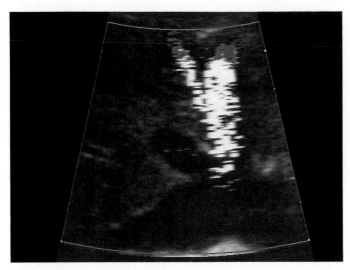

Plate 2   Pixels in the colour image. The pixels within CDI images are much larger than those in grey scale imaging and therefore give rise to jagged vessel margins and usually lead to inappropriately wide display of narrow vessels. This image has been magnified to demonstrate this. This figure is reproduced in colour in the colour plate section at the front of this volume.

poral resolution. The effects of some of these are discussed further in the section on artefacts below.

Extracting information from the Doppler signal

As discussed above the Doppler signal contains a spectrum of frequencies which vary to a greater or lesser extent with cardiac or respiratory changes. The range and magnitude of these frequencies and the way in which they change throughout the cardiac cycle embody much information concerning cardiac activity, the proximal vascular tree, the vessel at the site of interrogation and the state of the vascular bed or vessels distal to the examination site. A wide range of techniques and mathematical computations have been devised in attempts to extract this information[22] and, at the present time, only limited success has been achieved. However, a number of indices are used frequently all of which are applied to a graphical display of the frequency information. This is termed 'spectral analysis' and the means by which this is achieved should be understood before attempting to interpret any values derived from it.

Spectral analysis

Spectral analysis is the process by which the frequency content of the ultrasound signal, and the way in which it varies with time, is analysed and displayed. In practice measurement of the frequency content takes a significant amount of time and there are limitations both on the range of frequencies detectable and the resolution with which the

different frequencies can be separated. The way in which the analysis is performed varies somewhat from one make of equipment to another but usually a fast Fourier transform (FFT) is used.[23] It is not necessary to have a technical understanding of the principles of this in order to comprehend and interpret the results it produces.

The spectral analysis display takes the form of a graph of frequency on the vertical axis and time on the horizontal axis (Figs 17 and 18). Both frequency and time are divided into small but finite increments and the spectral tracing therefore consists of an array of tiny elements or pixels. The width of each pixel is determined by the time resolution available and is commonly 5, 10 or 20 milliseconds. The pixel height is determined by the frequency resolution of the system and is typically 25 or 50 Hertz. The clinical

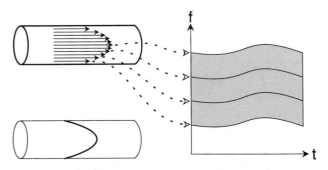

Fig. 17   Spectral analysis. Spectral analysis produces a graphic display of frequency (f) on the vertical axis and time (t) on the horizontal axis. The width of the displayed frequency band directly correlates with the range of velocities present within the vessel, the highest velocities corresponding to the highest frequencies and vice versa.

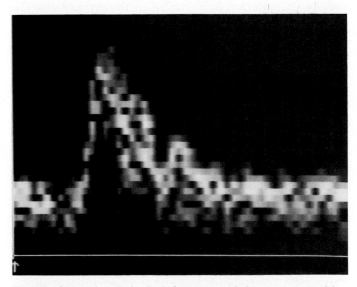

Fig. 18   Spectral analysis. Both frequency and time are measured in small increments and give rise to pixelation within the spectral display. In this example the equipment settings have been altered to maximise this effect.

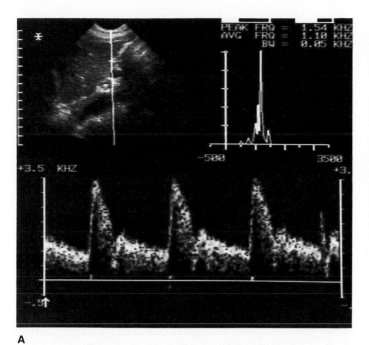
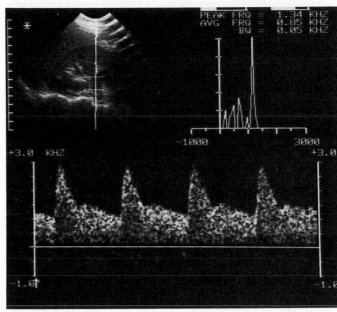

A   **B**

Fig. 19 Spectral analysis of plug and parabolic flow. A: During arterial systole, especially during the upstroke, all the blood is moving with a plug profile and a very narrow range of frequencies is displayed. **B:** During diastole in this renal artery there is a uniform spread of frequencies from peak to minimum indicating a parabolic velocity profile.

applications of spectral analysis are not generally affected by the restrictions in time resolution but the limitations of frequency resolution may become important when investigating very low velocity flows, particularly in the portal venous system and peripheral veins. In these clinical settings velocities below 5 cm/second may occur and would typically give rise to Doppler signals of approximately 200 Hertz. If the frequency resolution is 50 Hertz then clearly the mean frequency can only be calculated with an accuracy of ± 25%. The amplitude (brightness) of the signal within each pixel of the spectral analysis image is approximately proportional to the number of scatterers giving rise to signals within that particular frequency range during the appropriate time interval. It will be appreciated, therefore, that in plug flow, where most of the scatterers are moving with very similar velocities, there is a narrow range of frequencies in the Doppler signal and the spectral display is that of a narrow frequency band (Fig. 19A). Conversely, if parabolic flow is present, there is a wide frequency range giving rise to a broad spectrum of frequencies in the spectral analysis image (Fig. 19B). As a general rule, Doppler shift frequencies from blood flowing towards the transducer are displayed as positive (above the baseline) and vice versa. In several physiological and pathological circumstances there may be simultaneous flow towards and away from the transducer and this can be detected by simultaneous display of both forward and reverse flow in the spectral analysis image (Fig. 20).

Evaluation of the spectral Doppler trace is divided into

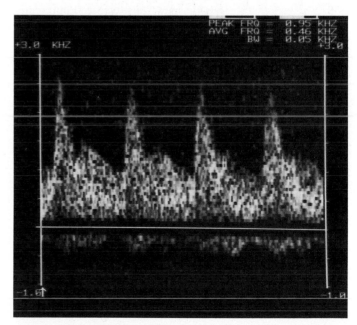

Fig. 20 Simultaneous forward and reverse flow. This tracing from an abnormal vessel shows infilling of the systolic frequency window and simultaneous display of flow in both forward and reverse channels confirming the presence of flow disturbance with vortex formation.

assessment of the waveform shape and analysis of the spectral content and each of these will be considered separately.

Waveform analysis For the purpose of waveform

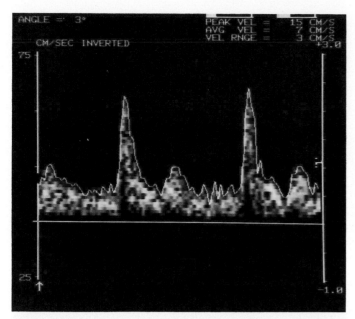

Fig. 21 Waveform analysis, peak frequency envelope. In order to permit calculation of the pulsatility index from this complex arterial waveform the equipment has automatically traced the outline of the peak frequency.

analysis the spectral content of the waveform is ignored and only the shape of the outline of the tracing is considered (Fig. 21).[24] In order to permit analysis of the waveform shape a number of end-points have to be identified (Fig. 22).[25] They include the peak end diastolic frequency, peak systole, the 'mean peak' value and, where relevant, the maximum negative deflection during diastole. From these end-points it is possible to calculate a wide range of values including systolic acceleration and deceleration, diastolic deceleration, various ratios of systole to diastole, including the A/B ratio and numerous simple indices including resistance index and pulsatility index.[22] Many more complex analyses have also been proposed but have not yet found regular clinical application.

Many of these values assume that it is possible to be certain about the exact moment at which diastole begins. This question has received little discussion in the literature though it is clear that many authors have made assumptions which are not proven by scientific investigation. For unidirectional arterial waveforms (Fig. 22A) the point of inflection on the curve from peak systole to end diastole is assumed to indicate the beginning of diastole. For bi-directional flows diastole is assumed to occur at the point where flow changes from forward to reverse (Fig. 22B) and for more complex waveforms various notches are assumed to indicate the commencement of diastole (Fig. 22C). It is probable that none of these end-points is actually valid and from a purely cardiological point of view diastole actually starts at the point of aortic valve closure which, to all intents and purposes, is at peak systole. The subsequent

deceleration is therefore not a true systolic deceleration and most, if not all, of the indices which compare or make use of the systolic and diastolic time intervals are probably invalid.

The A/B ratio This ratio was proposed by Gosling in 1976[26] specifically for assessing changes in common carotids and supra-orbital arteries. Spectral analysis of the signals from these vessels shows a secondary peak in early diastole which is termed the B peak and it is the ratio between this peak and the peak systolic amplitude which is calculated in this index (Fig. 22C). This index is not intended for generalised application but it has unfortunately been misquoted, misinterpreted and misused, most commonly by incorrect placement of the point of measurement for the B peak in waveforms derived from arteries other than those for which the technique was devised. This ratio has no specific advantages elsewhere in the arterial tree and is therefore not recommended for generalised use.

The resistance index The resistance index (RI)[27] was devised in 1973 for assessment of arterial waveforms where there is no reverse flow component. The value is

$$\frac{\text{peak systole} - \text{end diastole}}{\text{peak systole}}$$

and has the advantage that the value is independent of beam/vessel angle (cosine θ) and only requires the measurement of two precisely defined points in the spectral display (see Fig. 22A).

There is some confusion about the precise terminology both for this index and the pulsatility index (see below). The resistance index (sometimes incorrectly called the resistive index) was described by Pourcelot and is sometimes referred to as the Pourcelot index and given the abbreviation PI. This leads to confusion with the pulsatility index (also abbreviated to PI) and the situation is further confused by several authors, particularly amongst North American paediatricians, who use the resistance index but call it the pulsatility index. It is also important to be aware that the waveform is affected by many factors, several of which have nothing whatever to do with resistance to blood flow (see below).

The pulsatility index This index was devised by Gosling in 1971[3] to quantitate the energy in the oscillations of the waveform; the full equation is complex and therefore a simplified formula (the PI) is used in clinical practice.

$$\text{PI} = \frac{\text{peak systole} - \text{end diastole}}{\text{mean peak value}}$$

It is particularly valuable in arteries in which there is diastolic flow reversal and can be calculated from a frequency trace without the need to know the beam/vessel angle.

The PI requires the computation of the mean peak value throughout the cardiac cycle (see Fig. 22B). Manual tracing of complex waveforms may give rise to significant errors and automated tracings from technically inadequate Doppler signals may also give rise to erroneous values.

Despite these limitations, the PI has gained wide clinical acceptance, particularly in peripheral vascular disease. Again it is important to remember that the waveform shape may be influenced by a wide range of upstream, local and downstream factors and these should always be taken into consideration when using this or any other index.

The systolic/diastolic ratio The systolic/diastolic (S/D) ratio is effectively a variation of the resistance index and has found particular favour in obstetric applications (Fig. 22C).[28–30] The ratio is:

$$\frac{\text{peak systole}}{\text{end diastole}}.$$

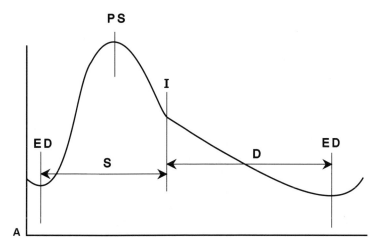

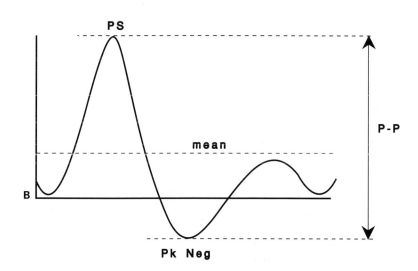

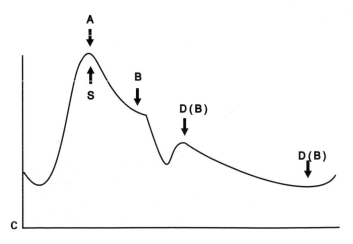

Fig. 22 Measurement of arterial waveform shape. A: For measurement of a 'low resistance' waveform the following values may be measured: end diastole (ED), peak systole (PS), systolic time interval (S), diastolic time interval (D), systolic/diastolic inflection (I). **B:** For bi-directional waveforms the peak to peak interval (P-P) from peak systole (PS) to peak negative deflection (Pk Neg) is measured together with a computed mean value throughout at least one (preferably more) cardiac cycles. **C:** For low resistance waveforms with a 'notch' there is agreement about the position of peak systole (S and A) but the diastolic values (D and B) vary from one author to another.

Unfortunately peak systole is frequently referred to as 'A' and end diastole as 'B' and this ratio is therefore also known as the A/B ratio though it is different from the previously mentioned A/B ratio. If there is also early diastolic flow reduction, this is sometimes incorrectly termed the dicrotic notch or just 'the notch'. Its presence and magnitude may correlate with the severity of vascular disease in the arterial bed of the pregnant uterus.

There is a later version of the S/D ratio which is the D/S ratio. Numerically this is usually indistinguishable from 1 minus the resistance index and is, of course, the inverse of the S/D ratio.

It is not clear which of the A/B, S/D or D/S ratios is most useful.

There are many other indices which have been devised to assess arterial waveform shapes, particularly in obstetrics.[31] The fact that so many exist tends to suggest that none is entirely satisfactory and this situation is not helped by the confusing terminology where different indices are given the same name and the same index is given different names. As a general rule it is probably safe to use the PI in peripheral vascular studies and the RI in all carotid and intra-abdominal studies.

Spectral breadth measurement The Doppler signal contains a spectrum of frequencies and the breadth of this spectrum is a measure of the range of velocities present within the vessel. During systolic flow in normal arteries with a diameter greater than 5 to 10 mm there is a narrow range of frequencies present but this range may become increased (broadened) by the presence of vascular disease. The degree to which the spectrum is broadened correlates roughly with the severity of the arterial disease[32] and it is, therefore, possible to give numerical values to the degree of spectral broadening. In small arteries the velocity profile is closer to parabolic and the normal spectrum is broad.

Unfortunately, as with waveform indices, a number of spectral broadening indices have been devised[33] and the majority are called the 'spectral broadening index' (SBI), although they are mathematically by no means identical. A simple and readily usable SBI compares the range of frequencies displayed at peak systole with the absolute peak systolic value and is expressed as a percentage (Fig. 23). The value of the SBI varies widely at different sites, at different phases in the cardiac cycle and with different equipment and control settings. Therefore normal values are not available and investigators wishing to use this index should assess their own range of normal values on their own patients and equipment and compare these values with those obtained in pathological cases.

Velocity information Using the Doppler formula it is, in theory, possible to calculate the instantaneous blood flow velocity, provided that the angle between the ultrasound beam and the direction of blood flow is accurately known and is less than 60°. In clinical practice there are a number

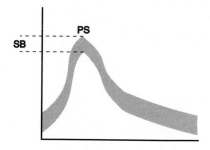

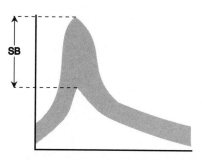

Fig. 23 Measurement of spectral breadth. The spectral broadening produced by arterial disease can be assessed by measuring the spectral breadth (SB) during peak systole and comparing this with the peak systolic value (PS).

of different specific values for velocity which may be useful in different clinical situations[34] including:

peak systole
peak end diastole
mean peak
instantaneous mean
time averaged mean

The values for peak systole and end diastole have already been discussed when considering the resistance index.

The mean peak value is the mean of the individual values comprising the peak velocity outline (Fig. 21). The instantaneous mean (Fig. 24) is difficult, and usually impossible, to calculate but in theory should be the mean value of the velocities of all the red cells moving throughout the vessel cross-section at any instant in time. Unfortunately this information is not generally available but the spectral content at any spectral analysis time interval contains information about both the range of velocities present and the approximate proportion of scatterers travelling with each individual velocity. If there is true plug flow there is, of course, a very narrow band of velocities with all red cells travelling at almost the same velocity. In true parabolic flow there is a uniform distribution of velocities from the peak down to zero resulting in an even grey scale in the display throughout the velocity range. In this situation the mean velocity is 50% of the peak, whereas in plug flow the mean is equal to the peak value.

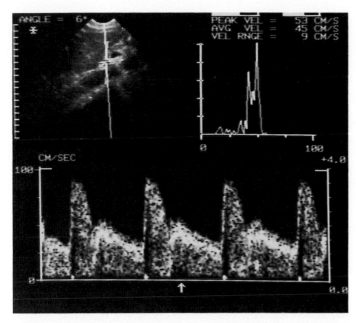

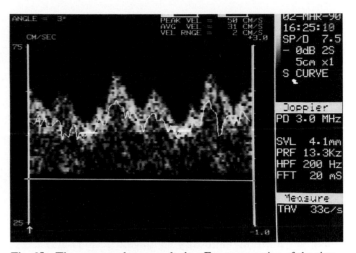

Fig. 25 Time averaged mean velocity. For computation of the time averaged mean velocity (TAV) the equipment has been set to measure the instantaneous mean velocity for every time interval throughout the trace (indicated by the thin white line) and to calculate the mean of these to give the TAV (33 cm/sec).

Fig. 24 Instantaneous mean velocity. The arrow below the spectrum analysis trace in this example indicates the time interval at which the instantaneous frequency spectrum has been assessed. The grey scale display in the spectrogram indicates that there are many more scatterers travelling with velocities close to the peak with relatively few low velocity scatterers at this time. This assessment is confirmed by the histogram (upper right) showing that most scatterers are travelling with velocities between 40 and 55 cm/sec. The instantaneous average velocity calculation above the histogram indicates a value of 45 cm/sec.

In the majority of clinical situations, the ratio between the true mean and the peak actually lies somewhere between 50% and 100% and, within arteries, varies throughout the cardiac cycle. It will be appreciated therefore that computation of the true instantaneous mean is both complex and inaccurate and a wide range of different mathematical approaches have been used by different equipment manufacturers.

To compute the volume of blood flowing through a vessel, or to calculate the mean velocity averaged over a significant time interval, it is necessary to calculate the time averaged mean velocity (Fig. 25).[35] Numerically this is simply the mean of a series of instantaneous mean velocities, usually averaged over one or more cardiac cycles. The accuracy of the ultimate value is limited by the same factors which influence the accuracy of the individual instantaneous mean calculations.[36-38] The time average mean velocity is frequently abbreviated to time averaged velocity (TAV).

Colour flow imaging

Colour flow imaging (CFI) is a rapid and easy to use technique for the detection of flow within the field of view and can be used for the rapid confirmation of vascular patency, for the assessment of the direction of flow and for the iden-

tification of areas of flow disturbance. The precise hues allocated to the colour Doppler overlay are under the user's control and have not, as yet, been standardised so that it is not possible to draw specific conclusions from the hues seen in the colour display and real velocity information cannot, therefore, be gauged from visual inspection of the display. However, the colour display is a useful 'road map' for identifying specific areas of interest and for guiding placement of the range gate for conventional spectral Doppler analysis for measurement of the various indices discussed above. Several modern colour flow imaging systems also permit the user to apply a contrasting colour, commonly green, to a variable and narrow range of frequencies, thus highlighting areas of flow which contain these specific frequencies. If the tagged frequency is progressively changed during imaging, it can be used to gauge the mean velocity present within a vessel segment, though the values obtained are much less accurate than those derived from spectral analysis.

Equipment requirements and selection

The characteristics of the equipment for performing Doppler examinations at different clinical sites vary and can conveniently be divided into four groups, namely: cardiac, peripheral, deep (abdominal) and trans-vaginal. The requirements for cardiac Doppler are discussed in the Cardiac Ultrasound volume and the other three categories are discussed below.

Peripheral

The majority of vascular surgeons use simple continuous wave (CW) pencil probe systems for assessing the patency of the palpable peripheral arteries (see Vol. 2, Ch. 49) and, with training, simple subjective analysis of the audio signal enables the operator to determine whether a vessel segment is healthy or not. These systems are simple and inexpensive and can be linked to a spectrum analyser to derive the conventional waveform indices. In skilled hands the combination of clinical assessment and CW pencil probe evaluation can predict or exclude clinically significant vascular disease with a high degree of accuracy.

The role of pulsed Doppler and duplex scanning is in the detailed evaluation of the major vessels, particularly the extracranial carotid, iliac, femoral and popliteal arteries (see Vol. 2, Chs 48 and 49). The combination of duplex and colour Doppler probably permits the detection of minor yet haemodynamically significant lesions and is essential for differentiating between the signals arising from adjacent vessels, e.g. internal from external carotid or superficial from deep femoral arteries, the signals from which are mixed in the CW Doppler output.

The frequency of the imaging component of a duplex system is determined by the depth of the vessel under investigation; but generally a 7.5 MHz transducer is appropriate.

The frequency of the pulses used for acquiring the Doppler information from deep vessels is ideally less than that used for imaging and is typically between 2 and 3 MHz. Attempts to use a higher frequency Doppler generally lead to significant loss in sensitivity and difficulty in acquiring an adequate Doppler trace. Equipment for peripheral vascular imaging and Doppler should therefore have the facility for using different frequencies for the imaging and the Doppler pulses.

Unfortunately the carotid and femoral vessels generally run roughly parallel to the skin surface and there may, therefore, be difficulty in positioning the transducer to give an adequate beam/vessel angle. This problem can to some extent be overcome by use of a steerable Doppler beam. Most modern array transducers permit beam steering through an angle of at least 20° (Fig. 26); this, together with minor degrees of probe angulation, generally permits a beam/vessel angle of 60° or less to be achieved. An alternative approach is to use a separate ultrasound crystal ('off-set Doppler') for acquiring the Doppler information (Fig. 27). If this crystal is placed at one end of the array, a satisfactory beam/vessel angle can almost always be achieved, although there is sometimes difficulty in obtaining satisfactory contact with both the imaging and Doppler transducers simultaneously.

An additional important factor is the range of Doppler shift frequencies which the equipment is capable of detecting and displaying. For arterial studies on pathological vessels accurate representation of frequencies above 8 kHz may be necessary to document stenoses adequately, whereas for venous studies in the lower limb, frequencies

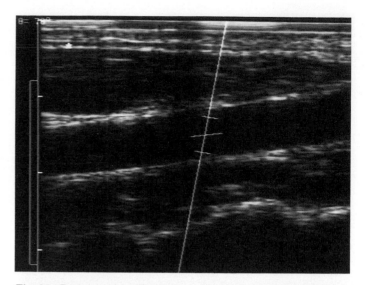

Fig. 26 Beam steering. The angle at which the ultrasound beam leaves a straight linear array transducer can be varied by about 20° in most modern machines. This function can be used to improve the beam/vessel angle and is particularly useful when the vessel under investigation lies approximately parallel to the skin surface.

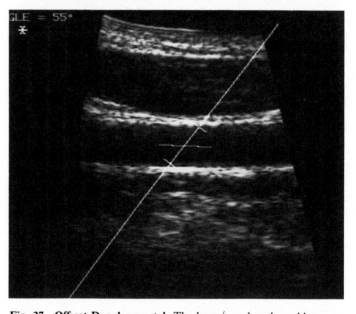

Fig. 27 Off-set Doppler crystal. The beam/vessel angle problem can also be overcome by use of a separate crystal mounted at the end of the imaging transducer. In this example the Doppler crystal is mounted on a swivel permitting the operator to optimise the beam/vessel angle further.

below 100 Hz should be detectable in order to demonstrate spontaneous venous flow.

Abdominal and obstetric applications (deep Doppler)

With the exception of fetal heart detection, continuous wave Doppler has no application in abdominal and obstetric applications. Duplex imaging with Doppler and colour flow imaging are essential prerequisites for these deeper investigations. The imaging frequency is determined by the depth of penetration required but is generally from 3.5 to 5 MHz. A transmitted Doppler frequency of 2 MHz is appropriate for the majority of deep investigations, though 3 MHz may be appropriate for more superficial structures, for example in paediatrics and transplanted kidneys.

Almost without exception all modern scanners designed for deep Doppler applications use 'in-line' Doppler where the imaging and Doppler pulses are transmitted and received by the same transducer (as shown in all the preceding duplex images). Mechanical systems using a single crystal generally have greater sensitivity allowing significantly lower ultrasound powers to be used in the Doppler mode than is possible with array transducers. However, mechanical scanners cannot perform true simultaneous 'duplex' imaging and Doppler and cannot be used for colour Doppler imaging (other than for very fast flow rates e.g. in cardiology).

Deep Doppler investigations are also compromised by the relationship between pulse repetition frequency and maximum detectable Doppler shift frequency. For imaging deep structures, the pulse repetition frequency must be limited to 5 kHz to avoid overlap between consecutive pulses and, because of the way the Doppler information is detected, this prevents the correct identification of Doppler frequencies greater than 2.5 kHz (see aliasing, p. 83). Whilst this is not a problem for venous studies, many deep arteries may give rise to Doppler shifts of higher frequency, particularly if the beam/vessel angle is small. There is inevitably a compromise between depth penetration and maximum detectable Doppler frequency and it is helpful if the equipment has the facility for the operator to control directly the pulse repetition frequency during Doppler investigations.

The range of Doppler frequencies which can be detected and displayed on the spectral analysis must be adequate to cover both portal venous and arterial investigations, though the upper frequency requirement is lower than that required for peripheral vascular work.

Trans-vaginal Doppler

Duplex and/or colour flow imaging are essential for the detection and correct identification of targets from which Doppler spectra are to be obtained.

As with other applications, the imaging frequency is limited by the depth of penetration required and is typically 5 to 7.5 MHz with a Doppler frequency of 3 to 5 MHz.

The construction of trans-vaginal transducers inevitably

constrains the Doppler to be 'in-line' with the imaging pulses.

The detectable velocity range need not be as wide as for other applications since extremely low venous flows and high velocity arterial flows are unlikely to be encountered in early pregnancy or in gynaecological investigations.

Scanning techniques

Peripheral arteries

The carotid arteries are best examined with the patient supine with the head and neck supported on a soft pillow. The head should be turned slightly away from the side being examined with the chin elevated a little but care must be taken to make sure that the neck muscles are relaxed and that the patient is comfortable. The trunk of the common carotid artery is best identified on longitudinal anterior scans but the bifurcation and internal and external vessels may be better seen via a postero-lateral approach from the posterior aspect of the sternomastoid muscle. This approach is particularly helpful if access to the bifurcation is impaired by limited neck movement, a prominent mandibular angle or a high bifurcation. If difficulties are experienced in obtaining adequate Doppler signals due to a limited beam/vessel angle it is often possible to obtain a more satisfactory signal with the transducer placed at right angles to the vessel and angled to look either upstream or downstream (Fig. 28).

Difficulties with identifying or differentiating the internal and external carotids may also be overcome by studying the colour flow image obtained with the transducer at right angles to the long axis of the vessel, but angled to give an adequate Doppler signal.

The external iliac vessels can be imaged through a full urinary bladder placing the probe on the opposite side of the pelvis to the vessel being studied and looking across the pelvic cavity. Although imaging of the vessel in this

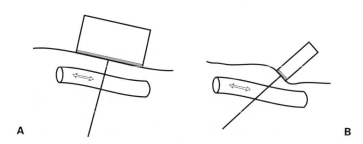

Fig. 28 Optimisation of beam/vessel angle on superficial vessels.
A: When a linear array transducer is used to image a superficial vessel the beam/vessel angle tends to be close to 90°. **B:** This can be overcome by rotating the transducer to image the vessel in cross-section and then angling the transducer to improve the beam/vessel angle.

plane is often excellent, it is difficult to obtain a good beam/vessel angle. To overcome this problem it may be necessary to place the probe just above the inguinal region and to attempt to look down the axis of the ipsilateral vessel.

The proximal and distal femoral arteries are easily seen with the patient lying supine, but investigation of the popliteal artery usually requires the patient to lie on their side with the leg under examination flexed by no more than 10° to 15°. It is usually possible to examine both popliteal arteries with the patient lying on their left side.

The deep veins of the leg exhibit extremely low velocity flow at rest and it may be necessary to augment this flow in order to produce a detectable Doppler signal (Fig. 29). Flow within the femoral and popliteal veins can be augmented by gentle manual compression of the calf and flow within the popliteal and calf veins can also be augmented by compression of the dorsum of the foot. In addition flow can be temporarily suspended by asking the patient to undertake the Valsalva manoeuvre and there is normally a compensatory transient increase in flow velocity on resumption of normal breathing. The pressure within the leg veins is very low and those which are superficial are extremely susceptible to compression by the examining transducer. Even modest pressure may completely obliterate the vessel lumen and prevent its detection. In patients where detection of any of the deep veins proves particularly difficult, especially the deep calf veins, it may be helpful to examine the patient standing. Although this

increases the diameter of the veins, there is usually a concomitant further reduction in flow velocity and some form of flow augmentation is required in order to produce a detectable Doppler signal.

Deep Doppler investigations

The portal vein is readily accessible to ultrasound imaging and is often best seen on transverse epigastric scans. However, in this position the vessel axis is at right angles to the ultrasound beam and this scanning approach is therefore usually inappropriate for Doppler studies. A satisfactory alternative approach is to use the right lateral intercostal

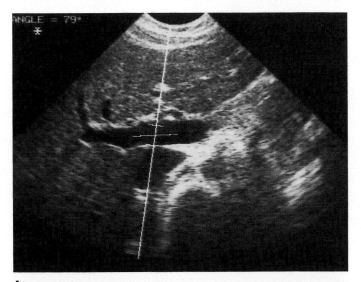

A

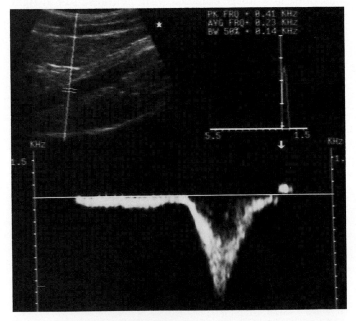

Fig. 29 Deep venous flow augmentation. The slow spontaneous flow velocity in this femoral vein has been briefly augmented by squeezing the patient's calf. This form of augmentation helps to confirm the patency of both the calf veins and those veins between the calf and point of Doppler examination.

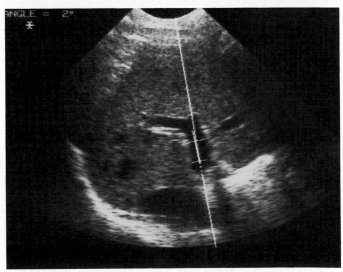

B

Fig. 30 Doppler study of the portal vein. A: The anterior approach to the portal vein is optimal for imaging but gives a poor beam/vessel angle (79°) for Doppler studies. **B:** The lateral intercostal approach optimises the beam/vessel angle (2° in this case).

window via which the main portal vein and its right branch are orientated almost directly along the line of the ultrasound beam (Fig. 30). If the vessel is being studied merely for the purpose of confirming its patency, colour flow imaging alone is adequate and the examination should be performed after a meal when the flow is maximal. If flow velocity information is required, the investigation should be performed under standard conditions, normally after a 6 to 8 hour period of fasting.

Similar considerations apply to the hepatic artery which is again best seen via the anterior approach but gives a better Doppler angle if the right lateral intercostal approach is used.

The approach utilised for Doppler investigation of the native kidney is determined by the nature of the information which is being sought. Colour flow imaging on lateral coronal scans gives a good overall view of renal perfusion and usually identifies the renal hilum with sufficient accuracy for a range gate to be positioned for detection of the main artery and vein at the hilum. However, if flow information is required from the main renal arteries, for instance for the detection of renal artery stenosis, it may be necessary also to take an anterior approach using colour Doppler to attempt to identify the origins and courses of the two vessels. This examination is ideally performed with the patient fasted.

For obstetric Doppler examinations the output power of the Doppler device is an important consideration. There is almost invariably a substantial increase in the transmitted ultrasound energy when Doppler examinations are performed and in many machines this is under the operator's control. Care should be taken to reduce the transmitted power to the lowest value consistent with obtaining an adequate examination and the total duration of the examination should be restricted to the shortest possible time. These restrictions are especially important when Doppler studies are being performed via the trans-vaginal route where the target tissue is much closer to the transducer and higher frequency transducers (which usually have a higher output power) are being employed.

Artefacts, errors and pitfalls

Beam/vessel angle

Problems associated with the angle between the ultrasound beam and the axis of flow within the vessel are probably the commonest source of difficulties and errors with Doppler investigations.[39] If the beam/vessel angle is significantly greater than 60° there is a marked reduction in the Doppler shift frequency and significant uncertainties arise concerning the accuracy of any derived velocity values. As the beam/vessel angle approaches 90° it is unlikely that any useful Doppler trace will be obtained. However, there is occasionally sufficient radial flow during the pulsatile expansion of the vessel in systole for a bi-directional Doppler signal to be detected. The outline of the waveform is obviously arterial in nature but this waveform is valueless for assessing the flow characteristics in the vessel or for measurement of any of the waveform indices.

Aliasing

The phenomenon of aliasing arises from the relationship between the maximum detectable Doppler shift frequency and the pulse repetition frequency (PRF) of the interrogating ultrasound beam. In pulsed Doppler ultrasound, the Doppler shift frequency is compiled from measurements taken from a large number of rapid sequential pulses. As the Doppler shift frequency approaches the PRF, there are insufficient samples to enable the waveform to be determined accurately (Fig. 31). Any Doppler shift frequency greater than half the PRF is underestimated and interpreted by the equipment as flow in the opposite direction. This situation most commonly occurs where the maximum systolic frequencies fall above the aliasing limit and the peak systolic component of the waveform appears on the wrong side of the baseline (Fig. 32A). Provided that the baseline has not been shifted from the middle of the display range the artefact will not be overlooked. However, when studying arteries with high velocity flow it is often necessary to move the baseline downwards to give a larger area for display of the forward flow component. This may result in the aliased peak information not being displayed in the image and the artefact may therefore go unrecognised (Fig. 32B). If any index measurements are taken from the waveform it is essential to be absolutely certain that the peak systolic information is correctly detected and displayed. A similar artefact may occur if the peak systolic frequencies fall above those which can be displayed in the selected frequency range of the equipment.

There are a number of steps which can be taken to attempt to overcome aliasing. Firstly, if the equipment permits it, the PRF may be increased. As this is done, range ambiguities may arise by virtue of the fact that echoes may still be received from one pulse after the subsequent pulse has been transmitted. These echoes will then be misrepresented as appearing from superficial structures. Equipment which permits the operator to increase the PRF to this level usually includes some indication on the screen to show the sites at which range ambiguities may appear (Fig. 33).

If the PRF cannot be raised sufficiently, there are a number of alternative approaches and these can be deduced from the Doppler formula. Given that the velocity of ultrasound and the blood flow velocity cannot be changed, the only way in which the Doppler shift frequency can be reduced is for the ultrasound frequency or the value of Cos

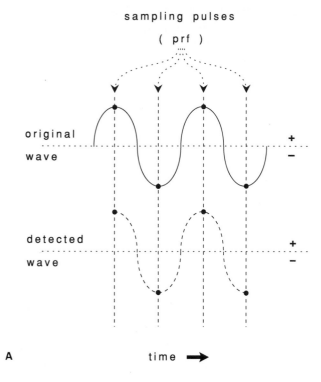

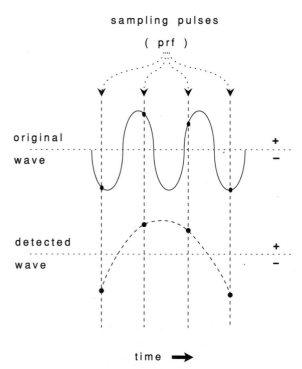

Fig. 31 Aliasing. A: The original ultrasound wave is sampled by pulses emitted at the pulse repetition frequency (PRF). In this example the wave is sampled at both the peak positive and peak negative points and the detected wave is an accurate representation of the original wave. **B:** If the frequency of the original wave increases but the PRF remains unchanged the frequency of sampling of the original wave is insufficient for the detected wave to reproduce correctly the frequency of the sampled wave. In this example the detected wave shows a gross artefactual reduction in frequency.

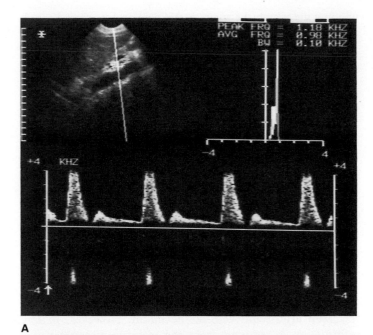

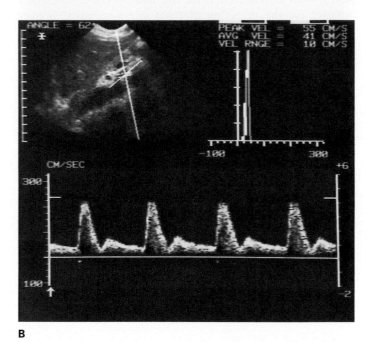

Fig. 32 Aliasing. A: The equipment examining this coeliac axis has a PRF of 8.5 kHz. The peak velocity detected exceeds 4.25 kHz and that component above this value is incorrectly displayed in the negative flow channel. **B:** This artefact may be overlooked if the display baseline is shifted downwards such that the aliased peaks no longer appear in the display. Any waveform indices measured from this display will be incorrect. This problem is overcome in some scanners by repositioning the aliased peak on top of the systolic complex.

θ to be reduced. The former can be achieved by using a lower Doppler transmission frequency, the latter may be achieved by increasing the beam/vessel angle and thereby decreasing the effect of cosine θ.

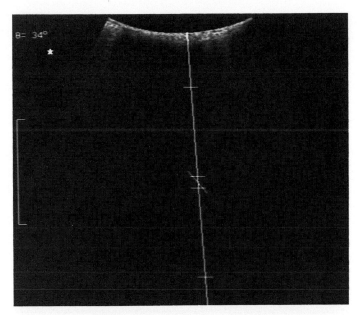

Fig. 33 High PRF range ambiguities. In this example the operator has chosen to increase the PRF to 15 kHz. This does not allow sufficient time between pulses for all the echoes from the deepest part of the image to be received before the next pulse is transmitted. Range ambiguities therefore occur and are displayed as additional single lines crossing the Doppler line of sight. Vessels at either of these sites would give rise to a Doppler signal which would be mixed with that from any vessel from within the actual range gate (see Plate 6).

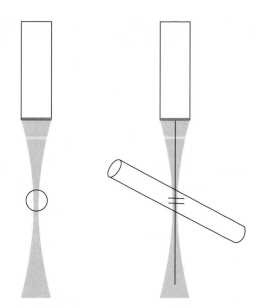

Fig. 34 Undersampling. The blood flow within a vessel may be inadvertently undersampled if the vessel diameter is significantly greater than the ultrasound beam width or if the range gate is narrower than the vessel diameter. Both of these situations lead to an overestimation of mean velocity.

Sample volume size and position

Doppler measurements assume that the vessel is uniformly insonated (p. 72) (Fig. 14) and that the range gate encompasses the whole of the cross-section of the vessel. In clinical practice these assumptions are seldom true with the result that the flow is usually undersampled,[32] though occasionally sampling of structures outside the vessel may occur.

Undersampling of the vessel cross-section occurs if the range gate is less than the vessel diameter and is likely to occur if the ultrasound beam width is significantly less than the vessel width (Fig. 34).[40] With single crystal ultrasound devices the beam width is fixed and cannot be altered by the operator but in array transducers the width of the beam in the scanned plane is variable and, if a large diameter vessel is being studied, it may be preferable to defocus the beam in order to minimise undersampling. Unfortunately some modern phased array scanners automatically focus the beam at the depth of the range gate position and do not permit the operator to undertake intentional defocusing. Annular array transducers would permit optimisation of the beam width in both planes but, at present, there are few, if any, scanners available in which good quality Doppler can be achieved via an annular array transducer.

A further and more complex cause of undersampling is due to vessel movement during the Doppler acquisition process. This is most likely to be a source of difficulty with vessels which undergo significant degrees of translocation during cardiac pulsations, for example the superior mesenteric artery and the umbilical arteries. If the translocatory movements cause the vessel to move in and out of the range gate throughout the cardiac cycle, there may be regular and reproducible loss of Doppler information during a specific phase of the cardiac cycle. If this occurs during systole a significant loss in signal strength is noted (Fig. 35A), whereas if it occurs during diastole artefactual reduction in diastolic flow is produced with potentially dangerous clinical consequences (Figs 35B and 35C). This artefact is difficult to identify when the umbilical artery is being studied and it is therefore advisable to undertake all umbilical artery studies with a range gate which is intentionally longer than the vessel diameter and to repeat the examination several times, preferably from different segments of the umbilical cord.

If a small range gate is placed within a large vein which contains a coarse vortex and the vein moves during respiration, a confusing spectral trace may result (Fig. 35D).

If the range gate or beam width are significantly greater than the vessel diameter it is unlikely that problems will arise unless an additional vessel or branch falls within the sample volume. This situation seldom leads to clinical confusion though, in theory, it might be possible for a segment of the umbilical vein to pass in and out of the beam width and give a false impression of transitory diastolic flow reversal. More often oversampling gives rise to helpful information, such as simultaneous detection of the renal

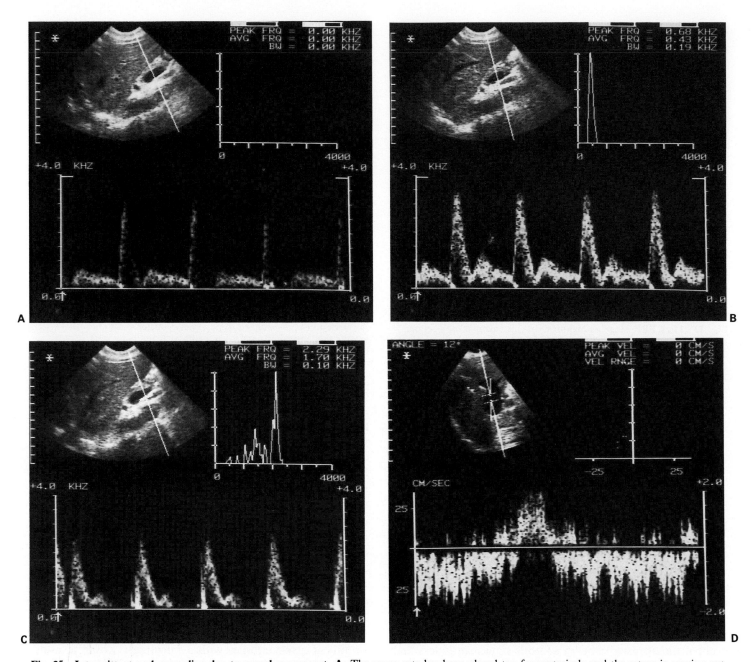

Fig. 35 Intermittent undersampling due to vessel movement. A: The range gate has been placed too far posteriorly and the artery is moving out of the sample volume during systole. **B:** Normal superior mesenteric artery trace. **C:** The range gate is too proximal with the artery only entering the sample volume during systole. **D:** Respiratory movement in a dilated portal vein in which there is a coarse vortex. The flow direction changes from forward to reverse as the vortex moves in and out of the sample volume.

artery and renal vein at the hilum, confirming correct location of the range gate when difficulty is experienced in detecting flow in one or other vessel, particularly in suspected renal vein thrombosis. Within the liver, detection of the hepatic artery signal can be used to confirm correct placement of the range gate in the region of the portal vein (Fig. 36). If no adjacent venous signal can be detected there is greater confidence in the diagnosis of absence of portal flow.

Velocity calculations

There is an increasing number of clinical applications of Doppler ultrasound in which calculation of one or more aspects of blood velocity is useful. The derived values always depend upon knowledge of the beam/vessel angle and are subject to numerous errors and uncertainties. The degree of error introduced by beam/vessel angle measurement is highly dependent upon the absolute value of the

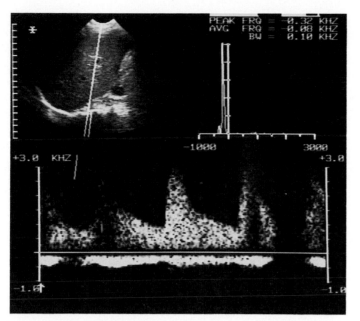

Fig. 36 Oversampling due to large range gate. A large range gate with consequent oversampling has been employed to advantage in this case with possible portal vein thrombosis to confirm the presence of a low velocity reversed flow portal venous signal alongside the intrahepatic arterial branches.

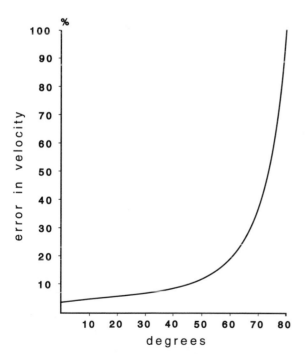

Fig. 37 Change in velocity calculation error with beam/vessel angle. This graph shows the percentage velocity error which occurs for a 5° error in beam/vessel angle measurement. For angles below 50° the error is insignificant but there is a very rapid increase for angles greater than 60°.

beam/vessel angle.[37] If this angle is less than 45° a 5° error in angle measurement gives rise to a velocity error of less than 10% (Fig. 37). However, for angles greater than 45° there is a very rapid increase in the error introduced by a 5° uncertainty, such that at 70° the error is 35% and at 80° 100%. This point again emphasises the importance of keeping the beam/vessel angle as small as possible.

In some scanners the spectral display is calibrated in velocity rather than frequency shift, even when no beam/vessel angle information has been entered. These displays assume a beam/vessel angle of 0°; unless a true beam/vessel angle has been indicated the velocity information is totally meaningless and users of such equipment must be aware of this inadequacy.

The mean peak value (as used for the pulsatility index calculation) should ideally be traced automatically from the waveform outline (see Fig. 21).[24] However, the operator must undertake this manually if the machine does not incorporate automatic waveform tracing or if the automatic tracing fails due to a noisy or interrupted waveform. Minor degrees of error may be introduced by manual tracing, particularly if the waveform is complex in shape. Both the manual and automatic techniques may also be subject to error if the waveform is inadequate, usually due to insufficient sensitivity or gain (Fig. 38).

Measurement of the instantaneous mean velocity and time averaged mean velocity are influenced by two major factors. The calculation of mean velocity has to make allowance for the different number of scatterers travelling at the different velocities present within the sampled volume. There is no precise way of doing this and different assumptions are made by different equipment manufacturers. Some merely take the mean peak value and multiply this by a constant, usually 0.6 to 0.7, assuming a standard velocity profile throughout the cardiac cycle in all vessels. Clearly this is an invalid assumption. An alternative and common approach is to assess the mode velocity (the most commonly occurring value during any time interval) or to determine the highest frequency detectable with a power level at a predetermined number of decibels less than that of the peak value. Typically this latter measurement may be taken at levels of −3, −6, −9 or −12 dBs from the peak value and each of these, of course, gives rise to a different mean value. There is as yet no uniform agreement concerning the ideal way of calculating the true mean velocity and the results vary by at least 50%. It is therefore essential that in any unit where velocity values are to be used clinically the range of normals must be established using the equipment available in that institution.

Blood flow velocity calculations always assume that the blood is flowing along the long axis of the vessel at the site of measurement. This situation only applies in the central axis of straight, non-branching vessels (see p. 67). In many clinical situations it may be difficult or impossible to obtain an ideally suited segment of vessel for study and the

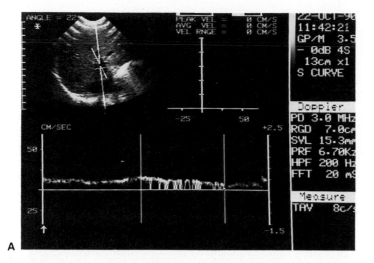

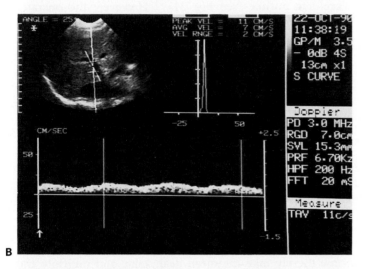

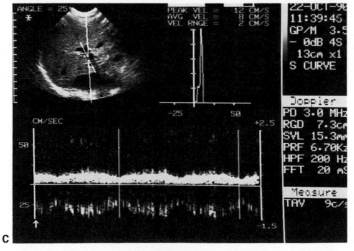

Fig. 38   Velocity errors due to incorrect gain settings. A: With the gain too low there are drop outs in the TAV measurement giving an inappropriately low value (8 cm/sec). **B:** With correct gain setting a true value of 11 cm/sec is obtained. **C:** With the gain too high there is signal breakthrough into the reverse flow channel with a resultant apparent decrease in the mean velocity value (9 cm/sec) (see also Fig. 42).

consequent distortion of the velocity profile in a suboptimal vessel segment may lead to significant velocity errors. This is particularly marked in the situation illustrated in Plate 1B in which the axis of flow in the left portal vein branch is clearly at approximately 45° to the long axis of the vessel owing to the presence of a coarse vortex within the vessel arising from the bifurcation of the left and right portal veins. It is quite possible for velocity profile distortions and non-axial flow to introduce velocity errors of a further 50%.

An additional significant factor influencing the derived velocity values relates to the relationship between the vessel size and the sample volume size as discussed above. If the vessel is significantly undersampled this may give rise to loss of low velocity peripheral flow and a consequent over-estimate of the mean velocity, whilst partial or complete movement of the vessel out of the range gate during the sampling period gives rise to loss of information causing a reduction in computed mean velocity.

Volume flow calculation

Volume blood flow is calculated by multiplying the time averaged mean velocity by the vessel cross-sectional area. The velocity calculation may have an error of at least 50% (see p. 87) and a further major error may be introduced by incorrect assessment of the vessel cross-sectional area.[37,38] In arterial studies the vessel area is usually computed from a one-dimensional diameter measurement and any error in this is squared during the calculation process. In addition, the arterial diameter normally varies by ± 10% through the cardiac cycle and, unless this is taken into account and a mean value obtained, a further potential error of 20% can arise. The vessel diameter must not be measured from a colour Doppler image as the resolution of these systems is poor and the spread of the colour overlay leads to an overestimate of several millimetres.

For veins, computation of the cross-sectional area from a single diameter measurement is not appropriate since very few veins are circular in cross-section. It is therefore

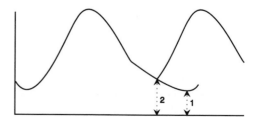

Fig. 39   Change in resistance index with heart rate. Measurement of the resistance index depends upon measurement of end diastole. When the heart rate is slow end diastole is late (1) and low. If the heart rate increases, end diastole apparently occurs earlier (2) giving a higher value and corrupting the RI calculation. The effect on PI would be much less.

essential to measure the cross-sectional area of a vessel directly. However, this must be done on an image at right angles to the vessel axis in order to prevent geometrical distortion: this is precisely the position in which Doppler information is inadequate and the Doppler signal must be obtained from a separate study with an appropriate beam/vessel angle. There is, therefore, often considerable doubt as to whether or not the cross-sectional area and Doppler information were obtained from the same site. This is especially important where a tributary joins between the sites of the two measurements and in vessels with an irregular cross-sectional area, such as the portal vein.

Waveform analyses

Calculation of the resistance index (RI) depends on measurements of both peak systole and end diastole. Although diastolic flow does decrease with increasing peripheral vascular resistance, the apparent value of the end diastolic flow is significantly altered by heart rate alone. At fast heart rates the onset of systole encroaches upon diastole resulting in an apparent rise in the end diastolic value, and vice versa (Fig. 39). It is in theory possible to compensate for this by extrapolating the diastolic flow deceleration and normalising the cardiac period to a standardised value. In practice, however, this form of normalisation is almost never undertaken. The significance of the heart rate on RI values must not be overlooked. For example changes in the RI in the fetal circulation have been attributed to 'circulatory maturation' but are probably a reflection of the changes in heart rate through gestation.

Computation of the pulsatility index (PI) is subject to the same uncertainties if there is continuous forward flow and the diastolic value used in the formula is end diastole. Difficulties in measuring the mean peak value have been discussed (see p. 87) and one piece of equipment has been marketed in which the mean value used in the PI calculation was, in fact, the time averaged mean and not the mean peak value. Once again it is important to be aware of the way in which the equipment in use calculates the various indices and ideally to establish one's own normal range wherever possible.

A further source of corruption of the RI and PI values is distortion of the waveform due to vessel movement with respect to the sample volume throughout the cardiac cycle. This may lead to significant error in index calculation (Fig. 35).

Finally, when using the waveform indices as diagnostic tools it is essential to remember that the actual waveform is determined not only by the state of the distal vascular tree but is influenced by a wide range of upstream, local and downstream factors including cardiac function, aortic valve function, the state of the arterial tree, upstream and downstream stenoses and blocks and the presence and efficacy of collateral circulations. Changes in any one of these variables may have a significant effect upon the numerical indices, though the source of this effect may not be evident from the Doppler trace alone. Cases of unsuspected right heart disease have been diagnosed by identification of abnormal central venous waveforms and patent ductus arteriosus has been detected by noting diastolic flow reversal in the renal arteries whilst undertaking investigation to exclude renal vein thrombosis in neonates.

Spectral information   The range of frequencies present within the Doppler spectrum may be adversely affected by a number of factors including under and oversampling as discussed above. Undersampling most commonly results from use of a too small a range gate, with consequent loss of low frequency information, but eccentric placement of a small range gate may also lead to underestimation of the higher velocities present in the centre of the vessel.

An additional artefact which may compromise the quality of the spectral trace is that produced by the low frequency but high amplitude Doppler signal arising from the pulsating arterial wall. Although the velocity of movement of the wall is low, it is an extremely efficient ultrasound reflector and therefore gives rise to a very high amplitude low frequency signal. This appears in the Doppler trace as 'wall thump' (Fig. 40A) and its presence corrupts measurements of the peak or mean frequencies. As the wall thump signal is of very low frequency, it can be selectively removed by a wall thump filter or 'high pass filter'. This allows the user selectively to reject the low frequency components of the Doppler signal. For arterial studies it may be necessary to increase the high pass filter to a value of 600 or even 800 Hertz in order to eliminate the wall thump (Fig. 40B). However, the filter also removes true low frequency Doppler shifts and when such a high filter frequency is applied, velocity calculations taken from the spectrum show an artefactual apparent increase in velocity. This is seldom of such magnitude to be important in arterial imaging but, if venous studies are performed with a wall filter set at a high value, much of the flow information may be lost or the presence of flow may even be overlooked.

In addition to the Doppler signal arising from arterial walls, any rapidly moving tissue gives rise to a Doppler shift. This is particularly noticeable with colour flow imaging when it may be annoying but seldom leads to diagnostic error. When using spectral Doppler, however, errors may easily occur if the operator is unaware of the possible origin of the Doppler trace (Fig. 41).

Mirror image artefacts

The mirror image artefact in spectral analysis is seen as a spurious flow signal on the wrong side of the baseline (Fig. 42). There are many causes for this effect, the commonest of which is probably related to inadequacies in the

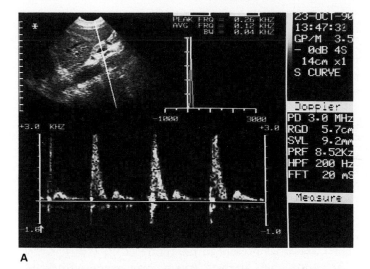

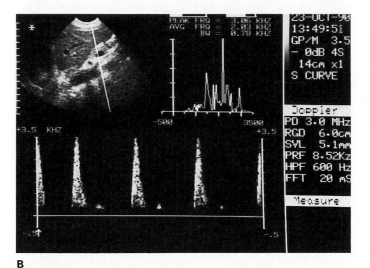

Fig. 40   Wall thump. A: The low velocity excursions of arterial walls give rise to a high amplitude low velocity signal seen in this example as a strong positive and negative peak overlying the beginning of systole. **B:** Increasing the high pass filter (HPF) from 200 to 600 Hz has eliminated the wall thump but also leads to loss of most of the true diastolic flow.

Colour flow imaging

Colour flow Doppler is subject to the same limitations and artefacts as conventional pulsed Doppler. However, the problem of aliasing is more likely to occur because, in order to prevent range artefacts in the image, the PRF is determined in the normal way by the time necessary to

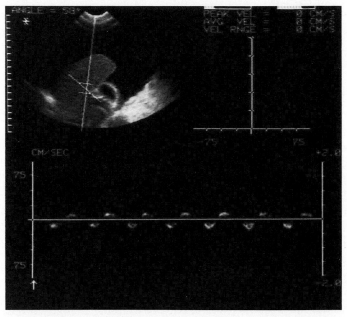

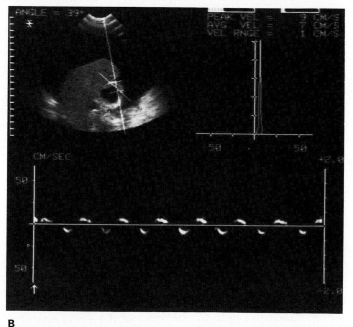

Fig. 41   Tissue movement. A: The Doppler trace from the portal vein in this patient with liver disease and ascites shows apparent oscillating flow. **B:** The range gate has been repositioned over the gallbladder wall and gives an identical trace. The Doppler signal is due to tissue movement induced by cardiac contractions and not to blood flow at all.

scanner's electronics; it is particularly prevalent with multi-element transducers. A similar artefact can be produced if the Doppler gain is too high (Fig. 38C) or if the beam/vessel angle is too small. In this case the artefact may be due to radial flow during the systolic expansion of the vessel. An alternative cause in certain circumstances may be the presence of a branch vessel or separate vessel included in the range gate but carrying blood in the opposite direction in which case the spectrum truly indicates the real flow situation.

Care must be taken to differentiate this appearance from that produced from true disturbance with flow reversal, either physiological or due to vessel disease.

allow all pulses to return from the deepest tissues to be imaged. However, in the majority of colour flow systems some of these pulses are used to produce the conventional grey scale information and the remainder are used for the colour flow Doppler. The effective PRF of the Doppler

pulses is thus markedly lower than the imaging PRF and the aliasing limit is therefore lower. As a result even moderate flow velocities present in normal arteries during systole often give rise to aliasing. In the colour flow display this appears as a reversal of the flow colour such that part

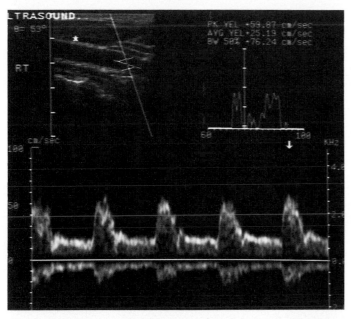

Fig. 42 Mirror image artefact. Flow in this common carotid artery is towards the probe and gives rise to the spectral analysis signal above the baseline. The similar low amplitude waveform below the baseline is a mirror image artefact. The cause is uncertain but in this case it could be due to simultaneous detection of flow within the superior thyroid artery if the sample volume is greater than that indicated by the range gates (see also Fig. 38C).

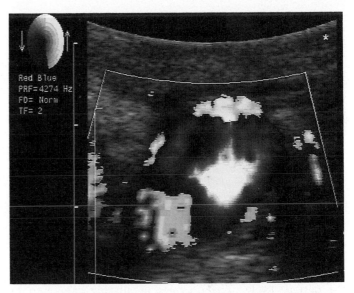

Plate 4 Apparent flow reversal due to aliasing. In this transverse scan of a large vein in which there is parabolic flow the flow velocity in the centre of the vessel exceeds the aliasing limit. The coding passes from blue through white to red without a break indicating that this is true aliasing. This figure is reproduced in colour in the colour plate section at the front of this volume.

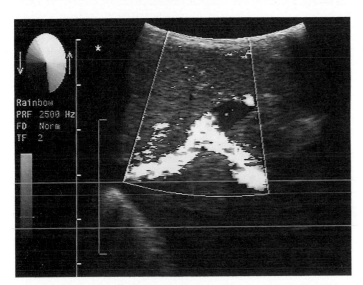

Plate 3 Mosaic artefact due to aliasing. The flow velocity in this patent ductus venosus exceeds the aliasing limit giving rise to the mosaic artefact. Normal velocity flow within the left branch of the portal vein gives rise to a correctly coded blue signal. This figure is reproduced in colour in the colour plate section at the front of this volume.

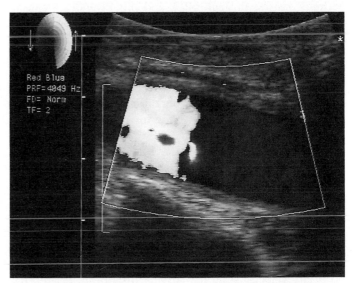

Plate 5 True flow reversal. Same case as Plate 4, longitudinal scan. There is a small area of aliasing within the red flow segment. The radial orientation of the imaging pulses arising from this curvilinear array gives rise to flow effectively towards the transducer in the red segment of the vessel and away from the transducer in the blue segment. At the point where the flow is at right angles to the beams there is a small black gap between the red and blue segments confirming true flow reversal at this point. This figure is reproduced in colour in the colour plate section at the front of this volume.

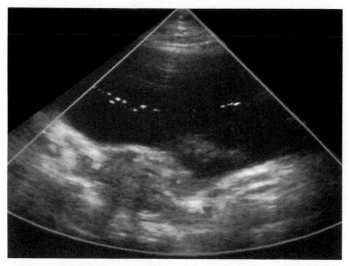

Plate 6 Colour range artefact. Imaging of these deep vessels within the pelvis required a low PRF. In order to overcome aliasing the PRF has been increased and has resulted in range ambiguities giving rise to artefactual colour signals within the bladder. This figure is reproduced in colour in the colour plate section at the front of this volume.

or all of a vessel may show transient colour reversal during the cardiac cycle. The presence of aliasing can often be inferred from the mosaic mixture of colours in an image (Plate 3). However there are occasions where the aliased segment of the image gives an appearance almost indistinguishable from true flow reversal (Plate 4). In this situation it can be seen that the colour flips directly from red to blue without passing through black and this provides a clue to the artefactual nature of the appearance. If there is true flow reversal, there is almost always a point in the image where the flow passes through a right angle to the beam as it changes from flow towards the probe to flow away from the probe. At this point there is a brief instant during which no Doppler signal is obtained and this produces a small black gap between the true forward and true reverse flow pixels (Plate 5).

If the operator increases the PRF to the point where range ambiguities occur, the true areas of colour flow may be duplicated at inappropriate sites within the image (Plate 6).

On many colour flow machines the PRF is controlled indirectly by setting the velocity scale. If high velocity flow is imaged with a low velocity scale setting, aliasing results (Plate 7A). When this is corrected by choosing a more appropriate velocity scale the aliasing disappears (Plate 7B).

A further and very important artefact in colour flow images results from the relatively poor spatial resolution compared with grey scale imaging. The colour picture elements are smaller in number and larger in size than the grey scale imaging elements and the Doppler pulses are often intentionally made longer than imaging pulses to improve the accuracy of Doppler frequency measurement.

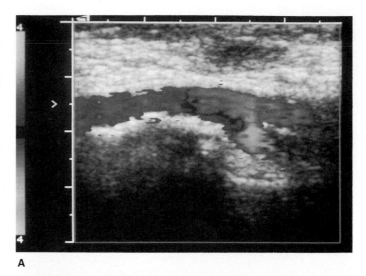

A

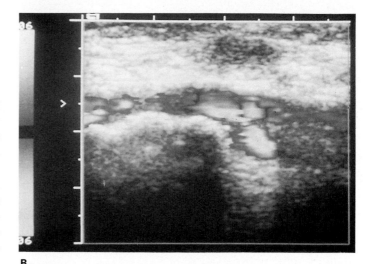

B

Plate 7 Aliasing and its correction. A: The axillary artery has been examined with an inappropriate velocity range and consequent low PRF. The colour flow image is corrupted by aliasing. **B:** The velocity range, and therefore PRF, have been markedly increased to overcome the aliasing. Note the apparent change in flow direction similar to that seen in Plate 5, in this case due to a curved vessel imaged with a straight linear array. This figure is reproduced in colour in the colour plate section at the front of this volume.

These two factors combine to degrade significantly both the axial and azimuthal resolution of the colour image. When large vessels are being displayed this is of little importance but, with small vessels (a few millimetres in diameter), there is almost always an overestimate of vessel diameter. This overestimate is likely to be of the order of at least 1 mm and, for very small vessels, may lead to an apparent overestimate of vessel diameter approaching 100%! The colour image must therefore never be used for vessel diameter measurements. In addition, many machines permit the colour image to be integrated over a variable period of several seconds. This enhances the resulting 'road map' appearance and may produce attractive colour images but the integrated vessel pulsations lead to yet further artefactual increase in the apparent vessel diameters.

Beam/vessel artefact The colour coding of blood flow in CDI is determined by the direction of flow 'with respect to the transducer'. If a long vessel segment is examined with a sector scanner, or a curved vessel is examined with a linear array, flow in part of the vessel may be towards the transducer whilst it is away from the transducer in another segment. There is thus a sudden reversal in colour coding at the point where the flow is at right angles to the beam (Plate 7B).

Colour mirror image artefact In anatomical situations where there is a strong specular reflector in the image (such as the diaphragm or bladder wall) a mirror image artefact may occur similar to that seen in conventional 2D imaging (see p. 89). This artefact is commonly observed during CDI of the subclavian artery as it crosses the apex of the lung (Plate 8).

Frame rate artefact The frame rate of CDI may be very low, especially when using a large region of interest or examining deep vessels (see p. 73). If a long vessel segment is being examined it is quite possible for information to be collected from one end of it during systole and the other end during diastole. This may lead to very confusing and rapidly changing colour hues in the image. This artefact can be simulated by rapid backwards and forwards longitudinal movement of the transducer during CDI scanning (Plate 9).

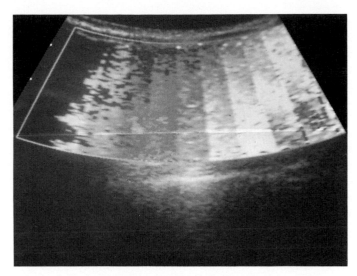

Plate 9 Frame rate artefact. Scan obtained during rapid backwards and forwards longitudinal movement of the transducer. The separate blocks of colour demonstrate the way in which the colour information is obtained during time blocks, each of which may be relatively long if a low frame rate is in use. This figure is reproduced in colour in the colour plate section at the front of this volume.

Safety considerations

The signals returning from red cells moving within blood vessels are extremely feeble, such that they are not usually detectable in conventional grey scale images. In Doppler studies it is the frequency of these feeble signals which we require to detect and the equipment therefore includes devices to enhance them. The simplest way of achieving this is to increase the power of the transmitted pulses during Doppler acquisition. It is almost an invariable rule that when the Doppler function is selected on a duplex system, the pulse power is increased by an order of magnitude or more. In addition, the ease and accuracy of frequency measurement of the returning Doppler shifted signal is improved by increasing the ultrasound pulse length. The combination of increased pulse power and pulse length results in an often huge increase in the ultrasound energy dissipated within the patient.[41,42]

In addition there is a trend towards the use of higher frequency transducers to improve imaging resolution. In an attempt to mitigate partially the increased attenuation of the higher frequency signals, there has been a concomitant increase in imaging power output levels in many scanners using these high frequency transducers.

The combination of these two factors has now raised ultrasound power levels into and, in some cases beyond, the range of powers typically used for therapeutic ultrasound procedures. If we believe that therapeutic ultrasound has a genuine effect then we accept that ultrasound at this power level is capable of producing biological changes. Whilst these may be beneficial in soft tissue injuries in adults, the effects of exposure of the ovum

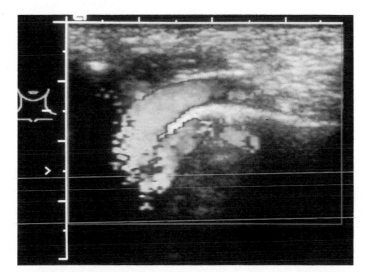

Plate 8 Mirror artefact. The subclavian artery has been imaged as it curves over the apex of the lung. The lung surface acts as a specular reflector and gives rise to a mirror image artefact with an apparent duplicate vessel lying beneath the lung surface. This figure is reproduced in colour in the colour plate section at the front of this volume.

and developing conceptus to these ultrasound power levels causes concern. This is especially so in trans-vaginal Doppler studies where these structures are much closer to the transducer, with less attenuation in the tissue path, and higher frequency, and therefore usually higher power, transducers are employed. The power levels now produced by many trans-vaginal transducers in Doppler mode are equal to or greater than those which have been shown in studies on pregnant small mammals to be capable of producing fetal damage.

These considerations place Doppler ultrasound in a similar position to conventional diagnostic radiography where there is a well-documented but small potential hazard from each exposure. The ALARA (As Low As Reasonably Achievable) principle should be applied in Doppler ultrasound as in radiography. The transmitted power should be under the operator's control and should always be set as low as possible, consistent with achieving a diagnostic result. In addition the duration of the examination and the duration during which the transducer is held stationary over any tissue volume should be reduced as far as possible consistent with obtaining the diagnostic information which was being sought. There must always be a genuine clinical indication for performing a Doppler ultrasound study in obstetrics, especially if this is being performed via the trans-vaginal route in early pregnancy.

REFERENCES

1 Franklin D L, Schlegel W, Rushmer RF. Blood flow measured by Doppler frequency shift of back-scattered ultrasound. Science 1961; 134: 564–565
2 Callaghan D A, Rowland T C, Goldman D E. Ultrasonic Doppler observation of the fetal heart. Obstet Gynecol 1964; 23: 637
3 Gosling R G, Dunbar G, King D H, et al. The quantitative analysis of occlusive peripheral arterial disease by a non-intrusive ultrasonic technique. Angiology 1971; 22: 52–55
4 Woodcock J P, Gosling R G, Fitzgerald D E. A new non-invasive technique for assessment of superficial femoral artery obstruction. Br J Surg 1972; 59: 226
5 Grant E C. Duplex ultrasonography: its expanding role in non-vascular diagnosis. Radiol Clin N Am 1985; 23: 563
6 McDonald D A. The viscous properties of blood. In: Blood flow in arteries. London: Edward Arnold. 1974: p 55–70
7 McDonald D A. Blood flow in arteries. London: Edward Arnold. 1974: p 95
8 Histand M B, Miller C W, McLeod F D. Transcutaneous measurement of blood velocity profiles and flow. Cardiovasc Res 1973; 7: 703–712
9 Hoecks A P G, Ruissen C J, Hick P, Reneman R S. Transcutaneous detection of relative changes in artery dimensions. Ultrasound Med Biol 1985; 11: 51–59
10 Hokanson D E, Strandness D E, Miller C W. An echo-tracking system for recording arterial wall motion. IEEE Trans Sonics Ultrasonics SU-17 1970; 130–132
11 Olsen C F. Doppler ultrasound: a technique for obtaining arterial wall motion parameters. IEEE Trans Sonics Ultrasonics SU-24 1977; 354–358
12 Batten J R, Nerem R M. Model study of flow in curved and planar arterial bifurcations. Cardiovasc Res 1982; 16: 178–186
13 Lee B Y, Assadi C, Madden J L, Trainor F S, McCann W J. Haemodynamics of arterial stenosis. World J Surg 1978; 2: 621–629
14 Zwiebel W J, Zagzebski J A, Crummy A B, Hirscher M. Correlation of peak Doppler frequency with lumen narrowing in carotid stenosis. Stroke 1982; 13: 386–391
15 Shung K K, Siegelmann R A, Reid J M. Angular dependence of scattering of ultrasound from blood. IEEE Trans Biomed Eng BME-24 1977; 325–331
16 Cobbold R S C, Veltink P H, Johnston K W. Influence of beam profile and degree of insonation on the C W Doppler ultrasound spectrum and mean velocity. IEEE Trans Sonics Ultrasonics SU-30 1983; 364–370
17 Barber F E, Baker D W, Nation A W C, Strandness D E, Reid J M. Ultrasonic duplex echo-Doppler scanner. IEEE Trans Biomed Eng BME-21 1974; 109–113
18 Fish P J. Multichannel, direction-resolving Doppler angiography. In: Kazner E, de Vlieger M, Muller H R, McCready V R. eds. Ultrasonics in medicine: Proceedings of the Second European Congress for Ultrasound in Medicine and Biology. Amsterdam: Excerpta Medica. 1975: p 153–159
19 Namekawa K, Kasai C, Tsukamoto M, Koyano A. Real-time blood flow imaging system utilising autocorrelation techniques. In: Lerski R A, Morley P. eds. Ultrasound '82. New York: Pergamon Press. 1982: p 203–208
20 Omoto R, Yokote Y, Takamoto S, Kyo S, et al. The development of real-time two-dimensional Doppler echocardiography and its clinical significance in acquired valvular heart disease. Jap Heart J 1984; 25: 325–340
21 Kasai C, Namekawa K, Koyano A, Omoto R. Real-time two-dimensional blood flow imaging using an autocorrelation technique. IEEE Trans Sonics Ultrasonics SU-32 1985; 458–464
22 Evans D H, McDicken W N, Skidmore R, Woodcock J P. Waveform analysis and pattern recognition. In: Evans D H, McDicken W N, Skidmore R, Woodcock J P. eds. Doppler ultrasound: physics, instrumentation and clinical applications. Chichester: John Wiley. 1989: p 162–187
23 Brigham E O. The fast Fourier transform. New Jersey: Prentice-Hall. 1974
24 Skidmore R, Follett D H. Maximum frequency follower for the processing of ultrasonic Doppler shift signals. Ultrasound Med Biol 1978; 4: 145–147
25 Gosling R G. Extraction of physiological information from spectrum analysed Doppler shifted continuous wave ultrasound signals obtained non-invasively from arterial systems. In: Hill D W, Watson B W. Eds. IEE Medical Electronics Monographs. Stevenage, Herts: Peregrinus. 1976: p 74–125
26 Gosling R G. Extraction of physiological information from spectrum analysed Doppler shifted continuous wave ultrasound signals obtained non-invasively from arterial systems. In: Hill D W, Watson B W. eds. IEE Medical Electronics Monographs. Stevenage, Herts: Peregrinus. 1976: p 73–125
27 Planiol T, Pourcelot L. Doppler effect study of the carotid circulation. In: de Vlieger M, White D N, McCready V R. eds. Ultrasonics in Medicine. New York: Elsevier. 1973: p 104–111
28 Stuart B, Drumm J, Fitzgerald D E, Duignan N M. Fetal blood velocity waveforms in normal pregnancy. Br J Obstet Gynaecol 1980; 87: 780–785
29 Trudinger B J, Giles W B, Cook C M, et al. Fetal umbilical artery flow velocity waveforms and placental resistance: clinical significance. Br J Obstet Gynaecol 1985; 92: 23–30
30 Trudinger B J, Giles W B, Cook C M. Uteroplacental blood flow velocity-time waveforms in normal and complicated pregnancy. Br J Obstet Gynaecol 1985; 92: 39–45
31 Pearce J F M. Uteroplacental and fetal blood flow. Clin Obstet Gynecol 1987; 1: 157–184
32 Van Merode B J, Hick P, Hoeks A P G, Renemam R S. Limitations of Doppler spectral broadening in the early detection

of carotid artery disease due to the size of the sample volume. Ultrasound Med Biol 1983; 9: 581–586

33 Evans D H, McDicken W N, Skidmore R, Woodcock J P. Spectral broadening indices. In: Doppler ultrasound: physics, instrumentation and clinical applications. Chichester: John Wiley. 1989: p 171–173

34 Evans D H. On the measurement of mean velocity of blood flow over the cardiac cycle using Doppler ultrasound. Ultrasound Med Biol 1985; 11: 735–741

35 Fish P J. A method of transcutaneous blood flow measurement – accuracy considerations. In: Kurjak A, Kratochwil A. eds. Recent advances in ultrasonic diagnosis 3. Amsterdam: Excerpta Medica. 1981: p 110–115

36 Gill R W. Accuracy calculations for ultrasonic pulsed Doppler blood flow measurements. Australas Phys Eng Sci Med 1982; 5: 51–57

37 Gill R W. Measurement of blood flow by ultrasound; accuracy and sources of error. Ultrasound Med Biol 1985; 11: 625–641

38 Evans D H. Can ultrasonic duplex scanners really measure volumetric flow? In: Evans J A. ed. Physics in medical ultrasound. London: IPSM. 1986: p 145–154

39 Johnston K W, Maruzzo B C, Cobbold R S C. Errors and artifacts of Doppler flowmeters and their solutions. Arch Surg 1977; 112: 1335–1341

40 Powalowski T, Borodzinski K, Nowicki A. Effect of ultrasonic beam width on blood flow estimation by means of C W Doppler flowmeter. Scripta Medica Univ Brno 1975; 48: 97–103

41 Duck F A, Starritt H C, Anderson S P. A survey of the acoustic output of ultrasonic Doppler equipment. Clin Phys Physiol Meas 1987; 8: 39–49

42 Duck F A. Output data from European studies. Proceedings of the second WFUMB symposium on safety and standardisation in medical ultrasound. Ultrasound Med Biol 1989; 15: Suppl 1, 61–64

6

Interventional techniques

Hans Henrik Holm, Jan Fog Pedersen, Søren Torp-Pedersen, Steen Karstrup, Christian Nolsøe and Anders Glenthøj

INTRODUCTION

Ultrasonically guided interventions are gaining widespread use, as scheduled procedures or as ad hoc extensions of the ultrasound examination. Such procedures are therefore described and discussed in many of this textbook's chapters. This section focuses on the general principles for ultrasound guided interventions. Furthermore, techniques that are not dealt with elsewhere in the text will be described in more detail.

Three levels of use of ultrasound for biopsy work may be identified. At the simplest level, suitable only for large or palpable lesions, the scan is used merely to plan the procedure, marking a suitable skin puncture site that avoids penetrating hazardous regions such as major blood vessels and indicates the approximate depth the needle needs to penetrate. A common example is in the drainage of a pleural effusion; similarly in ascites there is usually no need to involve the ultrasound scanner beyond the planning stage but the importance of avoiding bowel loops adherent to the parietal peritoneum makes a preliminary scan useful.

At the second level the scanner is used not only to plan the procedure but also to monitor the position of the needle in real time throughout the procedure. The transducer is simply positioned close to the puncture site so that the needle passes within the scan plane. This is known as the free-hand technique but may be called the 'three hand technique' because it is expedited by having an assistant hold the transducer while the operator uses both hands on the syringe. It is suitable for relatively simple procedures with lesions larger than 1 to 2 cm not too deeply located and has the advantage that no special transducer is required. However, the requisite hand-eye co-ordination makes it a skill-dependent method and not all operators find it easy to learn. A typical situation where free-hand guidance is sufficient is in the needling of breast masses. However, it is not suitable for small, deeply placed lesions.

The most precise method, using various forms of needle guide, forms the main subject of this chapter.

General principles

In 1969 Kratochwil described a hand held puncture transducer with a central canal for percutaneous needle insertion under A-scan guided control.[1] A few months later needle puncture guided by B-scanning was introduced in our laboratory using an off-axis puncture transducer mounted on the articulated arm of a static scanner (Fig. 2A).[2,3] Almost simultaneously Goldberg and Pollack began cyst punctures using A-scan guidance.[4] In 1974 the first dynamic puncture transducer – a 'home-made' linear array transducer with a needle steering attachment at the end of the transducer – was developed in our laboratory.[5]

Today interventional ultrasound has gained widespread use and the majority of manufacturers of medical ultra-

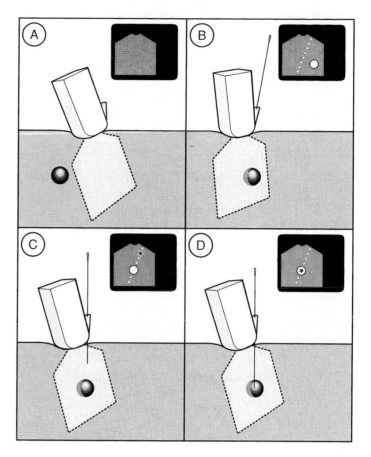

Fig. 1 Principle of an ultrasound guided puncture. A: Target non-visualised, outside image plane. **B:** Transducer moved and target now visualised in image plane, but not transected by puncture line. **C:** Transducer tilted, target transected by puncture line. Needle inserted through puncture attachment. Needle tip echo indicates actual needle position. **D:** Target hit.

sound equipment now supply special puncture transducers or puncture attachments for their ordinary transducers.

The basic principle of an ultrasound guided biopsy is that the rather complicated three-dimensional problem of hitting a small target is converted to a much simpler two-dimensional problem by use of a two-dimensional imaging technique (Fig. 1). A needle steering device restricts the movement of the needle to a predetermined path in the image plane. The needle will thus inevitably hit the target if inserted when the target is visualised and transected by the electronically generated puncture line which indicates the needle path.

Transducers

There are as many puncture guiding devices as there are different transducers. They can be divided in two main groups, namely dedicated puncture transducers which are equipped with an internal puncture canal (Figs 2A to C)

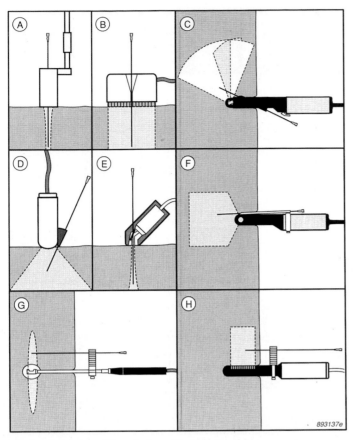

893137e

Fig. 2 Puncture guiding devices. Dedicated puncture transducers (A to C). Puncture attachments (D to H). **A:** Puncture transducer for static compound scanner. **B:** Linear array puncture transducer which allows perpendicular and oblique needle insertion. **C:** Trans-rectal multiplane scanner with oblique, built-in puncture canal for prostatic biopsies. **D:** Sector scanner with needle steering device attached. **E:** Conventional transducer placed in a puncture adapter in which the ultrasound field is reflected by an acoustic mirror. The needle is inserted through a puncture canal into the reflected sound field. **F:** Endoscanner with needle steering device for trans-rectal or trans-vaginal punctures attached (longitudinal scanning). **G:** Trans-rectal scanner with needle steering device for trans-perineal puncture (transverse scanning). **H:** Trans-rectal scanner with needle steering device for trans-perineal puncture (longitudinal scanning).

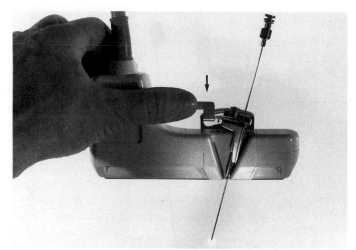

Fig. 3 Linear array puncture transducer (Aloka). The needle guide can be opened by activating spring loaded lever (arrow) allowing appropriate lining to be inserted. The puncture direction can be angulated and locked.

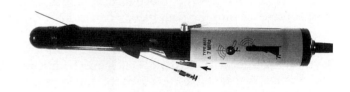

Fig. 4 Trans-rectal multiplane scanner with built-in oblique puncture canal (Bruel & Kjaer). The scan plane can be rotated by turning the lever (arrow).

and puncture attachments which are mounted on ordinary transducers (Figs 2D to H). It is generally an advantage to choose a system which enables the examiner to perform the puncture with the same transducer or at least the same type of transducer as used for the initial scan.

A typical puncture transducer is the linear array with a central canal or slot that enables the needle to enter the sound field through a hole or a slit in the sole (Figs 2B and 3). Such transducers are relatively expensive.

A multiplane endoprobe with an oblique internal puncture canal has been developed especially for prostatic scanning and biopsy (Figs 2C and 4). With this probe the examination is usually started with transverse scans, which

are preferable for the detection of focal lesions in most cases, but the actual biopsy is guided by longitudinal scans (Fig. 5). With this technique very accurately located biopsies can be obtained from ultrasonically visualised suspicious areas in the prostate.

Needle guide systems are available from most manufacturers of both mechanical and electronic scanners. Whatever type of needle guide is used it should fulfil two requirements: the puncture canal must be at least 3 to 4 cm long (to prevent the needle from deviating during the puncture) and the examiner must be able to release the needle easily. This is especially important when catheter procedures are to be carried out following the initial puncture.

Since needles of various sizes are used, guides of different calibres must be available. This problem can be solved in a variety of ways (Fig. 6). The attachment may be equipped with linings of various calibres, e.g. from gauge

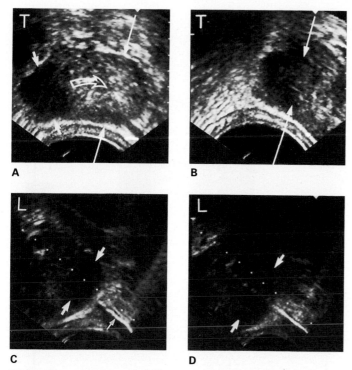

Fig. 5 Prostatic biopsy with multiplane scanner. A: Transverse rectal scan reveals a suspicious echo-poor lesion in the prostate (short arrows). The axis of image rotation indicated by long arrows. **B:** The probe is rotated to the right until the target area is intersected by the common axis of image rotation (arrows). **C:** By turning the lever the image plane is now shifted through oblique to truly longitudinal. The probe is tilted until the target (arrows) is intersected by the puncture line which indicates the needle path. The needle (small arrow) is inserted up to the lesion. **D:** Biopty-gun biopsy is performed, the needle track is faintly seen within the lesion.

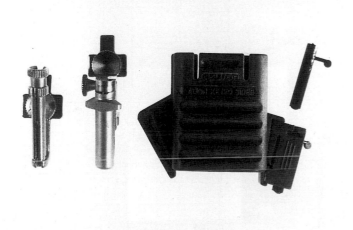

Fig. 6 Attachable needle steering devices. Left: In this version, two U-shaped cylinders which can be rotated independently allow 14 and 18 gauge puncture canals to be selected; they can be opened (Bruel & Kjaer). **Centre:** Due to a special design the calibre of this puncture canal, which can be opened, is adjustable to any needle size between gauge 14 and gauge 23 (Bruel & Kjaer). **Right:** Sterile disposable puncture attachment (Acuson).

Table 1 Conversion from 'gauge' needle dimension and 'french' catheter dimension to metric system

Needle gauge	Diameter (mm)	Catheter 'french'	Diameter (mm)
25	0.51	5	1.67
24	0.56	6	2.0
23	0.64	7	2.3
22	0.72	8	2.7
21	0.82	9	3.0
20	0.90	10	3.3
19	1.10	11	3.7
18	1.26	12	4.0
17	1.49	13	4.3
16	1.67	14	4.7
15	1.84	15	5.0
14	2.13	16	5.3
13	2.44	17	5.7
		18	6.0
		19	6.3
		20	6.7
		22	7.3
		24	8.0

14 to 23 (Table 1). Alternatively a needle steering device that can be adjusted to any calibre of needle from 12 to 20 gauge may be used.

Special puncture attachments are available for transrectal and trans-vaginal scanners (Figs 2F to H) either in the form of a long tube attachment to the probe, or as a multichannel puncture attachment for trans-perineal biopsies.[6] Special puncture equipment for trans-perineal treatment of prostatic cancer has been developed and is described later (Fig. 28).

Sterilisation An ultrasonically guided puncture should be regarded as a minor surgical procedure and sterilisation of the equipment should be in accordance with the department's normal practice for such procedures.

Ultrasound transducers do not tolerate autoclaving, while gas sterilisation is too time consuming for routine use. Sterility can be achieved by use of a sterile rubber covering for the transducer. Alternatively, provided the transducer and cable junctions are watertight, it can – together with the steering device and other necessary utensils – be sterilised by immersion in various fluids, e.g. glutaraldehyde (Cidex) or plain 70% alcohol.

Sterilisation in alcohol takes only a few seconds and is therefore very attractive from a practical point of view. However, alcohol is not effective against fungi, hepatitis or immunodeficiency viruses. Glutaraldehyde and Korsoline are both effective against a wide spectrum of bacteria as well as fungi and viruses. 10 minutes immersion kills vegetative pathogens including *Pseudomonas*, human immunodeficiency (HIV) and hepatitis B (HBV) viruses, while *Mycobacteria* require 1 hour's immersion. To kill resistant pathogenic spores 3 hours' immersion is needed. It is important that the equipment is mechanically cleansed of gel and debris before submersion.

Needles

A large variety of needles for aspiration and biopsy is available. However, for practical purposes of economy and operator familiarity it is generally advantageous to restrict the number of different types used to perhaps four or five (Fig. 7). Some of those should be available in more than one length.

In order to reduce the risk of complications it is advisable to use as thin a needle as possible.[7] To avoid contamination of the interior of the needle before it reaches the target use of a stylet is often appropriate. The majority of needles currently in use are disposable. If non-disposable sterilised needles are used, it is important that a needle with a very sharp tip is used.

When a needle is inserted under ultrasound control the shaft is generally invisible, but the needle tip is usually well-visualised as a relatively strong echo. The mechanisms for production of the one 'needle tip echo' are rather complex.[8] Attempts have been made to improve needle visualisation. Roughening the outer surface of the needle enhances its reflectivity in laboratory studies, but its clinical value is not as convincing. The contents of the needle can be made more reflective by roughening the stylet, introducing a guide wire or by filling the needle with air or an air-gel mixture. Apart from relatively rare cases of unexplained non-visualisation, a missing needle tip echo almost always results from deviation of the needle from the sound field.

Surprisingly almost all fluid collections, even those consisting of thick pus or debris, can be aspirated through an 18 gauge (1.2 mm) needle (Fig. 7A). This size of needle may therefore be routinely used for aspiration of all fluid collections, cysts and abscesses. The needle should contain a stylet to prevent obstruction of the lumen by blood clot or tissue during needle introduction. The only exception to the routine use of an 18 gauge needle is amniocentesis when a disposable 19 or 20 gauge needle is generally preferable.

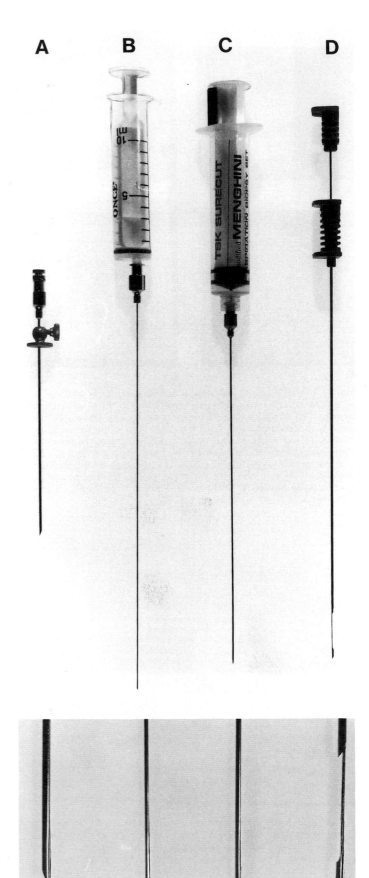

Fig. 7 Commonly used needles for interventional ultrasound. A: 18 gauge needle with adjustable stopscrew. Ideal for puncturing fluid collections and as a guide needle for fine needle punctures. **B:** 23 gauge fine needle without stylet mounted on 10 cc syringe for aspiration cytology. **C:** 21 gauge Surecut cutting needle with stylet. The syringe is equipped with a locking device to maintain the vacuum. **D:** Tru-cut type needle especially designed for Biopty-gun.

As a fine needle is flexible, the skin may prove a major obstacle to its insertion. However, an 18 gauge guide needle (as used for puncturing fluid collections (Fig. 7A)) with an inner diameter just large enough to take the fine needle, considerably facilitates skin puncture. The guide needle is advanced a few centimetres into the patient (depending on the thickness of the abdominal wall). Penetration to the correct depth may be secured by a stopscrew. A fine needle biopsy usually requires several passes, but with a guide needle only one skin puncture is needed.

The commonly used needle sizes for cytology are 22 and 23 gauge (0.7 mm and 0.6 mm) (Fig. 7B). They do not have a cutting tip but are bevelled to varying degrees. To establish a vacuum during biopsy the needle is mounted on a 10 ml syringe which may be fitted into a special aspiration handle which facilitates the procedure. These fine needles do not contain a stylet because the amount of tissue entering the needle during insertion is negligible compared to the amount obtained during aspiration.

These needles make it possible to obtain true tissue cores from the target tissue. Two types are commonly used (Fig. 7).

The Surecut needle (14 gauge to 25 gauge) is based on the Menghini principle. The needle, stylet and syringe are a unit (Fig. 7C). The stylet is attached to the plunger of the syringe and as the plunger is retracted it moves up in the needle, revealing the cutting tip. A locking device retains the plunger in the retracted position, thereby maintaining the negative pressure when the needle is advanced within the target. When the needle is removed the tissue core is not sucked into the syringe but, because of the stylet, is kept in the distal portion of the needle. When the locking device is deactivated the tissue core can be expelled. The Surecut system has the advantage that it can be operated by one hand. This is particularly important for ultrasound guided biopsy. The most commonly used size of Surecut needle for abdominal biopsies is 21 gauge (0.8 mm).

The conventional Tru-cut needle (14 gauge) has a biopsy chamber that can be opened and closed (Fig. 7D). The closed needle is inserted into the patient. When inserted to the correct depth the needle is opened by advancing its inner portion so that the surrounding tissue moves into the biopsy chamber. As the outer part of the needle is advanced, with the inner part fixed, the tissue in the chamber is separated from the surrounding tissue by the cutting edge of the outer needle. The closed needle can then be removed with a tissue core in the chamber.

The conventional Tru-cut needle must be manipulated by two hands and is therefore not well-suited for biopsy under ultrasound guidance. It can, however, be mounted in various automated biopsy gun systems which greatly facilitate use of this type of needle. The Biopty-gun is one such system (Fig. 8). Special disposable Tru-cut type nee-

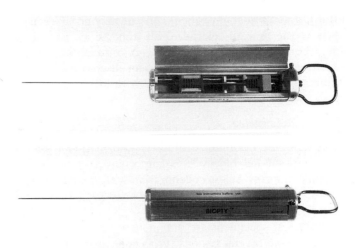

Fig. 8 Biopty-gun. Top: The specially designed Tru-cut type needle (Fig. 7D) is mounted in the spring loaded gun. **Bottom:** The closed gun ready for biopsy. When triggered, the spring mechanism activates the Tru-cut action and the biopsy is taken instantaneously.

dles (Fig. 7D) (gauge 14 to gauge 20) are placed in the spring-loaded gun which is then closed and ready for use. When the biopsy needle has been guided to the edge of the target the trigger is activated. The biopsy is taken automatically and instantaneously.

Patient preparation

Preparation of the patient before an ultrasound guided interventional procedure depends upon the nature of the intervention. For a fine needle biopsy (i.e. outer diameter of needle below 1 mm) no laboratory test or any other kind of preparation or post-puncture observation is required and the procedure can be done on an outpatient basis. Thus the puncture can be performed as an integral part of the ultrasound study, saving time for both the patient and the department.

If the patient's clinical condition or biochemical tests indicate a coagulation disorder, special precautions are taken. These guidelines are the same as those followed when the patient is to have a large bore needle biopsy and are as follows:

a) procedure only performed as an inpatient;
b) coagulation factors above 40 arbitrary units (normal range 70–130);
c) thrombocyte count above 40 000 per microlitre (normal range 150 000 to 400 000);
d) at least 1000 ml of blood available for transfusion.

Ideally the patient should be thoroughly informed about the nature and purpose of the procedure prior to the puncture. However, if the puncture is an integral part of the ultrasound examination, patient consent may not have been given at the time of referral. This may be an advantage since the patient is spared anxiety in anticipation of the puncture. In order to minimise patient discomfort it is advisable to infiltrate the puncture site with local anaesthetic.

Cytology and histology

To achieve the optimum diagnostic information from an ultrasound guided biopsy it is important that the interventionalist forms a close collaboration with the pathologist and understands the problems of specimen preparation and interpretation.

Cytological specimens are obtained by aspiration which should sample several regions, especially in the periphery of the lesion, since central areas often show necrosis and haemorrhage leading to non-diagnostic specimens. If Papanicolaou staining is used, immediate fixation in 95% alcohol is optimal, but a spray fixative may be used. Air drying is simpler, but in this case May-Grunwald-Giemsa staining will normally be used. Both techniques take about 30 minutes to carry out. If needed, rapid staining techniques on air dried smears are available and may be useful to check the adequacy of the aspirate and form a preliminary diagnosis. The slides should be restained by the May-Grunwald-Giemsa method for final diagnosis.

Histological fine needle biopsies are treated in the same way as ordinary biopsies (fixed in formaldehyde, dehydrated, cleared, embedded in paraffin, sectioned and stained).[9] If a 0.6 mm needle is used, fragmentation is often a problem and material can easily be lost during embedding. It is recommended that the specimen is placed between two pieces of gauze after fixation. Fragmentation is seldom a problem when the needle diameter is 0.8 mm or larger.

Both fine needle aspiration cytology (FNAC) and fine needle aspiration biopsy (FNAB) are reliable methods and complement each other.[10,11] FNAB provides excellent structural information, important in diagnosing both benign and malignant lesions, whereas FNAC provides little structural information (Fig. 9).

Special stains and immunostaining are more easily performed on FNAB specimens since many sections can be made from one biopsy. (Extra unstained sections should always be put aside in case these methods should be needed after evaluation of the routinely stained sections). With FNAC only a limited number of smears is available and immunostaining may be difficult to perform since cell membranes remain intact in a cytological smear.

Evaluation of a FNAB is very fast for a pathologist whose primary training is in histology. On the other hand FNAC allows a better evaluation of cellular detail, especially for small-cell tumours with fragile cells that are easily crushed during sectioning.

The processing of a FNAC specimen is much cheaper

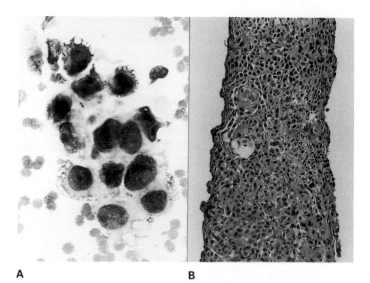

A   **B**

Fig. 9   Specimens from a retroperitoneal biopsy. A: Cytological fine needle aspiration showing poorly differentiated malignant cells. (May-Grunwald-Giemsa stain, ×550). **B:** Histological fine needle biopsy from same lesion showing poorly differentiated carcinoma, probably an epidermoid carcinoma. (Haematoxylin-eosin stain, ×125).

than that for FNAB and a cytological diagnosis can be made within 1 hour whereas a histological diagnosis usually has to be postponed until the following day.

Diagnostic accuracy

The ability of ultrasound to guide the insertion of a needle during a biopsy presumably improves diagnostic accuracy. This is, however, not necessarily the case and we need to quantify the diagnostic impact of interventional ultrasound with answers to basic questions such as: how often is a positive result true? how sensitive is the test? etc. The basic diagnostic accuracies are defined as follows.[12]

The success rate is the percentage of biopsy procedures resulting in sufficient material for microscopic evaluation. It is not always easy to classify biopsies into the two simple categories 'sufficient' and 'insufficient'. Three tissue cores from a liver lesion may contain only necrotic tissue and the procedure may erroneously be classified as insufficient, lowering the success rate, despite the fact that ultrasound correctly identified a lesion and that the biopsy needle cut three cores without a geographic miss. Likewise, an aspiration biopsy yielding only peripheral blood is not insufficient if the biopsied liver lesion is a haemangioma. Finally, the classification is at the mercy of the pathologist. A meagre specimen may be diagnostic for one pathologist and insufficient for another.

The sensitivity of the technique is the percentage of malignant lesions where the ultrasound guided biopsy material is diagnosed as malignant. In some biopsy series the sensitivity is boosted by excluding insufficient biopsies from calculation. In these cases sensitivity should be read as the percentage of malignant lesions with a sufficient biopsy where the ultrasound guided biopsy material is evaluated as malignant. The sensitivity of the biopsy procedure is affected by the quality of ultrasound, for example improved resolution may produce a paradoxical drop in success rate because biopsy of smaller lesions is attempted. Furthermore, the calculated sensitivity is highly affected by the choice of gold standard for diagnosis.

The gold standard reference must be an independent diagnostic technique against which the diagnoses obtained at biopsy are compared. The choice of 'gold standard' is important since it may skew the results. The gold standard in a liver biopsy series may be autopsy findings or operative diagnosis within 30 days of the ultrasound guided fine needle biopsy. This is only available for about 15% of biopsies and so the calculated sensitivities should be viewed with caution since this 15% represents a selected group. Furthermore, by using this type of gold standard it becomes impossible to separate the diagnostic abilities of ultrasound and ultrasound guided biopsy because gold standard refers to whether or not cancer is present in the liver and not to the nature of the biopsied lesion itself. For the ultrasound guided biopsy to be correct from a metastatic liver lesion two events must occur: a) ultrasound must select a malignant lesion for biopsy and b) the subsequent biopsy must be evaluated as malignant. Figure 10 illustrates that autopsy does not necessarily provide the truth.

The specificity of the technique is the percentage of non-malignant lesions where the ultrasound guided biopsy material is evaluated as non-malignant; sensitivity is the ability to diagnose cancer, specificity is the ability to diagnose non-cancer. Specificity seems to be more at the mercy of the gold standard than sensitivity because negative biopsy results are not as likely to be followed by operation or autopsy as are malignant results. A false positive result may lead to an operation, whereas a true negative result usually will not.

Sensitivity and specificity are useful indices when comparing different procedures, but are not very useful in the diagnostic situation where we wish to know the trustworthiness of a positive or negative biopsy result. The following indices are useful when we do not know the patient's disease, but do know the biopsy result.

The positive predictive value (PV-positive) is the percentage of malignant biopsy results that are true positives. A PV-positive of 90% tells us that a malignant biopsy result has a 90% probability of being correct. Since cancer is defined histologically the PV-positive of a histological biopsy is 100%. Therefore analysis of PV-positive is only meaningful in cytological biopsies. A cytological diagnosis of cancer is an indirect diagnosis and not necessarily true. Non-malignant conditions, especially inflammation, may give cellular changes which may be misinterpreted as cancer. PV-positive is affected by the prevalence of malignant

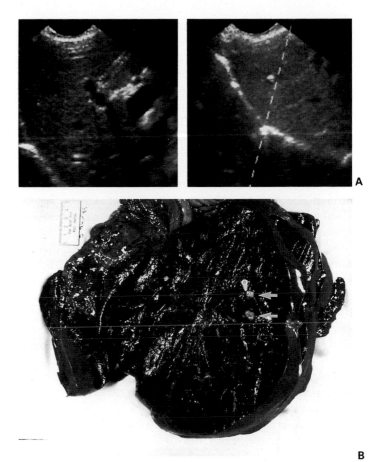

Fig. 10   A: **Ultrasound image of fine needle biopsy** of an echo-poor lesion in the right lobe of the liver (left). The needle tip is seen on the puncture line inside the lesion (right). The patient had a primary lung cancer and the biopsy was positive. **B:** 14 days later the patient died and autopsy was performed. Surprisingly, no metastasis was found and the pathologist speculated that perhaps the needle had passed through the liver into the right sided lung tumour, thus explaining the positive biopsy result. The department of ultrasound, however, disagreed with this explanation and insisted that the liver be sliced more finely: eventually the metastasis was found (the two halves are indicated by arrows).

lesions in the biopsy series, which again is determined by the quality of ultrasound (ability to find subtle lesions) and the patient population. If the only lesions biopsied are those with a high clinical and ultrasound suspicion of malignancy there will be very few benign lesions to create false positives and the PV-positive will be high. If, on the other hand, even regions with only slightly suspicious changes in echo pattern are sampled there will be a larger fraction of benign lesions, increasing the number of false positives and giving a lower PV-positive result.

PV-positive is one of the few diagnostic indices that can be measured reliably because a positive biopsy result will normally be verified by other means. It is an important index since it denotes the patient's risk of cancer when he has a positive biopsy. It is therefore a measure of the diagnostic impact of the ultrasound guided biopsy. This can be illustrated by a clinical example. A patient on chemotherapy for colonic cancer develops elevated liver enzymes (the risk for liver metastases may be 50%). Ultrasound of the liver shows a solid lesion in the liver (the risk for metastasis now increases to 90%). A cytological biopsy is positive (the risk for cancer is now 98%). As long as the PV-positive increases above the patient's risk before biopsy, there is a diagnostic impact.

The negative predictive value (PV-negative) is the percentage of non-malignant biopsy results that are true negatives. Its significance is parallel to a PV-positive, signifying the trustworthiness of a negative biopsy result. However, it is difficult to quantify since a negative biopsy result is rarely verified by the gold standard.

Sensitivity, specificity, PV-positive and PV-negative are intertwined as can be seen in Table 2. Sensitivity and specificity are the true characteristics of a test and do not change with changing patient environment (prevalence). PV-positive and PV-negative are the diagnostic outcomes and do change with prevalence. The problems with the gold standard are most often so great that only PV-positive can be calculated.

This synopsis of the basic diagnostic indices is important since they are used to compare procedures. It must therefore be kept in mind that, for instance, a PV-positive of 98% is determined by the sensitivity and specificity of ultrasound (do we select the right area for biopsy?), the geographic accuracy of the biopsy procedure (do we actually sample what we think we are sampling?), the success rate of the procedure (how good is the needle or the person manipulating the needle?), and the sensitivity and specificity of the microscopic evaluation (how good is the pathologist?).

Table 2 Diagnostic indices. The relationship between sensitivity, specificity, PV-positive, PV-negative, and prevalence. The bottom equation illustrates that a given test, i.e. constant S and SP, will have increasing PV-positive with increasing prevalence. Likewise, in a given population, i.e. constant prevalence, any increase/decrease in S or SP will result in an increase/decrease in PV-positive.

	Cancer	Non-cancer
Positive test	True positive (TP)	False positive (FP)
Negative test	False negative (FN)	True negative (TN)

Sensitivity (S): TP/(TP+FN)
Specificity (SP): TN/(TN+FP)
PV-positive: TP/(TP+FP)
PV-negative: TN/(TN+FN)

PV-positive = $(S \times p)/((S \times p) + ((1 - SP) \times (1 - p)))$, p = prevalence.

Safety and complications

Very few papers have been published about risks in ultrasound guided percutaneous techniques, and virtually none of them concerns ultrasound alone. In a large question-

Table 3 Distribution of punctures for the entire material

Type of puncture	Number of punctures
Fine needle biopsies (0.6 to 0.8 mm)	3500
Large bore biopsies (1.2 to 2.1 mm)	700
Punctures or catheter drainage (1.2 to 1.8 mm)	2800
Nephrostomy (1.8 to 3.2 mm)	1000
Total	8000

naire, including 63 108 cases of fine needle aspiration biopsies, Smith found a total of 101 complications (0.16%).[13] The data included four deaths, giving a mortality rate of 0.006%. In a literature survey of 11 700 cases Livraghi et al found a rate of major complications of 0.05% and a mortality rate of 0.008%.[14]

These data suggest that ultrasound guided interventional procedures carry a very low risk; however, in these surveys it was not specified to what extent ultrasound was the guiding modality.

In the period from 1969 to 1987 approximately 8000 ultrasound guided interventional procedures were performed in our department and a yearly report on the department's diagnostic and therapeutic activities generated. The complications related to puncture have been recorded continuously based on information from the clinical departments.[15]

Of the 8000 punctures 3500 were fine needle aspiration biopsies for cytology and/or fine needle cutting biopsies for histological evaluation (Table 3). Three passes with each needle type have routinely been used. 700 were large bore biopsies (needle diameter between 1.2 and 2.1 mm) from liver, kidney or prostate. 2800 were punctures of fluid collections – mainly in the abdomen – using a 1.2 mm spinal needle or a one step 5.7 F (1.8 mm) pigtail catheter. Finally there were 1000 percutaneous nephrostomies with insertion of either a one-step 5.7 F (1.8 mm) pigtail catheter or a 10 F (3.2 mm) Foley catheter using the Seldinger technique with dilation to 14 F (4.5 mm).

Unless the patient's clinical condition indicated coagulation disorders, all fine needle punctures, including those done on an outpatient basis, were performed without any preparation or laboratory test. Coarse needle biopsies were performed following the guidelines routinely used by the referring department.

Figure 11 shows the total number of punctures per year as well as the year by year changes in the number of the different puncture types for the period 1975 to 1987.

Complications were defined as post-puncture conditions which required treatment. This means that transient pyrexia, haematuria or pain which did not require treatment (except simple analgesics and observation) were not considered complications and consequently not included. Patients who have abscess drainage often develop fever

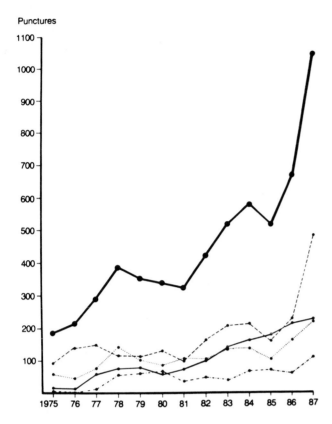

Punctures

Fig. 11 Annual changes in different types of punctures. The increase between 1975 and 1987 included all types of procedure.

—————————	= Total number of punctures
---------------	= Fine needle biopsies (0.6 to 0.8 mm)
—·—·—·—·—	= Large bore biopsies (1.2 to 2.1 mm)
—————————	= Catheter drainage or nephrostomy (1.8 to 3.2 mm)
················	= Puncture of fluid collections (1.2 mm)

Table 4 Registered complications after 8000 ultrasound guided punctures

No.	Complication	Puncture target	Needle	Treatment
1	bleeding	renal cyst	1.2 mm	1000 ml blood transfusion
2	bleeding	hepatic haemangioma	1.2 mm	1000 ml blood transfusion
3	bleeding	aneurysm (misinterpreted as pancreatic cyst)	1.2 mm	not instituted, pt. died
4	bleeding	pancreatic cancer		laparotomy (1000 ml haematoma)
5	bleeding	liver metastasis	FNB	2500 ml blood transfusion
6	bleeding	liver metastasis	FNB	1500 ml blood transfusion
7	bleeding	liver metastasis	FNB	not instituted, pt. died
8	abscess formation	pyonephrosis	cath*	ureteric stricture operation
9	septic shock	renal abscess	cath	antishock treatment
10	bile leak	gallbladder	1.2 mm	laparotomy (1500 ml bile)
11	bile leak	portal lymph node metastasis	FNB	laparotomy (200 ml bile)
12	bile leak	pancreatic cancer	FNB	laparotomy (2000 ml bile)
13	bile leak	liver metastasis portal lymph node metastasis	FNB	ultrasound guided intra-peritoneal catheter
14	abdominal pain	duodenal diverticulum	cath	laparotomy (choledocholithiasis) postop. complications. Pt. died
15	organ rupture	hydro-nephrosis	cath	nephrectomy (haematoma & laceration of the renal parenchyma)

FNB – fine needle biopsy
★ 5.7 F pig tail catheter

after the puncture and consequently receive antibiotic treatment to prevent severe septicaemia. In this group, therefore, fever and consequent antibiotic treatment was not considered a complication.

A total of 15 complications were registered (Table 4) of which three were fatal (numbers 3, 7 and 14). This gives an overall complication rate of 0.19% and a mortality rate of 0.04%. Patients having only fine needle aspiration have approximately the same rates of complications and mortality, 0.20% and 0.03%, respectively. It must be admitted that these rates are minimum estimates, since our data is based upon feedback from the clinical departments. However, it is our experience that in any case where complications occur feedback emerges immediately!

It is worth noting that three out of seven complications were intraperitoneal bleeding in patients who had hepatomegaly caused by multiple metastases, and that the only death after fine needle biopsy was in this group. Based on this experience we have changed our guidelines so that patients with enlarged livers due to multiple metastases are considered to be at increased risk of bleeding and will not

be biopsied routinely. If, for some reason, the clinician finds the microscopic diagnosis important to obtain, the biopsy will be performed only if special precautions are taken as appropriate for the individual patient's condition.

It is debatable whether or not fine needle biopsies of liver haemangiomas carry a high risk.[14] We have performed many such biopsies without observing any complication. (One patient (number 2) had intraperitoneal bleeding after biopsy of a liver haemangioma using a 1.2 mm cutting needle; he recovered fully after receiving a 1 litre blood transfusion.) We therefore consider it safe to perform fine needle biopsies of suspected liver haemangiomas.

Despite the complications experienced, we conclude that it is justifiable to perform fine needle biopsies on an outpatient basis and, since the complication rate is very low, we require coagulation studies only when clinically indicated.

The possible risk of spreading tumour cells is of major importance when biopsy of a suspected malignant lesion is performed. When a malignant mass is punctured there is a theoretical risk of seeding tumour cells along the needle tract and of spreading tumour cells into the blood or lymph. It is known that malignant cells may sometimes be found in the circulation after a needle biopsy.[16] It is, however, important to realise that the presence of tumour cells in the blood circulation of a patient with cancer does not mean that metastases are present or will occur at all.[17] In accordance with animal experiments and clinical experience the accepted concept is that such circulating cells are of no prognostic importance. 18 gauge needle biopsies of carcinomatous lymph nodes transplanted into rabbits has been reported to cause cells to escape through the capsular perforation. However, this did not result in local tumour growth.[16] Needle biopsy of transplanted adenocarcinomas in rats does not affect the average survival rate or the percentage of metastases.[18] Needle biopsies of breast cancer and renal cancer in humans do not appear to worsen the prognosis.[19,20]

These results agree with the clinical impression that tumour seeding attributable to needle biopsies is extremely rare. In a series of fine needle biopsies of 469 patients with prostatic cancer, there was no evidence of local tumour growth at the biopsy site.[16] In only one of almost 4000 fine needle biopsies of cancers of the lung was tumour growth from the needle tract demonstrated.[21] Livraghi et al found two cases of needle tract seeding in their literature study evaluating 11 700 fine needle biopsies,[14] and Smith in his large questionnaire found three cases of cancer seeding along the needle tract among 63 108 fine needle biopsies.[13] In our own material of 3500 fine needle biopsies with six needle passes per case we have never experienced seeding of cancer into the tract. Thus, it seems reasonable to conclude that there is little risk of spreading tumour cells by a fine needle biopsy and, even if spread to regional lymph nodes or along the needle path does occur, usually the immune response of the patient will eliminate these cells. We have never experienced complications such as pneumothorax, fistula formations, or pancreatic juice leak known to occur in other series.[13,14]

Our experience supplements the low complication rates of literature and questionnaire studies and we therefore conclude that this extremely useful technique has a very low risk as long as the guidelines described are followed.

Diagnostic procedures

Cytological fine needle aspiration biopsy (CFNAB)

For this procedure we use a 0.6 to 0.8 mm fine needle without a stylet, a 10 cm long 1.2 mm guide needle to accommodate the fine needle, 10 ml syringe, needle guide and sterile scanning gel, all on a sterile tray. An optional sterile cover for the transducer should be included, unless the transducer can be sterilised.

The transducer is positioned with the electronic puncture line on the scanner screen traversing the target and the entry point of the needle is marked on the skin. Scanning gel is then wiped off, skin sterilised, local anaesthetic applied, skin sterilised, and the area draped as for minor surgery (Fig. 12A). The puncture guide is mounted on the sterilised or draped transducer and sterile scanning gel is applied. The transducer is again positioned so that the puncture line traverses the target and the guide needle is inserted through the needle guide. The guide needle is only inserted 1 or 2 cm, depending on the thickness of the skin (Fig. 12B). If a sector scanner is used the guide needle is rarely visualised.

The fine needle attached to the 10 ml syringe is then inserted through the guide needle. It is seen moving along the puncture line as a bright spot indicating the position of the needle tip. Not uncommonly the needle deviates. If the pass seems likely to miss the target, the needle is retracted and reinserted. Deviation of the needle is indicated by loss of the tip echo in the scanning plane. The transducer is then tilted back and forth until the needle echo is found. When the needle echo is seen inside the target full suction is applied with the syringe. The needle is then moved in and out of the lesion several times and the suction is then gently released. The needle is removed and handed to an assistant who separates needle and syringe, fills the syringe with air, reconnects needle and syringe, and expels the contents of the needle onto a glass slide. The slide is then smeared with another glass slide. One needle pass thus produces two slides for microscopic evaluation. The procedure is repeated sampling different areas of the target, we normally perform three needle passes.

Histological fine needle biopsy (HFNB)

The equipment required is the same as for cytological FNA except that a cutting needle with an outer diameter of 0.6 to 0.8 mm is used and a sterile piece of paper is needed.

The cutting needle is inserted in the same way as the aspiration needle previously described. When the needle tip is seen just outside the target, the plunger is retracted. While the locking device holds the plunger retracted the needle is advanced into the target and a tissue core is cut into the needle. If the target is small the needle can be retracted and re-advanced since there is room for a 3 cm tissue core in the needle. The needle is removed and the

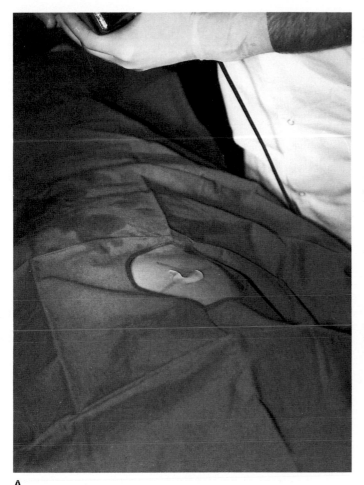

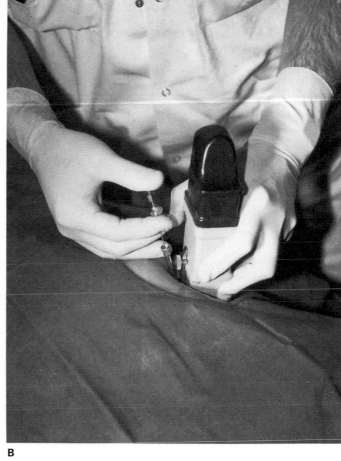

A **B**

Fig. 12 **A: Draping. B:** Guide needle inserted.

tip is placed on the sterile paper, the locking device deactivated, and the tissue core dislodged onto the paper.

Typically three needle passes are performed. The tissue cores can be seen with the naked eye so the adequacy of the samples can be evaluated immediately. The cores are placed in formalin and follow routine histological processing.

The skin is surprisingly resistant to a fine needle and if the guide needle is not to be used a minute incision is recommended. One benefit of the use of a guide needle is that there is only one skin penetration even when multiple fine needle insertions are made.

There are numerous makes and designs of fine needle available and it is not our aim to recommend any one type or make. We have described the Surecut needle since we have experience with this needle. Generally the requirement of a fine needle system is that it is designed as a one hand procedure. This rules out, in our opinion, any system that demands removal of a stylet and mounting of a syringe. Since it may be difficult to manipulate the syringe with one hand, we recommend an unorthodox grip or the use of an aspiration handle (Fig. 13).

We routinely perform three passes with a fine needle. If a patient has both a cytological and a histological fine needle biopsy he will undergo six needle insertions. A single needle pass is insufficient since only a minute fraction of the lesion is sampled. The optimum number of needle passes is not known.

Some investigators advocate the use of a quick stain performed in the biopsy room for immediate evaluation by a pathologist to ensure that representative material has been obtained. The biopsy can then be repeated immediately if necessary. This approach depends on skilled interpretation of the slides and therefore usually demands that a pathologist be present. To achieve this the biopsy procedures must be planned ahead.

Comparison of fine needle techniques

The two types of needles have the same outer diameter and they probably carry the same complication rate. The histological needle samples a smaller volume of the lesion so a slightly lower sensitivity is to be expected, but histological diagnosis is more reliable since false positives

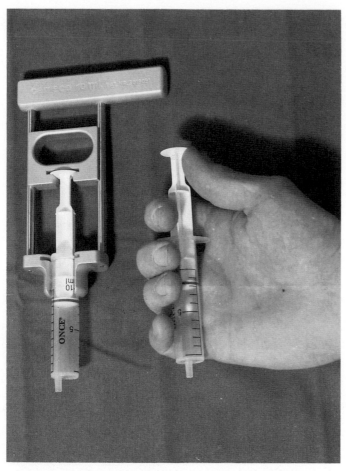

Fig. 13 Left: aspiration handle for a 10 ml syringe. Right: If a handle is not available, an unorthodox grip will allow the thumb to perform retraction of the plunger.

Table 5 Results of 0.6 mm cytological and 0.8 mm histological biopsies in 91 operated cases of solid or solid/cystic pelvic mass.

| | | Cytological diagnosis | | |
	Positive	Negative	Insufficient	Total
Malignant tumour	27	1	3	31
Benign condition	2	38	20	60
Total	29	39	23	91

Success rate: 68/91 = 75%
PV-positive: 27/29 = 93%
PV-negative: 38/39 = 97%

| | | Histological diagnosis | | |
	Positive	Negative	Insufficient	Total
Malignant tumour	23	3	5	31
Benign condition	0	45	15	60
Total	23	48	20	91

Success rate: 71/91 = 78%
PV-positive: 23/23 = 100%
PV-negative: 45/48 = 94%

Table 6 Results of 0.6 mm cytological biopsies in 301 cases of solid renal mass on ultrasound (first series).

| | | Cytological diagnosis | | |
	Positive	Negative	Insufficient	Total
Malignant tumour	185	25	8	218
Benign condition	14	61	8	83
Total	199	86	16	301

Success rate: 285/301 = 95%
PV-positive: 185/199 = 93%
PV-negative: 61/86 = 71%

theoretically do not occur. Furthermore, tumour typing is easier with tissue specimens.

The choice of needle depends on the type of patient and the target organ. If the patient has a known primary cancer and a lesion in the liver is identified only CFNAB is performed because the clinical problem is malignancy versus non-malignancy and the high sensitivity of CFNAB is advantageous. If a patient without a known primary has a lesion in the liver both CFNAB and HFNAB are performed, the latter to help in deciding the primary site. In these cases an extra tissue core for electron microscopy is added.

The liver is one of the easiest organs to biopsy: both CFNAB and HFNAB carry a success rate of 95%. Furthermore, interpretation of the material is not difficult since the demonstration of extrahepatic cells or tissue alone indicates the presence of tumour. Cytology alone will not usually permit the differentiation between primary and secondary liver tumours.

Other organ systems are not as easy to biopsy. Table 5 shows the results of a series of gynaecological fine needle biopsies.[22] Here, both needle types have a success rate of approximately 80%. Fortunately the two techniques are complementary and when performed together the success rate (the rate of at least one biopsy being sufficient) rises to 96%. The explanation for this is probably that soft tumours are easy to biopsy with CFNAB (the tissue is easily dislodged into the needle) whereas it is difficult to cut a core, while hard tumours give meagre cytological specimens but excellent cores, for instance uterine fibromyomas.

Fine needle biopsy of the kidney is especially troublesome (Table 6); our initial experience gave a PV-positive of 93%.[23] Table 7 shows a more recent experience with simultaneously performed CFNB and HFNB.[24] Because the false positive rate with cytology was no better we now rely on HFNAB almost exclusively for renal tumour diagnosis. Unfortunately, the tumours are often necrotic and soft so the success rate of HFNAB in the kidney is not impressive. Repeated biopsies are therefore sometimes necessary.

Table 7 Results of 0.6 mm cytological and 0.8 mm histological biopsies in 138 cases of solid renal mass on ultrasound (second series).

| | Cytological diagnosis | | | |
	Positive	Negative	Insufficient	Total
Malignant tumour	78	7	2	87
Benign condition	7	43	1	51
Total	85	50	3	138

Success rate: 133/138 = 96%
PV-positive: 78/85 = 92%
PV-negative: 43/50 = 86%

| | Histological diagnosis | | | |
	Positive	Negative	Insufficient	Total
Malignant tumour	63	8	16	87
Benign condition	0	39	12	51
Total	63	47	28	138

Success rate: 110/138 = 80%
PV-positive: 63/63 = 100%
PV-negative: 39/47 = 83%

Coarse needle biopsy

Needles with an outer diameter equal to or larger than 1 mm are by definition not fine needles. It seems reasonable to classify biopsy with these needles as 'coarse needle biopsy'. The Biopty system is the simplest and most effective method for using these needles. Needles with outer diameters of 1.2 mm and 2.0 mm (Fig. 7D) are available.

The patient is prepared in the same way as for a fine needle biopsy and the needle is mounted in the sterile firing device (Fig. 8). A small skin incision is made for the needle guide and the needle observed moving along the puncture line. The gun is fired when the needle tip is at the surface of the target. The action advances the inner needle 23 mm revealing the 17 mm biopsy chamber; immediately afterwards the outer cutting needle advances 23 mm, cutting a tissue core into the biopsy chamber. The two movements are so fast that they are perceived as one.

Since the system is automatic, the cutting action is always performed correctly ensuring a success rate close to 100%. The needle will always advance 23 mm during biopsy so care must be taken to ensure that no vital parts are in the needle path. A modification that limits the action to half the normal throw is available where a biopsy must be made close to blood vessels.

A large bore needle is required when the samples from a fine needle are not adequate. This is especially the case in non-neoplastic diseases in the liver and kidney. At our hospital all kidney biopsies for diffuse disease are performed under ultrasound guidance with the 2.0 mm Biopty needle though liver biopsies are only guided by ultrasound when the conventional blind Menghini technique has proved unsuccessful. For both types of biopsy one tissue core is sufficient. For large bore biopsies patients must be admitted and screened for coagulation disorders.

For many years prostatic biopsies have been performed with the 2.1 mm Tru-Cut needle via the trans-perineal or trans-rectal approach. In the past 2 years trans-rectal prostatic biopsy with the 1.2 mm Biopty needle has gained widespread use. Where the clinical problem is the question of malignancy the 1.2 mm needle serves this purpose well. The 100% success rate with this needle rules out the need for prostatic cytology, which carries a false positive rate that cannot be disregarded.

Cyst puncture

The equipment needed is: 1.2 mm needle (with stylet, long enough to reach the target), syringe (10, 20 or 60 ml depending on the size of the cyst), needle guide (with a slot for a 1.2 mm needle) and sterile gel, all on a sterile tray. The procedure is just as for fine needle biopsy. The skin puncture site is identified, local anaesthesia is applied and the area is cleansed and draped. No skin incision is necessary.

The needle is inserted and the tip is seen moving along the puncture line. Needle deviation is seldom a problem since the needle does not bend as easily as a fine needle. The tip of the needle is positioned in the cyst (Fig. 14), the stylet removed and the syringe is attached. Evacuation of the cyst is then monitored on ultrasound. As the cyst shrinks the needle is repositioned so that the tip remains in the fluid. The needle is then removed and the fluid sent for appropriate analyses.

Even multiloculated cysts can usually be emptied. It is common for the compartments to communicate so that evacuation can be accomplished with a single puncture. Where the loculi do not communicate the needle is repositioned until all compartments have been evacuated.

The standard technique must be modified for the puncture of two commonly encountered cysts, ovarian and thyroid.

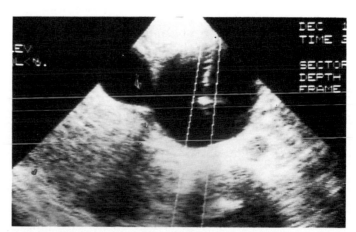

Fig. 14 Puncture of pancreatic cyst. Transverse scan shows pancreatic pseudocyst in the midline close to the gallbladder. The needle is seen in the cyst. Note the guide line.

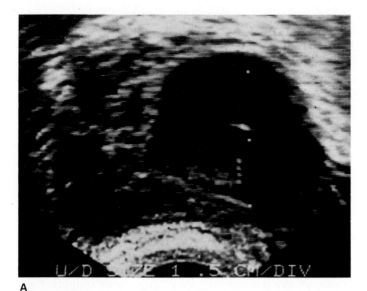

Fig. 15   A: Trans-vaginal puncture of an ovarian cyst. The echo from the needle tip is seen centrally in the cyst. **B:** The trans-vaginal scanner is a sector scanner at the tip of a finger shaped probe. The needle leaves the needle guide immediately outside the image.

Ovarian cysts may be punctured via the trans-vaginal route. The tip of the vaginal scanner can almost always be brought into contact with the cyst – separated from it only by the vaginal wall at the fornix. When a trans-vaginal needle guide is used, needle deviation is not a problem since the distance from the scanner to the cyst is usually only 1 cm (Fig. 15).

Thyroid cysts are very superficial and a free hand technique is recommended since they are almost impossible to miss. A 5 cm intramuscular needle (0.6 mm outer diameter, no stylet) mounted on a syringe is appropriate.

When large cysts are being aspirated it may be cumbersome to manipulate a large syringe at the same time as ensuring correct needle placement. This difficulty can be overcome by fitting a connecting tube between the needle

and syringe. An assistant can then apply suction while the examiner only has to handle the needle and transducer.

Occasionally what was thought to be a cyst turns out to be solid. When this happens the procedure is easily converted into a fine needle biopsy using the 1.2 mm needle positioned in the solid lesion as a guide needle for the fine biopsy needle.

Generally there is no need to puncture a cyst simply to verify its cystic nature, this can almost always be reliably established from ultrasound criteria. The most important indication for abdominal cyst puncture is to rule out an abscess.

Cytological examination of cyst fluid seldom reveals important information as the contents are nearly always acellular. Cyst puncture will therefore rarely distinguish malignant from benign pathology, though elevated lipid contents in renal cysts have been reported as an indirect sign of malignancy.[25] Since the diagnosis of hydatid disease is primarily serological, diagnostic puncture, though not contra-indicated, is seldom needed. However, ultrasound can be used to guide therapeutic instillation of 0.5% silver nitrate solution or antihelminthic agents. Where the origin of a cyst is unknown, puncture may be carried out simply to establish which organ system it belongs to. Amylase in the fluid establishes a pancreatic origin just as appropriate hormone analyses establish gynaecological origin.

Therapeutic cyst puncture is undertaken in the hope that the cyst will not recur after evacuation. This raises the question of whether to inject substances that will reduce the recurrence rate. So far no controlled trial in any organ system has shown that this is effective. For instance, a controlled trial with comparison between tetracycline and saline as sclerosing agents in thyroid cysts showed no difference and established that the benefit was in the puncture and flushing and not in the tetracycline.[26]

The indication for cyst puncture varies from organ to organ:

a) liver: therapeutic puncture is rarely indicated;

b) kidney: cyst puncture is only indicated if the patient has pain from the cyst or if it is causing obstruction. Both are very rare and the relevance of using various sclerosing agents, e.g. 96% alcohol, is not obvious;

c) pancreas: there are many optimistic reports of high cure rates after puncture of pancreatic pseudocysts. They share one common weakness, namely a very short follow up time. Reaccumulation during the first year brings the cure rate down to the spontaneous regression rate of approximately 7%;[27]

d) ovaries: the fear of overlooking neoplasm is the main reason for gynaecological cyst puncture. Some patients referred for cyst puncture have previously undergone surgery where a cyst of non-epithelial origin was removed. A prudent approach in non-operated patients is to select patients under the age of 40, with a simple unilocular cyst.

Table 8 Biochemical tests on cyst fluid

Test	Elevated in
Creatinine	Urinoma
Amylases	Pancreatic cyst
Protein (+)	Exudate, lymphocele
Protein, glucose (+) Urea	Renal cyst
Bilirubin (+)	Biloma
Potassium, chloride	Hydatid cyst

(+) Labstix

Granberg reports a cure rate of 70% in such patients;[28]

e) thyroid: these cysts are almost always cystic degeneration in an adenoma and the main problem for the patient is cosmetic. Hegedüs reports a cure rate of 43% to 47% in these patients.[26]

A fluid collection demonstrated on ultrasound can have a number of causes. The clinical history of the patient will often limit the possibilities to one or two. Diagnostic aspiration is indicated when the therapeutic strategy depends upon the nature of the fluid.

Many fluid collections are either large or superficially located, or both, and are easily punctured with a free-hand technique. However, if the collection is more deeply located or lies close to a structure that must not be punctured a guided puncture is highly recommended.

Inspection of the fluid will often reveal the presence or absence of blood, bacteria and bile. In Table 8 a number of simple analyses are listed.

Contrast studies

As described in the sections on nephrostomy and abscess drainage, the inserted catheters can serve not only a therapeutic but also a diagnostic purpose. Antegrade pyelography is frequently used to delineate a ureteric obstruction. Fistulography is a simple and effective way to monitor abscess cavity size and to disclose a communication between an abscess cavity and a hollow organ.

Two further diagnostic applications are ultrasound guided percutaneous trans-hepatic cholangiography (PTC) and ultrasound guided percutaneous pancreatography.[29] The typical indication for performing a PTC is to differentiate between a stone in the common bile duct and cancer or chronic pancreatitis of the head of the pancreas. Rather than relying on presumed normal anatomy it is an obvious advantage to perform the PTC under ultrasound guidance to delineate the actual anatomy. Usually only one puncture is needed and, if only part of the intrahepatic bile duct system is dilated, a selective PTC can be performed.

Percutaneous injection of contrast medium directly into a pancreatic duct is not possible without ultrasound guidance. This technique can be very useful in patients in whom ERCP is not possible, or where biopsy of a sus-

pected pancreatic mass is negative, or to define the extent of a malignancy before surgery.

Therapeutic procedures

Nephrostomy

Since the introduction of the ultrasound guided percutaneous nephrostomy in 1974[30] this technique has gained widespread use. Using ultrasound it is possible both to visualise the interventional procedure and subsequently control the correct placement of the inserted catheter. However, the majority of centres used a combined approach, ultrasound to guide the fine needle and radiological fluoroscopy for placement of the guide wire and catheter.

Two different nephrostomy techniques are generally used: a Seldinger technique with tract dilatation and subsequent balloon catheter placement (Fig. 16), and a one-step technique in which a pigtail catheter is introduced with a trochar inserter (Fig. 17).

If the nephrostomy is primarily for antegrade pyelography, or if the nephrostomy tube is expected to be left in place for only 2 or 3 days, a 5.7 F one-step pigtail catheter can be used. The relatively small diameter of the catheter and the speed of the procedure are easier for the patient. If a prolonged or permanent nephrostomy is planned a 10 F Foley balloon catheter is required. The soft silicone material causes less skin irritation than the rigid polyethylene of the one-step catheter. If the drainage lasts longer than 2 months the catheter should be exchanged to avoid concretions on the balloon and inside the catheter. This

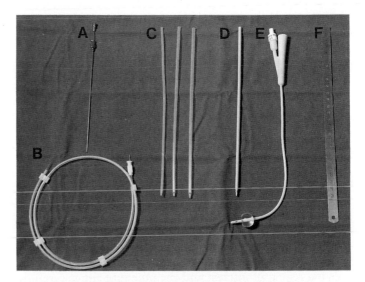

Fig. 16 Foley balloon catheter nephrostomy kit. A: 1.2 mm lumbar puncture needle with stylet. **B:** Soft-tip Lunderquist guide wire. **C:** 10, 12 and 14 F dilators for the three-step dilatation technique. **D:** 14 F one-step screw dilator. **E:** 10 F Foley balloon catheter with 3 ml sterile water in balloon. **F:** Ruler for measuring the distance to the calyx.

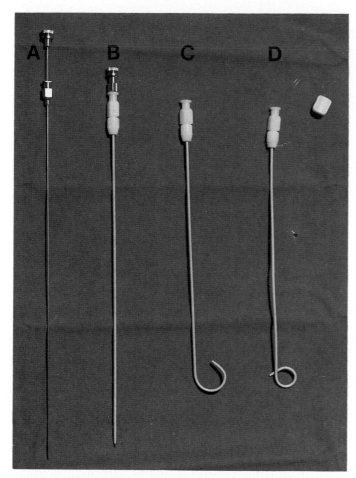

Fig. 17 Trochar nephrostomy catheters. A: Trochar with stylet. **B:** Trochar with catheter pulled over it. **C:** 5.7 F pigtail catheter. **D:** 5.7 F loop catheter.

can be done without any imaging technique since the tract is mature.

It is worth noting that the lumen of a 10 F balloon catheter actually measures 14 F at the site of the deflated balloon, and that the narrowest inner diameter of the 10 F catheter matches the inner diameter of the 5.7 F pigtail catheter.

Recently, a third type of catheter, the pigtail loop catheter has been introduced. This catheter combines the one-step technique with internal fixation (Fig. 26).

The patient is placed in the lateral decubitus or prone position to allow a retroperitoneal needle route. A sector scanner should be used in order to provide a small footprint with a large field of view. The transducer is placed over the region of interest and the puncture site is carefully chosen in order to make the needle path as close to perpendicular to the renal capsule as possible. Ideally the catheterisation should be performed via a lower or middle calyx. The depth of the calyx is measured in order to ensure that the dilators will be inserted far enough.

Local anaesthesia is applied, preferably under ultrasound guidance, to ensure that it is placed correctly. If the procedure is an elective balloon catheter nephrostomy, it is recommended that the patient be given systemic analgesics (e.g. 50 mg pethidine or 10 mg morphine) since the dilatation can be painful.

The puncture must be performed under sterile conditions. After skin disinfection an incision is made in order to allow passage of dilators and catheter. An 18 gauge spinal needle is introduced through the needle steering device along the electronically displayed puncture line to the centre of the renal pelvis. The stylet is removed and, if the needle has been placed correctly, urine is seen to escape.

A soft-tip Lunderquist guide wire is introduced through the needle which is then removed. From this stage on fluoroscopy is often a better means of monitoring the procedure. The dilator is inserted over the guide wire and passed through the tissues; penetration is easier if the dilator is rotated as it is inserted.

A three-step serial dilatation technique with 7 F, 10 F and 14 F dilators has proved effective (Fig. 16C). Recently a screw dilator that dilates to 14 F in one step (Fig. 16D) has been developed.[31] Regardless of the type of dilator it is mandatory to ensure that the length of the inserted part of the dilator corresponds to the previously measured distance to the centre of the calyx.

If the dilatation has been thoroughly performed the soft 10 F silicone Foley catheter can easily be introduced and the balloon inflated with 3 ml sterile saline. Usually the balloon is clearly seen inside the pelvis (Fig. 18). If any doubt remains concerning the correct placement of the catheter sterile saline can be injected through the catheter while observing the kidney with ultrasound. Microbubbles in the saline will 'light up' the pelvis if the catheter is correctly placed.

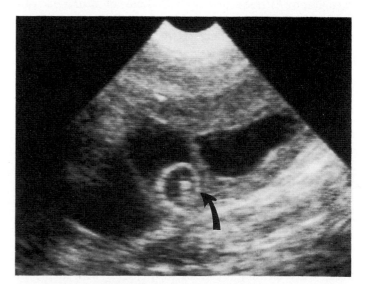

Fig. 18 Kidney with dilated pelvis and 10 F balloon catheter in the middle calyx. Arrowhead points at inflated balloon.

For the one-step method the trochar with the pigtail catheter pulled over it is introduced via the needle steering device. When the needle tip is seen inside the calyx the needle is held in position while the catheter is advanced over it. The catheter curls up inside the calyx and urine will be seen escaping through it. Simple catheters must be fixed to the skin with a suture while loop catheters need no skin fixation. If confirmation of the catheter position is needed an antegrade pyelogram can be performed.

Abscess drainage

Ultrasonography is well-suited for the detection of fluid collections in the upper abdomen and pelvis and ultrasound guided percutaneous aspiration is an effective tool for diagnosis and treatment. As a result of this, surgical drainage of intra-abdominal abscesses has been almost completely replaced by percutaneous insertion of catheters or needles into the infected cavities in many centres. The technique of percutaneous drainage differs from radiologist to radiologist and has been extensively described.[32–34] In principle two different methods may be used.[32]

a) puncture drainage. The pus is aspirated through a 1.2 mm needle. The abscess is irrigated with sterile saline until the returning fluid is clear. Follow up scanning is performed after approximately 2 days and the puncture is repeated if necessary;

b) continuous catheter drainage. A catheter is placed into the abscess cavity (Fig. 19). The cavity is irrigated repeatedly and the catheter is secured in place for drainage and daily irrigation until the infection has resolved.

Two basic techniques for introducing drainage catheters into fluid collections are available: the trochar method and the Seldinger technique. The usual catheter is a multihole soft pigtail measuring from 6 to 10 F. Catheters should not be inserted through the gastrointestinal tract or urinary bladder. Where this is unavoidable, puncture drainage should be performed. Antibiotics can be instilled into the abscess cavity, but the value of this approach has never been proven. Many antibiotics need to be metabolised before they are effective and may be locally irritant if used in high concentration. X-ray studies may be useful to demonstrate the placement of the catheter and to reveal fistulous communications.

Several reports have documented definitive cure rates of intra-abdominal abscesses of 80% to 90%. A marked clinical improvement can usually be observed a few hours after the drainage.

The most common complication, seen in less than 5% of patients, is rigors a few hours following the treatment, due to bacteraemia.[32–35] This problem can be avoided by giving the patient cover with an appropriate antibiotic. Bleeding following insertion of the catheter has been reported in a few patients.[33,34]

Pelvic abscesses may be difficult to access. Valuable alternatives to the transabdominal route are the trans-rectal, trans-vaginal, trans-perineal or trans-gluteal routes.[36] Ultrasound guided percutaneous drainage has also been described from the thorax, neck, brain, skin and breast (Fig. 30).[33,37]

Pleural effusions

Pleural effusions are most commonly seen in patients with malignancies. Effective control of recurrent malignant pleural effusions can improve the quality of life in the cancer patient.[38] Ultrasound is most often used to determine whether a loculated pleural radiographic opacity is due to consolidation or a pleural effusion and to locate the best site for thoracocentesis.[39] Ultrasound guided percutaneous thoracocentesis may be performed either for diagnostic or for therapeutic purposes. If possible the patient is examined in the sitting position. A small sector transducer facilitates intercostal scanning. For a diagnostic puncture, a short 19 or 21 G needle can be used.[40] A pigtail catheter can be inserted by the trochar technique for drainage. The catheter can be left in place and connected to a sealed system for continuous drainage.

Gastrostomy

Ultrasound guided percutaneous gastrostomy can be performed for nutritional support in patients with oesophageal or oropharyngeal malignancy. The procedure is performed under local anaesthesia and can be facilitated by distending the stomach with air or fluid through a nasogastric tube. Guided by ultrasound the safest access is chosen, special care being taken to avoid traversing the liver, the retroperitoneal vessels or the spleen. Both Seldinger and trochar methods have been described for puncture and insertion of catheters into the stomach.[41,42] A variety of catheters can be used. When the Seldinger technique is used, dilatation of a track can be performed and a soft balloon catheter inserted into the lumen of the stomach (Fig. 20).

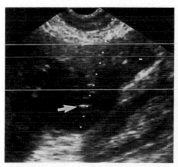 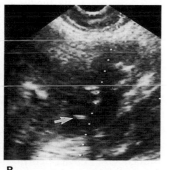

A   **B**

Fig. 19 A: Percutaneous drainage of a liver abscess. The echo from the tip of the trochar is seen inside the abscess (arrow). **B:** The pigtail catheter is seen inside the almost empty abscess (arrow).

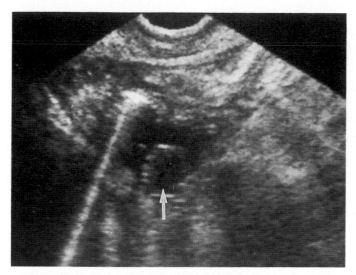

Fig. 20 Percutaneous gastrostomy. A soft balloon catheter (arrow) has been inserted into the the antrum of the stomach.

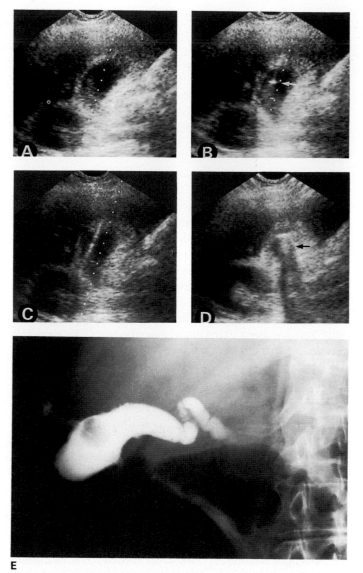

E

Fig. 21 The procedure of ultrasound guided percutaneous cholecystostomy. A: Infected gallbladder with thick wall. A trans-hepatic puncture route has been chosen. **B:** The echo from the tip of a puncture needle (arrow) is seen in the lumen of the gallbladder. **C:** The echo from a guide wire in the lumen of the gallbladder. **D:** An air filled balloon is seen inside an emptied gallbladder (arrow). **E:** Cholecystogram showing the catheter with the balloon centrally in the fundus of the gallbladder.

Cholecystostomy

The gallbladder is readily accessible for needle puncture and catheterisation. Several reports have documented the usefulness and safety of ultrasound guided percutaneous cholecystostomy both for diagnosis and for treatment.[43-46] In the treatment of poor operative risk patients with acute cholecystitis percutaneous cholecystostomy may replace surgical cholecystostomy (Fig. 21A to D). The technique has also proved useful in the diagnosis and treatment of patients with distal common bile duct obstruction.

Theoretically the safest approach is a trans-hepatic puncture route, entering the gallbladder where it is adherent to the liver, to avoid bile leaks. However, several authors have treated patients with acute cholecystitis using the transperitoneal route without encountering significant bile leakage.[47] Two basic techniques have been described, the trochar and the Seldinger technique. Soft pigtail (Fig. 2) or soft balloon catheters are most frequently used because they secure the catheter (Fig. 21E).

Other suggested indications for ultrasound guided puncture of the gallbladder include diagnostic aspiration of fluid for chemical or bacteriological examination, diagnostic cholecystocholangiography and fine needle biopsy. Furthermore, it is possible, via a percutaneous cholecystostomy, to remove gallstones or to infuse solvents for dissolution.

Pancreatic pseudocysts

Pancreatic pseudocysts typically develop in patients with pancreatitis. They can be punctured either for diagnostic or therapeutic purposes (Fig. 22).[48,49]

For diagnostic aspiration a 0.9 mm or a 1.2 mm needle might be used, depending on the size of the cyst and on the amount of debris. The aspirated material is routinely sent for amylase determination, culture and cytology. If the aspirate is purulent, percutaneous drainage should be undertaken. Other common indications for therapeutic drainage include pain, biliary and gastric outlet obstruction and cases with large cysts which are not resolving spontaneously.

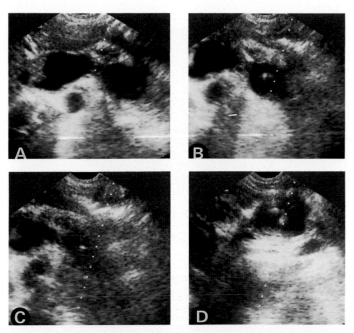

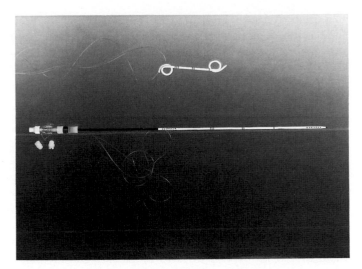

Fig. 23 **Top: Double pigtail catheter for pancreatic cysto-gastrostomy. Bottom:** Catheter mounted on trochar needle.

Fig. 22 **Puncture drainage of two pancreatic pseudocysts. A:** Cysts are seen in the head and body of the pancreas. **B:** A needle has been inserted into the cyst in the tail, traversing the stomach. **C:** The cyst has been emptied. **D:** Puncture drainage of the cyst in the pancreatic head.

A pseudocyst may be drained using either a repeated 'short-term' puncture drainage or a 'long-term' continuous catheter drainage. Short-term puncture drainage seems to be indicated in the acutely ill patients, hopefully to avoid spontaneous rupture of the cysts. Puncture drainage is also performed in non-acute cysts and can, in some patients, provide pain relief. However, cysts very often recur following puncture drainage, even after repeated punctures.

Long-term catheter drainage is indicated in patients with cysts which cannot be controlled by repeated punctures. The catheter drainage is most simply performed using the trochar technique with pigtail catheters varying in size from 6 to 10 F. The puncture route is typically trans-peritoneal, but a retroperitoneal or trans-gastric route might also be used. Success rates ranging from 70% to 90% have been reported, on average drainage takes about 3 weeks, but may range from a few days to about 3 months.[48,49] A potential risk of long-term catheter drainage is infection of a previously non-infected cyst. Rare complications such as pneumothorax and pleural effusion have been reported.

A new technique for internal drainage of pancreatic pseudocysts has been suggested by Hancke & Henriksen.[50] A special double pigtail catheter (Fig. 23) is introduced percutaneously and trans-gastrically into the cyst cavity. Under gastroscopy the catheter is positioned with one curved end in the cyst and the other in the stomach.[50,51]

Tumour therapy

Methods Ultrasound guided percutaneous destruction of tumours seems to be an obvious approach since a needle can be placed in any tumour visible on the ultrasonic image. Thus it is possible to apply therapeutic agents accurately into a tumour.[52]

In principle there are three different means of tissue destruction: a) chemical, b) radiation, c) heat.

a) chemical agents
Application of chemical agents in order to destroy tissue is already an accepted treatment in certain highly selected patients. As outlined later in this section, in patients in whom surgery for some reason is contra-indicated, parathyroid adenomas may be treated with ultrasound guided injection of ethanol.[53] In the same way liver tumours have been treated with some success.[54] Injection of caustic and antineoplastic drugs offer another possibility.[55] However, at present selection of the correct chemical and definition of the indications for this approach are not clear.

A different application is the use of adhesive agents to treat cysts in various sites, e.g. kidney, liver, thyroid. Alcohol has been used with limited success; fibrin seems to be a promising possibility.

b) radiotherapy
Interstitial radiotherapy provides an alternative to external radiation in selected tumours. The advantage over the conventional external radiotherapy are twofold. Firstly, radiation can be confined to the tumour thereby avoiding side effects and complications due to normal tissue being damaged. Secondly, as a consequence of the precise control of the radiated volume, a higher total tumour dose can be delivered, increasing tumour destruction.

Radioactive seed implantations have occasionally been used in the treatment of otherwise untreatable abdominal cancers,[56] but the results have not been promising. As discussed in detail later, another application for interstitial radiotherapy is prostatic cancer,[57] as an alternative to radical prostatectomy.

c) heat

Hyperthermia as a treatment for cancer has been applied both systemically and locally with limited success.[58] The problem is to achieve a sufficiently high temperature inside the tumour without damaging the surrounding healthy tissue. To reach this goal the heat should ideally originate from within the tumour, so called interstitial or local hyperthermia. This has been achieved by various implantable energy sources such as microwave antennae, coils and filaments. If the treatment is to be performed percutaneously, the device has to be small enough to pass through a needle with an acceptably small diameter.

Recently a new approach using a low power neodynium yttrium aluminium garnet (Nd-YAG) laser as the energy source has been suggested.[59,60] Nd-YAG laser light has the potential of destroying tumour tissue by means of phototoxicity and thermoradiation. It can be applied directly into solid tissue since the light conducting fibres can be introduced through a needle. An attractive possibility therefore, is to combine interventional ultrasound with laser therapy. Since most tumours are spherical, the fibre optics should be arranged to spread the light in a sphere; a system which meets this demand has been manufactured.[60] The size of the lesion produced depends on the energy delivered, the maximum diameter achieved was 44 mm (4 watts for 30 min). Macroscopically the lesions have a central cavity delineated by a charred rim of tissue and beyond this a zone of coagulation (Fig. 24A). On ultrasound the lesions appeared as highly reflective circles (Fig. 24B).

By means of a purpose-made multiple steering device it is possible to place microthermocouples interstitially at predetermined distances from the laser fibre tip to allow temperature measurements and thus prediction of the extent of thermo-destruction (Fig. 24B). Ultrasound appears to be a suitable method for monitoring the lesions produced by interstitial Nd-YAG laser hyperthermia. Animal experimental work is currently being carried out to investigate the biological effects and the possible complications of the method. Ultrasonically monitored percutaneous interstitial Nd-YAG laser hyperthermia is promising for the treatment of liver metastases, prostate cancer, parathyroid adenomas, CNS tumours and other well-demarcated neoplasms.

Prostatic cancer Trans-perineal insertion of ^{125}I seeds into the prostate, guided by trans-rectal ultrasound, was described in 1983.[57] The technique is a modification of the method described by Whitmore.[61] The rationale is that

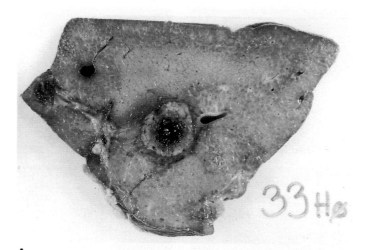

A

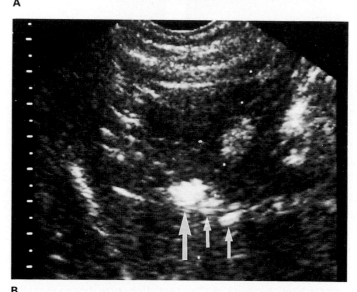

B

Fig. 24 A: Section of pig liver 8 days after interstitial laser coagulation with 4 W for 600 s. The charred wall of the central cavity is seen surrounded by a light zone of heat necrosis. **B:** In vivo ultrasound scan of pig liver following laser coagulation (large arrow). Two microthermocouples are seen close to the lesion (small arrows).

radioactive sources distributed uniformly throughout the prostate will deliver a radiation dose sufficient to destroy all tumour tissue – a radiation dose higher than can be safely administered by external beam therapy. [125]I initially has ideal physical characteristics for the treatment of prostatic cancer as its half life of approximately 60 days is well-suited for a slow growing cancer. The choice of this isotope is now being questioned (see below).

A trans-rectal transducer with a rotating 7 MHz transducer is used for planning and insertion (Fig. 25). The transducer is mounted in a rigid fixture that can be manipulated in the x, y and z planes. A needle guide matrix with multiple channels spaced 1 cm apart is mounted on

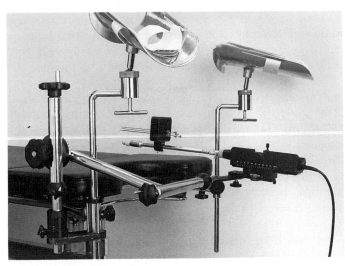

Fig. 25 Equipment for trans-perineal seed implantation. The rectal transducer is mounted in a fixture that can be positioned accurately in the x, y and z planes. The multichannel puncture guide is mounted on the rectal tube. For illustration, needles are inserted in the guide.

the rectal tube outside the patient. Needles inserted through the canals will cross the sound field at specific points which are indicated on the ultrasound image by an electronically generated grid.

At a planning session the patient is placed in the lithotomy position and the fixture is manipulated until the lower row of needle canals is a constant and preselected distance from the rectal wall as the transducer is moved in and out of the rectum (Fig. 26). In this position needle insertion will be parallel to the rectum. Furthermore this position of the transducer is well-defined and can be reproduced on the day of insertion.

Parallel transverse images of the prostate spaced 5 mm

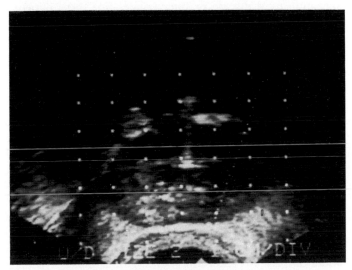

Fig. 26 Transverse image of the prostate with superimposed electronic needle matrix. Each dot corresponds to a canal in the puncture guide. The bottom row of dots has a constant distance to the rectal wall as the scanner is moved in and out.

apart are obtained from apex to base. On each image the prostate is outlined with a light pen and the electronic needle grid is superimposed. The prostatic volume is obtained with serial planimetry.[62] The appropriate number of seeds is calculated from the volume of the gland and the activity of the radioactive seeds. Using the serial images, longitudinal drawings of the prostatic outline with the needle canals are produced. A uniform three-dimensional seed distribution plan is then constructed and the position of the seeds within each needle determined. An isodose curve for each transverse ultrasound image is then drawn to ensure that an adequate minimal peripheral tumour dose is obtained while the rectal wall is spared.

The needles (1.3 mm with a blunt stylet) are then loaded with seeds. The needle tips are sealed with a silicone plug after which a combination of seeds and teflon spacers are introduced. Finally the stylet is inserted. Each needle is prepared for a specific canal in the seed matrix and the spacers ensure that the seeds maintain their position in the prostate. The needles are then sterilised.

For the implantation procedure the patient is again placed in the lithotomy position. Spinal anaesthesia may be used or, if the procedure follows staging lymphadenectomy, general anaesthesia is employed. The fixture is manipulated until the parallel transverse images from base to apex match the planning images. The perineum is cleansed and draped and the sterilised needle guide is mounted on the transducer. Two anchoring needles are inserted to stabilise the prostate.

The transducer is positioned at the most superior scanning plane and all needles designed to be inserted this far are introduced. The needles are then emptied one after the other. A stopper is swung behind the stylet and the needle is retracted over the stylet leaving the row of seeds and spacers in the prostate (Fig. 27). The scanner is then retracted 5 mm and the procedure is repeated for the needles designed to have their tip placed in this scanning plane, and so forth.

Correct position of each needle is ensured ultrasonically. When the needle enters the sound field it is seen as a bright echo. If necessary the needle is repositioned until its position corresponds to the canal through which the needle has been inserted.

The original technique has the major drawback that needle insertion is not visualised longitudinally making it difficult to correct for any superior displacement of the prostate by the needles. This problem has been overcome by the development of multiplanar imaging during insertion (Fig. 28). The scanner can move freely in relation to the needle guide so that any needle can be visualised longitudinally. As with the conventional technique, the needle insert is monitored by transverse imaging and correct position is ensured in this plane. The scanning plane is then changed to longitudinal and correct insertion depth is ensured before the needle is emptied.

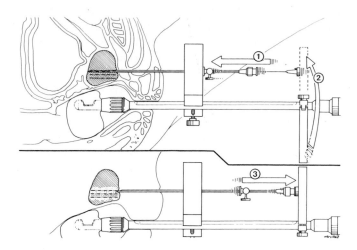

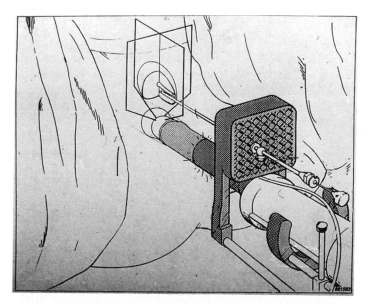

Fig. 27 Top: When the needle is correctly positioned the seeds and spacers have correct position in the prostate but are still in the needle. **Bottom:** As the needle is withdrawn over the immobile stylet, the row of seeds and spacers is left in the prostate.

Fig. 28 Apparatus for trans-perineal seed implantation guided by multiplanar imaging. The multiplanar probe is mounted in a fixture which allows the transducer to be rotated. When the transducer is locked, the electronic matrix corresponds to the multichannel needle guide. When the transducer is rotated away from the locked position the needle guide does not follow the movement. Thereby any needle can also be visualised longitudinally.

The newest needle guide has canals spaced 5 mm apart. This quadruples the number of needle canals and increases the freedom of choice in the three-dimensional dose distribution.

Despite its ideal physical properties ^{125}I may not be the best isotope; recent reports have raised doubts on its ability to control prostatic cancer. For example, Lee et al found residual cancer in 87% of patients followed up after a conventional Whitmore implant.[63] Although these patients did not benefit from the higher accuracy of ultrasound guidance the results are so discouraging that it is possible that the isotope itself is to blame. Iversen et al found 50% persistent cancer after ultrasound guided seed implantation.[64] This study, which covered a 5 year period, also reported a significant number of major radiation side effects. There is ongoing work with ^{198}Au as well as a combination of ^{192}Ir with interstitial heating as alternative methods.

Multiplanar imaging ensures very accurate placement of multiple needles into the prostate via the trans-perineal route. It seems probable that an almost ideal insertion technique has been developed before the optimal therapeutic agent has been identified. The work by Lee et al[63] (87% positive biopsies) and that by Kabalin et al[65] (93% positive biopsies) suggest that irradiation may not be an effective therapy. Percutaneous laser treatment, however, seems promising. Theoretically, it is possible to destroy all prostatic tissue with a laser fibre inserted through an array of needles. If this is feasible in practice, percutaneous treatment may become an alternative to radical prostatectomy.

Liver cancer The increasing use of ultrasonic screening of the liver has resulted in the detection of more and more early stage hepatocellular carcinomas (HCC). This is especially true in Asian countries where the prevalence of HCC is considerably higher than in the rest of the world. The large majority develop in chronically diseased livers. Previously, non-surgical treatment of HCC has included methods such as trans-catheter arterial embolisation, chemotherapy and radiotherapy.

Because these procedures have not proved curative, liver resection has come to be considered the method of choice. However, a high proportion of patients with HCC are not candidates for surgery either because of severe cirrhosis, age, multifocal disease or tumour site. For these patients, as well as for selected patients with a limited number of liver metastases, ultrasound guided percutaneous treatment is a promising alternative form of therapy.

A number of authors have injected 96% alcohol in hepatocellular carcinoma.[54,66–70] Their techniques have only differed slightly. In the largest series 32 lesions in 23 patients were treated.[67] Requirements for treatment were that the lesions had a diameter of less than 4.5 cm, were focal and detectable ultrasonically, preferably solitary and showed no evidence of metastases or portal thrombosis. The baseline study included ultrasound, fine needle biopsy, dynamic CT and serum alfa-fetoprotein assay. Depending upon the lesion diameter and consistency, and the compliance of the patient, 1 to 4 ml of 96% alcohol was injected under ultrasound control once or twice weekly on an outpatient basis (a total of 271 injections). The echo pattern of the HCC changes considerably during the alcohol injection, generally becoming increasingly reflective (Fig. 29). With the exception of one intraperitoneal haem-

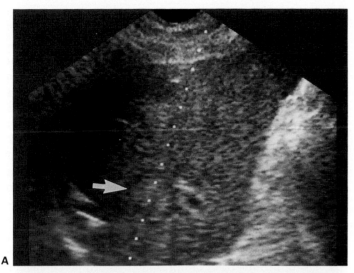

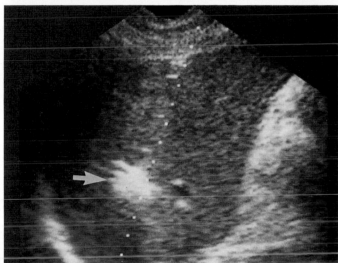

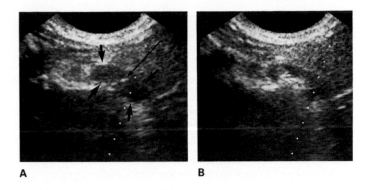

Fig. 30 A: longitudinal scan of the neck. A parathyroid tumour (short arrows) is seen close to the thyroid gland. The echo from a fine needle is seen centrally in the parathyroid tumour (long arrow). **B:** The parathyroid tumour has become echogenic following injection of ethanol.

Fig. 29 Ultrasound guided alcohol injection in liver cancer. A: A 2 cm echo-poor liver lesion proved to be an HCC at histological fine needle biopsy. **B:** A fine needle has been inserted along the puncture line and 4 ml of 96% alcohol injected. The lesion has become echogenic corresponding to the distribution of the alcohol.

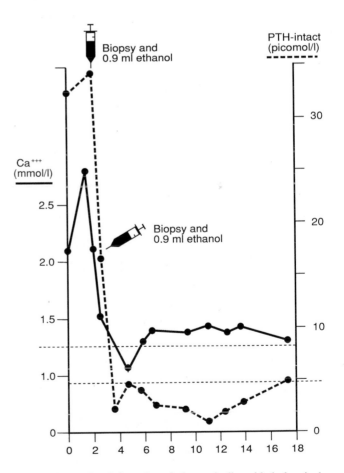

Fig. 31 Example of the value of ultrasonically guided chemical parathyroidectomy in a patient in hypercalcaemic crisis. The serum concentration of ionised calcium (continuous line) is normalised following injections of ethanol (syringes). The serum concentration of intact parathyroid hormone (PTH-intact) (dotted line) decreases dramatically after injections. (Same patient as in Figure 2A).

orrhage,[69] no significant complications have occurred in the 100 patients treated so far. Moderate pain is common, as is a transient fever and slight increase in liver enzyme levels.

At present there are no randomised studies available but the results are promising. In Livraghi's series all lesions were smaller after 6 to 27 months follow up and no evidence of HCC was present at fine needle biopsy or dynamic CT.

In the series of Livraghi,[67] Ohto[68] and Shiina[69] a total of 14 patients had histopathological follow up. In 10 of these the tumour was totally necrotic and in the remaining four approximately 90% of the tumour was necrotic.

There is general agreement that ultrasonically guided

alcohol injection is an important alternative in the treatment of small HCC when surgery is contra-indicated. With increased experience and improved technique the indications for alcohol injection may expand, though it may be that destruction of focal liver cancer will be simpler with laser coagulation (see above).

Parathyroid adenoma   Ultrasonography has proved to be a useful technique for localising enlarged parathyroid glands in the neck. However, it is difficult to distinguish parathyroid tumours from thyroid nodules, especially if they protrude from the posterior surface of the gland. Less commonly, lymph nodes or deeply localised muscular tissue have been misinterpreted as being parathyroid tissue.[71] To improve the reliability of the diagnosis of ultrasonically

suspected parathyroid lesions the use of ultrasound guided fine needle biopsy has been introduced.

Fine needle aspiration (0.6 mm) for cytological examination is one of the methods used. However, most investigators have found a cytological distinction between thyroid and parathyroid cells difficult.[72] In a randomised blind study it was possible to diagnose 56% of parathyroid tumours correctly and 70% of thyroid lesions correctly using specific cytological criteria.[73] An alternative to cytology is immunochemical measurement of the parathyroid hormone content in the aspirate.[74,75] Finally, it has been possible by means of a 0.8 mm cutting needle (Surecut) to obtain small tissue cores for reliable histological diagnosis.[76]

The ability to place a needle precisely in an often small parathyroid adenoma, and obtain a reliable tissue diagnosis, has formed the basis of ultrasound guided percutaneous inactivation of parathyroid tumours using intraglandular injection of 96% ethanol (ultrasound guided chemical parathyroidectomy).[77–79]

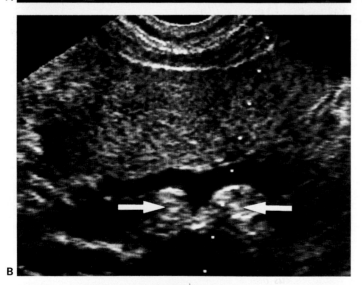

Fig. 32   Localisation of the coeliac trunk prior to coeliac block. **A:** Longitudinal scan through the aorta. Arrow indicates coeliac trunk. Inferiorly to the trunk is the superior mesenteric artery. **B:** Transverse scan through the coeliac trunk. Arrows indicate the two locations where 10 ml of 96% alcohol are injected to inactivate the coeliac plexus.

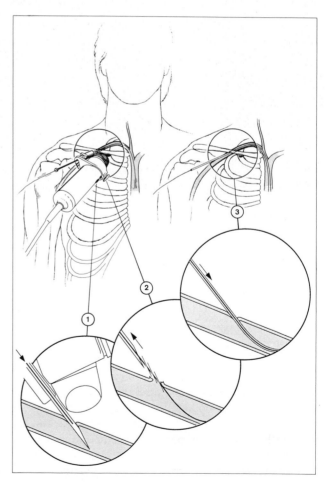

Fig. 33   Principle of the one-hand one-step technique for ultrasound guided subclavian vein catheterisation. 1) The spinal needle with the guide wire serving as a stylet punctures the vein. 2) The needle is withdrawn leaving the guide wire inside the vein. 3) The catheter is inserted over the guide wire.

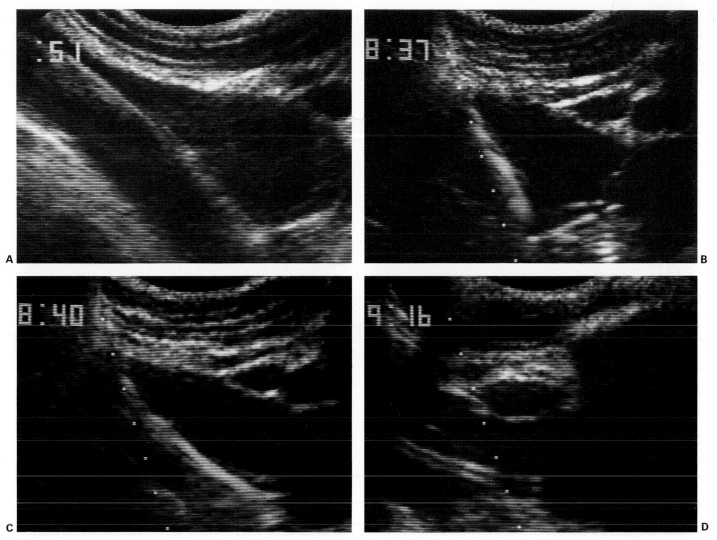

Fig. 34 A: Subclavian vein is compressible with the transducer. **B:** Needle is seen inside the vein. **C:** Highly echogenic guide wire is clearly visible inside the vein. **D:** Catheter correctly placed in subclavian vein.

The injections of ethanol can be performed on an outpatient basis with local anaesthesia under complete ultrasound control. The dose of ethanol is estimated individually, depending on the lesion size but should not exceed half of the volume of the tumour. The dispersion of the ethanol inside the gland is marked by the appearance of fine, dotted echoes spreading through the gland (Fig. 30).

In a prospective study, including treatment of 18 patients with primary hyperparathyroidism, a significant biochemical improvement was observed in 12 patients, with obvious clinical improvement seen in eight.[78] Similar figures were found in a later study in which eight of 12 patients with primary hyperparathyroidism and a high surgical risk became normocalcaemic after treatment.[79] Furthermore, three of four patients with severe acute hypercalcaemic symptoms were treated successfully in this study.

A rare complication is vocal cord paralysis due to damage to the recurrent laryngeal nerve.[78,79]

Ultrasound guided chemical parathyroidectomy is an attractive alternative to surgery. However, at present the treatment should be limited to patients with severe or life threatening hypercalcaemia and who are poor surgical candidates (Fig. 31).

Coeliac plexus block

Patients with severe chronic upper abdominal pain, most often caused by pancreatic cancer, may be relieved permanently by blocking the coeliac plexus using a number of agents including alcohol injection. This can easily be performed under ultrasound control.[80,81] On the basis of transverse and longitudinal scans, the location of the coeliac axis is determined. The coeliac nerve plexus surrounds the origin of the axis (Fig. 32). Under ultrasound guidance a fine needle is placed as close as possible on each side of the origin of the coeliac axis. A test injection of 10 ml local anaesthetic on each side may be attempted. If the test block proves effective (i.e. relief of pain for 6 hours) permanent coeliac ganglion neurolysis by injection of 10 ml 96% alcohol on each side is performed.

The published results are almost identical.[80,81] Complete or almost complete pain relief was obtained in one third of approximately 150 patients. In another third there was obvious pain reduction and in the remaining third there was no effect of the procedure.

The treatment has proved to be less effective in chronic relapsing pancreatitis and ultrasonically guided plexus block should probably be reserved for chronic pain caused by pancreatic cancer.

Subclavian vein catheterisation

Subclavian vein catheterisation is a commonly utilised procedure for administering fluid, blood and drugs as well as for monitoring central venous pressure.[82] Despite widespread use the conventional technique of catheter placement is quite frequently associated with complications, some of which can be serious and even lethal.[83]

These include pneumothorax, arterial puncture, haemothorax and pneumomediastinum. The reason for most complications is probably that the puncture is performed blindly.

To circumvent the problems associated with the conventional method ultrasonic guidance has been suggested.[84] In the technique we have developed for ultrasonically guided subclavian vein catheterisation[85] both vein puncture and insertion of the guide wire can be performed with one hand as a one-step technique (Fig. 33).

The patient is placed in the Trendelenburg position. The transducer is placed lateral to the costoclavicular ligament and the vein is identified by the fact that it is compressible with the transducer (Fig. 34A). A spinal needle with the guide wire inserted as a stylet (Fig. 33) is introduced and will follow the electronically displayed puncture line.

When the needle tip is seen inside the vein (Fig. 34B) the highly reflective guide wire is gently pushed forward by the hand holding the needle. This confirms intravenous placement (Fig. 34C). This procedure eliminates the risk of air embolism while exchanging the stylet with a guide wire. When the guide wire is correctly placed the needle is withdrawn and the catheter threaded over the guide wire (Figs 33 and 34D).

Using this technique we have to date performed 75 subclavian vein catheterisations of which 70 were successful. The only complications experienced were two small haematomas which resolved spontaneously.

REFERENCES

1 Kratochwil A. Presentation: First World Congress on Ultrasonic Diagnostics in Medicine. Vienna: 1969

2 Gammelgaard P A, Holm H H, Kristensen J K, Rasmussen S N. Ultrasound in renal diagnosis. Film presented at the American Institute of Ultrasound in Medicine, Annual meeting. Cleveland: 1970

3 Holm H H, Kristensen J K, Rasmussen S N, Northeved A, Barlebo H. Ultrasound as a guide in percutaneous puncture technique. Ultrasonics 1972; 10: 83–86

4 Goldberg B B, Pollack H M. Ultrasonic aspiration transducer. Radiology 1972; 102: 187–190

5 Pedersen J F. Percutaneous puncture guided by ultrasonic multitransducer scanning. JCU 1977; 5: 175–177

6 Holm H H, Gammelgaard J. Ultrasonically guided precise needle placement in the prostate and the seminal vesicles. J Urol 1981; 125: 385–387

7 Menghini G. One-second biopsy of the liver – problems of its clinical application. N Engl J Med 1970; 283: 582–584

8 Hjelmroth H E. Puncture needles and ultrasonic wave propagation in ultrasonically guided puncture. In: Holm H H, Kristensen J K. eds. Ultrasonically guided puncture technique. Copenhagen: Munksgaard. 1980

9 Torp-Pedersen S, Juul N, Vyberg M. Histological sampling with a 23 gauge modified Menghini needle. Br J Radiol 1984; 57: 151–154

10 Glenthøj A, Sehested M, Torp-Pedersen S. Diagnostic reliability of cytological and histological fine needle biopsies from focal liver lesions. Histopathology 1989; 15: 375–383

11 Glenthøj A, Sehested M. Histological and cytological fine needle biopsies from focal liver lesions. Intra- and interobserver reproducibility of diagnoses. APMIS 1989; 97: 611–618

12 Wulff H R. Rational diagnosis and treatment. Oxford: Blackwell. 1986

13 Smith E H. The hazards of fine needle aspiration biopsy. Ultrasound Med Biol 1984; 10: 629–634

14 Livraghi T, Damascelli B, Lombardi C, Spagnoli I. Risk in fine needle abdominal biopsy. JCU 1983; 11: 77–81

15 Nolsøe C, Nielsen L, Torp-Pedersen S, Holm H H. Major complications and deaths due to interventional ultrasound: A review of 8000 cases. JCU in press.

16 Engzell V, Esposti P L, Rubio C, et al. Investigation on tumor spread in connection with aspiration biopsy. Acta Radiol Ther Phys Biol 1971; 10: 385

17 Engell H C. Cancer cells in the circulating blood. Acta Chir Scand 1955; suppl 201

18 Main M E, Dunning W F. Is the biopsy of neoplasms dangerous? Surg Gynecol Obstet 1946; 82: 567

19 Robbins G F. Is aspiration biopsy of breast cancer dangerous to the patient? Cancer 1954; 7: 774

20 von Schreeb T, Arner O, Skovsted. Renal adenocarcinoma: is there a risk of spreading tumour cells in diagnostic puncture? Scand J Urol Nephrol 1967; 1: 270–276

21 Nordenström B, Björk V O. Dissemination of cancer cells by needle biopsy of lung. J Thorac Cardiovasc Surg 1973; 65: 671

22 Larsen T, Torp-Pedersen S T, Bostofte E, Bentzen M, Sehested M S G, Rank F. Ultrasonically guided fine needle biopsy of gynecologic tumors – experience with histology and cytology. Submitted to Gyn Oncol.

23 Juul N, Torp-Pedersen S T, Grønvall S, Holm H H, Kock F. Ultrasonically guided fine needle aspiration biopsy of renal masses. J Urol 1985; 133: 579–581

24 Juul N, Torp-Pedersen S, Glenthøj A. US-guided biopsy of solid renal masses. 5th International Congress on Interventional Ultrasound. Herlev, Denmark: August 1989

25 Kleist H, Jonsson O, Lundström S, Nauclér J, Nilson A E, Petterson S. Quantitative lipid analysis in the differential diagnosis of cystic renal lesions. Br J Urol 1982; 54: 441–445

26 Hegedüs L, Hansen J M, Karstrup S, Torp-Pedersen S T, Juul N. Tetracycline for sclerosis of thyroid cysts. A randomised study. Arch Intern Med 1988; 148: 1116–1118

27 Hancke S, Holm H H, Koch F. Ultrasonically guided puncture of pancreatic mass lesions. In: Holm H H, Kristensen J K. eds. Interventional Ultrasound. Copenhagen: Munksgaard. 1985

28 Granberg S: Ultrasound in the diagnosis and treatment of ovarian tumors. Thesis. Kompendiet Lindome, Gothenburg, Sweden: 1989

29 Makuuchi M, Bandai Y, Ito T, Wada T. Ultrasonically guided percutaneous transhepatic cholangiography and percutaneous pancreatography. Radiology 1980; 134: 767–770

30 Pedersen J F. Percutaneous nephrostomy guided by ultrasound. J Urol 1974; 112: 157–159

31 Nielsen L. Quick step screw dilatator. WFUMB meeting, Washington DC: October 1988

32 Gronvall S. Diagnostic and therapeutic puncture of intraabdominal fluid collections. In: Holm H H, Kristensen J K. eds. Interventional Ultrasound. Copenhagen: Munksgaard. 1985

33 Casola G, vanSonnenberg E. Sonographic guidance for percutaneous drainage of abscesses and fluid collections. In: vanSonnenberg E. ed. Interventional ultrasound. New York: Churchill Livingstone. 1987

34 Pruett L T, Simmons L R. Status of percutaneous catheter drainage of abscesses. Surg Clin North Am 1988; 68: 89–105

35 Bagi P, Dueholm S, Karstrup S. Percutaneous drainage of appendiceal abscess. Dis Colon Rectum 1987; 30: 532–535

36 Nosher L J, Winchman K H, Needell S G. Transvaginal pelvic abscess drainage with US guidance. Radiology 1987; 165: 872–873

37 Karstrup S, Nolsøe C, Branrand K, Nielsen K R. Ultrasonically guided percutaneous drainage of breast abscesses. Acta Radiol 1989 (in press)

38 Austin H E, Wayne F. The treatment of recurrent malignant pleural effusion. Ann Thorac Surg 1979; 28: 190–203

39 Marks M W, Filly A R, Callen W P. Real-time evaluation of pleural lesions: New observations regarding the probability of obtaining free fluid. Radiology 1982; 142: 162–164

40 Simeone F J. Interventional ultrasound of the thorax. In: vanSonnenberg E. ed. Interventional ultrasound. New York: Churchill Livingstone. 1987

41 vanSonnenberg E, Wittich G R, Cabera O A, et al. Percutaneous gastrostomy and gastroenterostomy. II. Clinical experience. AJR 1986; 146: 581–586

42 Ho C S, Gray R R, Goldfinger M, Rosen I E, McPerson R. Percutaneous gastrostomy for internal feeding. Radiology 1985; 156: 349–351

43 Lohela P, Soiva M, Suramo I, Taavitsainen M, Holopeinen O. Ultrasound guidance for percutaneous puncture and drainage in acute cholecystitis. Acta Radiol 1986; 27: 543–546

44 vanSonnenberg E, Wittich R G, Casola G. Diagnostic and therapeutic percutaneous gallbladder procedures. Radiology 1986; 160: 23–26

45 Vogelzang L R, Nemcek A A. Percutaneous cholecystostomy. Diagnostic and therapeutic efficacy. Radiology 1988; 168: 29–34

46 Bandai Y. Percutaneous transhepatic gallbladder drainage (PTGBD). In: Watanabe H, Makuuchi M. eds. Interventional real-time ultrasound. Tokyo: Igaku-Shoin. 1985

47 Gronvall S, Stage G J, Boesby S, Sobye A. Transperitoneal US-guided cholecystostomy in acute cholecystitis. Abstract. 5th International Congress on Interventional Ultrasound. Copenhagen: 1989

48 vanSonnenberg E, Wittich R G, Casola G, et al. Percutaneous drainage of infected and noninfected pancreatic pseudocysts: experience in 101 cases. Radiology 1989; 170: 757–761

49 Torres E W, Evert B M, Baumgartner R B, Bernardino E M. Percutaneous aspiration and drainage of pancreatic pseudocysts. AJR 1986; 147: 1007–1009

50 Hancke S, Henriksen W F. Percutaneous pancreatic

cystogastrostomy guided by ultrasound scanning and gastroscopy. Br J Surg 1985; 72: 916–917

51 Sacks B, Greenberg J J, Porter H D, et al. An internalised double-j catheter for percutaneous transgastric cystogastrostomy. AJR 1989; 152: 523–526

52 Holm H H, Juul N. Interventional ultrasound in cancer therapy. In: Holm H H, Kristensen J K. eds. Interventional ultrasound. Copenhagen: Munksgaard. 1985

53 Karstrup S, Holm H H, Torp-Pedersen S, Hegedüs L. Ultrasonically guided percutaneous inactivation of parathyroid tumours. Br J Radiol 1987; 60: 667–670

54 Livraghi T, Festi D, Manti F, Salmi A, Vettori C. US-guided percutaneous alcohol injection of small hepatic and abdominal tumors. Radiology 1986; 161: 309–312

55 Guarnieri A, Canale M. Ultrasonically guided fine needle drug-infiltration of liver metastases. Third Interventional Congress on Interventional Ultrasound. Copenhagen 1983

56 Holm H H, Strøyer I, Hansen H, Stadil F. Ultrasonically guided percutaneous interstitial implantation of Iodine 125 seeds in cancer therapy. Br J Radiol 1981; 54: 665–670

57 Holm H H, Juul N, Pedersen J F, Hansen H, Strøyer I. Transperineal ^{125}I seed implantation in prostatic cancer guided by transrectal ultrasonography. J Urol 1983; 130: 283–286

58 Bleehen N M. Hyperthermia in the treatment of cancer. Br J Cancer 1982; 45: 96–100

59 Matthewson K, Coleridge-Smith P, O'Sullivan J P, Northfield T C, Bown S G. Biological effects of intrahepatic neodynium: yttrium-aluminium-Garnet laser photocoagulation in rats. Gastroenterology 1987; 93: 550–557

60 Nolsøe C, Torp-Pedersen S, Oldag E, Holm H H. Nedynium-YAG laser induced interstitial hyperthermia. Development of a diffuser tip. Comparison of ultrasonic and macroscopic measurement of the thermal lesions produced. 8th Congress of Interventional Society for laser surgery and medicine. Taipei: 1989

61 Whitmore W F, Hilaris B, Grabstald H. Retropubic implantation of Iodine 125 in the treatment of prostatic cancer. J Urol 1972; 108: 918–920

62 Hastak S M, Gammelgaard J, Holm H H. Transrectal ultrasonic volume determination of the prostate: A preoperative and postoperative study. J Urol 1982; 127: 1115–1118

63 Lee F, Torp-Pedersen S T, Meiselman L, et al. Transrectal ultrasound in the diagnosis and staging of local disease after I-125 seed implantation for prostate cancer. Int J Radiat Oncol Biol Phys 1988; 15: 1453–1459

64 Iversen P, Bak M, Juul N, et al. Ultrasonically guided 125 Iodine seed implantation with external radiation in management of localised prostatic carcinoma. Urology 1989; 34: 181–186

65 Kabalin J N, Hodge K K, McNeal J E, Freiha F S, Stamey T A. Identification of residual cancer in the prostate following radiation therapy: role of transrectal ultrasound guided biopsy and prostate specific antigen. J Urol 1989; 142: 326–331

66 Shinagawa T, Ukaji H, Iino Y, et al. Intratumoral injection of absolute ethanol under ultrasound imaging for treatment of small hepatocellular carcinoma: attempts in three cases. Acta Hepatol Jpn 1985: 26: 99–103

67 Livraghi T, Salmi A, Bolondi L, et al. Small hepatocellular carcinoma: Percutaneous alcohol injection – results in 23 patients. Radiology 1988: 168: 313–317

68 Ohto M, Sugiura N, Ebara M, Kimura K, Isomura S, Watanabe Y. Treatment of hepatocellular carcinoma by alcohol injection into the tumor and irradiaton of the tumor. Gan To Kagaku Ryoho 1986; 13: 1625–1634

69 Shiina S, Yasuda H, Muto H, et al. Percutaneous ethanol injection in the treatment of liver neoplasms. AJR 1987; 149: 949–952

70 Sheu J C, Huang G T, Chen D S, et al. Small hepatocellular carcinoma: Intratumor ethanol treatment using new needle and guidance system. Radiology 1987; 163: 43–48

71 Butch R J, Simeone J F, Mueller P R. Thyroid and parathyroid ultrasonography. Radiol Clin North Am 1985; 23: 57–71

72 Söderström N. Identification of normal tissue by aspiration cytology. In: Linsk J A, Franzen S. eds. Clinical aspiration cytology. Philadelphia: J. B. Lippincott. 1983

73 Glenthøj A, Karstrup S. Parathyroid identification by ultrasonically guided aspiration cytology. Is a correct cytological identification possible? APMIS 1989; 97: 497–502

74 Doppman L J, Krudy A G, Marx J S, et al. Aspiration of enlarged parathyroid glands for parathyroid hormone assay. Radiology 1983; 148: 32–35

75 Karstrup S, Glenthøj A, Torp-Pedersen S, Hegedüs L, Holm H H. Ultrasonically guided fine needle aspiration of suggested enlarged parathyroid glands. Acta Radiol 1988; 29: 213–216

76 Karstrup S, Glenthøj A, Hainau B, Hegedüs L, Torp-Pedersen S, Holm H H. Ultrasound-guided, histological, fine-needle biopsy from suspected parathyroid tumours: Success-rate and reliability of histological diagnosis. Br J Radiol 1989 (in press)

77 Solbiati L, Giangrande A, De Pra L, Bellotti E, Cantu P, Ravetto C. Percutaneous ethanol injection of parathyroid tumours under US guidance: treatment of secondary hyperparathyroidism. Radiology 1985; 155: 607–610

78 Karstrup S, Transbøl I, Holm H H, Glenthøj A, Hegedüs L. Ultrasound-guided chemical parathyroidectomy in patients with primary hyperparathyroidism: a prospective study. Br J Radiol 1989; 62: 1037–1042

79 Karstrup S, Holm H H, Glenthøj A, Hegedüs L. Ultrasonically guided chemical parathyroidectomy in a highly selected series of patients with primary hyperparathyroidism. Accepted for publication AJR, 1989

80 Gammelgaard J, Jensen F. Ultrasonically guided celiac plexus block in intractable pain. Abstract: 4th European Congress on Ultrasonics in Medicine. Dubrovnik, Yugoslavia: 1981

81 Greiner L, Ulatowski L, Prohm P. Sonographisch gezielte und intraoperative alkoholblockade der z liakalganglien bei konservativ nicht beherrschbaren malignombedingten oberbauchschmerzen. Ultraschall Med 1983; 4: 57–59

82 Eerola R, Kaukinen L, Kaukinen S. Analysis of 13 800 subclavian vein catheterisations. Acta Anaesthesiol Scand 1985; 29: 193–197

83 Mitchell E S, Clark A R. Complications of central venous catheterisation. AJR 1979; 133: 467–476

84 Machi J, Takeda J, Kakegawa T. Safe jugular and subclavian venipuncture under ultrasonographic guidance. Am J Surg 1987; 153: 321–323

85 Nolsøe C, Nielsen L, Karstrup S, Lauritsen L. Ultrasonically guided subclavian vein catheterisation. Acta Radiol 1989; 30: 108–109

Safety of diagnostic ultrasound

Gail ter Haar

INTRODUCTION

The increasingly widespread use of diagnostic ultrasound techniques means that safety considerations have become more important. The main applications for which safety is of paramount importance are those in obstetrics and neonatology. It seems probable that the most sensitive targets that are exposed to ultrasound are those in the embryo or fetus, and thus the potential for inducing adverse effects will be greatest here.

Although the bio-effects literature is apparently very extensive, the overwhelming majority of studies reported concern the interaction of therapeutic ultrasound with biological systems and very few deal with 'diagnostic' exposures, let alone diagnostic machines used in clinical practice.

Therapeutic ultrasound uses either continuous or tone burst exposures whereas diagnostic ultrasound employs short pulses. It can be seen from Table 1, in which a number of important exposure parameters are compared, that there is some overlap in the amount of acoustic power emitted during a pulse, even though the time averaged intensities are lower for therapy devices. It is clear that therapy devices can induce changes in biological systems, (albeit beneficial) and so we must ascertain whether or not diagnostic devices can also induce changes, in this case unwanted.

It is now generally accepted that the two main mechanisms that may produce biological change are heat and cavitation. These two mechanisms will be discussed, and methods of minimising their potential effects will be suggested.

Biological effects

As outlined above, the two main mechanisms by which ultrasound may cause damage to biological systems are heat and cavitation. These two effects will be considered separately.

a) Biological effects of heating

Although it is known that therapeutic ultrasound can raise tissue temperatures significantly, very few measurements of the temperature rises induced by diagnostic exposures have been made. ter Haar et al[1] have reported biologically insignificant temperature rises measured in liver tissue in vitro following pulse echo exposures (I_{SPPA} 183 Wcm^{-2}; I_{SPPA} Wcm^{-2}; 3.3 MHz), but rises up to 1.9°C following 1 minute's exposure to Doppler ultrasound (I_{SPPA} 190 Wcm^{-2}; I_{SPTA} 6.2 Wcm^{-2}). However, higher temperatures have been measured at bone surfaces. For example, using the pulsed Doppler exposures detailed above, temperature rises of 4.7°C have been registered at the surface of mature bone with an overlying 8 mm of muscle in vitro. The greatest temperature rise occurs when the Doppler beam meets the bone surface at normal incidence (ter Haar unpublished data). Uncalcified fetal bone is unlikely to show these temperature rises.

Tissue heating is likely only to be a significant biological problem in obstetric applications. Here, some data on the effects of supra-normal temperatures on the well-being of the fetus or embryo is available. Although there is very little information about the effect of hyperthermia on humans during pregnancy, all other mammalian species

Table 1 Ultrasound exposure for therapy, imaging and Doppler.

	Therapy	Imaging	Pulsed Doppler
Pulse length	1–10 ms	~1 μs	~10 μs
Frequencies	0.75–3 MHz	3–7 MHz	3–7 MHz
Pulse repetition frequencies	100–300 Hz	~1 kHz	~10 kHz
Peak intensity in the pulse I_{SPPA}	0.25–3 Wcm^{-2}	21–933 Wcm^{-2}★ (mean 267 Wcm^{-2})	1.1–710 Wcm^{-2}★ (mean 213 Wcm^{-2})
Time averaged peak intensity I_{SPTA}	25–300 mWcm^{-2}	0.3–166 mWcm^{-2}★ (mean 16.1 mWcm^{-2})	110–9500 mWcm^{-2}★ (mean 1943 mWcm^{-2})
Total power	~1 W:	0.5–80 mW★ (mean 22.8 mW)	3.2–500 mW★ (mean 81 mW)
Peak positive pressure p+	0.25 MPa	0.8–8.8 MPa★ (mean 4.08 MPa)	0.2–6.3 MPa★ (mean 3.43 MPa)
Peak negative pressure p−	0.25 MPa	0.8–3.9 MPa★ (mean 1.99 MPa)	0.2–6.3 MPa★ (mean 1.71 MPa)
Beam widths	~1 cm	~2 mm	~2 mm

★ Data taken from Duck[2]

that have been studied appear to be susceptible to heat damage.

The effect of a hyperthermic insult depends on the stage of embryonic or fetal development and on both the temperature rise, and the time for which it is imposed. Thermally induced embryonic death is possible at any stage, but is most likely during the pre-implantation stage. The uterus and its secretions change significantly at this stage and are vitally linked to the stage of development of the embryo. If embryonic development is delayed, it may be put out of phase with the nutrient uterine secretions. It appears that hyperthermia during this stage either kills the embryo outright or the embryo goes on to develop normally. Death, resorption or abortion may, however, occur at any stage of development.

Abortion is a well-known consequence of elevated temperatures. There may be a number of causes for this, including increased uterine activity, or severe cellular damage that is incompatible with the continued development of the fetus or embryo.

Hyperthermia is known to be a teratogen in 'a number of mammalian species e.g. rats, mice, sheep, pigs and monkeys.[3] Adverse effects may be found if the temperature is elevated during a crucial stage in organogenesis. It appears that the central nervous system is most susceptible to damage. Examples of defects found are neural tube defects, microphthalmia, microcephaly and micrencephaly.

Research indicates that it is the temperature elevation above normal that is important in producing effects rather than the actual temperature reached. Temperature rises above normal that can produce death, resorption, abortion or teratogenesis in the mammalian species that have been studied, are in the range 1.5 to 2.5°C.

Thus, it is known that death and teratogenic effects are possible outcomes of raised temperatures in utero. Early embryos are more likely to show lethal effects than are late embryos or fetuses. Teratogenic effects are most likely during early stages of organogenesis, the central nervous system being most at risk. The most sensitive stages are those when cell proliferation is most intense. It should be noted that adult proliferative tissues may also be at risk (e.g. testis and bone marrow).

Diagnostic ultrasound that heats the embryo or fetus by less than 1°C can be used without reservation for any length of time. At higher temperature rises, the risk of causing adverse effects increases with the length of exposure time. It should, however, be noted that hyperthermia research has in general heated the whole body of the fetus. The consequences of selective heating, as would be achieved for example from a Doppler beam, have not been studied.

It seems likely that pulse echo imaging can be used safely as far as thermal considerations are concerned, whereas some degree of caution should be exercised, where Doppler examinations are to be used, although if examina-tions are kept as short as possible, it is unlikely that the elevated temperatures produced will lead to significant biological damage.

b) Biological effects of cavitation

Cavitation is the term used to describe the activity of microscopic gas bodies when they are influenced by an ultrasonic field. The behaviour of a bubble depends on its size and on the characteristics of the acoustic field with which it interacts. For every ultrasonic frequency there is a bubble diameter that is 'resonant'. If the acoustic amplitude is sufficiently high, these bubbles oscillate violently in the ultrasonic field and may undergo a cycle of rapid growth and implosion, resulting in very high local temperatures and shear stresses. For lesser amplitudes and for smaller bubbles, the bubble may be set into forced oscillations, setting up streaming motions around it. These small bubbles may grow to resonant size and undergo collapse. Large bubbles may also oscillate and may disintegrate, thus seeding the population of smaller bubbles. (For more detailed information, see reference[4]).

This bubble activity requires that stabilised microscopic gas bodies exist in tissue, or that the nuclei from which they may be formed (nucleation sites) exist. It has been shown that such bubbles do exist in tissues[5] and that therapeutic ultrasound exposures can cause these to grow to a detectable size. Very little is known about nucleation sites in tissues, but it seems likely that the same tissue type in different individuals or even in different sites within one individual, may have significantly different gaseous content and therefore different likelihood of cavitation.

It has not been demonstrated that diagnostic pulses of ultrasound can induce cavitation in mammalian tissues, although effects have been seen in Drosophila[6] and in agar gels.[1]

The biological consequences of cavitation activity due to diagnostic ultrasound are not well-understood. It is known from work at therapeutic output levels that tissue immediately around the site of a collapse cavitation event is completely disrupted. Cell lysis is seen, but on a very localised scale, a few microns across. Bubbles that are oscillating in a stable fashion, without collapsing, set up streaming patterns around themselves.

In fluids, the shear stresses associated with the liquid's movement may be quite considerable, and cells in the vicinity may be lysed. In more structured tissues, such fluid movement may not be possible and the effect of oscillating bubbles will be considerably damped.

The greatest hazard from diagnostic ultrasound lies in the possibility that a cavitation event may occur in amniotic or body fluids close to a developing organism, lysing a cell or group of cells such that irreparable damage may occur. Cavitation may occur in blood plasma, but no reports of thrombus formation have been published.

c) Biological effects from other mechanisms

There are a number of other ways in which ultrasound may interact with tissues, but the biological consequences of these are even more poorly understood than those of cavitation. In particular, for diagnostic ultrasound where there may be significant non-linear propagation effects, nothing is known about the biological effects of non-linearity on tissues.

Epidemiological surveys

There are few published epidemiological studies of the effects of in utero ultrasound examinations on children, and these are on small populations. The literature has been extensively reviewed by Ziskin and Petitti.[7]

Effects that have been studied are birthweight;[8–10] structural fetal anomalies;[8,10–12] neurological effects;[9,10] incidence of childhood cancer[13,14] and hearing in children.[10]

No conclusive evidence has been presented that ultrasound can produce any abnormalities in any of these studies. In fact, in only one study was there any indication of an effect, namely in the birthweight study of Moore et al, but Stark et al[10] were unable to support this finding in an analysis of the same data base.

Although it is reassuring that all the epidemiological evidence to date is negative, and it is certainly true that if diagnostic scanning in obstetrics were producing obvious fetal abnormalities in large numbers they would have been picked up by now, it should be remembered that all the published surveys have covered relatively small sample populations. In addition, there has been no attempt to quantify the doses of ultrasound used. No epidemiological surveys have been carried out to date on Doppler ultrasound.

Minimising the possibility of harm

What has gone before has been somewhat theoretical and hypothetical. We need to know the answer to the question: how can the user minimise the probability of producing biologically significant heating or cavitational effects using the controls provided on the machine?

We know that the amount of heating obtained increases with acoustic output intensity, exposure (or dwell) time, and with ultrasonic frequency. If the time averaged intensity is increased, for example by increasing the pulse repetition frequency without altering pulse amplitude, then the amount of heating may be expected to increase. Important quantities for determining whether cavitation may be produced are peak negative pressure, pulse length, pulse repetition frequency and exposure time. Thus, for example, for all modes of operation of diagnostic scanners we can deduce that increasing the exposure time and output power will increase both the amount of heating obtained and the probability of cavitational effects, while increasing the transducer frequency increases the probability for biologically significant thermal effects because of the increased absorption, but decreases the probability of cavitational effects.

Table 2 illustrates the way in which thermal and cavitational effects may vary when different machine settings are altered for different operating modes. Where possible settings that minimise the possibility of producing significant heat or cavitation should be used. It should be noted that this is a broad generalisation as there are probably as many ways of driving transducers as there are machines available, highlighting the need for a good understanding of each individual machine and for good exchange of information between manufacturer and user.

General guidelines

In conclusion, a few general recommendations may be made to ensure the continued safe use of ultrasound.

a) Machine default output conditions should be set to give low output power and high receiver gain.
b) The time that a transducer is in contact with the skin while transmitting should be kept to a minimum.
c) The acoustic output should be kept to the minimum level consistent with good clinical accuracy and performance.

Appendix

There have been a number of statements issued by national and international bodies concerning the safe use of medical ultrasound. The most recent is a statement issued by the European Federation of Societies for Ultrasound in Medicine and Biology (EFSUMB) in 1989:

Ultrasound imaging for diagnostic purposes in obstetrics has been in extensive clinical use for more than 25 years. Numerous investigations of various degrees of sophistication have been undertaken in an endeavour to detect adverse effects. None of these studies has proved that ultrasound at diagnostic intensities as used today has led to any deleterious effect to the fetus or mother. In view of the current lack of well-designed, controlled, long-term prospective epidemiological studies, it is necessary to resort to evidence culled from laboratory studies in vitro and in vivo. Diverse effects of potential clinical significance have been reported from a variety of biological systems subjected to either pulsed or continuous wave diagnostic ultrasound. Those effects that have been chosen for further study have either not been confirmed or have given conflicting results. Routine clinical scanning of every woman during pregnancy using real time B-mode imaging is not contra-indicated by the evidence currently available from biological investigations and its performance should be left to clinical judgement. As new instrumentation using higher acoustic outputs, and new clinical procedures become more widespread, thus giving the potential for higher tissue exposures, it will be necessary to continually

Table 2 Table showing in general terms how variation of machine controls may alter the probability of producing biologically significant thermal or cavitational effects.

	Probability of biologically significant –		
	thermal effects	cavitation effects	
ALL OPERATING MODES			
Exposure time ↑	↑	↑	These lead to greater acoustic energy absorption.
Output power ↑	↑	↑	
Transducer frequency ↑	↑	↓	Absorption increases with frequency increase. Cavitation threshold decreases with increasing frequency.
Switching to freeze frame	↓/0	↓/0	Some transducers continue to operate although the picture is frozen.
IMAGING + M-MODE			
Selection of M-mode from imaging mode	↑	↑	This gives repeated exposure of the same small tissue volume.
Sector format	↑	?	Line density is increased near transducer
Choice of narrow sector angle or high resolution	↑	↑	Increase in line density
Focal zone depth ↑	↑	↑	For some machines the power is increased to account for attenuation losses.
Receiver gain	0	0	These are "receive" variables not "transmit"
Grey scale	0	0	
M-mode time base	0	0	
PULSED DOPPLER			
Range gate length ↑	↑	↑	In some machines power is increased to account for attenuation losses.
Range gate depth ↑	↑	↑	
Velocity range ↑	↑	↑	
Receiver gain	0	0	These are "receive" variables not "transmit"
Doppler audio gain	0	0	
Doppler time base	0	0	

Key
↑ indicates an increase
↓ indicates a decrease
0 indicates no change expected

re-evaluate the safety of these diagnostic procedures. The committee (The Ultrasound Radiation Safety Committee of EFSUMB) endorses the clinical safety statement made by the AIUM (1988), while emphasising the need for further investigations into bio-effects from physical, biological and clinical standpoints.

REFERENCES

1 ter Haar G R, Duck F A, Starritt H, Daniels S. Biophysical characterization of diagnostic ultrasound equipment – preliminary results. Phys Med Biol 1989; 34: 1533–1542
2 Duck F A. Output data from European studies. Ultrasound Med Biol 1989; 15 Suppl 1: 61–64
3 Edwards M J. Hyperthermia as a teratogen: a review of experimental studies and their clinical significance. Teratogenesis, Carcinogeneous and Mutagenesis 1986; 6: 563–582
4 ter Haar G R. Ultrasonic biophysics. In: Physical principles of medical ultrasound 1986; 379–435
5 Daniels S, ter Haar G. Bubble formation in guinea pigs and agar gels during ultrasonic irradiation. Proc I O A 1986; 8: 147–157
6 Child S Z, Carstensen E L, Smachlo K. Effects of ultrasound on Drosophila III. Exposure of larvae to low temporal average intensity, pulsed irradiation. Ultrasound Med Biol 1981; 7: 167–173
7 Ziskin M, Petitti D. Epidemiology of human exposure to ultrasound – a critical review. Ultrasound Med Biol 1988; 14: 91–96
8 Bakketeig L S, Eik-Nes S H, Jacobsen G, et al. A randomized controlled trial of ultrasonographic screening in pregnancy. Lancet 1984; 2: 207–210
9 Scheidt P D, Stanley F, Bryla D A. One year follow-up of infants exposed to ultrasound in utero. Am J Obstet Gynecol 1978; 121: 742–748
10 Stark C R, Orleans M, Haverkamp A D, Murphy J. Short- and long-term risks after exposure to diagnostic ultrasound in utero. Obstet Gynecol 1984; 63: 194–200
11 Hellman L M, Duffus G M, Donald I, Sunden B. Safety of diagnostic ultrasound in obstetrics. Lancet 1970; 1: 1133–1135
12 Bernstine R L. Safety studies with ultrasonic Doppler technique: a clinical follow-up of patients and tissue culture study. Obstet Gynecol 1969; 34: 707–709
13 Cartwright R A, McKinney P A, Hopton P A, et al. Ultrasound examination in pregnancy and childhood cancer. Lancet 1984; 2: 999–1000
14 Kinnier-Wilson L M, Waterhouse J A. Obstetric ultrasound and childhood malignancies. Lancet 1984; 2: 997–999

The normal pancreas

Steven Garber and William R. Lees

INTRODUCTION

Its retroperitoneal position and the proximity of overlying bowel gas has traditionally prevented adequate ultrasound visualisation of the pancreas, especially of the tail region. However, recent improvements in ultrasound equipment and techniques have meant that, in skilled hands, a diagnostic examination can be achieved in over 95% of patients.[1]

Much has been written of the relative merits of ultrasound and computed tomography (CT) in evaluating the pancreas, although diagnostic results are similar in the majority of patients. Their roles should be seen as complementary and now, together with magnetic resonance imaging (MRI) and pancreatography, they provide powerful tools for the assessment of pancreatic disease.

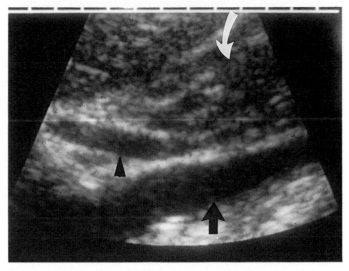

Fig. 2 Normal pancreas. Longitudinal scan showing the pancreas (curved arrow) and its relation to the portal vein (arrowhead) and inferior vena cava (arrow).

Anatomy

The pancreas lies transversely across the abdomen in the anterior pararenal space, extending from the concavity of the duodenum to the splenic hilum. Anatomically it is divided into a head, neck, body and tail, which is the most cephalad part of the gland.[2]

The pancreas is readily located using vascular landmarks (Figs 1 and 2). The head lies anterior to the inferior vena cava and caudal to the portal vein (Fig. 3). It relates closely to the duodenal curve and is the broadest part of the gland. The uncinate process extends posteriorly from the head to pass behind the superior mesenteric vessels. Between the

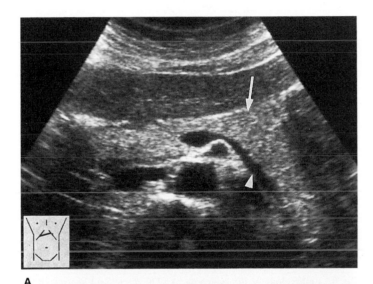

A

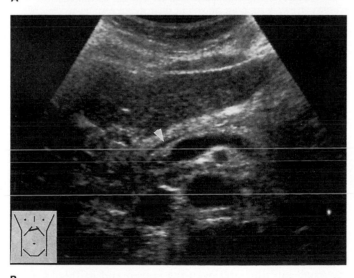

B

Fig. 1 Normal pancreas. A: The pancreatic body (arrow) is shown lying anterior to the splenic vein (arrowhead). **B:** The pancreatic duct (arrowhead) is shown in the head of the pancreas.

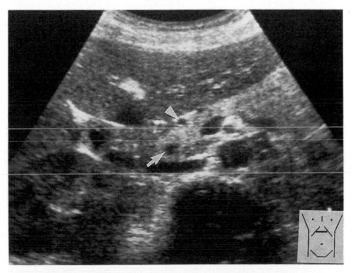

Fig. 3 Head of pancreas. The pancreatic head is shown in relation to the common bile duct (arrow) and gastroduodenal artery (arrowhead).

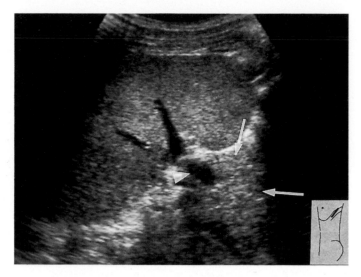

Fig. 4 Tail of pancreas. The normal pancreatic tail (arrows) is shown in relation to the splenic vein (arrowhead).

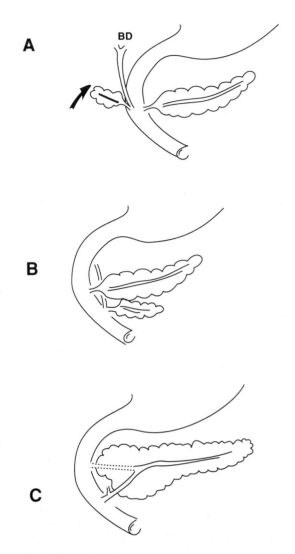

Fig. 5 Embryology of the pancreas. A: The dorsal and ventral (curved arrow) anlagen are shown in their initial relation to the bile duct (BD). **B:** The ventral pancreas lies adjacent to the dorsal segment following its migration around the duodenum. **C:** The normal adult configuration. The head of the pancreas has components from both the dorsal and ventral anlagen while the uncinate process derives exclusively from the ventral anlage.

head and body there is a slight tapering of the pancreas, the neck, which lies posterior to the gastric antrum. The body of the pancreas passes across the midline anterior to the superior mesenteric vessels and aorta.

The splenic artery and vein run along its posterior border, the latter providing a useful location marker for ultrasound. The left renal vein passes between the superior mesenteric vessels and aorta and is also a posterior relation of the pancreas. The tail forms the left lateral portion of the gland and is often the hardest part to visualise on ultrasound; its tip may lie within the lieno-renal ligament remaining anterior to the splenic vessels (Fig. 4).

The pancreatic duct runs the length of the gland.

The position of the gland, its size and degree of obliquity vary greatly from person to person.

Embryology

The pancreas is formed from the union of dorsal and ventral anlages (Fig. 5). The former arises from the posterior wall of the duodenum and the latter from the common bile duct. The ventral bud initially develops with two lobes; normally, the left fails to develop and the ventral pancreas is formed from the right lobe. When the bile duct migrates around the duodenum the ventral pancreatic bud follows, fusing with the dorsal bud in the seventh week of intra-uterine life.

The uncinate process and part of the head develop from the ventral bud, the remainder of the gland from the dorsal anlage. The duct of the dorsal pancreas fuses with the ventral duct to form the main pancreatic duct (duct of Wirsung) which opens into the duodenum with the common bile duct at the ampulla of Vater. The proximal portion of the dorsal duct may disappear or may remain as the acces-

sory pancreatic duct (duct of Santorini), opening into the duodenum a few centimetres proximal to the ampulla.

Congenital anomalies

Ectopia

Pancreatic tissue can be found anywhere in the gut but rarely distal to Meckel's diverticulum. The stomach wall, the small intestine and even the spleen and gallbladder can all contain ectopic tissue.

The commonest form of pancreatic ectopia is the annular pancreas (Fig. 6).[3] Pancreatic tissue encircles the bowel,

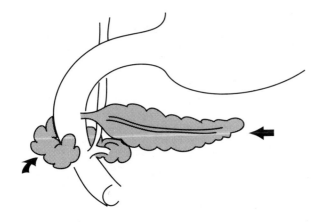

Fig. 6 Annular pancreas. The ventral anlage (curved arrow) encircles the duodenum and may lead to obstruction.

usually the second part of the duodenum, lying within the muscularis mucosa.[4] Patients present in early life (50% in the first year) with proximal small bowel obstruction. Sometimes only partial encirclement is seen and these patients may be symptom-free. Annular pancreas is thought to be persistence of the left lobe of the ventral pancreas. Associations have been demonstrated with duodenal atresia, malrotations, tracheo-oesophageal fistulae and imperforate anus.[5]

Pancreas divisum

In a small percentage of cases (1% to 5%) dorsal and ventral anlagen fail to fuse and their duct systems remain separate; this is termed 'pancreas divisum', an anomaly that is most often diagnosed by ERCP.[6] On cannulation of the duct of Wirsung, contrast only fills the ventral segment of the gland; the accessory duct of Santorini must be cannulated separately to delineate the pancreatic body and tail. It can also be recognised with high resolution ultrasound (Figs 7 and 8).

Pancreas divisum is thought to predispose to pancreatitis in the dorsal pancreatic segment because of inadequate drainage.[6] However, despite pancreatic duct pressure monitoring, the precise association remains uncertain.

Cysts

Solitary or multiple congenital cysts may be found in the pancreas. In cystic fibrosis these contain inspissated secretions.

Lipomatosis

In this condition the exocrine components of the gland are replaced by fat.

Size

The usefulness of pancreatic measurement is often questioned because of its irregular shape. This is particularly true of the pancreatic tail which, as well as varying in size, may also vary in position. Using CT the position of the pancreatic tail is seen to range from antero-lateral to

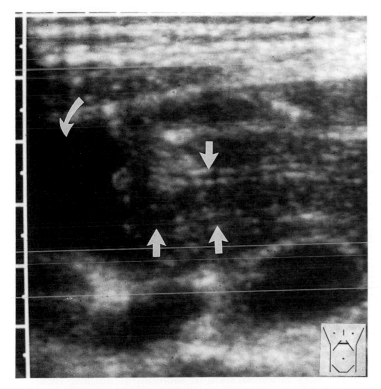

Fig. 7 Pancreas divisum. The two non-communicating pancreatic ducts (arrows) open into the fluid filled duodenum (curved arrow).

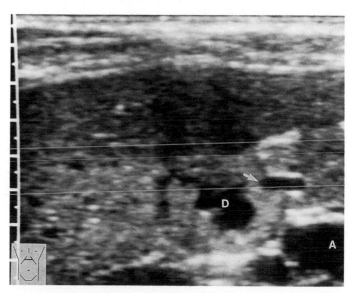

Fig. 8 Pancreas divisum. A dilated duct of Santorini (arrow) at its opening into the duodenum (D). A – aorta.

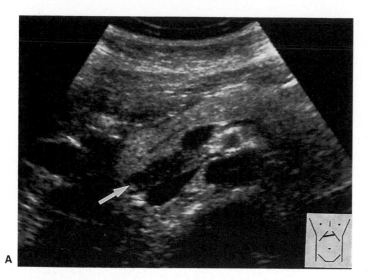
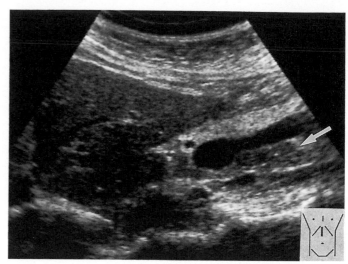

Fig. 9 Normal ventral pancreas. A: transverse and **B:** longitudinal scans. The decreased reflectivity of the ventral pancreas (arrows) compared with the rest of the gland is shown.

antero-medial to the left kidney. In one study the classically described cranial curving of the gland was only seen in 50% of normal cases.[7] Several studies have however, looked at pancreatic size. Ultrasound derived figures of 25 mm and 15 mm as maximum AP diameters for the head and body respectively are quoted.[8–10] Though inadequate visualisation of the tail has often prevented its inclusion in these measurements, one study reported a maximum diameter of 35 mm in the normal gland.[11]

These wide variations in size of the normal pancreas are in part age related. The fact that the pancreas tends to atrophy with age must be borne in mind: a pancreas of normal size for a young patient may, in the elderly, represent a diffusely enlarged gland.[11] Not all pancreatic disease results in an increase in gland size, for instance, in diabetes mellitus the pancreas may be smaller than normal.[12]

Reflectivity

The normal pancreas is homogeneous with a reflectivity greater than or equal to adjacent liver.[13] Correlation with CT shows that variations in reflectivity probably relate to the degree of fatty infiltration.[14] After 60 years of age, fatty accumulation in pancreatic tissues is common; it is also increased in the obese,[15] in Cushing's disease and in patients on corticosteroids.[16] Fat is deposited along the pancreatic septa.[14] On CT this is recognised by a change from a gland with a smooth contour to one divided into discrete lobules. As its fat content increases, the reflectivity of the pancreas increases and the gland may then become indistinguishable from surrounding retroperitoneal fat, causing overestimation of pancreatic size. A grading method for pancreatic reflectivity has been proposed[17] but, as a generalised increase in reflectivity is probably not of clinical significance,

its practical value is doubtful. It seems likely that intra-lobular fat can also contribute to reflectivity: the ventrally-derived portion of the gland (uncinate and posterior part of the head) is relatively echo-poor in 28% of subjects (Fig. 9)[18] and this correlates with a lack of intra-parenchymal adipocytes on histology. It is important to recognise that this is a normal variant.

Pancreatic duct

Visualisation of the pancreatic duct constitutes an important part of imaging the pancreas. Ductal enlargement occurs in a wide range of pancreatic disease so that an appreciation of the upper limit of normal is vital. The duct is best assessed in the region of the pancreatic body where it lies perpendicular to the ultrasound beam and follows a relatively straight course.[19] In the pancreatic head its course and position are variable. The calibre of the duct increases with age but in subjects younger than 60 years its maximum diameter, in the region of the body, should be no more than 2 mm.[19] With modern ultrasound equipment the duct can be adequately visualised in almost 90% of patients. It is seen as a tubular structure with reflective walls.

If more precise information is required, particularly in the pancreatic head region, secretin can be administered to stimulate pancreatic secretion. This has two main effects: firstly the duct dilates, so aiding its visualisation and secondly pancreatic juice outflow into the duodenum improves definition of the pancreatic head.[20] In normal subjects Bolondi demonstrated a mean duct diameter of 1.1 mm in the fasting state, increasing to 2.7 mm 3 minutes after administration of secretin. If outflow from the pancreatic duct is obstructed, dilatation following secretin may be even more marked.

Imaging techniques

Several different ultrasound methods may be used to visualise the pancreas:

> transabdominal ultrasound imaging
> Doppler (spectral and colour flow mapping)
> endoscopic ultrasound
> intra-operative ultrasound.

The technical constraints differ for each of these.

Transabdominal ultrasound

For pancreatic imaging both sector and linear array probes are useful with ultrasound frequencies of between 3 and 7.5 MHz. Scanning techniques to overcome the problem of intestinal gas have been developed. Overnight fasting ensures an empty stomach and reduces peristalsis. The head and body of the gland can usually be imaged through the liver, particularly with the patient upright.[21]

Several methods to move intervening bowel gas away have been developed. Firm pressure with the ultrasound probe displaces overlying bowel loops and is often sufficient alone to achieve adequate access to the pancreas. Standing the patient upright or turning the patient obliquely causes the bowel loops to descend relative to the fixed pancreas. The pancreatic tail can often be visualised through the spleen but it is helpful to give a fluid load, producing an acoustic window through the stomach.[22] Up to 500 ml of any non-gassy fluid may be needed.[23] The fluid is given with the patient on the left side to fill the stomach body. Scanning is delayed a few minutes to allow the fluid to settle. The body and tail of the gland are best seen in this position. Turning the patient onto their right side allows fluid to pass into the antrum and duodenum facilitating examination of the head and uncinate process. In the fasted patient the fluid load in the stomach may all pass into the duodenum within a few minutes with the patient in this position. Duodenal paralysis greatly enhances visualisation of the ampulla and ventral segment of the pancreas but is not often required.

Doppler

Doppler blood flow studies are now an integral part of the ultrasound examination of the abnormal gland. Doppler insonation frequencies of 2.5 to 5 MHz are used with a high pass filter to reduce the effects of vessel wall and other non-vascular movements. The normal Doppler time velocity (spectral) waveform signals for all the major intra-abdominal vessels have been well-documented.[24] Although understanding of abnormal signals is incomplete, changes in the time velocity waveform do reflect the effect of pancreatic disease on surrounding vasculature (Fig. 10). In addition, pancreatic neoplasms have specific Doppler

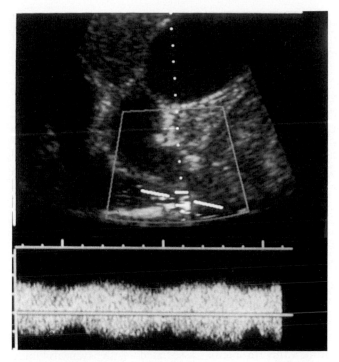

Fig. 10 Spectral Doppler. Trace of high velocity flow in the portal vein at a stenosis produced by a compressing pancreatic mass. Note the reversed flow component indicating flow disturbance.

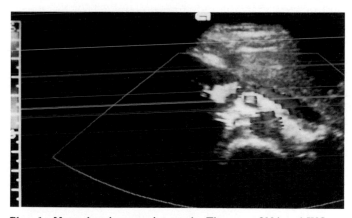

Plate 1 Normal peripancreatic vessels. The aorta, SMA and IVC are seen in transverse section with the splenic vein and proximal portal vein crossing transversely anterior to the SMA. This figure is reproduced in colour in the colour plate section at the front of this volume.

signals which can aid differentiation from benign disease.

Colour flow mapping (colour Doppler) complements spectral Doppler with useful anatomical information on the position of flowing blood and the relationships with masses (Plate 1).

Endoscopic ultrasound

Endoscopic ultrasound provides another means of over-

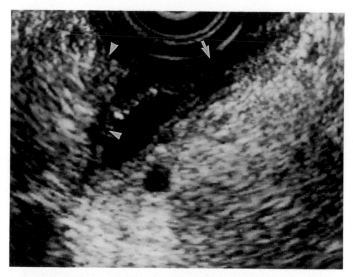

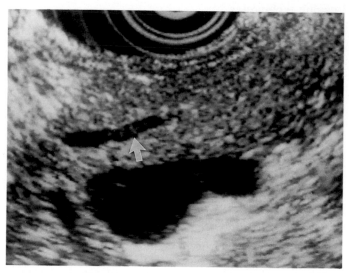

Fig. 11   Ampullary tumour. Endoscopic ultrasound showing tumour invading the bile duct (arrowheads) and duodenal wall (arrow).

Fig. 12   Duct dilatation. Endoscopic ultrasound image of a minimally dilated pancreatic duct (arrow).

coming the problems associated with transabdominal ultrasound. Conventional duodenoscopes have been modified to incorporate an ultrasound transducer at or near their tip. Both linear array and transverse radial scanners have been used. The linear array systems have a smaller field of view than the radial transducers which produce a 360° image. The latter are shorter in length and therefore impede scope flexibility to a lesser degree. They are covered by a rubber balloon which, when distended with fluid, ensures good contact with the bowel wall for acoustic transmission. As with intra-operative scanning, the close proximity of the target organ to the transducer allows a high frequency transducer to be used.

The duodenoscope is passed under visual control to the third part of the duodenum, after distension of the bowel with air. The air is then removed, the balloon distended and the scope slowly withdrawn. The head of the pancreas and uncinate process can be imaged through the duodenal wall, the body and neck through the gastric antrum and the tail through the stomach body. Resolution is much better than with transabdominal scanning so that small lesions not previously seen may be identified (Figs 11 and 12). It is more sensitive in identifying peripancreatic adenopathy and a better assessment of ductal anatomy can be made.[25]

It may be also possible to obtain biopsy specimens with this technique.

Intra-operative ultrasound

For intra-operative ultrasound linear array probes of up to 10 MHz are used to provide good resolution of structures close to the probe face. The transducer may be gas sterilised but covering with a sterile plastic drape or sheath is more practical and generally satisfactory. The surgically exposed pancreas is examined directly. To improve superficial resolution the lesser sac may be part-filled with saline and the probe held just above the tissue surface.[26]

Manipulation of the probe is best performed by the radiologist who is more familiar with ultrasound landmarks. If possible the patient should be scanned from the right side. Many intra-operative probes have a very short focus and the scanning technique should aim to bring the target into the focal zone. Intra-operative ultrasound is of value in searching for small tumours, such as insulinomas, and in defining the pancreatic anatomy, particularly of the ductal system, prior to surgery. Small calculi, cysts and vascular abnormalities are well-demonstrated.

REFERENCES

1 Lees W R. Pancreatic ultrasonography. Clin Gastroenterol 1984; 13(3): 763–789

2 The pancreas. In: Gray's anatomy. 37th edition. Williams P L, Warwick R, Dyson M, Bannister L H. Edinburgh: Churchill Livingstone. 1989: p 1380–1384

3 Ravitch M M. The pancreas in infants and children. Surg Clin North Am 1975; 55: 377–385

4 Hyden W H. The true nature of annular pancreas. Ann Surg 1963; 157: 71–77

5 Seifert G. Congenital anomalies. In: Kloppel G, Heitz P U. eds. Pancreatic pathology. New York: Churchill Livingstone. 1984: p 22–26

6 Cotton P B. Congenital anomaly of pancreas divisum as a cause of obstructive pain and pancreatitis. Gut 1980; 21: 105

7 Neumann C H, Hessel S J. CT of the pancreatic tail. AJR 1980; 35: 741–745

8 Niederau C, Sonnenberg A, Muller J, Erkenbrecht J, Scholten T, Fritsch W. Sonographic measurements of the normal liver, spleen, pancreas and portal vein. Radiology 1983; 149: 537–540

9 Weill F, Schraub A, Eisenscher A, Bougoin A. Ultrasonography of the normal pancreas: success rate and criteria for normality. Radiology 1977; 123: 417–423

10 De Graff C, Taylor K J W, Simmonds B, Rosenfield A. Gray scale echography of the pancreas. Reevaluation of normal size. Radiology 1978; 129: 157–161

11 Donovan P J. Technique of examination and normal pancreatic anatomy. In: Siegleman S S. ed. Computed tomography of the pancreas. New York: Churchill Livingstone. 1983: p 1–32

12 Goldberg B. The pancreas. Clin Diagn Ultrasound 1988; 23: 165–193

13 Filly R A, London S S. The normal pancreas: acoustic characteristics and frequency of imaging. JCU 1979; 7: 121–124

14 Marks V M, Filly R A, Callen P W. Ultrasonic evaluation of normal pancreatic echogenicity and its relation to fat deposition. Radiology 1980; 137: 457–459

15 Kreel L, Haertal M, Katz D. Computed tomography of the normal pancreas. J Comput Assist Tomogr 1977; 1: 290–299

16 Gupta A K, Arenson A M, Mckee J D. Effect of steroid ingestion on pancreatic echogenicity. JCU 1987; 15: 171–174

17 Worthen N J, Beaubeau D. Normal pancreatic echogenicity: relation to age and body fat. AJR 1982; 139: 1095–1098

18 Donald J, Shorvon P, Lees W R. A hypoechoic area within the head of the pancreas. Clin Radiol 1990; 41: 337–338

19 Bryan P J. Appearance of normal pancreatic duct. JCU 1982; 10: 63–66

20 Bolondi L, Gaiani S, Casanova S, Testa P, Priori P, Labo G. Improvement of pancreatic ultrasound imaging after secretin administration. Ultrasound Med Biol 1983; 9: 497–501

21 Lee J K T, Stanley R J, Melson G L, Sagel S S. Pancreatic imaging by ultrasound and computed tomography: a general review. Radiol Clin North Am 1979; 16: 105–117

22 Warren P S, Garret W J, Kossoff G. The liquid filled stomach: an ultrasonic window to the upper abdomen. JCU 1978; 6: 295–302

23 Vuoria P, Suramo I, Hyvarinen S. Transmission media for ultrasonography. Radiology 1980; 135: 520–522

24 Taylor K J W, Burns P T, Woodcock J P, Wells P N T. Blood flow in deep abdominal and pelvic vessels: ultrasonic pulsed Doppler analysis. Radiology 1985; 154: 487–493

25 Rifkin M D. Endoscopic ultrasonography of the gastrointestinal tract. Clin Diagn Ultrasound 1987; 23: 167–189

26 Charboneau J W, Gorman B, Reading C C, James M E, Grant C S. Intraoperative ultrasonography of pancreatic endocrine tumours. Clin Diagn Ultrasound 1987; 23: 123–134

Pancreatic inflammatory disease

Steven Garber and William R. Lees

Acute pancreatitis

Aetiology

The incidence of alcoholic pancreatitis is increasing in most countries of the Western world. Nevertheless, over 60% of cases in the United Kingdom are caused by gallstones and are more likely to be fatal, probably because of early bacterial contamination of necrotic pancreatic tissue.[1,2]

The mumps virus, hyperlipidaemia and hypercalcaemia can all cause acute pancreatitis and, although many other aetiologies are listed in the medical literature, these are relatively uncommon and clinically unimportant, being largely based on anecdotal case reports.

Many different experimental models of acute pancreatitis have been constructed but only three features of relevance to the disease in man can be derived from animal studies: reflux of bile or duodenal contents into the pancreatic duct system, an increase in intraduct pressure, and bacterial contamination of the interstitial spaces of the pancreatic parenchyma.

The most consistent experimental cause is elevation of the pressure in the pancreatic duct system. Above a pressure of 60 cm of water the basement membranes of alveoli rupture allowing duct contents to escape into the interstitium. This alone is enough to cause acute pancreatitis, but the presence of bile or duodenal content, particularly enterokinase, accelerates enzyme activation. Bacterial contamination leads to early infection of necrotic material.

The mechanism of alcohol induction of pancreatitis remains subject to debate (see below).

Definition

An accepted international definition of acute pancreatitis is 'an acute condition typically presenting with abdominal pain and usually associated with raised pancreatic enzymes in blood or urine, due to inflammatory disease of the pancreas.' The vagueness of this definition reveals the poverty of our understanding of the underlying pathology.[3]

Most of our knowledge of the progress of acute pancreatitis is based on radiological studies; the separation of acute pancreatitis into acute interstitial and necrotising varieties is of practical value. Acute interstitial pancreatitis (AIP) is a mild disease characterised by rapid recovery and complete restitution of the pancreas to normal whereas in necrotising pancreatitis there is irreversible destruction of the gland; it may be subclassified as mild (less than 50% of the pancreas necrosed) or severe. Mortality is much higher in the severe form.[4]

Pathomorphology

Histopathological studies of acute pancreatitis are difficult to perform because of the rapid autodigestion that occurs in pancreatic tissue after death. Despite this, all cases of severe and long-standing pancreatitis show a common feature: large and confluent foci of peripancreatic fat necrosis. These foci extend along the interstitial septa into the parenchyma of the pancreas itself and are associated with necrosis of contiguous acini.

Venous thrombosis, haemorrhage and infarction characterise advanced parenchymal damage; involvement of the parenchyma is irregular with necrosis often being very localised. These observations indicate that acute pancreatitis advances mainly through progression of fat necrosis across the surface of the gland, with subsequent patchy vascular damage leading to infarction.[5]

This theory is consistent with the available imaging evidence, where glandular tissue can appear well-perfused with normal architecture in the first 24 hours, patchy or confluent necrosis only becoming evident beyond 48 hours.

Clinical grading

Two clinical methods are commonly used for early assessment of the severity of acute pancreatitis. A cumulative score of clinical features can be used. On admission the key factors are: age over 55 years, white blood cell count >16 000, blood glucose >10 mmol/l, serum LDH >700 IU, and an AST >250 units. Other important prognostic factors within the first 48 hours of admission are a rising blood urea nitrogen (BUN) >5 mg%, PaO_2 <60 mm/mg and a serum calcium <2 mmol/l. Prognostic factor analysis provides a reliable method of identifying patients at risk of severe disease early in the course of the illness.[6,7]

Alternatively, a simple analysis of peritoneal lavage fluid has been proposed. This can be performed at the bedside and has similar accuracy in discriminating severe from mild pancreatitis. Dark coloured fluid with the appearance of prune juice is a strong indication of pancreatic necrosis with extension of the inflammatory process into the peritoneal cavity.[8]

Radiological grading methods based on morphological criteria have also been developed (see below).

Despite the increasing incidence of acute pancreatitis, mortality rates have steadily reduced over the past 10 years. This improvement can be attributed to improved metabolic maintenance (particularly with total parenteral nutrition), better management of patients in respiratory failure and active radiological monitoring of acute pancreatitis and its complications, especially the detection of pancreatic necrosis or abscess, leading to earlier intervention.

Acute interstitial pancreatitis Mild acute interstitial pancreatitis (AIP) causes swelling of the parenchyma of the gland, which may be focal or lobular in distribution. The duct system is compressed. Oedema accumulates in the peripancreatic fat spaces and there may also be a small transudate into the lesser sac or adjacent peritoneal recesses (Figs 1 to 3).

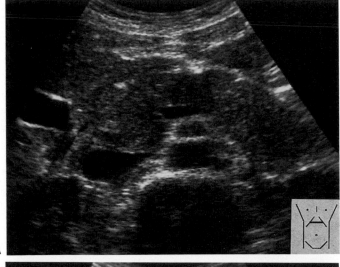

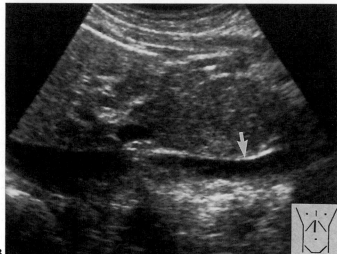

Fig. 1 Mild acute interstitial pancreatitis. A: Transverse section. **B:** Longitudinal section. There is generalised enlargement of the gland with a slightly heterogeneous parenchyma and an overall reduction in reflectivity. Note the indentation of the cava (arrow) by the swollen pancreatic head in B.

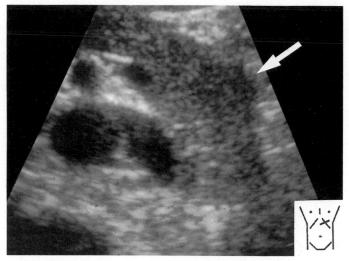

Fig. 2 Focal acute interstitial pancreatitis. A single lobule is enlarged and of reduced reflectivity (arrow).

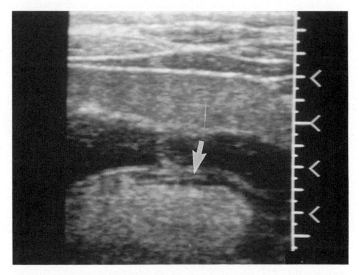

Fig. 3 Moderate acute interstitial pancreatitis. The pancreas is swollen with a small fluid collection in the lesser sac (arrow).

Ultrasound is highly specific in the diagnosis of AIP, typically showing pancreatic enlargement, a generalised reduction in parenchymal reflectivity and a relative increase in the reflectivity of the walls of a normal or narrowed duct system. Small fluid accumulations are easy to recognise but oedema in the surrounding fat may obscure the pancreatic boundaries. It is important to note that the changes in mild AIP may be focal: patchy oedema or necrosis can be confined to one or more individual pancreatic lobules which are 7 to 8 mm in diameter and are divided from one another by fine fibrous septa. Intrapancreatic oedema may render the septa visible as thin, bright lines radiating from the centre to the periphery of the gland. Colour Doppler frequently shows hyperaemia in and around the poorly reflective foci of acute pancreatitis.

CT is less sensitive in showing the intrapancreatic changes in mild AIP but demonstrates the effects on the surrounding tissues better.[9] Oedema in peripancreatic fat results in a density midway between fat and fluid and small fluid collections are easily recognised. Thickening of the peritoneum and Gerota's fascia are specific for retroperitoneal inflammation but, if these are the sole features on CT, they do not necessarily indicate the presence of active disease.[10]

The diagnosis of acute pancreatitis is usually made on clinical grounds together with a serum amylase elevated above 1000 IU/l. However, even in severe pancreatitis, the rise in serum amylase may be transitory and unrecorded so the diagnosis may be unclear. The majority of patients recover with conservative management. Imaging studies are not needed at this stage but it is very important that an ultrasound scan of the gallbladder and biliary tree be performed during recovery to detect gallstones. Over 30% of patients with gallstone pancreatitis will have further attacks of pancreatitis within 6 months and the recurrences are often more severe. Virtually all these can be prevented by interval cholecystectomy. The scan is best performed immediately prior to discharge when visualisation is better than during the acute stage, because of meteorism.

Complications are uncommon following AIP, but significant pseudocysts can follow even mild attacks and should be excluded by ultrasound or CT scanning prior to discharge.[11]

Necrotising pancreatitis For patients with clinically severe acute pancreatitis, the initial ultrasound examination should concentrate on the biliary tree; significant dilation (CBD >6 mm) is considered to be an indication for urgent endoscopy and biliary sphincterotomy with removal of any choledochal stones.[12]

A scan of the pancreas performed too early in the disease process may be misleading as the gland can appear to be remarkably normal in the first 24 hours. Meteorism, abdominal tenderness and other problems of the acute abdomen often preclude satisfactory ultrasound visualisation, although scans of the head and tail of the pancreas can usually be obtained through the flanks (Figs 4 and 5).

Respiratory failure from respiratory distress syndrome is the most common cause of death early in the disease, particularly in patients with fulminant necrosis. This is potentially reversible provided the patient can be adequately ventilated. Renal failure is particularly prevalent in older patients.

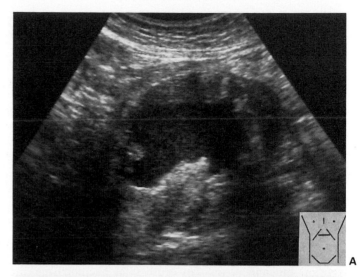

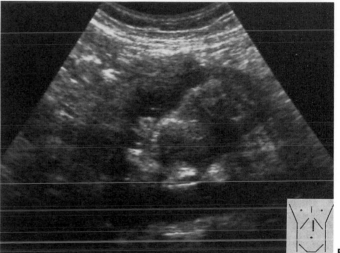

Fig. 5 Severe necrotising pancreatitis. A: Transverse section. **B:** Longitudinal section. The pancreas has been replaced by a heterogeneous mass with no discernible anatomical features.

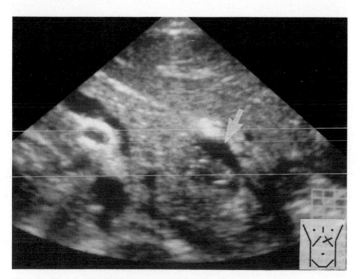

Fig. 4 Focal necrotising pancreatitis. A small focus of parenchymal necrosis in the tail is associated with leakage of juice into the peripancreatic fat space (arrow).

Septic pancreatitis Septic complications are the other major causes of death from pancreatitis. These include cholangitis (especially when the biliary tree is obstructed), infected pancreatic necrosis and infection of the peripancreatic spaces.[6] Infected pancreatic necrosis still carries a mortality of over 90% and the only effective treatment is resection of the necrotic tissue. Neither CT nor ultrasound scanning can diagnose infection reliably in the absence of gas formation, which is uncommon (about 10%),[13] diagnosis requiring biopsy guided by CT or ultrasound. The demonstration of infection on an immediate Gram stain (about 50% of cases[14]) is an indication for urgent surgery.

Percutaneous catheter drainage of infected pancreatic necrosis is rarely effective because of the viscid nature of the fluid, although percutaneous lavage may have some value. However, infection of a pseudocyst or a peripancreatic space is a less urgent complication which does not always require formal surgical intervention and can often be managed solely by catheter drainage.[15] Complications include haemorrhage, usually self-limiting, and empyema. However, resolution is often slow (up to 6 months) and cutaneous or enteric fistulae may develop.

Complications of acute pancreatitis The important complications of acute pancreatitis are:

- biliary obstruction;
- obstruction to the gastrointestinal tract;
- pancreatic ascites;
- renal obstruction;
- aneurysm formation;
- pseudocyst formation.

Most of these are minor and require no active intervention but aneurysms can cause fatal haemorrhage and should be searched for by colour Doppler or dynamic CT scanning in any case of severe necrotising pancreatitis. It is important to note that they take 2 to 3 weeks to develop.[10]

Pseudocysts Pathologically a pseudocyst is defined as a collection of pancreatic fluid with a high amylase content surrounded by a fibrous wall. The thickness of the wall depends on the duration of the cyst (Figs 6 to 8). Virtually all patients with clinically significant acute pancreatitis develop peripancreatic fluid collections in the first week of the disease, though only a few form true pseudocysts;[16,17] the majority resolve within 6 weeks but those that persist longer rarely resolve spontaneously.[18]

If the pancreatic duct system is disrupted, large quantities of pancreatic juice may leak. If this involves a small branch duct, the breach may heal, closing the communication between the cyst and the pancreatic duct but, when

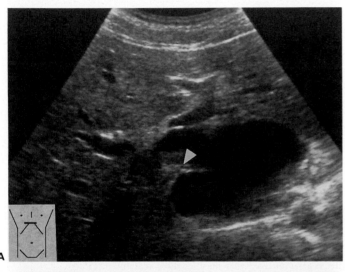

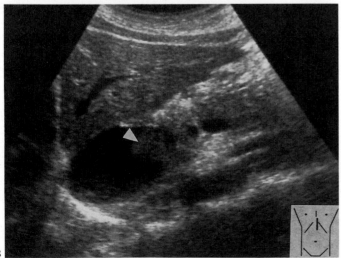

Fig. 6 Pseudocyst. A: Transverse, **B:** longitudinal scans in the upper abdomen show a small pseudocyst above the pancreas, probably lying in the lesser sac. The wall is thin (indicating that it is recent) and irregular in parts (arrowheads).

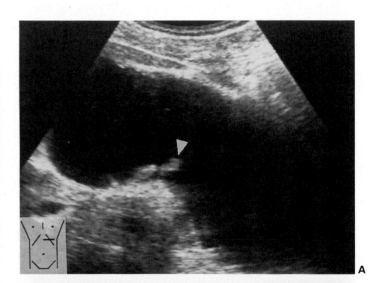

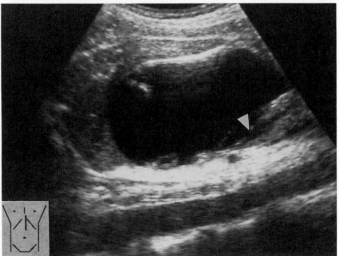

Fig. 7 Pseudocyst. A: Transverse, **B:** longitudinal scans in the epigastrium show a large pseudocyst extending to the left of the midline, along the lie of the lesser sac. Note the debris in the sac (arrowheads); its walls are thicker than in the case illustrated in Figure 6.

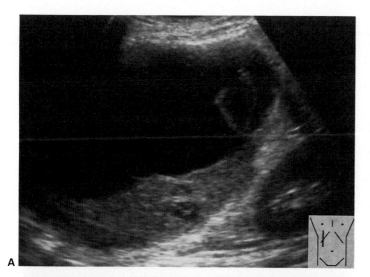

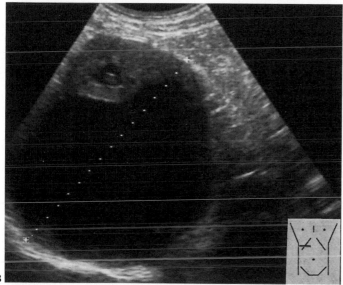

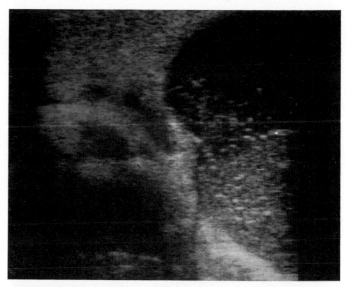

Fig. 9 Infected pseudocyst. An intra-operative scan showing low level echoes in the cavity.

Fig. 8 Large pseudocyst. A: Longitudinal, **B:** transverse scans of a 15 cm pseudocyst extending over the right kidney. Its wall is well-defined.

the main pancreatic duct is disrupted, oedema and fibrosis in the cyst wall may temporarily occlude the communication. Percutaneous drainage of the cyst often reveals the underlying communication once the pressure in the cyst has been relieved.

The surgical and radiological literature is replete with descriptions of chronic pseudocysts which have dissected through various tissue planes to unusual locations.[19] With prompt diagnosis and early treatment few cysts are now allowed time to dissect into remote locations and the vast majority lie close to the pancreas, most in the lesser sac.[13]

Pseudocysts develop in up to 50% of patients 2 to 3 weeks after a severe attack of acute pancreatitis (Figs 9 and 10). In the early stages considerable regression and healing may occur but, if there is no early response (a 6

week limit is recommended by Bradley[18]), percutaneous drainage is required and can be curative. This simple, well-tolerated procedure allows pseudocysts to be adequately drained through catheters as small as 5.5 F – it is rarely necessary to use catheters of larger than 7.5 F. Once the pseudocyst is decompressed and evacuated, an improvement in the patient's general condition can be expected and the choice then lies between early surgery and continued catheter drainage.

With non-communicating cysts, drainage ceases promptly after evacuation and the catheter can be safely removed after a few days, following a check ultrasound. If the cyst communicates with the duct system, pancreatic juice continues to flow at 30 to 200 ml daily. The communication may be demonstrated by ERCP which, though ordinarily contra-indicated in the presence of a pseudocyst, carries a minimal risk of rupture with a drainage catheter in situ.

Percutaneous drainage of pseudocysts after acute pancreatitis is curative in approximately one third of cases.[20] Thus it seems reasonable to continue percutaneous drainage for 2 to 3 weeks; but, if drainage persists, the pancreas distal to the duct disruption should be resected after mapping pancreatography (endoscopic or antegrade).

Surgical cyst-gastrostomy, the conventional surgical method, is most successful in long-standing pseudocysts with a thick and fibrous wall to which a suitable enterostomy can be made. It is less successful in the acute phase with underlying duct disruption, whereas a simple distal pancreatectomy is almost always effective. Virtually all cyst-gastrostomies will have closed after 6 to 8 weeks, and the advantage of this procedure over catheter drainage is unproven.

Pseudocysts often lie close to the spleen and its pedicle so that splenic vein thrombosis and splenic infarction are

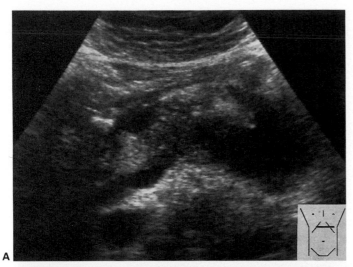

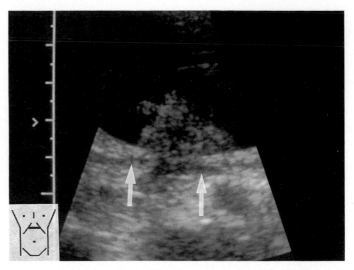

Fig. 11 Traumatic pancreatitis. A transverse view through the cyst shows a blood clot attached at the point of disruption of the gland. The main pancreatic duct can be seen to run through the disrupted segment (arrows).

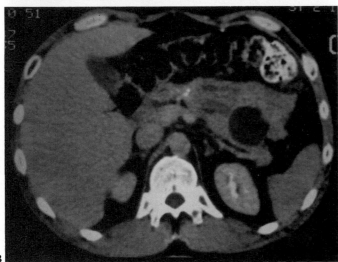

Fig. 10 Acute pancreatitis. A: Ultrasound, **B:** CT of a complex phlegmon arising from the tail of the pancreas and extending into the splenic pedicle. There is a small associated pseudocyst.

common complications. The thrombosis may extend to include the superior mesenteric and portal veins also. Damage to the splenic artery by a pseudocyst is the most common cause of aneurysm formation. Subsequently gastric varices may develop and the patient may re-present with a haematemesis.

Traumatic pancreatitis Severe pancreatic trauma almost always disrupts the duct, spilling pancreatic juice into the peripancreatic spaces resulting in pseudocysts that are often very large. With penetrating injuries, the disruption can occur at any point and there is usually also traumatic necrosis (Fig. 11).[21] The neck of the pancreas is most vulnerable to blunt injury, the duct being ruptured where it is compressed against the aorta and spine. Even complete transection of the pancreas can be clinically silent until the development of pancreatic ascites or a large pseudocyst. Distal pancreatectomy is required if there has been

complete disruption of the main pancreatic duct. A pancreatogram is essential in planning surgery.

As with communicating pseudocysts, percutaneous decompression of the fluid collection improves the general wellbeing of the patient and allows a contrast study of the distal pancreas.

Relapsing pancreatitis The concept of a relapsing form of acute pancreatitis was originally proposed in Marseilles in 1960, but it is no longer recognised as a distinct entity.[22] Repeated attacks of acute pancreatitis are common in patients with gallstones and in cases of untreated hypercalcaemia and hyperlipidaemia.

Acute pancreatitis can also occur as an exacerbation of chronic pancreatitis. It is this latter group of patients that has caused most of the confusion in classification. Recurrent attacks of acute pancreatitis in patients with underlying chronic pancreatitis vary from bouts of abdominal pain to full-blown attacks of pancreatitis. Careful ultrasonography usually reveals a focus of reduced reflectivity confined to a small portion of the pancreas or even to a single lobule. This may also be associated with a small localised peripancreatic effusion or an intrapancreatic collection. These small foci of acute pancreatitis are usually hypervascular on colour Doppler. Similar bouts of focal acute pancreatitis may follow percutaneous biopsy procedures and ERCP if the injection pressure has been too high.

Obstructive pancreatopathy Pancreatic fibrosis and atrophy of the parenchyma follow partial or complete obstruction of the main pancreatic duct. On histology this is a desmoplastic reaction most commonly seen surrounding infiltrating pancreatic carcinomas but also found with any intraduct lesion that interferes with free flow of pancreatic juice.[23] The lesion may be a small tumour, neurofibroma, smooth muscle tumour and even heterotopic pancreatic tissue infiltrating the major or minor papilla and is often obscured by the surrounding fibrosis and can be difficult to find, even in resected specimens.[24]

Many cases of pancreatitis secondary to congenital abnormalities of the pancreas have their origin in incomplete drainage. Pancreas divisum has an incidence of approximately 6% but is seen in a higher proportion of patients with acute pancreatitis or obstructive pancreatopathy; whether it is a genuine aetiological factor or simply reflects selection bias of patients for ERCP has never been satisfactorily resolved. Careful ultrasonography often reveals the main pancreatic continuing towards the cranial

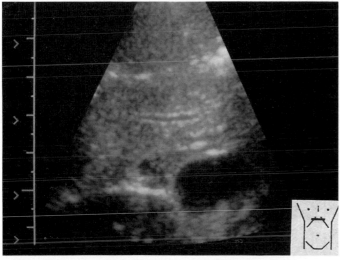

Fig. 12 Pancreas divisum. Transverse section through the head of the pancreas. The duct runs ventral to the more usual course.

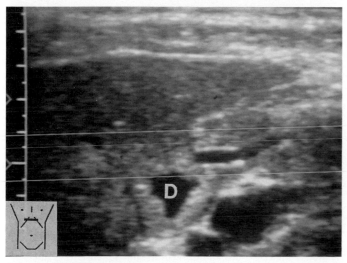

Fig. 13 Obstructive pancreatopathy. There is dilatation of the dorsal duct caused by poor drainage via the accessory papilla. The duct is visible as it enters the fluid filled duodenum (D).

and ventral aspect of the duodenal loop, a sign of dominant drainage via the duct of Santorini (Figs 12 and 13). The ventral segment of the gland is relatively echo-poor because it does not contain fat in the form of intracellular vacuoles which are a feature of the dorsal anlage; it can be distinguished from the more reflective dorsal segment in up to one third of normal subjects (see Ch. 8, p. 138).

The pancreas divisum anomaly can modify the distribution of disease. For example, in gallstone pancreatitis only the ventral pancreas may be affected while, because drainage via the minor papilla is more precarious, obstructive pancreatopathy may be confined to the dorsal portion.

Other congenital anomalies of pancreatic drainage are rare and, with the exception of the annular pancreas, usually asymptomatic. Drainage of the annular pancreas may be so poor that it results in pancreatic fibrosis with subsequent duodenal stenosis.

Chronic pancreatitis

Aetiology and pathomorphology

Chronic pancreatitis is a relatively uncommon disease whose incidence varies from 0.2% to 3% in autopsy series. It seems to have become more common in the past 20 years and this is believed to be a real change rather than merely the result of better diagnosis. The rise has probably been caused by an increase in alcohol consumption. The pathogenesis of chronic pancreatitis is still unclear: it is even uncertain whether chronic pancreatitis is a discrete entity and how it relates to acute pancreatitis.

The morphological features of advanced chronic pancreatitis are irregular scarring of the pancreatic parenchyma (typically on a lobular scale), strictures of the main pancreatic duct and stenosis of the side branches (usually at their junctions with the main duct). Intraductal protein plugs are a common finding and these frequently calcify in severe disease. Many cases show focal necrosis with intrapancreatic pseudocyst formation.

Two explanations of the mechanism of alcohol damage have been proposed. An alteration of the pancreatic juice such that proteins precipitate out to form plugs that obstruct the pancreatic ducts is one suggestion.[23] Focal obstructive pancreatitis with degeneration and fibrosis of the pancreatic parenchyma would follow and the causal plugs may calcify. An alternative proposal is that alcohol directly damages the pancreatic parenchyma, producing focal necrosis. Healing by fibrosis causes strictures of the duct system which interfere with the flow of pancreatic secretions leading to precipitation of protein plugs upstream from the stenoses.[25] It is probable that both mechanisms operate in the majority of patients with alcoholic pancreatitis. The first theory explains the phenomenon of idiopathic calcific chronic pancreatitis; the second explains the predominantly parenchymal changes in the alcoholic, with severe pancreatic pain but minimal duct changes on pancreatography.

An understanding of the evolution of chronic pancreatitis is important for the interpretation of the morphological changes.[26]

Early chronic pancreatitis

The morphological features of early chronic pancreatitis are:

a) parenchymal damage with fibrosis;
b) periductal fibrosis predominantly at bifurcations of the duct system;
c) irregularities of the main pancreatic duct;

d) increase in bulk of the pancreatic parenchyma;
e) intraduct protein plugs.

A combination of imaging techniques is required to demonstrate all of these features. Pancreatography is the most sensitive for duct changes and is generally regarded as the most specific method of diagnosis.[27] In non-calcific chronic pancreatitis CT scanning has a sensitivity of no better than 50% and may be misleading unless there is significant duct dilatation or cyst formation.[28] High resolution ultrasonography is capable of demonstrating parenchymal changes involving the main pancreatic duct and, under good conditions of visualisation, can demonstrate the side branches. However, ultrasonography is notorious for being operator- and patient-dependent and has a lower success rate than CT scanning in visualising the entire pancreas (Fig. 14).

Severe chronic pancreatitis

Severe chronic pancreatitis is easy to diagnose by ultrasound, CT or even plain film radiography. The morphological features are:

a) strictures of the main pancreatic duct with upstream dilatation;
b) calculi within the duct system;
c) confluent parenchymal fibrosis;
d) cavities;
e) involvement of surrounding structures by inflammation (Figs 15 and 16).

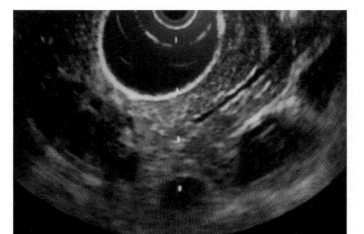

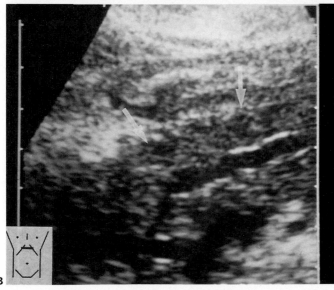

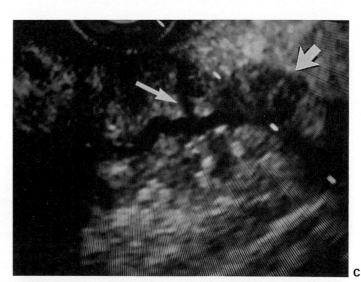

Fig. 14 Chronic pancreatitis. A: An endoscopic ultrasound of mild chronic pancreatitis. The parenchyma is normal but there is an increase in the reflectivity of the walls of the main duct. **B:** A section through the head and mid-body showing a dilated duct with irregularly reflective walls. The parenchyma contains some echo-poor lobules (arrows). **C:** Moderate chronic pancreatitis. An endoscopic scan shows dilatation of the main duct and of a side branch (arrow) which drains a poorly reflective lobule. Another inflamed lobule is seen with prominent intralobular septa (broad arrow). Highly reflective foci are seen throughout the parenchyma.

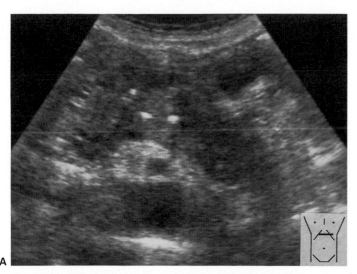

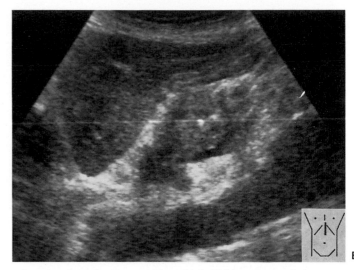

Fig. 15 Calcific pancreatitis. A: Transverse, **B:** longitudinal section of a moderately enlarged pancreas with multiple highly reflective foci representing calcification.

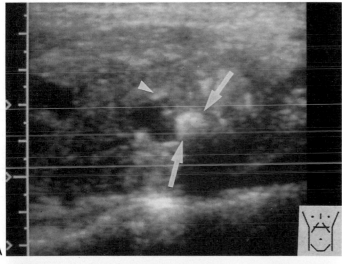

Fig. 16 Chronic calcific pancreatitis. A: Oblique section through the head of the pancreas showing a large calculus dilating the duct (arrows). The whole gland is bulky with small calculi within the parenchyma (arrowhead). **B:** Transverse section through the pancreatic body shows an obstructing calculus (arrow) causing duct dilatation (7 mm). The surrounding parenchyma is atrophic. **C:** Endoscopic ultrasound scan showing small calculi within the duct in the ventral segment (arrow). Note the difference in reflectivity between the ventral segment and the surrounding dorsal gland.

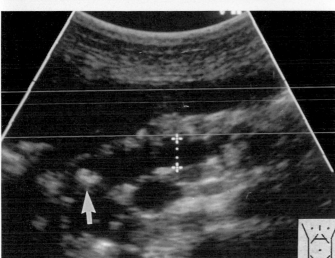

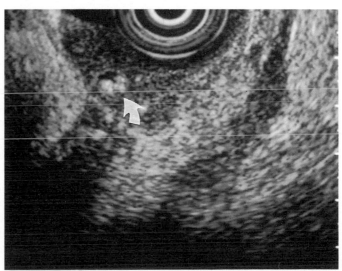

Grading of chronic pancreatitis

The various imaging techniques view the same morphological features in slightly different ways. In order to establish a common descriptive base, a grading scheme for the morphology of chronic pancreatitis was proposed at the Classification Meeting in Cambridge in 1983.[3,29] This is summarised in Table 1.

Table 1   Grading of chronic pancreatitis

Ultrasound and CT signs of chronic pancreatitis:
   Main duct dilated (>4 mm)
   Gland enlarged (2 × N)
   Cavities (<10 mm)
   Irregular ducts
   Focal acute pancreatitis
   Parenchymal heterogeneity
   Duct wall echoes increased
   Irregular head/body contours

	ERCP	Ultrasound and CT
1. Normal	Quality study demonstrating whole gland to be normal	
2. Equivocal	< 3 abnormal branches	One sign only
3. Mild	> 3 abnormal branches	Two or more signs
4. Moderate	Abnormal main duct and branches	Two or more signs
5. Marked	Abnormal main duct and branches, with one or more of: large cavities (> 10 mm) gross gland enlargement (> 2 × N) intraduct filling defects or calculi duct obstruction, stricture or gross irregularity contiguous organ invasion	

The diagnosis of chronic pancreatitis cannot be made on the basis of a single morphological characteristic, except where there is stricture of the main pancreatic duct or calculi. The diagnosis can be made if two features are present, but with limited confidence; if three or more are present, the diagnosis is highly specific.

From pancreatography, non-calcific chronic pancreatitis can be classified into mild and moderate forms, depending on whether there is involvement of the main pancreatic duct system. Demonstration of at least three abnormal side branches is required for diagnosis of mild chronic pancreatitis, and evidence of narrowing or irregularity of the main pancreatic duct for a diagnosis of moderate disease.

Fluid filled cavities are frequently seen. These are pancreatic or peripancreatic collections which fill with contrast medium on pancreatography. They represent cysts, pseudocysts, or even abscesses and it is impossible to infer their true nature from the pancreatogram. Cavities may be large, but if smaller than 10 mm in diameter are rarely of major significance and are considered a feature of mild or moderate disease.

Common bile duct narrowing may be caused by fibrosis in the head of the pancreas. This is uncommonly seen in mild or moderate pancreatitis but occurs in up to 25% of patients with severe disease.

The features of severe chronic pancreatitis are intraduct calculi, strictures of the main pancreatic duct with upstream dilatation, cavities of greater than 10 mm in diameter and extension of the inflammatory process to involve contiguous structures. Any one of these signs is sufficient to alter the grade from moderate to severe, provided that there is also involvement of the main pancreatic duct and its side branches.

Chronic pancreatitis may be a focal disease involving small segments of pancreatic tissue. The descriptive term 'groove pancreatitis' has recently been proposed for the common type of focal pancreatitis, which affects the segment of pancreas lying between the common bile duct and the duodenum. This may result in dense focal fibrosis, indistinguishable from a desmoplastic tumour.[30]

The value of a grading system is that the underlying morphology can be described in the same terms by different imaging techniques, each of which shows only some of the features. This leads to repeatable description that allows populations to be compared and individual patients to be systematically followed up.[29] There is good correlation between ERCP and ultrasonography using this scheme.[31]

The natural history of chronic pancreatitis is still not adequately understood. In patients with alcoholic chronic pancreatitis who continue to drink, the disease appears to progress inexorably to calcific chronic pancreatitis with duct obstruction, fibrosis and atrophy of functioning pancreatic tissue.[32,33] Paradoxically, the pain of chronic pancreatitis may remit when all functioning pancreatic tissue has been destroyed and hence chronic pancreatitis may 'burn out' in its end stages.[34]

Complications of chronic pancreatitis

The principal complications of chronic pancreatitis are pseudocyst formation, biliary obstruction, portal vein thrombosis and duodenal obstruction. Pseudocysts in this condition are almost always secondary to complete duct obstruction by a calculus and rarely respond to conservative measures or percutaneous drainage.[15]

The peribiliary fibrosis of chronic pancreatitis typically leads to the classical 'rat tail' stricture in the distal common bile duct but short strictures indistinguishable from their malignant equivalent are frequently seen. Evidence of previous portal vein fibrosis is commonly seen on colour Doppler imaging, with visualisation of varices or portal venous collaterals after occlusion of the main portal vein. The portal vein thrombosis has usually been clinically silent with full physiological compensation via collaterals.[35] Local high velocity flow can often be demonstrated by spectral (duplex) or colour Doppler in regions where the vein is compressed.

Surgery and chronic pancreatitis

Indications for pancreatic surgery are intractable pain with duct dilatation or focal fibrosis, recurrent pseudocyst formation and biliary or duodenal obstruction.

Focal pancreatitis with fibrosis can be impossible to distinguish from pancreatic cancer with a desmoplastic reaction, and biopsy is essential to establish a diagnosis prior to surgical intervention. Guided fine needle aspiration cytology has traditionally been used but has sensitivity of no better than 82% in a large series.[36] More recently cutting biopsy needles of 1.2 mm diameter have been employed to give true histology. These have a slightly higher complication rate but are more sensitive in the diagnosis of cancer and can give a specific histological diagnosis of chronic pancreatitis.

Percutaneous pancreatography

Provided the pancreatic duct is larger than 3 mm in diameter, puncture with a fine needle under ultrasound control for pancreatography is relatively simple. The technique appears to be safe and is successful in 90% of cases. Because a complete map of the pancreatic duct system is essential for adequate surgical planning, it is extremely useful in the 20% to 30% of cases of chronic pancreatitis where the pancreatogram provides inadequate information, either through failure to cannulate or because of a complete block in the main pancreatic duct.

Endoscopic ultrasonography

Commercial devices are now available that incorporate high resolution, high frequency (7.5 or 10 MHz) ultrasound probes mounted on the end of conventional side-viewing duodenoscopes. They are capable of resolution of the order of 0.2 mm. A tip-mounted ultrasound probe is placed into the second part of the duodenum using endoscopic techniques, and the probe is withdrawn past the ampulla of Vater, around the duodenal loop into the gastric antrum and then along the greater curve of the stomach. The entire pancreas can be visualised in over 70% of patients, and over 75% of the pancreas in 90%. The soft tissue display is very much better than that obtained by conventional ultrasound or CT scanning, showing the anatomy of the side branches of the pancreatic duct system together with high contrast resolution of the surrounding parenchyma.

Endoscopic ultrasonography is useful in discriminating the normal from the abnormal pancreas in patients with pain of suspected pancreatic origin, and for differentiating focal pancreatitis from pancreatic carcinoma. 10% to 15% of patients with pancreatic disease cannot be adequately evaluated with conventional imaging methods, and this technique is the most specific diagnostic method currently available, next to biopsy. It is as well-tolerated as any simple upper gastrointestinal endoscopy, carries no significant hazard, and can be performed as an outpatient procedure. The very small field of view obtained by the instrument and the invasive nature of the technique limit its application in the early stages of evaluation of pancreatic disease, but it is finding increasing acceptance in specialist pancreatic centres for the investigation of difficult pancreatic problems.

REFERENCES

1 Trapnell J E, Duncan E H L. Patterns of incidence in acute pancreatitis. BMJ 1975; 2: 179–183
2 Imrie C W, White S. A prospective study of acute pancreatitis. Br J Surg 1975; 62: 490–494
3 Sarner M, Cotton P B. Classification of pancreatitis. Gut 1984; 25: 756–759
4 Banks S, Wie L, Gersten M. Risk factors in acute pancreatitis. Am J Gastroenterol 1983; 78: 637–640
5 Gyr K, Heitz P U, Berlinger C. Pancreatitis. In: Kloppel G, Heitz P V. eds. Pancreatic pathology. Edinburgh: Churchill Livingstone. 1984: p 44–72
6 Ranson J H C. Acute pancreatitis: pathogenesis, outcome and treatment. Clin Gastroenterol 1984; 13: 843–863
7 Imrie C W, White S. A prospective study of acute pancreatitis. Br J Surg 1975; 62: 490–494
8 McMahon M J, Playforth M J, Pickard I R. A comparative study of methods for the prediction of severity of attacks of acute pancreatitis. Br J Surg 1980; 67: 22–25
9 Balthazar E J, Robinson D L, Megibow A J, Ranson J H. Acute pancreatitis: value of CT in establishing prognosis. Radiology 1990; 174: 331–336
10 Freeny P C. Computed tomography of the pancreas. Clin Gastroenterol 1984; 13: 791–818
11 Donovan P J, Sanders R C, Siegelman S S. Collections of fluid after pancreatitis: evaluation by computed tomography and ultrasonography. Radiol Clin North Am 1982; 20: 653–665
12 Safrany L, Cotton P B. A preliminary report: urgent duodenoscopic sphincterotomy for acute gallstone pancreatitis. Surgery 1981; 89: 424–428
13 Vernacchia F S, Jeffrey R B, Federle M P, et al. Pancreatic abscess: predictive value of early abdominal CT. Radiology 1987; 162: 435–438
14 Gerzof S G, Banks P A, Robbins A H, et al. Early diagnosis of pancreatic infection by computed tomography-guided aspiration. Gastroenterology 1987; 93: 1315–1320
15 Freeny P C, Lewis G P, Marks W M. Percutaneous catheter drainage of infected pancreatic fluid collections and abscesses. Radiology 1986; 161: 89
16 Hill M C, Barkin J, Isikoff M B, Silverstein W, Kalser M. Acute pancreatitis: clinical vs CT findings. AJR 1982; 139: 263–269
17 Sarti D A. Rapid development and spontaneous regression of pancreatic pseudocysts documented by ultrasound. Radiology 1977; 125: 789–793
18 Bradley E L, Clements L J. Spontaneous resolution of pancreatic pseudocyst: implications for timing operative intervention. Am J Surg 1976; 129: 23–28

19 Sankaran S, Walt A J. The natural and un-natural history of pancreatic pseudocysts. Br J Surg 1975; 62: 37–44

20 Barlin J S, Smith F R, Pereiras R. Therapeutic percutaneous aspiration of pancreatic pseudocysts. Dig Dis Sci 1981; 26: 585–586

21 Vallon A G, Lees W R, Cotton P B. Grey-scale ultrasonography and endoscopic pancreatography after pancreatic trauma. Br J Surg 1979; 66: 169–172

22 Singer M V, Gyr G E, Sarles H. Revised classification of pancreatitis. Report on the second international symposium on the classification of pancreatitis in Marseille, France 28–30 March 1984. Gastroenterology 1985; 89: 683–690

23 Sahel J, Sarles H. Chronic calcifying pancreatitis and obstructive pancreatitis – two entities. In: Gyr K, Singer M V, Sarles H. eds. Pancreatitis; concepts and classification. Amsterdam: Elsevier. 1984: p 47–49

24 Lowes J R, Lees W R, Cotton P B. Pancreatic duct dilatation after secretin stimulation in pancreas divisum. Pancreas 1989; 4: 371–374

25 Klopel G, Adler G, Kern H F. Pathomorphology of acute pancreatitis in relation to its clinical course and pathogenesis. In: Malfertheiner P, Ditschuneit H. eds. Diagnostic procedures in pancreatic disease. Berlin: Springer Verlag. 1986: p 135–139

26 Nagata A, Homma T, Tamai K, et al. A study of chronic pancreatitis by serial endoscopic pancreatography. Gastroenterology 1981; 81: 884–891

27 Cotton P B, Lees W R, Vallon A G. Grey-scale ultrasonography and endoscopic pancreatography in pancreatic diagnosis. Radiology 1980; 134: 453–459

28 Malfertheiner P, Buchler M. Correlation of imaging and function in chronic pancreatitis. Radiol Clin North Am 1989; 27: 51–64

29 Axon A T R, Classen M, Cotton P B, Creemer M, Freeny P C, Lees W R. Pancreatography in chronic pancreatitis: international definition. Gut 1984; 36: 1107–1112

30 Nix G A, Schmitz P I. Diagnostic features of chronic pancreatitis distal to benign and to malignant pancreatic duct obstruction. Diagnostic Imaging 1981; 50: 130–137

31 Jones S N, Frost R A, Lees W R. Diagnosis and grading of chronic pancreatitis by morphological criteria derived by ultrasound and pancreatography. Clin Radiol 1988; 39: 43–48

32 Ammann R W, Muench R, Otto R, Buehler H, Freiburghaus A U, Siegenthaler W. Evolution and regression of pancreatic calcification in chronic pancreatitis. A prospective long-term study of 107 patients. Gastroenterology 1988; 95: 1018–1028

33 Kalthoff L, Layer P, Clain J E. The course of alcoholic and non-alcoholic chronic pancreatitis. Dig Dis Sci 1984; 29: 953

34 Bornman P, Marks I N, Girdwood A H. Mechanism of pain in chronic alcohol induced pancreatitis (CAIP). In: Gyr K, Singer M V, Sarles H. eds. Pancreatitis; concepts and classification. Amsterdam: Elsevier. 1984: p 193–195

35 Ferrucci J T Jnr, Wittenberg J, Mueller P R. Computed body tomography in chronic pancreatitis. Radiology 1979; 130: 175–182

36 Hall-Craggs M A, Lees W R. Fine-needle aspiration biopsy: pancreatic and biliary tumours. AJR 1986; 147: 399–403

Pancreatic malignancy

Steven Garber and William R. Lees

INTRODUCTION

Carcinoma of the pancreas accounts for 10% of all cancers of the digestive system and is the fifth commonest cause of cancer-related death in the United States. It is a highly lethal malignancy with a 5 year survival of only 1% to 2%.[1] Its incidence has increased sharply over recent years: in England and Wales it has doubled since 1930.[2] Despite advances in imaging techniques attempts at early diagnosis have been unsuccessful and less than 10% of cases are suitable for resection.[3] The overall mean survival time from presentation remains unchanged at 6 months.

Pancreatic cancer is more common in men (male to female ratio of 1.5:1) but over the years this difference has decreased. The incidence of pancreatic cancer is age-related, being uncommon below 45 but becoming increasingly common with age and markedly so in the seventh and eighth decades. There is no significant geographical distribution and no important genetic, familial or social class factors have been identified.[2] An association between pancreatic cancer and smoking has been established but no other carcinogens have been convincingly defined.[4] Chronic alcoholism, a Western diet and pre-existing diabetes mellitus have been implicated as aetiological factors in some studies but the evidence for all of these remains inconclusive.

Clinical features

The most common presentation is with weight loss, abdominal pain and jaundice. Often these symptoms have been present for several months.[5] Pain is most often epigastric and radiates to the back in 60% of patients. Jaundice occurs at some time in the condition in 90% of cases and is progressive, although initially it may fluctuate in severity.

Pathology

Primary non-endocrine pancreatic tumours can be classified by their cell type into ductal, acinar and connective tissue types (Table 1). Metastases constitute up to 7% of pancreatic tumours in some studies, lymphoma being the most common.

Ductal adenocarcinoma

Ductal adenocarcinoma is the commonest type of pancreatic malignancy and most epidemiological research data relate to this type of lesion. On surgical specimens the majority of tumours range between 1.5 and 5 cm.[6] The mean tumour mass at presentation is 30 g and most patients die by the time it has grown to 75 g. Its rapid growth (mean volume doubling time around 60 days)

Table 1 Classification of non-endocrine pancreatic carcinoma

Cancer type	Relative incidence
Ductal cell origin	
Ductal adenocarcinoma	80%
Giant cell carcinoma	5%
Adenosquamous carcinoma	4%
Mucinous adenocarcinoma	2%
Microadenocarcinoma	3%
Cystadenocarcinoma	2%
Acinar cell origin	
Acinar cell carcinoma	1%
Uncertain origin	
Pancreatoblastoma	
Papillary cystic carcinoma	All
Anaplastic carcinoma	rare
Connective tissue origin	

means that the tumour has been present for over 5 years before it can be detected by current imaging techniques.

Histology Ductal hyperplasia is frequently seen in tissue adjacent to tumours of ductal origin whereas this is not the case with acinar cell carcinomas. This, and evidence from mucin histochemistry, points to atypical ductal hyperplasia as a precancerous lesion in the development of ductal adenocarcinoma.[7]

Ultrasound appearances Pancreatic cancer arises in the head of the pancreas in 61% of cases, the body in 13%, the tail in 5% and is found in a combination of sites in 21%.[8] Dilatation of the pancreatic or bile ducts is readily demonstrated (Figs 1 and 2) so that tumours as small as 1 cm can be identified in the head of the pancreas.[9] Tumours elsewhere in the gland are harder to detect and may only be manifest by a change in the overlying pancreatic contour (Fig. 3). Patients with non-obstructing lesions present relatively late with tumours larger than 5 cm.

The majority of pancreatic cancers are poorly reflective and attenuating, in part related to their high connective tissue content which may constitute over 99% of the total mass. Small pancreatic tumours are homogeneous because their uniform internal structure presents few interfaces to the ultrasound beam (Fig. 4). Larger lesions are more heterogeneous because their internal structure becomes increasingly disorganised (Fig. 5) but uniformly strongly reflective adenocarcinomas are rare. Pancreatic carcinomas are usually well-defined with irregular or lobulated margins. Pre-existing chronic pancreatitis, surrounding inflammation, a multifocal carcinoma or a tumour of similar reflectivity to the surrounding parenchyma may all impair tumour definition on ultrasound. If the pancreatic duct becomes obstructed, it initially dilates smoothly with atrophy of the surrounding parenchyma (Fig. 6) but progressive dilatation results in elongation of the duct (associated with shrinkage of the parenchyma) that leads to kinking of the main pancreatic duct[10] and the 'chain of lakes' appearance. Different histological types may have

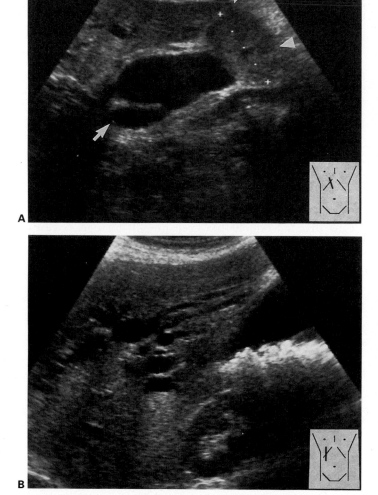

Fig. 1 Pancreatic carcinoma. A: A 4 cm echo-poor mass (arrowheads) is obstructing the lower end of the common bile duct. A dilated cystic duct (arrow) is also seen. **B:** Scan through the right lobe of the liver showing the dilated biliary tree and gallbladder which contains incidental calculi. Gallbladder calculi are very common and must not be assumed to be the cause of the obstruction.

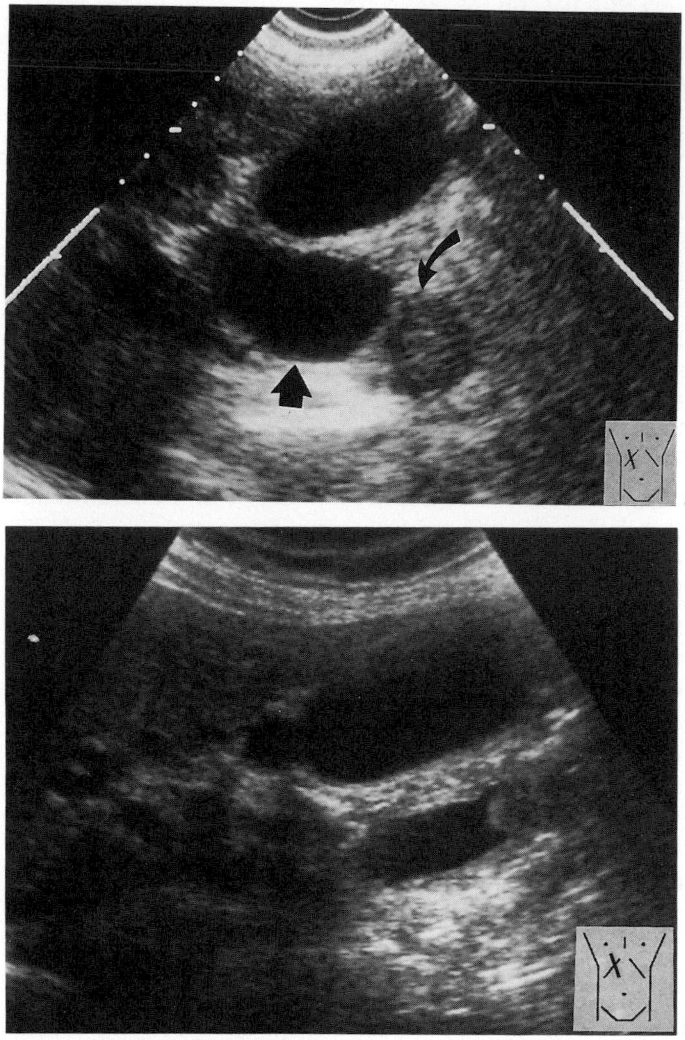

Fig. 2 Pancreatic carcinoma. A: A markedly dilated common bile duct (arrow) ends in a small, irregular pancreatic tumour (curved arrow). The gallbladder is also shown. **B:** A similar tumour, extending into the lumen of the duct.

different appearances, the most common variation being cystadenocarcinoma.

Staging In tumour staging tumour size and location, invasion of surrounding tissues, lymph node involvement and the presence of metastases must be assessed (Figs 7 and 8). There is no generally accepted staging scheme for pancreatic cancer as yet. Tumour size is taken as the maximum transverse diameter and is an important prognostic indicator, tumours smaller than 2 cm being particularly favourable. Whether a tumour is surrounded by parenchyma, is adjacent to the capsule, or has actually breached the capsule must be assessed.[11] An enlarging mass within the head of the pancreas may produce obstruction of the common bile duct early in its development. As

local invasion continues infiltration of the duodenum often occurs, distorting its mucosal outline and eventually leading to complete duodenal obstruction. Invasion of retroperitoneal fat occurs early, with tumour tracking along perineural sheaths and lymphatics (Fig. 6).[11]

Retroperitoneal invasion fixes the pancreas to the adjacent blood vessels (splenic and portal veins) which it may then invade (Fig. 9). Tumour may extend up to or invade the vessel wall or even obstruct its lumen. Vascular invasion is detectable on conventional ultrasound as distortion of the vessel structure, however it is better evaluated with duplex Doppler studies (Fig. 10). Flow in the hepatic and gastroduodenal arteries may also be affected by a pancreatic tumour. Typically these vessels become encased by tumour, resulting in stenosis. Early spread to surrounding lymph nodes is common. Nodes in

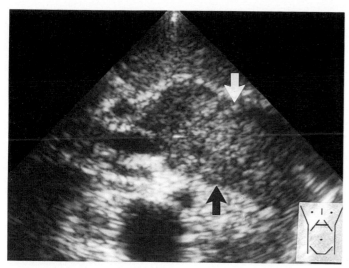

Fig. 3 Pancreatic carcinoma. The whole of the pancreatic tail is expanded by tumour (arrows).

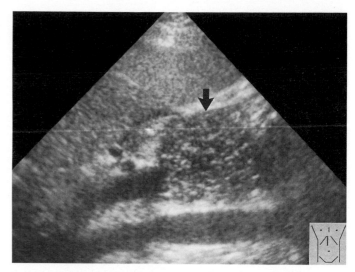

Fig. 5 Highly reflective pancreatic carcinoma. This tumour is heterogeneous with widespread areas of increased reflectivity unlike the common poorly reflective type.

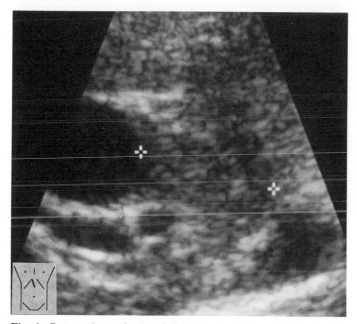

Fig. 4 Pancreatic carcinoma. A 2 cm tumour (calipers) is shown obstructing the common bile duct.

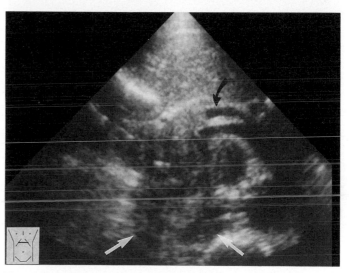

Fig. 6 Pancreatic carcinoma. The large tumour is infiltrating posteriorly into the retroperitoneum (arrows). The pancreatic duct is dilated (curved arrow).

the pancreatico-duodenal region, the inferior pancreatic body, the hepatoduodenal region and coeliac axis may all be involved. Metastases and ascites are only seen at a late stage.

Doppler studies Malignancy can affect portal vein blood flow in several ways. Compression of the vein produces a high velocity jet through the narrowed area. Just distal to this, vortices cause chaotic or tubulent flow (Fig. 10). The Doppler sonogram shows spectral broadening, in extreme cases with signals above and below the baseline. Invasion of the vessel wall produces local chaotic

flow. Portal vein occlusion obliterates the Doppler signal but collateral vessels may be demonstrated and there may be flow through small channels around the occlusion.[12] An occlusion may be missed without the use of Doppler because fresh thrombus is very poorly reflective. Colour Doppler facilitates the assessment by enabling small vessels to be located more rapidly and better demonstrating local flow disturbances. The imaging of flow allows more precise angle correction thus improving the accuracy of flow velocity measurements with spectral Doppler. Involvement of the portal vein by tumour is common, occurring in 65% of pancreatic and 40% of bile duct tumours. In assessing this complication Doppler analysis is probably more sensi-

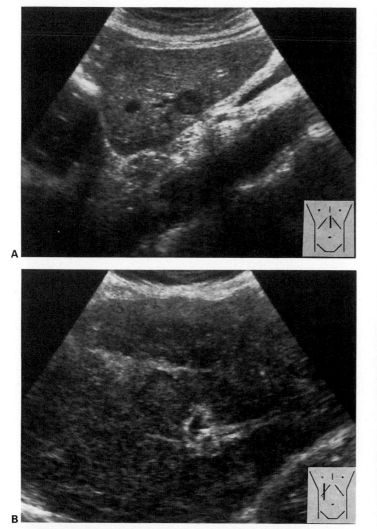

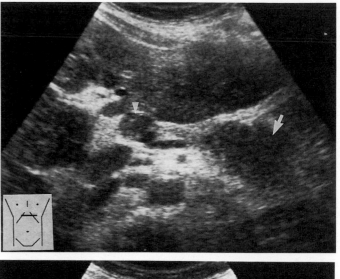

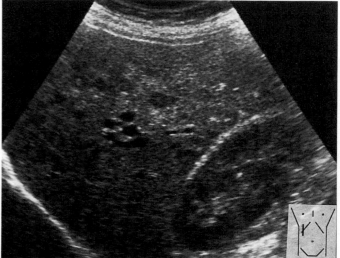

Fig. 7 **Liver metastasis.** Small, poorly reflective metastases from a carcinoma of the pancreas (same patient as Figure 2B).

Fig. 8 **Metastases. A:** Transverse scan showing a poorly defined carcinoma in the pancreatic body (arrow) and an enlarged peripancreatic node (arrowhead). **B:** Multiple liver metastases in the same patient.

tive than ultrasound imaging alone. Duplex Doppler offers the advantage over angiography of providing an assessment of the haemodynamic disturbances at the same time as the surrounding soft tissue anatomy. In addition to changes in the surrounding vasculature characteristic tumour Doppler signals have been detected from neoplastic lesions, including pancreatic tumours (Fig. 11).[13]

The neovascularisation associated with neoplasia is well-documented. Strickland described tumour vessels as wandering, with no diminution in calibre.[14] Histologically these tumour vessels are thin walled with little smooth muscle. Flow is characteristically slow and with low distal impedance, depicted on the Doppler spectrum as continuous forward flow throughout diastole. Also seen are high frequency Doppler shift signals, thought to represent arteriovenous shunts in the tumour. These are signatures of malignancy.

Doppler studies greatly enhance ultrasound examination

of pancreatic tumours and are very sensitive for portal vein involvement.

Differential diagnosis The most important differential diagnosis is from chronic inflammation (Fig. 12) but other lesions such as non-endocrine tumours, metastatic tumours (Fig. 13), malignant islet cell tumours and acute focal inflammation also must be considered.

Some tumours (e.g. mucinous cystic neoplasms) are predominantly cystic, distinguishing them from the relatively homogeneous ductal adenocarcinoma, though cysts may also form in inflammatory lesions. Endocrine tumours are often small with a reflective capsule. Pancreatic lymphoma may be large, multifocal and is not usually associated with massive or widespread lymphadenopathy. The demonstration of cysts, calcification or irregular duct dilatation favours chronic pancreatitis; however, an

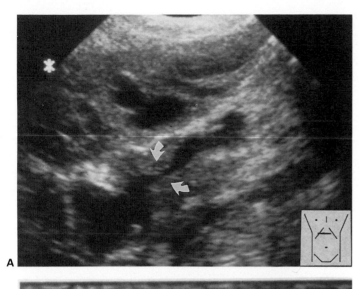

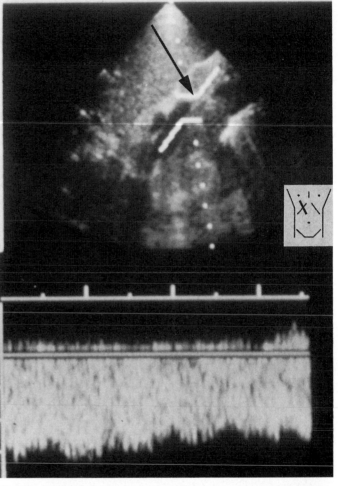

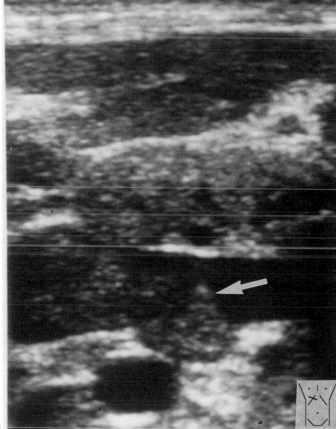

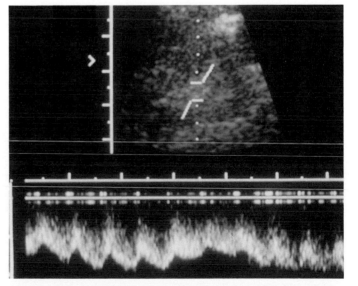

Fig. 10 Doppler of portal vein stenosis. Duplex Doppler study of high flow velocity in the portal vein just distal to a stenosis produced by tumour invading through the vein wall (arrow).

Fig. 9 Splenic/portal vein involvement. A: Pancreatic tumour compressing the portal vein (arrows). **B:** Pancreatic tumour invading through the wall of the portal vein (arrow).

Fig. 11 Tumour Doppler signal. Continuous flow pattern recorded from within a heterogeneous pancreatic tumour.

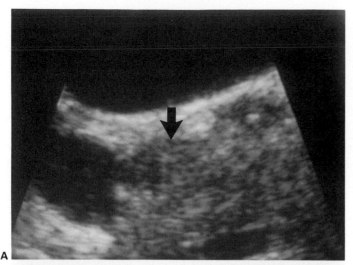

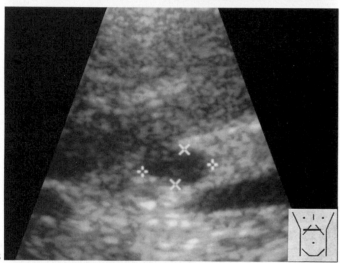

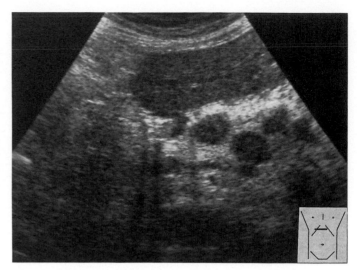

Fig. 13 Metastases to the pancreas. Multiple metastases to the pancreas in a patient with melanoma.

Fig. 12 Focal pancreatitis. A: An inflammatory mass involving the pancreatic head (arrow). No evidence of malignancy was found on biopsy and the patient remained well on follow up. **B:** A small, well-defined poorly reflective area is seen in the pancreatic head. Tubercle bacilli were cultured from a biopsy of this lesion.

underlying malignancy may be difficult to exclude. In acute biliary obstruction focal inflammation typically affects the pancreatic head to form apparent echo-poor masses; differentiation from ductal adenocarcinoma may be impossible.

Although adenocarcinoma is by far the commonest pancreatic malignancy, a range of other tumours must be considered, most of which carry a much better prognosis and some of which are curable. Accurate tissue diagnosis is therefore essential in the management of patients with a pancreatic mass.

Pancreatic biopsy

Pancreatic fine needle aspiration cytology has been widely used since its introduction at the beginning of the 1970s.

In large unselected series, although false positives are very rare, the sensitivity of the method is disappointing at around 75%.[15,16] This low detection rate is probably partly explained by the extensive desmoplastic reaction that pancreatic tumours excite; the fibrous tissue may deflect the biopsy needle leading to a sampling error. More recently immuno-cytochemical techniques have improved specificity; however, as only small tissue samples are obtained, only one or two stains can be performed.

In an attempt to improve both sensitivity and tissue specificity mechanical cutting devices have been developed. The Biopty Gun®, developed by Lindgren in Sweden, uses a Trucut needle modified with a spring powered trigger. Release of the trigger drives the stylet 2 cm into the lesion and this is quickly followed by a cutting sheath which is driven forward to trap a core of tissue in the stylet groove. Other self-firing devices have subsequently been introduced. In our series of 234 patients the sensitivity for diagnosing adenocarcinoma of the pancreas was 91.4% and a wide range of other tumours were successfully diagnosed (Table 2).

With this technique tissue penetration is predictable, the high cutting speed reduces both crush artefact and the time the needle spends within the patient and manipulation is

Table 2 Histologies encountered in pancreatic biopsies

Adenocarcinoma	213
Neuro-endocrine	7
Lymphoma	7
Adenoma	2
Pancreatoblastoma	1
Small cell	1
Clear cell	1
Leiomyoma	1
Colloid carcinoma	1

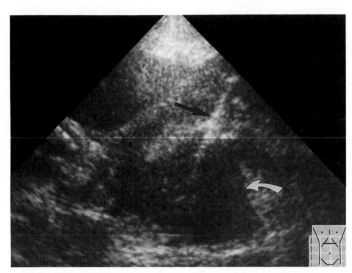

Fig. 14 Pancreatic biopsy. The tract from a percutaneous biopsy (arrow) of a pancreatic mass (curved arrow) is still seen up to 1 minute after the biopsy needle has been removed.

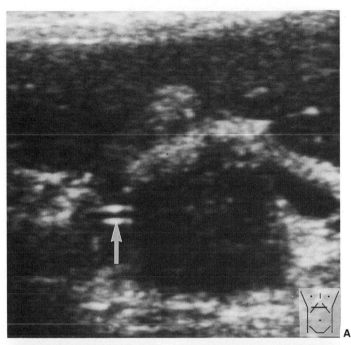

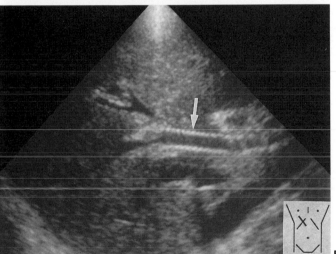

Fig. 15 Pancreatic carcinoma. A: A biliary stent (arrow) has been placed through the tumour. **B:** An expanding metal stent (arrow) is shown in the common hepatic duct.

one handed, ideal for ultrasound guidance. In addition, the high needle velocity induces cavitation in adjacent tissues which persists for long enough to highlight the sample volume, thus confirming that the desired region has been sampled (Fig. 14). Disadvantages are few: soft tissues may fragment, the gun makes a noise which may startle the patient and there is a theoretical risk of injury from the larger needle. However, the complication rate is very low with serious complications (e.g. pancreatic ascites) encountered in only three of our 234 patients.

Treatment

Surgical excision offers the only possible cure for carcinoma of the pancreas, yet is possible in less than 10% of cases. Even with surgery 5 year survival rates of only 5% to 18% are achieved.[3] Some Japanese studies[17] report 5 year survival rates of over 30% but these have not been confirmed elsewhere and may be explained by favourable histological types.

Contra-indications to resection include tumours larger than 3 cm, site other than the head, invasion of the portal vein or retroperitoneum and the presence of metastases. Little difference in patient survival is seen when pancreato-duodenectomy (Whipple's procedure) is compared with total pancreatectomy,[18] despite the inevitable diabetes in the latter. Intra-operative radiotherapy improves short-term survival.[19] Unresectable tumours may be treated with chemotherapy (BCNU, 5FU) or radiotherapy; results however, are disappointing with mean survival prolonged by around 6 months.

More important is palliation of the troublesome pruritis and jaundice. This may be achieved by stenting or by surgical bypass (Fig. 15). Ultrasound is useful for follow up of these patients to assess biliary duct dilatation and drainage and also to monitor tumour growth and spread.

Comparison of ultrasound and CT

Both ultrasound and CT are excellent imaging methods for pancreatic carcinoma (Fig. 16). In a patient with suspected pancreatic malignancy the sensitivity of ultrasound for detecting a pancreatic mass is of the order of 90%, approaching 98% with high resolution equipment and good

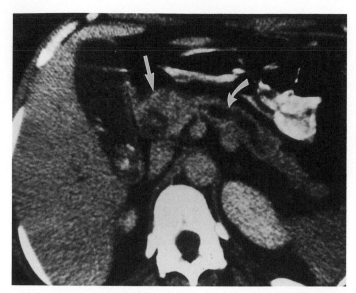

Fig. 16 Pancreatic tumour. CT showing a tumour in the head of the pancreas (arrow) with dilatation of the pancreatic duct (curved arrow).

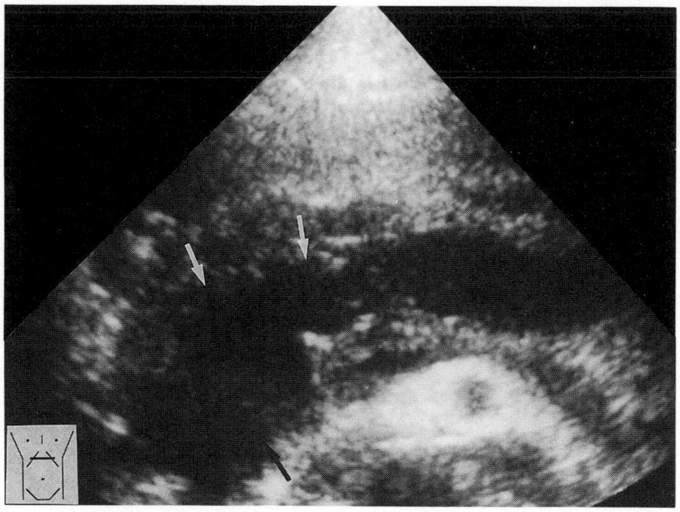

Fig. 17 Intraductal mucinous adenocarcinoma. The poorly reflective material filling the pancreatic duct is mucin secreted by the tumour (arrows).

technique.[20,21] This is limited by the small number of technical failures where overlying bowel gas or patient obesity prevent adequate visualisation of the pancreatic tail. Ultrasound is the best means of assessing the biliary tree in suspected biliary obstruction and in some 90% of patients both the level and cause of obstruction can be defined.[22] In a review of 27 patients with a suspected pancreatic mass and an equivocal appearance on CT, ultrasound, with its ability to detect parenchymal changes, successfully resolved the diagnostic dilemma in all cases.[22]

Ultrasound is also useful in staging pancreatic malignancy, with remarkably high accuracy for predicting non-resectability[20] though prediction of resectability is less good. The addition of Doppler and endoscopic ultrasound might improve this. The advantages of CT include fewer technical failures and its ability to detect other abdominal abnormalities.[23] The pancreatic tail is more reliably seen on CT, though, in the thin patient, fascial planes around the pancreatic head may be difficult to define. Using current generation CT scanners and state of the art techniques, the positive predictive value for tumour resectability is 78% and for non-resectability is 100%.[24,25]

The wide availability of ultrasound, together with the adjuvant techniques of Doppler and endoscopic scanning and the ability to obtain a biopsy specimen, suggest that ultrasound should be the initial test in the investigation of a patient with suspected pancreatic malignancy.

Other non-endocrine tumours

Giant cell carcinoma

Bizarre giant tumour cells and sarcomatous cells characterise this lesion. The cells are anaplastic with marked pleomorphism. Epithelial glandular elements and mucin may also be present.[26] Patients present late and the tumour, by this stage, is often a large echo-poor mass with a necrotic centre and metastases have occurred. The prognosis is poor with median survival around 2 months.

Adenosquamous carcinoma

This neoplasm is a mixture of adeno- and squamous carcinoma, probably arising from a stem cell capable of differentiating into both.[27] On ultrasound they are similar to ductal adenocarcinomas, though, if the squamous components predominate, they may undergo necrosis forming large cystic regions.[28] The prognosis is slightly worse than average for pancreatic cancers.

Mucinous adenocarcinoma

This well-recognised tumour is characterised by marked mucin production. It consists of well-differentiated clumps of columnar epithelium lying within mucinous spaces which are echo-free. Calcification may be seen. The pancreatic duct may be dilated and contain mucin of varying reflectivity (Fig. 17). ERCP demonstrates the mucin as filling defects and typically shows mucus flowing from a patulous papilla.[29] The prognosis is relatively good with long survival after pancreatectomy being reported.[2]

Microadenocarcinoma

Microadenocarcinomas are often large and elicit less desmoplastic reaction than ductal adenocarcinomas. They are composed of solid cellular regions with fine fibrous septa. The cells have uniform nuclei and form small mucin filled glands.[30] This tumour presents in a slightly younger age group than ductal adenocarcinomas; however, survival is poor.

Mucinous cystic neoplasms

These cystic tumours are now thought of as frankly or potentially malignant at presentation. They predominantly occur in middle-aged women and the majority are located in the body or tail of the pancreas (Fig. 18).[31] They are irregular in shape with a smooth outline. Unilocular or multilocular the cysts are lined by columnar epithelium and their surface often displays shaggy excrescences. On ultrasound the cystic elements can be clearly identified with internal septa and nodular or papillary projections. Mucinous tumours are cured by complete resection and, even if this is not possible, the prognosis is much better than for ductal adenocarcinoma. The mucinous duct-ectatic type is a variant, predominantly occurring in the head and uncinate process. It is due to a localised dilatation of a duct side branch.

Microcystic adenoma

The other main cystic pancreatic neoplasm is the microcystic adenoma. It is a well-defined, vascular tumour composed of innumerable small cysts with a fibrous stroma that may partially calcify (Fig. 19). It is non-invasive but may compress adjacent structures.[32] If the cysts are small (2 mm or less) the lesion is predominantly reflective; however, if they are larger, it is seen as a multiloculated cystic mass. The differential diagnosis is from the following pancreatic cystic lesions:

Pseudocyst
Mucinous cystic neoplasm
   mucinous duct ectatic type
Microcystic adenoma
Papillary cystic tumour
Congenital cyst
Cystic islet cell tumour
Vascular tumours
Cystic metastases
Hydatid disease
Pancreatic sarcoma.

Pancreatoblastoma

This rare tumour arises in the ventral pancreas, affecting

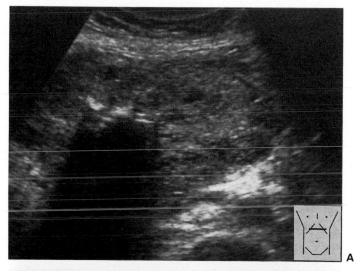

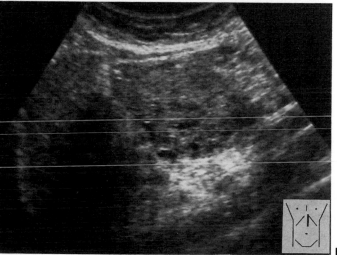

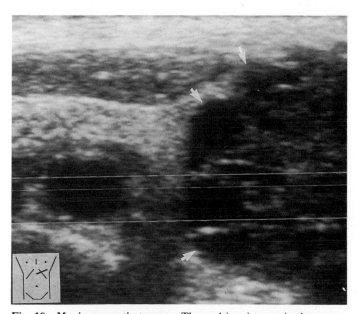

Fig. 18 Mucinous cystic tumour. The multicystic mass in the pancreatic tail (arrows) is the typical pattern of a mucinous cystic neoplasm.

Fig. 19 Microcystic adenoma. A well-defined heterogeneous tumour containing numerous very small cysts together with a central region of calcification that casts an acoustic shadow.

children under 7 years of age and is thought to result from a failure in organogenesis.[33] The tumours are often large and composed of sheets of epithelial cells interspersed with mesenchymal tissue. They appear on ultrasound as well-defined predominantly reflective masses.

Anaplastic carcinoma

This group of undifferentiated malignant tumours is similar clinically to ductal adenocarcinomas. On ultrasound they appear as large solid tumours.

Acinar cell carcinoma

These lesions are solid grey tumours with necrotic centres. Acinar formation occurs. Survival is similar to ductal adenocarcinomas.

Benign tumours (Fig. 20), papillary cystic tumours and tumours of connective tissue origin are all very rare.

Endocrine tumours

At least five types of islet cell are found in the normal pancreas, each producing a distinct peptide or amine; beta cells produce insulin, α cells glucagon, δ cells somatostatin, F cells pancreatic polypeptide and enterochromaffin cells serotonin. Tumours may arise from each of these cell types but, in addition, pancreatic endocrine tumours may develop from tissues found in the fetal pancreas or other glands. For example gastrinoma, VIPoma and tumours producing combinations of different peptides all occur.

Insulinoma is the commonest pancreatic endocrine tumour and, in contrast to other tumours described, it is almost always benign. Gastrinoma is the second most com-

mon; 60% or more are malignant. Insulinoma, gastrinoma, glucagonoma and VIPoma all produce recognisable clinical syndromes as a result of their excess hormone production. These symptoms mean that they present much earlier than other pancreatic neoplasms and so they are usually small, often less than 1.5 cm. Somatostatinomas and pancreatic polypeptidomas produce few if any clinical symptoms and at presentation the tumour bulk may be considerable.

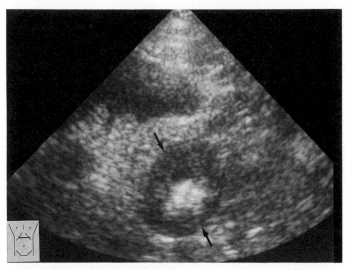

Fig. 21 Benign neuro-endocrine tumour. The mass in the pancreatic head (arrows) proved to be a benign neuro-endocrine tumour. The central area of high reflectivity represents calcification.

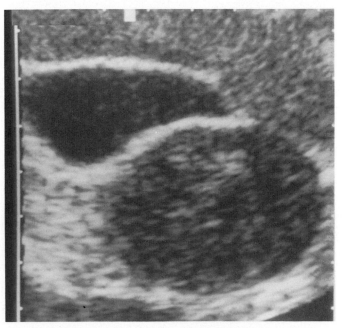

Fig. 22 Benign pancreatic tumour. This well-defined, homogeneous and poorly reflective tumour remained unchanged during follow up over several years.

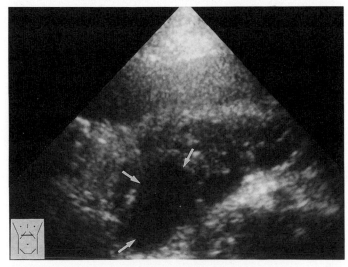

Fig. 20 Benign tumour in the pancreatic head. The tumour (arrows) is well-defined, poorly reflective and homogeneous.

Localisation of islet cell tumours can be extremely difficult because of their small size. Several imaging techniques may be required including ultrasound, ERCP, CT, MRI and angiography with venous sampling. Ultrasound is used as the initial localising investigation and has an important role as an intra-operative guide for the surgeon. Most published data relate to insulinomas. 90% of these tumours are small, well-defined oval masses with a homogeneous, poorly reflective pattern. In young patients (under 30 years of age), the normal pancreas is relatively echo-poor, making the tumour difficult to distinguish from normal parenchyma (Figs 21 and 22). Detection rates for small insulinomas with modern equipment and techniques compare favourably with both CT and angiography (all approximately 60%). The pancreatic tail remains an area of particular difficulty. The role of endoscopic ultrasound in detecting these lesions is under assessment. In our series of over 30 cases the sensitivity of detection approaches 95% for tumours over 5 mm in diameter but smaller lesions have not been detected. Intraoperative ultrasound is able to detect small adenomas not palpable by the surgeon with an overall detection rate for insulinomas of around 85% (Figs 23 and 24). The relations of the tumour to pancreatic blood vessels and the duct can be demonstrated, helping the surgeon decide whether enucleation is safe or whether partial pancreatectomy is required. Experience with endoscopic and intra-operative ultrasound for gastrinomas has been disappointing as these are frequently multiple, extremely small and may even be extra-pancreatic.

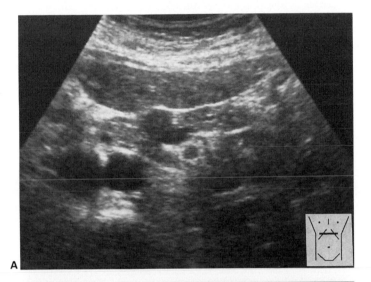

A

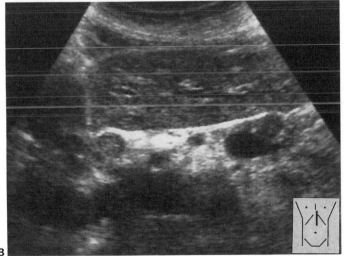

B

Fig. 23 Insulinoma. A: Longitudinal and **B:** transverse scans. The lesion is detectable by virtue of its lower reflectivity compared to the adjacent parenchyma and the distortion of the gland outline.

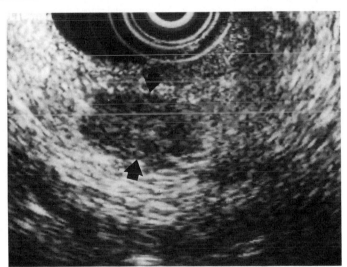

Fig. 24 Insulinoma. Endoscopic ultrasound showing a small, poorly reflective tumour in the pancreatic head (arrows).

REFERENCES

1 Axtell L M, Asire A J, Myers M Y. Cancer patient survival. End results in cancer. Report No.5 1976; 130–135
2 Russel R C G. Carcinoma of the pancreas and ampulla of Vater. In: Misiewicz J S, Pounder R E, Venebles C W. eds. Diseases of the gut and pancreas. Oxford: Blackwell Scientific Press. 1987
3 Warshaw A L, Swanson R S. Pancreatic cancer in 1988. Ann Surg 1988; 208: 541–553
4 Wynder E L. An epidemiological evaluation of the causes of cancer of the pancreas. Cancer Res 1975; 35: 2228–2233
5 Malagelada J R. Pancreatic cancer: an overview of epidemiology,

clinical presentation and diagnosis. Mayo Clin Proc 1979; 54: 459–467

6 Kloppel G, Mailler B. Classification of pancreatic nonendocrine tumours. Radiol Clin North Am 1979; 27: 105–120

7 Chien J, Baithun S I, Ramsay M. Histogenesis of pancreatic cancer: a study based on 248 cases. J Pathol 1985; 146: 65–76

8 Cubilla A L, Fitzgerald P J. A clinical pathological study of 380 patients. In: Pathology annual part 1. New York: Appleton Century Crofts. 1978: p 241

9 Lees W R. Pancreatic ultrasonography. Clin Gastroenterol 1984; 13: 763–789

10 Ohto M, Saotome N, Saisho H, et al. Real time ultrasonography of the pancreatic duct: application to percutaneous pancreatic ductography. AJR 1980; 134: 647–652

11 Kloppel G, Maillet B. Classification and staging of pancreatic non-endocrine tumours. Radiol Clin North Am 1989; 27: 105–119

12 Kane R A, Katz S G. The spectrum of sonographic findings in portal hypertension; a subject review and new observations. Radiology 1982; 142: 453–458

13 Taylor K J W, Ramos I, Carter D, Morse S S, Shower D, Fortune K. Correlation of Doppler ultrasound tumor signals with neovascular morphological features. Radiology 1988; 166: 57–62

14 Strickland B. The value of angiography in the diagnosis of bone tumour. Br J Radiol 1959; 32: 705–713

15 Hanke S, Holm H H, Koch F. Ultrasonically guided puncture of solid pancreatic mass lesions. In: Holm H H. ed. Interventional ultrasound. Copenhagen: Munksgaard. 1985: p 100–105

16 Hall-Craggs M A, Lees W R. Fine needle aspiration biopsy: pancreatic and biliary tumours. AJR 1986; 147: 399–403

17 Tsuchiya R, Noda T, Harada N. Collective review of small carcinomas of the pancreas. Ann Surg 1986; 203: 71–81

18 Van Heerden J A. Pancreatic resection for carcinoma of the pancreas. World J Surg 1984; 8: 880–888

19 Gunderson L L, Martin J K, Kirols L K. Intraoperative and external beam irradiation ± 5FU for locally advanced pancreatic carcinoma. Int J Radiat Oncol Biol Phys 1987; 13: 319–329

20 Campbell J P, Wilson S R. Pancreatic neoplasm: how useful is evaluation with ultrasonography? Radiology 1988; 167: 341–344

21 Lees W R, Vallon A G, Denyer M E. Prospective study of ultrasonography in pancreatic disease. BMJ 1979; 162–164

22 Ormson M J, Charboneau J W, Stephens D H. Sonography in patients with a possible pancreatic mass on computed tomography. AJR 1987; 148: 551–555

23 Freeny P. Radiology of the pancreas. Current opinion in Radiology 1989; 1: 81–93

24 Ross C B, Sharp K W, Kaufman A J, Andrews S A, Williams L F. Efficacy of computerised tomography in the preoperative staging of pancreatic cancer. Am J Surg 1988; 54: 221–226

25 Freeny P C, Marks W M, Ryan J A, Traverso L W. Pancreatic ductal adenocarcinoma; diagnosis and staging with dynamic computed tomography. Radiology 1988; 166: 125–133

26 Cubilla A L, Fitzgerald P J. Cancer (non-endocrine) of the pancreas (a suggested classification). Mayo Clin Proc 1979; 54: 449–458

27 Chen J, Baithun S I. Morphologic study of 391 cases of exocrine pancreatic tumours with special reference to the classification of exocrine pancreatic carcinoma. J Pathol 1985; 146: 17–29

28 Friedman A C. Radiology of the liver, biliary tract, pancreas and spleen. Baltimore: Williams and Wilkins. 1987: p 837–860

29 Itau Y, Kokul T, Atom Y, et al. Mucin hypersecreting carcinoma of the pancreas. Radiology 1987; 165: 51–55

30 Friedman A C, Edmonds P R. Rare pancreatic malignancies. Radiol Clin North Am 1989; 27: 177–190

31 Friedman A C, Lichtenstein J E, Dachman A M. Cystic neoplasms of the pancreas. Radiological-pathological correlation. Radiology 1983; 149: 45–50

32 Compagno J, Oerto J E. Microcystic adenomas of the pancreas (glycogen-rich cystadenomas). A clinico-pathologic study of 34 cases. Am J Clin Pathol 1978; 69: 289–298

33 Home A, Yano Y, Kotoo Y, et al. Morphogenesis of pancreatoblastoma; infantile carcinoma of the pancreas. Cancer 1977; 39: 247–254

Gallbladder and biliary tree

Henry C. Irving and Jane Bates

Normal anatomy of the biliary tree

Bile drains from the liver via the intrahepatic bile ducts which run in the portal tracts alongside the portal vein radicles and hepatic artery branches. The ducts gradually increase in diameter towards the porta hepatis, finally anastomosing to form the right and left hepatic ducts which drain the functional right and left hepatic lobes and are up to 2 mm in diameter in the normal non-distended state (Fig. 1). At the porta hepatis, the right and left hepatic ducts join to form the common hepatic duct which passes inferiorly for approximately 3 cm before being joined by the cystic duct to form the common bile duct.

The common bile duct continues caudally for approximately 7 cm lying anterior to the right margin of the portal vein and lateral to the hepatic artery (Fig. 2). It runs parallel with both vessels for a short distance before passing behind the first part of the duodenum. Distally, the common duct lies in a deep groove on the posterior aspect of the head of the pancreas, often completely surrounded by pancreatic tissue.

Within the posterolateral part of the pancreatic head, the distal end of the common bile duct passes laterally accompanying the pancreatic duct into the second part of the duodenum. Here the two ducts join and open into a conical shaped protuberance – the duodenal papilla (ampulla of Vater), which is situated on the medial wall of the duodenal lumen.

The lower end of the duct is surrounded by a circular muscle – the sphincter of Oddi, which controls the egress of bile and pancreatic juices into the duodenum.

Gallbladder

The gallbladder serves as a reservoir for bile secreted by the liver; thus its size varies according to digestive requirements throughout the day.

The gallbladder is a pear-shaped sac which lies in a fossa on the undersurface of the right lobe of the liver. It has a thin smooth wall, up to 2 mm in thickness (Fig. 3),[1] composed of an outer serosal layer, a middle fibromuscular layer and an inner mucosa. The bulbous distal portion of the gallbladder, the fundus, is generally in the most caudal and anterior position, often projecting below the inferior margin of the liver. The fundus tapers into the body and finally into the neck – the narrowest portion – which often curves abruptly posterocaudally before becoming continuous with the cystic duct (Fig. 4).

The wall of the gallbladder is at its thickest in the region of the neck – normally up to 3 mm (Fig. 5). A small pouch may be seen projecting caudally and posteriorly – Hartman's pouch, which often becomes more marked in cases of gallbladder dilatation. (In fact the loss of a normal tapering shape of the gallbladder and its replacement by a rounded shape is often a more reliable indicator of dilatation than overall measurements, which may be within normal limits).[2]

Cystic duct

The cystic duct, 3 to 4 cm in length, is composed of folds which project into the lumen in a spiral arrangement – hence the term 'spiral valve'. It is not in fact a true valve, and bile can flow in both directions through the duct determined by differences in pressure between the gallbladder and common bile duct. Its importance to the sonographer is that there may be an acoustic shadow beyond the valve falsely suggesting the diagnosis of a stone in the cystic duct (Fig. 6).[3]

Normal anatomical variants

Ducts

Normal variations in the anatomy of the ducts are common. The point at which the cystic duct joins the common hepatic duct is particularly variable; usually they unite just beyond the porta hepatis, but the cystic duct may join the right hepatic duct or the join may be much lower – occasionally within the head of the pancreas itself. The cystic duct may pass medially either posteriorly or anteriorly to the common hepatic duct, then curving laterally to join its medial border.

On ultrasound scans it is not usually possible to recognise the exact point of union of the cystic and common hepatic ducts, and it has therefore become accepted convention to refer to the extrahepatic bile duct as 'the common duct'.[4]

Gallbladder

The shape, size and position of the gallbladder are highly

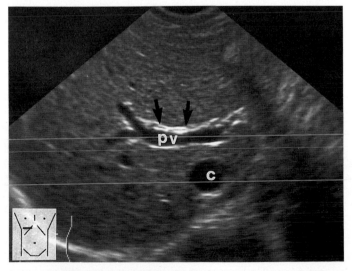

Fig. 1 Right hepatic duct. Transverse scan through liver showing a normal calibre right hepatic duct (arrows), anterior to the right branch of the portal vein (pv). (c – inferior vena cava).

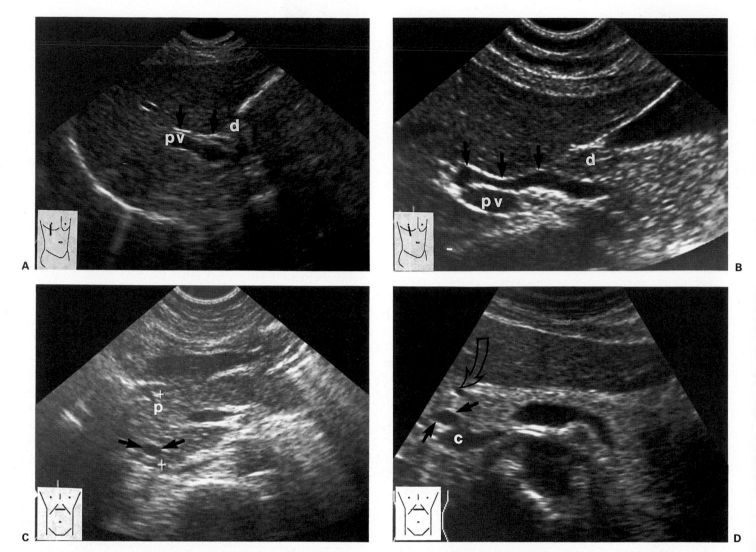

Fig. 2 Normal common duct. A: Longitudinal scan showing duct (arrows) anterior to portal vein (pv), and passing posterior to gas filled duodenum (d). **B:** Longitudinal scan showing duct passing posterior to fluid filled duodenum (d). **C:** Transverse scan showing duct (arrows) within head of pancreas (p). **D:** Transverse scan showing duct (arrows) about to enter duodenal papilla. (open arrow – gastroduodenal artery, c – inferior vena cava).

variable. In some cases the gallbladder fossa lies deep within the liver and the gallbladder appears to be surrounded by hepatic tissue – the so-called 'intrahepatic gallbladder' – which may mimic an intrahepatic cyst (Fig. 7). At the other end of the spectrum, the gallbladder may be attached to the porta only at the neck forming a very mobile structure which may be found in the right iliac fossa or even in the pelvic region, depending upon patient position.

In some subjects the fundus of the gallbladder is folded over – the 'Phrygian cap' – which can make examination of the lumen difficult.[5] Often patient positioning can unfold the gallbladder making it more accessible to full ultrasound interrogation (Fig. 8). Failing this, a more pro-

longed fast may dilate the gallbladder sufficiently for a successful study to be performed.

Folding of the gallbladder is a common variation which may mimic septation. The protuberance of the mucosa at the apex of the fold has led to false diagnoses of stones, but scanning in both longitudinal and transverse axes should help avoid this pitfall (Fig. 9).[6] True septa are rather less common and not usually of clinical significance. They can be distinguished from folding of the gallbladder by scans in both longitudinal and transverse planes with the patient both supine and in the left decubitus position. Septa can lead to errors in diagnosis when the sonographer reports one portion of the gallbladder as free of stones and misses a stone in the distal portion (Fig. 10).[7]

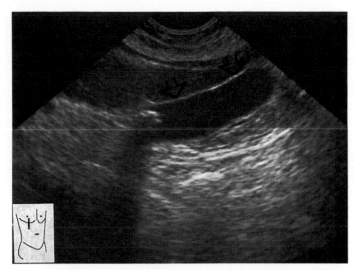

Fig. 3 Gallbladder. Normal gallbladder wall seen only as a thin line (arrows) when the gallbladder is filled (compare with Fig. 14). Note the stone in the neck of the gallbladder.

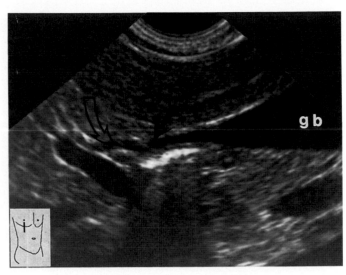

Fig. 4 Neck of gallbladder. Body of gallbladder tapers down to neck (arrow) which becomes continuous with the cystic duct (open arrow).

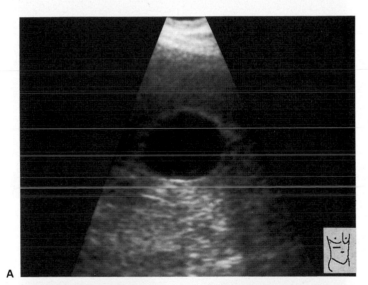

A

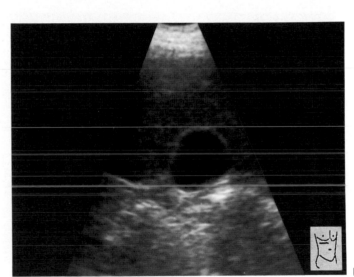

B

Fig. 5 Neck of gallbladder. Transverse scans through gallbladder showing how the wall becomes thicker in the neck. **A:** Fundus. **B:** Body. **C:** Neck.

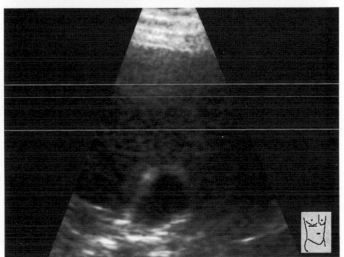

C

The gallbladder may be totally absent, or there may be double or even triple gallbladders with either a single cystic duct or with multiple separate cystic ducts – these anomalies are extremely rare.

Hepatic artery

Usually, the hepatic artery arises from the coeliac axis and runs for a short distance to the right before turning superiorly. At this point the artery lies anterior to the portal

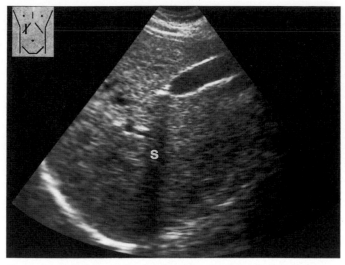

Fig. 6 Shadow from neck of gallbladder. Acoustic shadow (s) from normal neck of gallbladder.

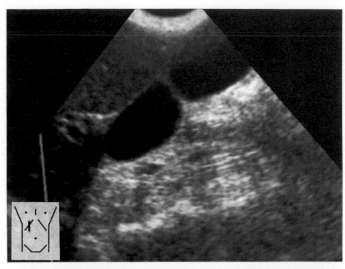

A

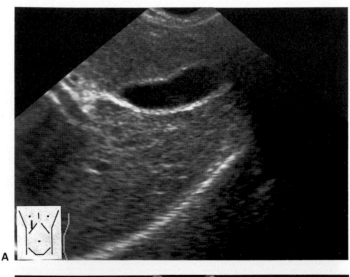

A

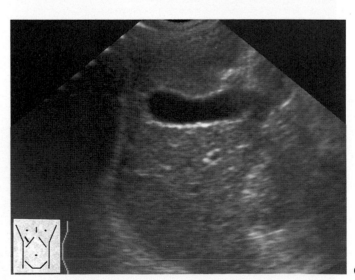

B

Fig. 8 Phrygian cap. A: Patient is supine. **B:** Patient is in right anterior oblique position.

B

Fig. 7 Intrahepatic gallbladder. A: Longitudinal scan. **B:** Transverse scan. **C:** Oblique scan.

C

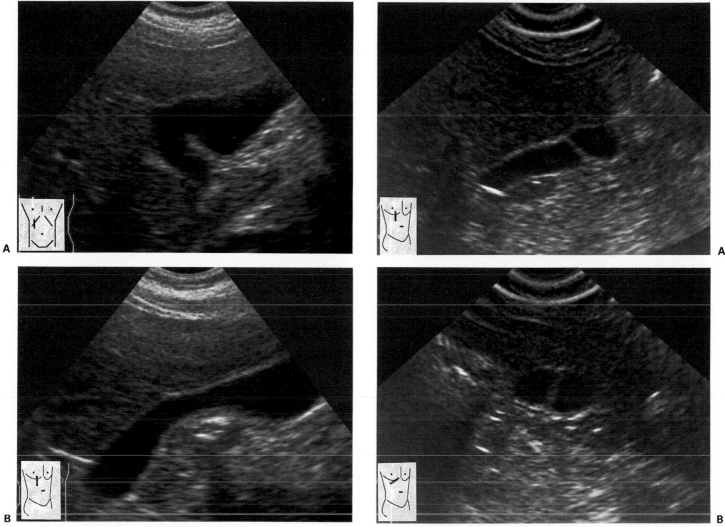

Fig. 9 Golded gallbladder. A: Patient is supine. B: Patient is in right anterior oblique position.

Fig. 10 Septated gallbladder. A: Longitudinal scan. B: Oblique scan.

vein with the common duct to the right. Just proximal to the porta hepatis the artery branches, and the right hepatic artery crosses to the right, posterior to the common hepatic duct before entering the substance of the liver (Fig. 11).

In about 15% of subjects, the right hepatic artery passes anteriorly to the common hepatic duct, and in a smaller proportion (approximately 5%), the right hepatic artery originates from the superior mesenteric artery – the replaced right hepatic artery – and passes posteriorly to the superior mesenteric vein before turning anteriorly to the portal vein.[8] Doppler (duplex or preferably colour) ultrasound may be useful in sorting out the anatomy in these cases,[9] although it is usually possible to identify the vessels by tracing them back to their point of origin (Fig. 12).

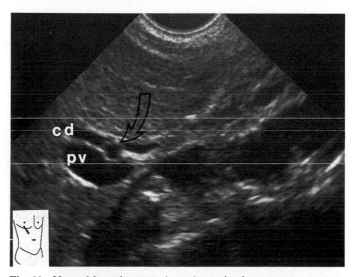

Fig. 11 Normal hepatic artery (arrow) crossing between common duct (cd) and portal vein (pv).

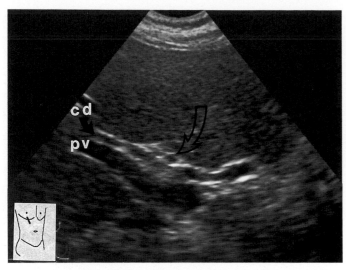

Fig. 12   Anomalous hepatic artery (open arrow) crossing anterior to common duct (cd).

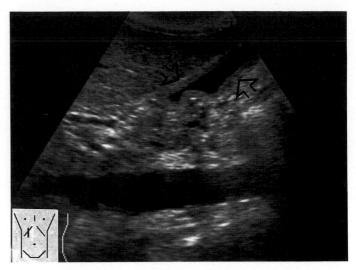

Fig. 14   Normal contracted gallbladder. Normal wall thickness of physiologically contracted gallbladder (open arrows).

Technique and ultrasound appearance

The biliary system should be examined after the patient has fasted – not only does this distend the gallbladder with bile to allow investigation of its lumen, but it helps to reduce the contents of the stomach and duodenum which may obscure the common duct and pancreas.

In some patients, the posterior wall of the gallbladder is closely adjacent to the duodenum and distal acoustic shadowing from the latter may simulate gallbladder pathology (Fig. 13). In such cases, giving the patient a drink of water usually helps to outline the duodenum and display the gallbladder wall more clearly.

The normal gallbladder in its non-fasted state is contracted and thick walled (Fig. 14). This is generally indistinguishable from pathological contraction and care should always be taken to ensure that the patient has adhered to the correct preparation if the gallbladder is small or not visualised on ultrasound.[10]

The equipment of choice for examination of the gallbladder and biliary tree is a sector or convex transducer which allows good acoustic access both subcostally and intercostally. A frequency of 5 MHz with a focal zone at the appropriate depth generally provides sufficiently good resolution to detect even small stones within the gallbladder. The penetration at this frequency may, however, not be adequate in large or obese patients; a 3.5 MHz transducer is then necessary. With the lower frequency the width of the beam is greater and small stones may not be demonstrated due to lack of acoustic shadowing (see Ch. 12, Fig. 4).[11] Similarly, if the stone is outside the focal zone of the transducer, in the near or far fields, acoustic shadowing from a stone may be lost because the beam is wider.[12] With electronic focusing the position of the focal zone is under user control, and this applies in all planes with annular arrays, which are particularly helpful in this type of problem.

For very superficial gallbladders in thin patients, a stand-off medium such as silicone gel often helps to place the gallbladder in the focal zone of the transducer, at the same time reducing reverberations and other near field artefacts. Another advantage of this manoeuvre is that it allows the gallbladder to be displayed in the wider part of the sector field of view for easier viewing.

A comprehensive examination of the biliary system naturally includes the demonstration of both liver and pancreas. The normal intrahepatic bile ducts are rarely

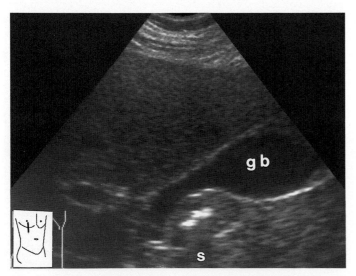

Fig. 13   Bowel indenting posterior wall of gallbladder (gb) with intraluminal gas casting an acoustic shadow (s).

visualised during routine scans but it is not uncommon to display the main right and left hepatic ducts as thin tubular structures running parallel to the main branches of the portal vein (Fig. 1).[13]

An initial survey of the gallbladder with the patient supine is usual. It is helpful to align the transducer along the long axis of the gallbladder to include neck, body, and fundus, and then the transducer can be angled both laterally and medially so that the entire volume of the gallbladder is interrogated by the ultrasound beam. A subcostal approach is often possible using suspended deep inspiration to bring the liver down so that the right lobe provides an acoustic window. However, an intercostal approach is the most successful technique in the majority of patients, allowing the gallbladder to be imaged through the right lobe of the liver in quiet respiration, with the minimum of artefact due to scattering and reverberation from adjacent bowel.

The normal gallbladder has an echo-free lumen and is surrounded by a smooth, moderately reflective wall. Since there is little attenuation of the ultrasound beam, the time-gain compensation used on most equipment will result in acoustic accentuation. However, this may not be apparent if gas filled bowel lies immediately posteriorly (Fig. 15). In transverse scans, the gallbladder appears circular, increasing in diameter towards the fundus. If possible, the transducer should be maintained at right angles to the long axis, as an oblique section may give a spurious impression of gallbladder wall thickening (Fig. 16).[14]

The gallbladder must be examined with the patient in at least two different positions if small mobile stones or non-mobile polyps are to be correctly diagnosed. Following initial scans in the supine position, the patient is turned

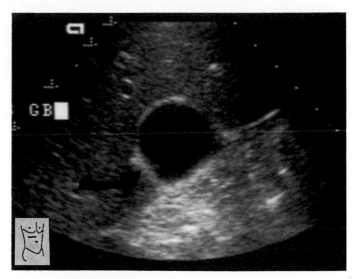

Fig. 16 Spurious gallbladder wall thickening (arrow) due to angulation of the beam.

into the left decubitus position. This allows the liver and gallbladder to fall away medially from the ribs, unfolding the gallbladder, and may also be useful in moving overlying bowel from the region of interest. Other patient positions may sometimes be necessary, for example erect scans with the patient either sitting or standing.

The right anterior oblique or left decubitus positions are indispensable for examining the common duct, which can then be traced distally running from the porta hepatis to the head of the pancreas as an immediate anterior relation of the portal vein (Fig. 17).[15] The lower end of the duct is best demonstrated on transverse scans through the head of the pancreas (Fig. 18) and, while a supine position is

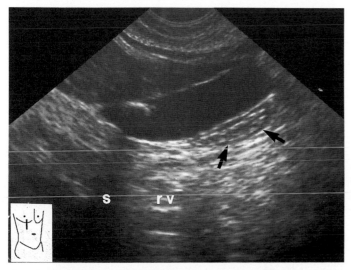

Fig. 15 Shadowing – stone versus gas. Posterior to the gallbladder there is shadowing beyond a stone, reverberation (rv) beyond gas-containing bowel, and transmission of sound beyond empty bowel (arrows).

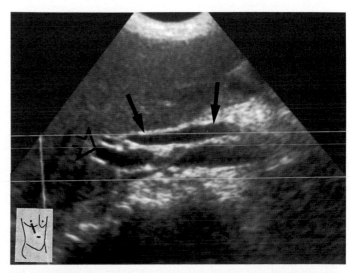

Fig. 17 Normal common duct (arrows) anterior to portal vein (open arrow). Note how the duct widens as it travels in the free edge of the lesser omentum.

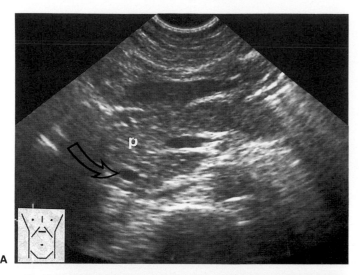

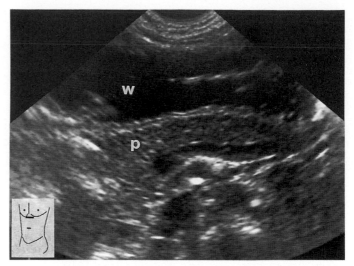

Fig. 19   Water load for pancreatic scanning. Water in stomach (w) as acoustic window improves visualisation of the pancreas (p).

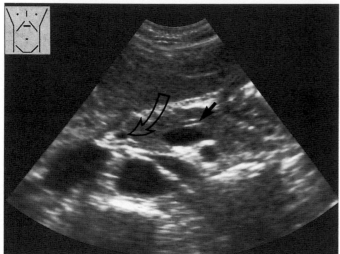

Fig. 18   Normal common duct in head of pancreas on transverse scans. **A:** Duct (open arrow) is within pancreatic substance (p). **B:** Duct (open arrow) is entering the duodenal papilla. (The pancreatic duct is also seen (solid arrow).)

usually adequate, a semi-erect position with the left side raised is recommended by some.[16] A water load may be helpful in allowing visualisation of the lower end of the common duct by displacing gas from the gastric antrum and duodenum in the left anterior oblique position, and it may also act as an acoustic window (Fig. 19).

Measurement of the common duct

As discussed in Chapters 13 and 18, when considering the investigation of the patient with jaundice, the ability of ultrasound to discriminate between a normal and a dilated common duct is vital in the management of the jaundiced patient. This facility for the distinction between 'surgical' and 'medical' causes of jaundice depends on knowing the upper limit of normal for the duct diameter.

However, a clear value dividing normal from abnormal

is not in fact easily attainable. In a normal population the values for the diameter of the common duct will be distributed around a mean,[4] as happens with all biological measurements. The level at which the upper limit of normal is placed will be a value judgement and conventionally the '95% limit' or '2 standard deviations from the mean' levels are used. By definition, therefore, some normals will fall outside the normal range, and conversely, some abnormals will fall within it.

In the case of the ultrasound derived measurement of common duct diameter, there are particular factors to be considered:

a) Level of the measurement – the duct is most consistently demonstrated in its proximal portion via the right anterior oblique longitudinal view and measurements are most often made just caudal to the porta hepatis.[15] Care must be taken not to let the indentation into the posterior wall of the duct, made by the right hepatic artery crossing between duct and portal vein, interfere with the measurement. Also, the duct usually widens slightly as it passes caudally in the free edge of the lesser omentum and after it receives the cystic duct (Fig. 17).

b) The walls of the duct are highly reflective, and 'blooming' of the echoes from the walls may reduce the apparent duct lumen.[13,17] The overall gain and swept gain controls should be optimally adjusted to minimise this artefact (Fig. 20).

c) The cross-sectional shape of the duct is oval rather than circular, and thus measurements may differ according to which diameter is demonstrated on a particular scan plane (Fig. 21).[15]

d) In the elderly there is a generalised loss of elasticity of the tissues and the normal duct diameter increases with advancing age.[18]

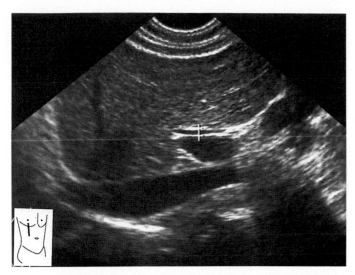

Fig. 20 Measurement of the common duct. Calipers on sharply defined walls of common duct.

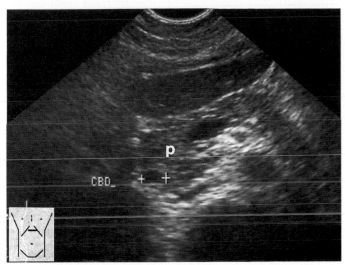

Fig. 21 Oval shape of common duct. False measurement of duct diameter due to oval shape in cross-section (p – pancreas).

e) The diameter of the duct is often increased in patients who have had a cholecystectomy. Ducts that were normal pre-operatively tend to remain normal post-operatively, while ducts that were acutely obstructed usually decrease in size post-operatively following stone removal or drainage procedure. However, ducts which were chronically dilated or in which there has been chronic infection often remain permanently dilated after surgery or non-operative drainage, or may even increase slightly in diameter.[19–21] Inflammation presumably reduces the elasticity of the duct wall so that it becomes incapable of recoiling back down, and the resultant floppy duct will distend with minimal pressure or volume increases as the duct assumes some of the original gallbladder reservoir function.[22,23]

f) There is a discrepancy between the ultrasound mea-surement of common duct calibre, and measurements made at cholangiography (oral, intravenous or direct). A radio-graphic magnification factor must be taken into account, the choleretic effect of intravenous cholangiography, and the direct pressure injection of contrast medium into the duct at both percutaneous transhepatic and endoscopic ret-rograde cholangiography all contribute to the discrepancy, and act in combination with factors a, b and c above.[15,17,19]

Bearing all the above in mind, a useful working rule is that the diameter of the normal common duct as measured on ultrasound scans is less than 5 mm in its upper portion, although this figure can be increased to 6 mm for a mea-surement at its lower end, 8 mm in the elderly, and 1 cm in patients who have had a cholecystectomy.

Using the 'less than 5 mm' limit, the sensitivity of ul-trasound for the diagnosis of extrahepatic obstruction has been shown to be 99% with a specificity of 87%,[24] while moving the limit to 5 mm would have decreased the sen-sitivity to 94% without significantly altering the specificity.

Function studies

While ultrasound scanning enables the display of excellent structural detail of the gallbladder (see Ch. 12), the images give little functional information. However, ultrasound can be used in combination with various pharmacological agents so that the dynamics of gallbladder filling and emptying can be studied in health and disease. Essentially the methods consist of estimating gallbladder volume and monitoring that volume at regular intervals over a period of time.

Gallbladder volume is calculated by first measuring the long axis (H), and then rotating the transducer by 90° until the maximum cross-sectional (width), and anteroposterior (AP) diameters can be measured.

Volume (V) is then estimated by one of the following methods:

a) the single cylinder method[25] in which,

$$V = 0.196 \, H \, (AP + width)$$

b) the ellipsoid method[26] in which,

$$V = \frac{\pi}{6} \, (H \times AP \times width)$$

(For practical purposes this equals half the product of the diameters in centimetres.)

c) the sum of cylinders method[25] in which the gallbladder image is divided into a series of cylinders of equal height and the volumes are summed. This method is cumbersome and time consuming to perform, although it can be automated by using a computer.[27]

It has been shown that while the single cylinder and sum of cylinders methods correlate well, the former consistently overestimates the true gallbladder volume.[25] It has also been shown that measurement of gallbladder volume by the ellipsoid method closely approximates the true volume, and was nearly identical to volume calculated by the sum of cylinders method.[26] Since the ellipsoid method is simple and quick, it is recommended for clinical use.

Gallbladder contraction can be provoked by giving a standard 'fatty meal' as in oral cholangiography, intravenous cholecystokinin, or even intraduodenal instillations, although it has been demonstrated that the use of intravenous cholecystokinin does not offer any advantage over the ingestion of fatty meals.[28]

Serial measurements of gallbladder volume then enable gallbladder function to be defined by four features: fasting gallbladder volume, residual gallbladder volume after maximal contraction, rate of emptying, and maximal percent emptied. Gallbladder emptying dynamics have been meticulously studied with these techniques in smokers, in pregnancy,[29] in patients with coeliac disease[30] and spinal cord injuries,[31] and in response to various drugs.

Recently, the assessment of gallbladder function has increased in importance as a result of the availability of the newer non-invasive methods of gallstone therapy.[32] Prior to embarking upon either gallstone dissolution therapy or extracorporeal shock wave lithotripsy, it is necessary to demonstrate that the cystic duct is patent. Ultrasound, before and after fatty meal, is able to provide this information;[33] the oral cholecystogram need not be resurrected for this purpose.

The response of the diameter of the common duct to a fatty meal has also provided considerable material for study. The fatty meal causes release of cholecystokinin from the duodenal mucosa and this promotes gallbladder contraction, relaxation of the sphincter of Oddi and an increase in the flow of bile from the liver. In a normal subject the bile duct diameter will either reduce or remain unchanged, but if there is partial or complete obstruction, the diameter will usually increase, though occasionally it remains unchanged.[34] Thus a reduction in duct diameter is normal, enlargement indicates obstruction while lack of change is indeterminate, although 84% of such (unresponsive) ducts actually turn out to be normal.[35] It has therefore been recommended that all ducts with a diameter of between 4 and 12 mm, when obstruction is suspected but not proven, should undergo a physiological stimulation test by the administration of a fatty meal, and that this significantly improves diagnostic accuracy.[36] Other workers have confirmed these findings, and concur with the recommendations that 'fatty meal sonography' is a useful test for identifying patients with partial common duct obstruction.[37]

Endosonography

Conventional transabdominal ultrasound is accurate at detecting dilatation of the biliary tree and in localising the site of obstruction (see Ch. 13). However, defining the nature of the pathology is more difficult, while delineation of the extent of spread of bile duct tumours is also difficult. Endoscopic ultrasonography enables a high frequency transducer to be placed in close proximity to the lower end of the bile duct and thus gives more detailed visualisation of lesions in this vicinity.[38]

For endoscopic ultrasonography a high frequency ultrasound transducer is incorporated into a fully functional fibre optic endoscope with both light and optical bundles and air/water channels together with controllable tip movement. Either mechanical sector scanners or electronic arrays (phased or linear) can be used. This specially adapted equipment is both difficult to use and expensive; it has therefore only been used in a few centres around the world.

By placing the ultrasound transducer in contact with the wall of the lesser curve of the stomach at the antrum, the extrahepatic bile ducts can be demonstrated from the bifurcation in the porta hepatis downwards. For evaluation of the lower end of the common bile duct, the transducer has to be moved onwards into the second part of the duodenum, and the rigidity that the ultrasound component imparts to the endoscope makes this a difficult manoeuvre. Once in position, the portal or splenic veins are used as landmarks to identify the common duct.

Endoscopic ultrasound is able to distinguish stones from tumour at the lower end of the common duct and is helpful in the staging of cholangiocarcinomas, particularly of Klatskin tumours at the porta hepatis. A recent prospective comparative study of endosonography, transabdominal ultrasound and CT scanning in the diagnosis of extrahepatic obstruction and in the evaluation of local spread of neoplastic obstructions, has shown endosonography to be significantly more sensitive, accurate and effective than the other two methods.[39]

Intra-operative ultrasound

Intra-operative ultrasound scanning can assist the surgeon during biliary tract surgery (see Ch. 15). Initial reports of its use to detect calculi in the common duct at operation[40] were not met with any enthusiasm – principally because the A-mode traces obtained with the early equipment were difficult to interpret. However, the advent of real time imaging has led to the resurgence of this technique, which has been shown to be as accurate as per-operative cholangiography for the detection of common duct stones,[41] so that in some centres intra-operative ultrasound has become established as a routine adjunct to per-operative cholangiography.[38]

A high frequency transducer is necessary (7.5, 10, or even 12 MHz) and the scan head should be small. Some manufacturers produce probes that can be sterilised in ethylene oxide gas or in various sterilising liquids, but the easiest method is to place the probe within a sterile cover which can then be placed directly in the operative field. Sterile saline is used to provide acoustic coupling.

The three main uses of intra-operative ultrasound of the biliary tract are:

a) in helping to locate the common bile duct where the anatomy has been distorted by previous surgery or inflammatory disease;

b) in assessing the presence of stones within a gallbladder that has a thickened wall or is surrounded by adhesions that preclude adequate palpation and;

c) in the detection of stones within the common duct.

It is for this latter application that surgeons are advised to use the technique alongside operative cholangiography in patients who are at high risk for common duct stones (e.g. patients who have had jaundice, pancreatitis, small stones in the gallbladder, or dilatation of the common duct) in order to select which patients should undergo operative exploration of the bile duct. In low risk patients, it is suggested that intra-operative ultrasound should be used to screen the common duct for stones, thus reducing the requirement for operative cholangiograms and duct explorations.[43]

REFERENCES

1 Finberg H J, Birnholz J C. Ultrasound evaluation of the gallbladder wall. Radiology 1979; 133: 693–698

2 Slovis T L, Hight D W, Philippart A I, Dubois R S. Sonography in the diagnosis and management of hydrops of the gallbladder in children with mucocutaneous lymph node syndrome. Pediatrics 1980; 65: 789–794

3 Taylor K J W, Carpenter D A. The anatomy and pathology of the porta hepatis demonstrated by gray scale ultrasound. JCU 1975; 3: 117–119

4 Parulekar S G. Evaluation of common bile duct size. Radiology 1979; 133: 703–707

5 Edell S. A comparison of the 'Phrygian cap' deformity with 'bistable and gray scale ultrasound. JCU 1978; 6: 34–35

6 Sukov R J, Sample F, Sarti D A, Whitcomb M J. Cholecystosonography – the junctional fold. Radiology 1979; 133: 435–436

7 Cooperberg P L, Gibney R G. Imaging of the gallbladder, 1987. Radiology 1987; 163: 605–613

8 Marchal G, Kint E, Nijssens M, Baert A L. Variability of the hepatic arterial anatomy: a sonographic demonstration. JCU 1981; 9: 377–381

9 Berland L L, Lawson T L, Foley W D. Porta hepatis: sonographic discrimination of bile ducts from arteries with pulsed Doppler with new anatomic criteria. AJR 1982; 138: 833–840

10 Marchal G, Van de Voorde P, Van Dooren W, Ponette E, Baert A. Ultrasonic appearance of the filled and contracted normal gallbladder. JCU 1980; 8: 439–442

11 Filly R A, Moss A A, Way L W. In vitro investigation of gallstone shadowing with ultrasound tomography. JCU 1979; 7: 255–262

12 Jaffe C C, Taylor K J W. The clinical impact of ultrasonic beam focussing patterns. Radiology 1979; 131: 469–472

13 Dewbury K C. Visualisation of normal biliary ducts with ultrasound. Br J Radiol 1980; 53: 774–780

14 Lewandowski B J, Winsberg F. Gallbladder wall thickness distortion by ascites. AJR 1981; 137: 519–521

15 Behan M, Kazam E. Sonography of the common bile duct: value of the right anterior oblique view. AJR 1978; 130: 701–709

16 Laing F C, Jeffrey R B, Wing V W, Nyberg D A. Biliary dilatation: defining the level and cause by real time ultrasound. Radiology 1986; 160: 39–42

17 Sauerbrei E E, Cooperberg P L, Gordon P, Li D, Cohen M M, Burhenne H J. The discrepancy between radiographic and sonographic bile duct measurements. Radiology 1980; 137: 751–755

18 Wu C-C, Ho Y-H, Chen C-Y. Effect of aging on common bile duct diameter: a real time sonographic study. JCU 1984; 12: 473

19 Graham M F, Cooperberg P L, Cohen M M, Burhenne H J. The size of the normal common hepatic duct following cholecystectomy: an ultrasonic study. Radiology 1980; 135: 137–139

20 Mueller P R, Ferrucci J T Jnr, Simeone J F, et al. Post-cholecystectomy bile duct dilatation: myth or reality? AJR 1981; 136: 355

21 Wedmann B, Borsch G, Coenen C, Paassen A. Effect of cholecystectomy on common bile duct diameters; a longitudinal prospective ultrasonographic study. JCU 1988; 16: 619–624

22 Glazer G M, Filly R A, Laing F C. Rapid change in caliber of the non-obstructed common duct. Radiology 1981; 140: 161–162

23 Mueller P R, Ferrucci J T, Simeone J F, vanSonnenberg E, Hall P D A, Wittenberg J. Observations on the distensibility of the common bile duct. Radiology 1982; 142: 467–472

24 Cooperberg P L, Li D, Wong P, Cohen M M, Burhenne H J. Accuracy of common duct size in the evaluation of extrahepatic biliary obstruction. Radiology 1980; 135: 141–144

25 Everson G T, Braverman D Z, Johnson M L, Kern F. A critical evaluation of real time ultrasonography for the study of gallbladder volume and contraction. Gastroenterology 1980; 79: 40–46

26 Dodds W J, Groh W J, Darweesh R M A, Lawson T L, Kishk S M A, Kern M K. Sonographic measurement of gallbladder volume. AJR 1985; 145: 1009–1011

27 Hopman W P M, Brouwer W F M, Rosenbusch G, Jansen J B M J, Lamers C B H W. A computerized method for rapid quantitation of gallbladder volume from real time sonograms. Radiology 1985; 154: 236–237

28 Hopman W P M, Rosenbusch G, Jansen J B M J, de Jong A J L, Lamers C B H W. Gallbladder contraction: effects of fatty meals and cholecystokinin. Radiology 1985; 157: 37–39

29 Braverman D Z, Johnson M L, Kern F. Effects of pregnancy and contraceptive steroids on gallbladder function. N Engl J Med 1980; 302: 362–364

30 Delamarre J, Capron J-P, Joly J-P, et al. Gallbladder inertia in celiac disease: ultrasonographic demonstration. Dig Dis Sci 1984; 29: 876–877

31 Nino-Murcia M, Burton M, Chang P, Stone J, Perkash I. Gallbladder contractility in patients with spinal cord injuries: a sonographic investigation. AJR 1990; 154: 521–524

32 Simeone J F, Mueller P R, Ferrucci J T. Non-surgical therapy of gallstones: implications for imaging. AJR 1989; 152: 11–17

33 Bellamy P R, Hicks A. Assessment of gallbladder function by ultrasound; implications for dissolution therapy. Clin Radiol 1988; 39: 511–512

34 Simeone J F, Mueller P R, Ferrucci J T, et al. Sonography of the bile ducts after a fatty meal: an aid in the detection of obstruction. Radiology 1982; 143: 211–215

35 Wilson S A, Gosink B B, vanSonnenberg E. Unchanged size of a dilated common bile duct after a fatty meal: results and significance. Radiology 1986; 160: 29–31

36 Simeone J F, Butch R J, Mueller P R, et al. The bile ducts after a fatty meal: furthur sonographic observations. Radiology 1985; 154: 763–768

37 Darweesh R M A, Dodds W J, Hogan W J, et al. Fatty meal sonography for evaluating patients with suspected partial common duct obstruction. AJR 1988; 151: 63–68

38 Amouzal P, Palazzo L, Amouzal G, et al. Endosonography:

promising method for diagnosis of extrahepatic cholestasis. Lancet 1989; ii: 1195–1198

39 Tio T L. Endosonography in gastroenterology. Berlin: Springer Verlag. 1988

40 Knight R P, Newell J A. Operative uses of ultrasonics in cholelithiasis. Lancet 1963; i: 1023–1025

41 Lane R J, Glazer G. Intra-operative B-mode ultrasound scanning of the extrahepatic biliary system and pancreas. Lancet 1980; ii: 334–337

42 Sigel B, Coelho J U C, Spigos D G, et al. Real time ultrasonography during biliary surgery. Radiology 1980; 137: 531–533

43 Sigel B, Machi J, Beitler J C, et al. Comparative accuracy of operative ultrasonography and cholangiography in detecting common duct calculi. Surgery 1983; 94: 715–720

Gallbladder pathology

Henry C. Irving

INTRODUCTION

Ultrasound is now firmly established as the primary imaging investigation in all cases of suspected gallbladder disease.[1] The contents of the gallbladder lumen and the structure of its wall can be examined with accuracy and ease, while the rest of the hepatobiliary system and other surrounding structures can also be studied.[2]

Since the early days of ultrasound, there have been many studies comparing the accuracy rates, physical limitations, availability and relative costs of the various imaging techniques that are available for studying the gallbladder.[3-6] These, and many others, have recently been reviewed with the intention of providing clear diagnostic guide-lines for assessing gallbladder disease,[7] and after many years of pre-eminence, the oral cholecystogram has been relegated to a secondary role while intravenous cholangiography has become extinct!

In patients who present with acute right upper quadrant pain, ultrasound has an unsurpassed ability to demonstrate lesions of the gallbladder, can be performed rapidly at low cost and may show other causes for the patient's pain. Cholescintigraphy, using a ^{99m}Tc labelled derivative of iminodiacetic acid, is useful as a second line test for confirmation of cystic duct obstruction, either when ultrasound has failed to show stones, or when the origin of the symptoms remains in doubt in the presence of stones. Ultrasonically guided percutaneous aspiration of the gallbladder may be used on rare occasions for diagnosing acute acalculous cholecystitis.

When a patient presents with recurrent or chronic right upper quadrant pain, ultrasound will almost always solve the diagnostic problem posed by chronic gallbladder disease. The oral cholecystogram can be used when the ultrasound is technically unsatisfactory, e.g. in an obese patient, or when the result of the ultrasound is equivocal. Endoscopic retrograde cholangiography may be employed on the rare occasions when convincing symptoms persist despite negative findings on both ultrasound and oral cholecystography.

However, advances in the range of non-surgical therapies of gallstone disease are posing further demands on imaging techniques, and it is no longer enough for the imaging test simply to distinguish disease from absence of disease.[8] Selection of patients for oral bile acid therapy, extracorporeal shock wave lithotripsy, percutaneous dissolution or percutaneous cholecystolithotomy requires not only assessment of cystic duct patency, but also detailed information concerning gallbladder and duct morphology, as well as characterisation and quantification of gallbladder contents.[9] While ultrasound may be capable of providing most of this data,[10,11] it is likely that plain X-rays, oral cholecystography and perhaps also computed tomography will also be needed.

Because of its proven accuracy, speed of examination, low cost, and lack of toxicity or irradiation, ultrasound is an ideal tool for population screening,[12] and has been thus employed in several epidemiological studies for the assessment of the incidence of gallstone disease. The results of such studies tell us that the prevalence of gallstones in developed societies is approximately 10%, and that as many as two thirds of gallstone carriers are asymptomatic.[13,14] But, since the probability of developing biliary symptoms for subjects with silent stones has been shown to be only 18% in 24 years,[15] the increasing use of ultrasound in patients with symptoms which suggest the presence of gallstones, as part of routine physical examinations, or in screening studies, will unmask many previously undiagnosed stones and thus create both ethical and economic dilemmas for physicians and health care planners,[16] an uncomfortable penalty of improved diagnostic methods.

Stones

The composition, size, shape and number of stones vary widely from patient to patient. To these variations in chemical composition and physical characteristics must be added the variations in the effect that these stones have on the structure of the gallbladder itself. Thus it is not surprising that gallbladder stones present a myriad of ultrasound appearances.

Classical appearances The most commonly encountered ultrasound appearance of a stone in the gallbladder is that of a highly reflective intramural structure which is gravity-dependent and casts an acoustic shadow (Fig. 1). When all these features are present, the diagnostic accuracy is 100%.[4] It is useful to analyse each of these ultrasound features more closely so that the limitations of the method are appreciated, thus enabling scan technique and machine settings to be adjusted intelligently.

The size of a structure that can produce an echo from within the gallbladder lumen is not a limitation since it has been shown that particles as small as 5 to 10 μ will produce echoes within bile.[17] Such tiny particles are not considered to be 'stones', and indeed they will not fulfil the diagnostic criteria given above since they will not produce acoustic shadows.

The production of an acoustic shadow beyond a reflecting structure depends upon both the absorption and reflection of sound by the structure, and the resulting shadow should be sharp and 'clean' (Fig. 2). This is in contradistinction to the shadowing beyond bowel gas, which is caused purely by reflection of sound and is therefore usually less well-defined and 'dirty' due to reverberation artefacts (Fig. 3)[18] – a useful practical point in sorting out whether shadows are due to gallstones or to bowel gas (see Ch. 4). Shadowing beyond a stone is not affected by the chemical composition of the stone, the presence of calcium within the stone, or the shape and sur-

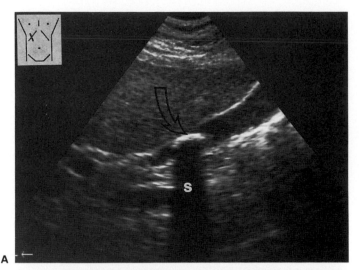

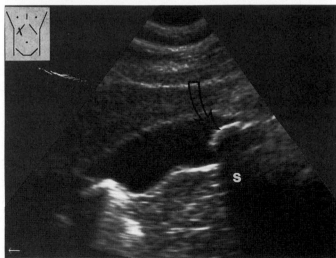

Fig. 1 Gall stones. 'Classical' appearances of stones in the gallbladder. A: With patient supine there is an echo from the stone within the gallbladder lumen (arrow) and there is an acoustic shadow (s) distally. B: With the patient upright, the stone (arrow) moves with gravity and drops into the fundus of the gallbladder.

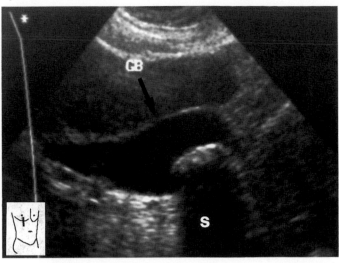

Fig. 2 Gall stone shadowing. 'Clean' shadowing (s). The acoustic shadow beyond the stone is free of reverberations.

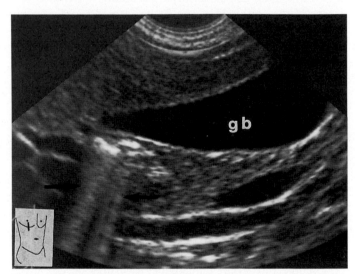

Fig. 3 Reverberative shadow. 'Dirty' shadowing (s). There are reverberation artefacts (arrows) distal to bowel gas (gb – gallbladder).

face characteristic of the stone,[19] but is dependent upon the geometric relationship between the ultrasound beam and the stone.[20] The beam width needs to be as small as possible since unless the stone occupies the full width of the beam, shadowing will not occur (Fig. 4). Beam width is reduced by focusing methods and by using transducers of higher frequency (see Ch. 2).

A further practical consideration concerning the demonstration of stones in the gallbladder relates to signal processing methods.[21] Currently available TV display units have limited dynamic range (less than 20 dB) and this necessitates the use of compression amplification. When this is combined with the use of time-gain compensation curves, the distinction between acoustic shadow and sur-

rounding tissues may be imperceptible.[22] This may be the most important limiting factor in real life scanning, but good quality modern equipment which is optimally adjusted should be capable of demonstrating stones in the gallbladder as small as 1 mm in diameter (Fig. 5).

Contracted gallbladder In the description of the 'classical' appearances of stones in the gallbladder, it will be appreciated that the gallbladder lumen contains fluid bile within which the echoes reflected by the stone or stones can be detected. In situations where the lumen is totally filled by stones, or where the gallbladder wall has been chronically inflamed and become fibrotic, or where the cystic duct has been obstructed, there may be no fluid bile within the lumen.

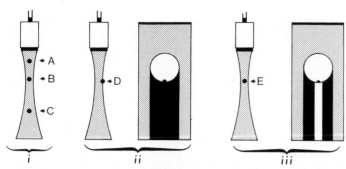

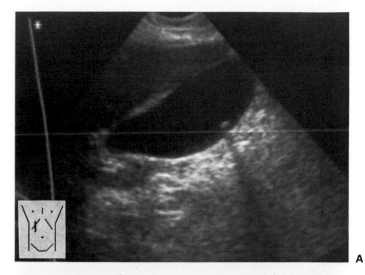

Fig. 4 Beam width and shadowing. Diagram to show the effect of beam width and incidence on the production of an acoustic shadow beyond a stone. (i) Stone B is in the focal zone of the beam and will give rise to an acoustic shadow, while stones A and C in the near and far fields of the beam are less likely to shadow (after Jaffe and Taylor).[21] (ii) and (iii) Diagrams to show the effect of positioning of a stone in relation to the beam; a linear array is viewed end on on the left and in the scanning plane on the right. Stone D (ii) at the periphery of the beam will not occupy a sufficient proportion of the beam width to cast a shadow, while the same size stone E (iii) at the centre of the beam will shadow (after Filly et al[20]).

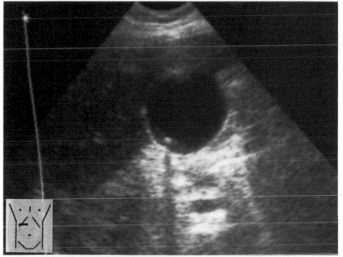

Fig. 5 Tiny stones with acoustic shadowing. A: Longitudinal scan. **B:** Transverse scan.

These 'contracted' or 'sclero-atrophic' gallbladders were initially recognised on ultrasound as a 'non-visualised' gallbladder lumen and this was shown to be a good indicator of pathology with an accuracy rate of 88%.[23] The findings become more reliable if distal acoustic shadowing can be seen to emanate from the gallbladder fossa (96% accuracy),[4] and the ability to locate the gallbladder fossa in different scan planes is crucial (Fig. 6) (see Ch. 11).[24]

Refinement of scanning technique can further improve the accuracy rates (to almost 99%), using movement of the patient during the study[25] to observe differences in movement between bowel gas in the duodenum or hepatic flexure and a contracted gallbladder full of stones. Diagnostic specificity is also aided by the observation of the wall-echo-shadow (WES) triad,[26] otherwise known as the 'double-arc-shadow sign'.[27] This complex consists of the reflective anterior wall of the gallbladder separated by a thin echo-poor rim (representing either a small amount of residual bile or an echo-poor portion of the thickened gallbladder wall) from the reflective anterior surface of the stone which casts a complete acoustic shadow (Fig. 7).

Persistent acoustic shadowing emanating from the gallbladder fossa may also be produced by a porcelain gallbladder, which is the term given to calcification of the gallbladder wall.[28] This condition is associated with gallstones in over 95% of cases, but the particular importance of recognising this entity lies in the increased incidence of both gallbladder carcinoma and cholangiocarcinoma (in 10% to 20% of cases), prophylactic cholecystectomy is usually advised (see section on gallbladder carcinoma, p. 202).

Movement/layering/floating of stones Gravity dependence of stones can be demonstrated by moving the patient during the ultrasound examination. Usually this is achieved by turning the patient into the left decubitus or right anterior oblique positions, but erect scans with the patient sitting or standing may also be performed. In this way, previously hidden stones lying in the neck of the gallbladder may come into view and the distinction between polyps and stones is facilitated (Figs 8 and 9).

Movement may also help when there are small stones from which it is proving difficult to demonstrate acoustic shadowing. If these stones can be collected into a group then the shadow may become more readily visible.[29]

Similarly, if small stones form a thin layer on the posterior wall of the gallbladder, the echoes from the stones may be erroneously ascribed to the wall itself. Shadowing from small stones lying on the posterior wall of the gallbladder may be obscured by the high reflectivity of the wall itself or of the immediately adjacent bowel gas causing a 'blooming' effect (Fig. 10). If such stones can be encour-

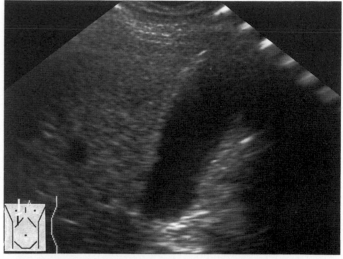

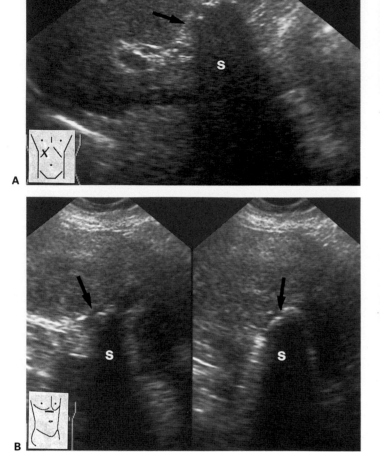

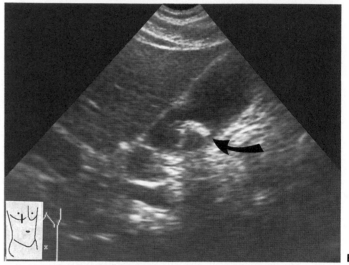

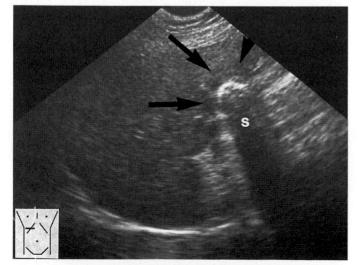

Fig. 6   Contracted gallbladder full of stones (arrows), with distal acoustic shadowing (s): **A:** Longitudinal scan. **B:** Transverse scans.

Fig. 8   Stone in the gallbladder. A: With the patient supine there is no evidence of any stone. **B:** A stone (arrowed) comes into view when the patient is turned right side up.

Fig. 7   Double-arc shadow sign. Echoes and acoustic shadow (s) emanate from the gallbladder fossa (arrows). Detection of an echo-poor anterior rim improves diagnostic specificity.

aged either to float across the gallbladder lumen or to clump together, the shadowing becomes obvious.

Floating stones which are of lower density than the surrounding bile give pathognomonic appearances, and this phenomenon has been utilised in clinical practice by iatrogenically increasing the density of the bile with radiographic contrast material.[30] Difficulties can sometimes arise when stones float up to the anterior wall so that the gallbladder lumen is not visualised, but once again, movement of the patient is crucial in avoiding this pitfall (Fig. 11).

Milk of calcium bile is another instance where gravity dependence is an aid to ultrasound diagnosis. The appearances here are predominantly those of echoes and shadowing from the gallbladder fossa, but layering out of the milk of calcium will be evident on the erect scans.[31,32]

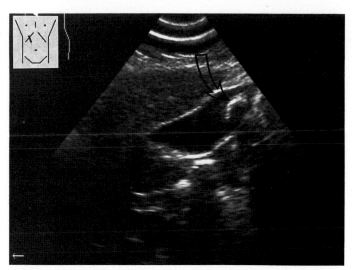

Fig. 9 Stone in the fundus. A stone (arrow) is clearly seen in the fundus of the gallbladder when the patient is scanned in the erect position.

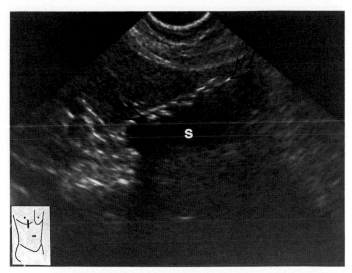

Fig. 11 Floating stones. The gallbladder lumen may be masked by the shadow (s) from stones (arrows) which float up to the anterior wall.

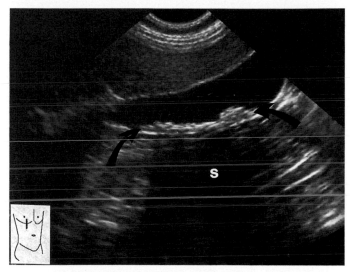

Fig. 10 Layered stones. A layer of stones on the posterior wall (arrows) is difficult to separate from the wall echoes, but note the distal shadowing (s).

Echogenic bile/biliary sludge

Non-shadowing, gravity-dependent echoes within the gallbladder are variously referred to as 'biliary sludge' or 'echogenic bile'. Several different pathological and physiological entities can result in these ultrasound appearances and, since neither of the above terms specifies a particular cause, there is considerable confusion about the significance of these findings.

Echogenic bile may be due to pus or blood in the bile as a result of infection or trauma, or it may be seen in association with obvious stones in the gallbladder (Fig. 12).[33] In these cases, the appearances are incontrovertibly

pathological, and when taken in conjunction with the patient's history, physical signs and other ultrasound features, the diagnosis can be quite specific.

However, echogenic bile may also be seen when there is bile stasis in the absence of stone disease, and this may be due to either pathological biliary obstruction or for physiological reasons, such as prolonged fasting,[34] in patients who are on parenteral nutrition[35] and after surgery on the gastrointestinal tract.[36] If the obstruction is relieved or if the gallbladder is rescanned after a normal diet has been resumed, the echoes will usually have disappeared from the bile. Occasionally the echoes may persist while all other investigations such as the oral cholecystogram and HIDA scintiscan are normal, but the significance of these findings has not yet been clarified (Fig. 13).

It has been pointed out that some non-shadowing echoes within the gallbladder are due to slice thickness artefacts. Clues that should alert the sonographer to this possibility include non-dependence on receiver gain and lack of change in height of debris between scans performed in transverse and longitudinal planes (Fig. 14).[37]

Occasionally non-shadowing echoes within the gallbladder may clump together giving the so-called 'sludge balls' or 'tumefactive sludge' (Fig. 15). This may give rise to a diagnostic dilemma since the appearances may mimic a soft tissue mass projecting into the gallbladder lumen resulting in a false diagnosis of gallbladder tumour (Fig. 16).[38] Movement of the echoes with gravity should be the key to differentiating these conditions, but the bile in these cases may be thick and viscid so that movement of the echoes may be imperceptibly slow. A repeat scan with a normal diet in the interim should reveal the true nature of the problem.[39]

In vitro studies have shown that the echoes in 'biliary

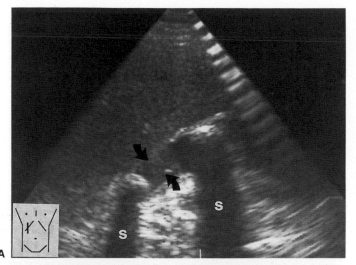

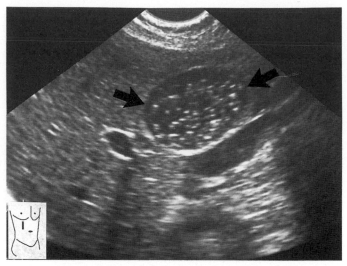

Fig. 13 **Echogenic bile.** The gallbladder contains non-shadowing echogenic material in this patient who had been on intravenous feeding. A rescan after normal diet had been resumed showed identical appearances but the patient was asymptomatic and both oral cholecystography and ^{99m}Tc-HIDA scans were normal.

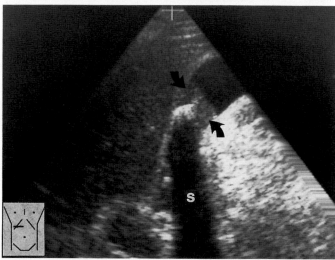

Fig. 12 **Stones and echogenic bile.** Stones giving rise to shadows (s) and non-shadowing echogenic bile (arrows). **A:** Longitudinal scan. **B:** Transverse scan.

sludge' are caused by particles of 5 to 10 μ size, and chemical analysis revealed that these were mainly calcium bilirubinate granules together with some cholesterol crystals.[17] It has been postulated that the so-called 'sludge balls' may represent an early stage of evolution of gallbladder stones,[40] but the relationship between the ability to form 'echogenic bile' on fasting and lithogenicity of bile remains largely speculative at present.

Gallbladder wall thickening

In the fasting state, the normal gallbladder is distended and has a wall thickness of less than 3 mm.[41] The normal anterior wall appears as a single smooth well-defined reflecting structure and its thickness can be measured accurately while the posterior wall can be more difficult to

measure because this wall is frequently in contact with air-containing bowel and the end point is indistinct (Fig. 17).

When the gallbladder contracts in response to a fat-containing meal or injection of cholecystokinin, the wall becomes thicker[42] and three distinct zones can then be identified – a strongly reflecting outer contour, a reflecting inner contour, and an echo-poor layer between the reflecting structures (Fig. 17).[43]

The method of measurement of gallbladder wall thickness is an important consideration since the ultrasound beam should be perpendicular to the wall so that measurements are truly axial. This may mean that measurements of both anterior and posterior wall thicknesses cannot be made on the same scan section.

It has been shown that minor angulation or decentring of the beam can cause 'pseudothickening' of the gallbladder wall[44] and recognition of this artefact fuelled an interesting debate. It had been observed that the gallbladder wall appeared to be thickened in the presence of ascites (Fig. 18)[45] and this was thought to be due to oedema of the gallbladder wall. It had also been shown that chronic alcoholics with hypoalbuminaemia had thickened gallbladder walls (Fig. 19), and in the majority of the cases under study there was no ascites in contact with the gallbladder.[46] It was therefore suggested that gallbladder wall thickening in the presence of ascites was due either to the underlying hypoalbuminaemia with shift of fluid from the intravascular to extravascular space, or to the artefactual pseudothickening which was particularly liable to occur when static B-scanners were used to examine gallbladders floating in ascites.

However, subsequent experience does show that gall-

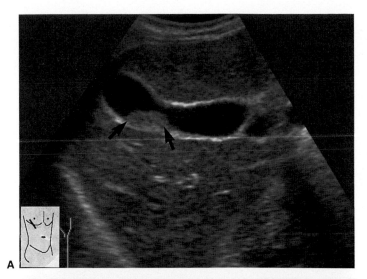

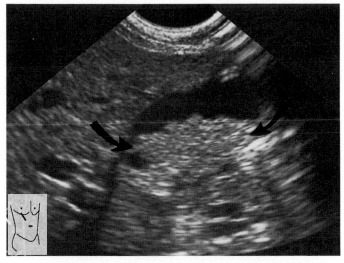

Fig. 16 Lumpy bile. Sludge gives the impression of a soft tissue mass (arrows) which led to the erroneous diagnosis of gallbladder carcinoma.

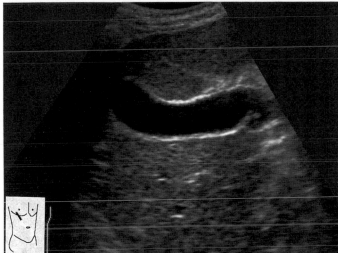

Fig. 14 False echogenic bile. **A:** Slice thickness artefact causing echoes within the gallbladder (arrows). **B:** The bile is echo-free after slight readjustment of transducer angulation.

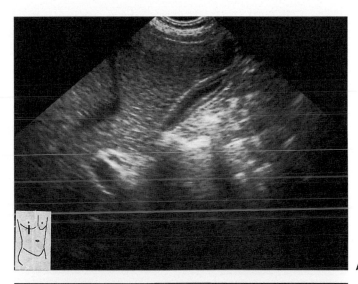

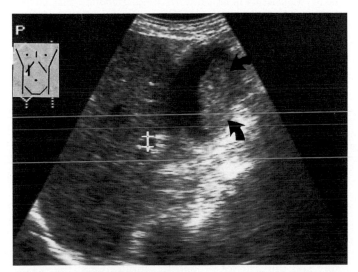

Fig. 15 Tumefactive sludge (arrows).

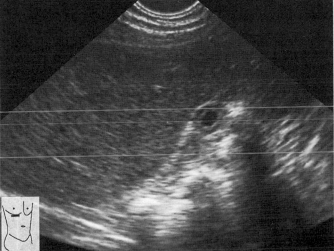

Fig. 17 Non-fasting gallbladder. Normal non-fasting gallbladder wall. **A:** Longitudinal scan. **B:** Transverse scan.

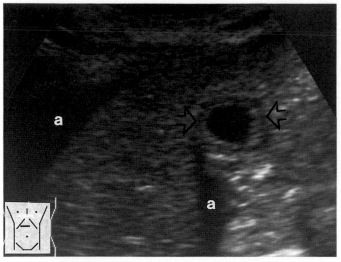

Fig. 18   Gallbladder in ascites. Thickened gallbladder wall (arrows) in the presence of ascites (a).

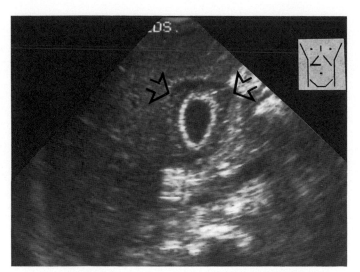

Fig. 20   Gallbladder in leukaemia. Grossly thickened gallbladder wall (arrows) in leukaemia.

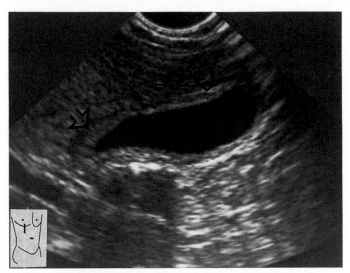

Fig. 19   Gallbladder wall in hypoalbuminaemia. Thickened gallbladder wall (arrows) in a patient with hypoalbuminaemia but no ascites.

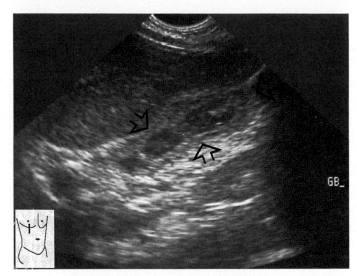

Fig. 21   Gallbladder in hepatitis. Thickened gallbladder wall (arrows) in acute viral hepatitis.

bladder wall thickening can be seen in the presence of ascites even when the serum albumin level is normal and care is taken over transducer angulation[47] and that in these cases the wall thickening is caused by ascites per se, presumably due to passive diffusion of fluid. A further twist to the tale has been provided recently by the observation that in patients with cirrhosis of the liver, portal hypertension can give rise to thickening of the gallbladder wall – 'congestive cholecystopathy' due to venous dilatation – in the absence of either hypoalbuminaemia or ascites.[48]

The gallbladder wall thickens in response to a wide range of pathological processes (Fig. 20) which are listed below, and is thus a very non-specific sign when used in isolation.[49] However, several of the conditions listed result in other ultrasound findings; the detection of gallbladder wall thickening may then provide useful contributory or confirmatory evidence.

Ultrasound signs may, of course, have uses other than purely diagnostic. In acute viral hepatitis, gallbladder wall thickening has not only been observed,[50] but has also been shown to correlate well with the degree of liver cell necrosis[51] and thus carries prognostic implications (Fig. 21).

Causes of gallbladder wall thickening
Physiological:
> Post-prandial

Inflammatory disease of the gallbladder:
> Acute cholecystitis
> Chronic cholecystitis
> Sclerosing cholangitis[52]
> AIDS[53]
> Crohn's disease[54]

Non-inflammatory disease of the gallbladder:
> Adenomyomatosis
> Carcinoma of gallbladder
> Leukaemia
> Multiple myeloma

Oedema of the gallbladder wall:
> Ascites
> Hypoalbuminaemia
> Heart failure
> Portal hypertension
> Renal disease
> Malignant lymphatic obstruction[55]/lymphoma

Nearby inflammatory disease:
> Acute viral hepatitis
> Alcoholic hepatitis[56]
> Acute pancreatitis
> Pericholecystic abscesses
> Hepatobiliary schistosomiasis[57]

Acute cholecystitis

The current therapeutic approach to patients who present with acute cholecystitis is to give immediate medical support in the form of analgesics and intravenous fluids, antibiotics if necessary, and to perform a cholecystectomy as soon as the patient is fit for operation, usually within the first 12 to 72 hours after admission.[58]

This modern trend for urgent cholecystectomy demands that the diagnosis must be made quickly, and therefore for patients who present with acute right upper quadrant pain, ultrasound is the initial imaging procedure of choice because of its ability to demonstrate anatomically defined gallbladder disease, it can be performed more rapidly and at lower cost than other tests such as HIDA scanning, and it enables a search to be made for other causes of the patient's pain.[1]

There is no single ultrasound sign that is specific for the diagnosis of acute cholecystitis; rather there is a range of findings which are conveniently discussed as either 'major' or 'minor' signs (Table 1).

Most studies have indicated that the sensitivity for a major sign of acute cholecystitis is 81% to 86%, and the specificity is 94% to 98%. The addition of a minor sign increases the sensitivity of ultrasound to 90% to 98%.[7] Not reflected in these figures for sensitivity and specificity is the ability to diagnose non-biliary sources of right upper

Table 1 Ultrasound signs of acute cholecystitis

Major	Minor
Stones in the GB	Pericholecystic fluid
Oedema of GB wall	Thickening of GB wall
Non-visualisation of GB	GB tenderness
Gas in GB wall	Intraluminal changes
	GB enlargement
	Round GB shape

quadrant pain – in as many as 35% of the patients without gall bladder disease.[59]

Increased thickness of the gallbladder wall (Fig. 22) is well-documented in acute cholecystitis,[60,61] but as discussed above, it is found in many other conditions, and is thus a minor sign. However, more obvious oedema of the gallbladder wall, which is recognisable by either a continuous echo-poor rim around the gallbladder or by a focal echo-poor zone in the wall, is a major sign of acute cholecystitis, providing that other causes of gallbladder wall oedema such as hypoalbuminaemia, heart failure, and other local inflammation have been excluded (Fig. 23). The echo-poor zones probably represent accumulation of oedema, inflammatory exudate, and/or haemorrhage. The echo-poor 'halo' is most easily demonstrated between the liver and the anterior wall of the gallbladder since the echo-poor bowel wall that is often adjacent to the posterior gallbladder wall may give a false positive 'halo sign'.[62]

Gallbladder tenderness is popularly known as the 'ultrasonic Murphy's sign',[63] but it does differ significantly from the clinical sign described by Murphy and modified by Moynihan.[64] In the clinical sign, the left hand of the examiner is placed on the costal margin in such a manner that the thumb lies over the fundus of the gallbladder. The thumb exerts moderate pressure and the patient is asked to take a deep breath. The sign is positive if the patient 'catches their breath' when the descending diaphragm

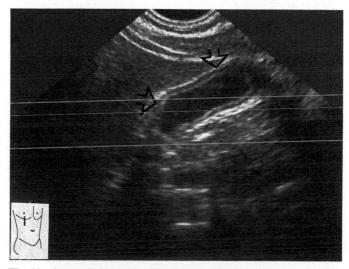

Fig. 22 Acute cholecystitis. Thickened gallbladder wall (arrows) with an echo-poor central zone due to acute cholecystitis.

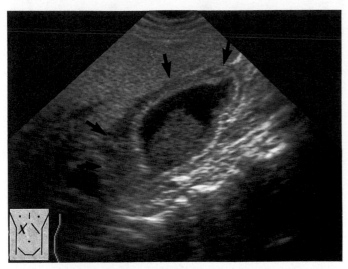

Fig. 23   Acute cholecystitis. Thickened gallbladder wall with an echo-poor 'halo' (arrows) due to acute cholecystitis. Note also the 'lumpy bile' giving echoes in the lumen.

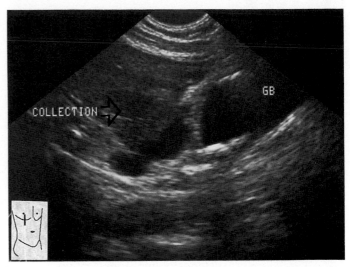

Fig. 25   Pericholecystic collection. The fluid within a pericholecystic leak contains non-shadowing echoes due to pus (arrow).

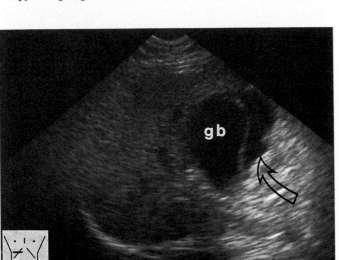

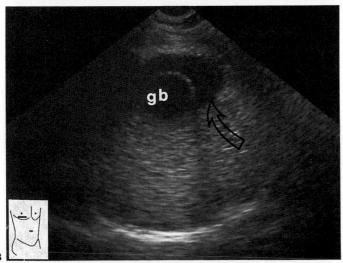

Fig. 24   Gangrene. Gangrenous gallbladder wall with small pericholecystic leak (arrow). **A:** Patient supine. **B:** Patient in right anterior oblique position (gb – gallbladder).

causes the inflamed gallbladder to impinge on the thumb. A positive ultrasonic Murphy's sign is present when the tenderness is maximal over the ultrasonically localised gallbladder,[65] thus ensuring that the pain is elicited only during image verified deformation of the gallbladder.[42] The combination of stones in the gallbladder and a positive ultrasound Murphy's sign are highly specific for acute cholecystitis (92%).[66]

Acute cholecystitis may progress to gangrenous cholecystitis which may perforate resulting in a pericholecystic abscess (Figs 24 and 25) or peritonitis. The morbidity and mortality associated with this condition are considerably higher than with uncomplicated acute cholecystitis and it is important to look for ultrasound signs that may expedite diagnosis and emergency surgery. Marked irregularity or asymmetrical thickening of the gallbladder wall reflect the pathological changes of ulceration, haemorrhage, necrosis and intramural micro-abscesses.[67]

Empyema of the gallbladder is difficult to recognise on ultrasound because the typical finding of sludge (non-shadowing gravity-dependent echoes) may be caused by many processes other than debris or pus (Fig. 26).[68,69] Intraluminal membranes, due to fibrinous strands of exudate and sloughing of gallbladder mucosa are features of gangrene of the gallbladder (Fig. 27).[70] Interestingly, only 33% of patients with gangrenous gallbladders are said to have a positive ultrasonic Murphy's sign[71] compared with the 95% prevalence in patients with acute non-gangrenous cholecystitis.[65] Perhaps the lack of pain is due to necrosis of the nerves in the muscular and serosal layers of the gallbladder.

Pericholecystic fluid collections may be due to localised peritonitis or to leaks from perforation of the gallbladder wall. These latter may vary in size and complexity from a small bile collection as a result of a microperforation to a

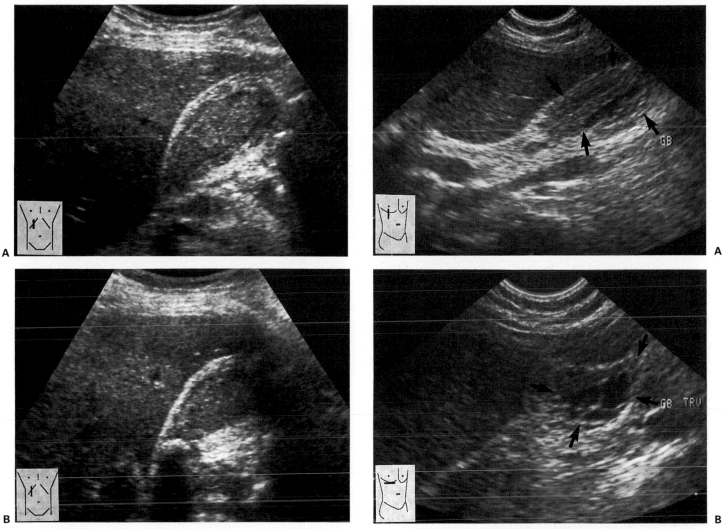

Fig. 26 Empyema of the gallbladder. A: Thickened wall and low level echoes filling the lumen. **B:** The same case showing a stone in the neck of the gallbladder.

Fig. 27 Gangrenous cholecystitis. Gangrenous gallbladder wall and typical intraluminal membranes representing desquamated mucosa:[62] **A:** Longitudinal scan. **B:** Transverse scan.

true pericholecystic abscess (Fig. 28).[72] The ultrasound appearances of such abscesses can be quite variable ranging from predominantly echo-free to predominantly highly reflective, although increased through transmission of sound should remain apparent.[73]

Gas in the gallbladder wall, the hallmark of emphysematous cholecystitis, is due to gas forming organisms in the bile, and is one of the major ultrasound signs of acute cholecystitis. It may be recognised by highly reflective areas within a thickened and oedematous gallbladder wall with shadowing and reverberations distally (Fig. 29).[74-76] There may also be gas within the gallbladder lumen which may make it difficult to distinguish the gallbladder from a loop of bowel. Repositioning the patient may help, and it has been documented that the gas in the gallbladder wall may shift with gravity,[77] and that the gas in the lumen may be seen to 'effervesce' on real time observation.[78] Although

this is an extremely rare condition, it is important to recognise because of its strong association with gangrene and perforation of the gallbladder.[79] Plain X-rays or CT scan are always recommended for confirmation because of the possibility of bowel gas or a porcelain gallbladder causing confusingly similar ultrasound features. Emphysematous cholecystitis may occur in the absence of gallstones – usually in diabetics – it is postulated that ischaemia of the gallbladder wall may be a primary factor in these cases.

Acute cholecystitis is acalculous in approximately 5% to 10% of all patients with acute cholecystitis.[80] It frequently occurs as a complication of a prolonged or severe illness such as recent major surgery, burns, sepsis, prolonged hypotension, general debility and diabetes.[81] Histologically, the changes in the gallbladder wall are similar to calculous cholecystitis, although gangrene and perforation are more common in the acalculous variety – presumably because of

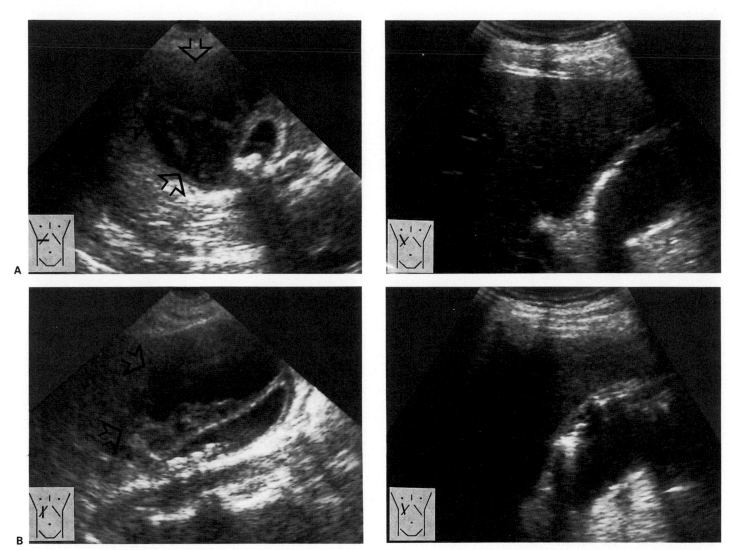

Fig. 28 Large pericholecystic abscess (arrows) extending into the liver from the thick walled gallbladder which is seen to contain stones. **A:** Longitudinal scan. **B:** Transverse scan.

Fig. 29 Emphysematous cholecystitis. Thickened gallbladder wall containing an area of high reflectivity with distal shadowing due to gas.

delayed diagnosis and treatment. The lack of stones and the inability to elicit the ultrasonic Murphy's sign in a comatose patient contribute to the diagnostic difficulty, although thickening of the gallbladder wall in association with a lack of response of the gallbladder to cholecystokinin, distension of the gallbladder and the presence of sludge are helpful signs (Fig. 30).[82] Diagnostic specificity may be improved by ultrasound guided percutaneous aspiration of the gallbladder so that bacteria and/or leukocytes can be detected in the bile,[83] but initial enthusiasm for the technique has become tempered by the limitation that a negative result does not excluded acute cholecystitis.[84] This is only to be expected when it is remembered that in patients coming to surgery for acute cholecystitis, only approximately half have infected bile from which aerobic or anaerobic organisms may be cultured.[58]

Chronic cholecystitis

In patients with recurrent right upper quadrant pain, chronic gallbladder disease has to be considered. Chronic cholecystitis is almost always found in association with gallstones although the exact aetiology is unclear and the classic 'chicken and egg' debate continues to rage. In association with the stones there is a chronic inflammatory cell infiltrate throughout all the layers of the wall which becomes thickened with fibrosis in both the subserosal and muscular layers, resulting in overall shrinkage of the viscus and reduction of the lumen. In this clinical context, the ultrasonic demonstration of stones in the gallbladder, with or without thickening of the gallbladder wall, is usually taken to be diagnostic (Fig. 31).

If the presence of ultrasonically demonstrated gallstones is taken as an indicator of chronic gallbladder disease as

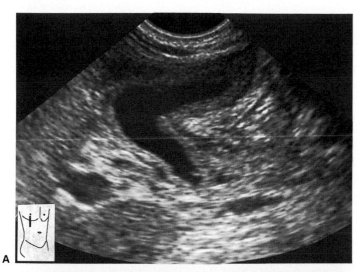

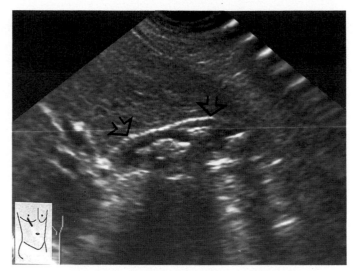

Fig. 31 **Chronic cholecystitis** with stones in a thick walled gallbladder (arrows).

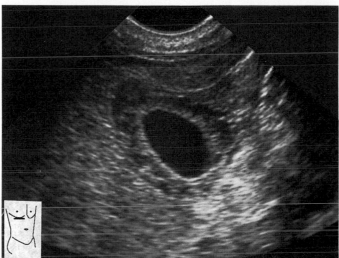

Fig. 30 **Acalculous cholecystitis.** Thickened gallbladder wall in acalculous cholecystitis. **A:** Longitudinal scan. **B:** Transverse scan.

defined by surgery, then ultrasound has been found to have a sensitivity ranging from 90% to 98%, with specificity consistently in the 94% to 98% range.[7] In addition, non-visualisation of the gallbladder at ultrasound has been shown to be highly predictive of gallbladder disease.[23]

Oral cholecystography is now generally held in reserve for patients in whom an adequate ultrasound cannot be performed for technical reasons, such as obesity, or when there is a strong clinical suspicion of cholecystitis despite a negative ultrasound, whilst endoscopic retrograde cholangiography has been recommended on the very rare occasions when both ultrasound and oral cholecystography are negative but convincing symptoms persist.[1]

Hyperplastic cholecystoses

In some cases of chronic cholecystitis, the lining epithelium of the gallbladder extends as downgrowths between the muscle bundles giving rise to deeply situated gland-like structures, known as Rokitansky-Aschoff sinuses. These diverticula may be extensive forming numerous gland-like spaces lined by epithelial cells not only in the inner part of the thickened and fibrous wall, but throughout its entire thickness and even extending beneath its serous coat where they may become dilated. Focal increase in wall thickness may result in localised narrowing of the gallbladder lumen, giving rise to the appearance of a stricture. The term 'cholecystitis glandularis proliferans' has been applied to such a condition.

However, the 'hyperplastic' changes in the gallbladder wall described above may occur in the absence of either gallstones or inflammatory infiltrates, when the condition is known as adenomyomatosis.[85] This is considered to be quite distinct from chronic cholecystitis, and although excessive intraluminal pressure has been suggested as the cause, the exact aetiology remains unclear.

The ultrasound features of adenomyomatosis are now well-recognised.[86] There is diffuse or segmental thickening of the gallbladder wall, with intramural diverticula which may be echo-free if they contain fluid bile, or highly reflective if they contain bile concretions. Segmental and eccentric wall thickening may produce mid-cavity strictures, and the high amplitude periluminal foci (due to aggregates of solid bile elements in the Rokitansky-Aschoff sinuses) give a typical 'diamond ring' appearance on transverse sections of the gallbladder (Fig 32).[87]

The clinical significance of adenomyomatosis of the gallbladder is controversial since it may be found in asymptomatic individuals. However, a significant proportion of patients with adenomyomatosis do improve after cholecystectomy, especially if the symptoms were more suggestive of biliary colic than of vague dyspepsia, or if gallstones are found in association with the adenomyomatosis.[85]

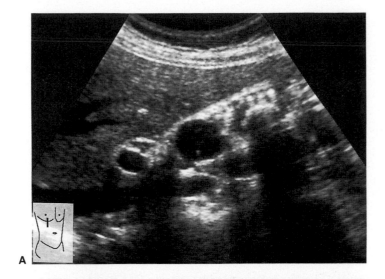

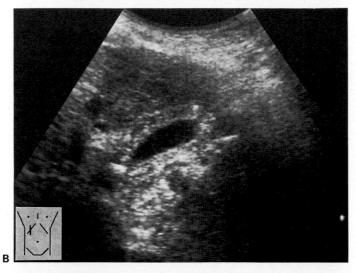

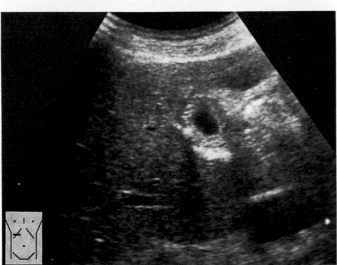

The 'strawberry gallbladder' of cholesterolosis is another non-inflammatory condition of the gallbladder and is the result of the accumulation of lipids in the mucosa of the gallbladder wall. The resulting surface nodules are usually less than 1 mm in diameter and cannot therefore be recognised on ultrasound. However, larger polypoid excrescences forming cholesterol polyps sometimes develop, and these can be detected as small reflective foci attached to the wall of the gallbladder. They may be single or multiple, generally do not cast acoustic shadows, and will not move with changes in patient position (Fig. 33).[88]

The aetiology of cholesterolosis is not fully understood although it is suggested that the mucosal changes might arise simply because of increased cholesterol uptake from bile containing extra cholesterol.[89] Whilst cholecystectomy is unlikely to benefit patients with vague dyspeptic symptoms, it is likely to help patients in whom the history

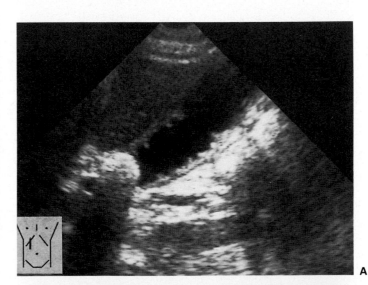

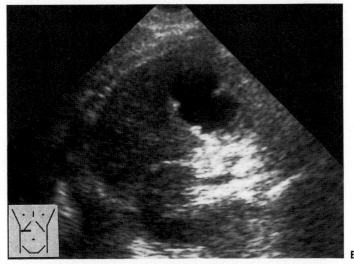

Fig. 32 Adenomyomatosis. A: Localised adenomyomatosis confined to the gallbladder fundus showing the typical 'diamond ring' appearance due to concretions in the dilated sinuses. Note the solitary large gall stone. **B:** Generalised adenomyomatosis, longitudinal and **C:** transverse scan in another case.

Fig. 33 Multiple cholesterol polyps projecting into the lumen of a gallbladder with a stone impacted in the neck. **A:** Longitudinal scan. **B:** Transverse scan.

suggests biliary colic, or when there are associated gall-stones.[85,89]

Polyps

Polyps of the gallbladder include pseudotumours such as inflammatory polyps, cholesterol polyps and adenomyomas, the localised form of adenomyomatosis. The typical ultrasound appearance of these polyps is of a small intraluminal reflective structure which is fixed to the gallbladder wall and does not cast an acoustic shadow (Figs 34 and 35). They are common, and in the absence of accompanying gallstones are probably not clinically significant.

The commonest type of true benign neoplasm is the adenoma which can be either sessile or papillary and is usually solitary.[90] Adenomatous gallbladder polyps have been described in Peutz-Jeghers syndrome,[91] 10% are

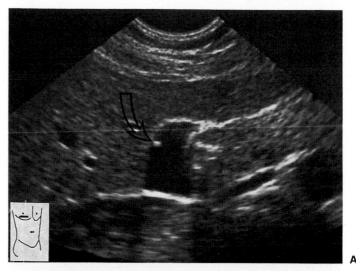

A

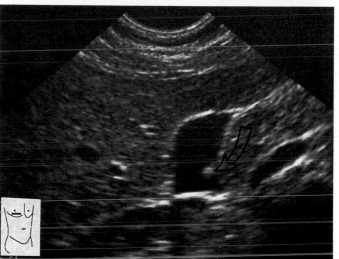

B

Fig. 35 **Two hyperplastic polyps** (arrows) within the same gall-bladder. **A:** Transverse scan near the neck of the gallbladder. **B:** Transverse scan near the fundus.

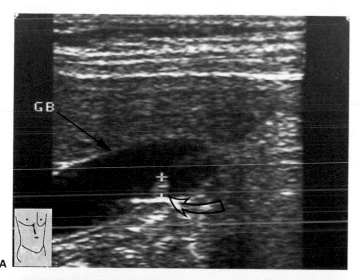

A

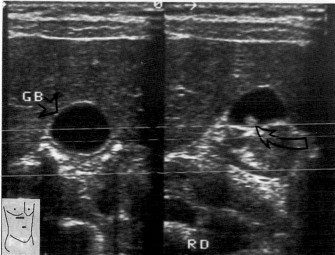

B

Fig. 34 **Hyperplastic gallbladder polyp** (curved arrows) in the gallbladder. **A:** Longitudinal scan. **B:** Transverse scans.

multiple, and 10% show evidence of carcinoma in situ.[92] Intestinal metaplasia can be found in large adenomas and may be a premalignant change[93] and, as in the intestinal tract, it is probably the larger adenomas that undergo malignant transformation. Adenomas are usually incidental findings, but they can cause biliary colic.

The typical ultrasound appearance is of a soft tissue consistency mass projecting into the gallbladder lumen. It remains fixed to the gallbladder wall despite movement of the patient and does not cast an acoustic shadow (Fig. 36). Because of the probability of an adenoma/carcinoma sequence, cholecystectomy is advisable, even for asymptomatic polyps.[94]

There are other benign neoplasms of the gallbladder including fibroma, lipoma, myoma, carcinoid, and haemangioma, but they are all extremely rare.[95]

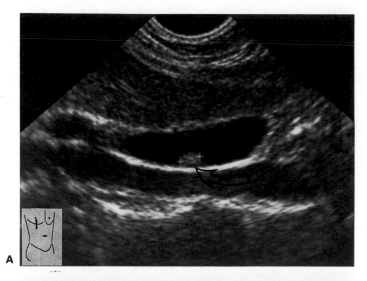

A

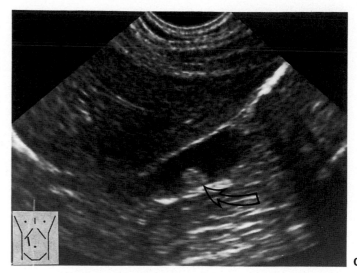

C

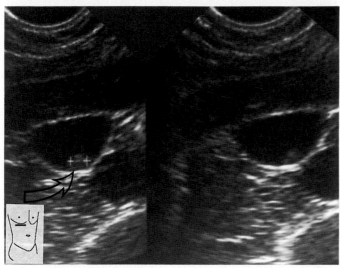

B

Fig. 36   Adenomatous polyp 7 mm in diameter (arrows).
A: Longitudinal scan. **B:** Transverse scans. **C:** Scan with patient upright.

Carcinoma

Carcinoma of the gallbladder is a highly malignant tumour characterised by early metastases and a rapidly downhill clinical course. It is the fifth most common malignancy of the gastrointestinal tract, comprising 1% to 3% of all cancers, affecting females four times as commonly as males, and its prevalence increases with age. There is a high correlation with gallstones (80% to 90%) and chronic cholecystitis suggesting that chronic inflammation of the gallbladder mucosa may result in a dysplasia which goes on to neoplastic transformation.

Diagnosis of this tumour is usually not made until local spread and metastases have occurred, but the ultrasound detection of gallbladder wall irregularities,[96] or of a complex reflective mass obliterating the gallbladder lumen[97] may enable the diagnosis to be made pre-operatively.

The various ultrasonic appearances of gallbladder carcinoma[98-101] have been well-described. The most common finding is of a large solid mass filling the gallbladder bed (Fig. 37). This appearance is non-specific and the underlying nature of the mass has to be guessed at by the lack of visualisation of a separate gallbladder lumen or the presence of stones within the mass. The tumour may also be detected as an irregular polypoid mass within the gallbladder lumen, or as irregular thickening of the gallbladder wall which may be focal or diffuse, or as a combination of the two.

Approximately 25% of patients with a porcelain gallbladder (calcification of the gallbladder wall) will have associated carcinoma and the lesion may be obscured by the acoustic shadow arising from the calcified anterior wall. Differentiating a porcelain gallbladder from a gallbladder full of stones is important because of this high risk of malignancy. With careful scanning, the non-calcified anterior wall of the gallbladder can be seen in the case of stones,[26,27] while the calcified posterior wall of a porcelain gallbladder may be seen, giving diagnostic appearances of a biconvex curvilinear reflective structure (Fig. 38).[28] The development of a carcinoma within a porcelain gallbladder can be detected if there is local or diffuse thickening of the gallbladder wall external to the calcified portion, an eccentric mass arising from the gallbladder wall, or if there is evidence of biliary obstruction, porta hepatis or peripancreatic lymphadenopathy, or liver metastases.[62]

Although the overall prognosis for this tumour remains bleak with a mean survival of less than 5 months from the time of diagnosis, ultrasound may facilitate treatment of early and curable carcinomas by the fortuitous detection of tumours in patients who are asymptomatic or who have symptoms attributable to the coexistent stones.[102] In countries where the rate of cholecystectomy for cholelithiasis has increased, there has been a corresponding decrease in the mortality from gallbladder carcinoma.[103]

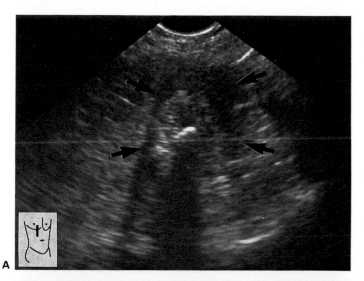

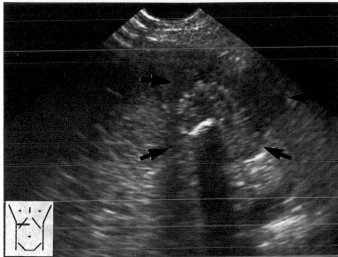

Fig. 37 Carcinoma of the gallbladder producing a large, ill-defined solid mass (arrows) in the gallbladder fossa – note the stone within the mass. **A:** Longitudinal scan. **B:** Transverse scan.

As with any other abdominal viscus, blood-borne metastases may find their way to the gallbladder, albeit rarely, and asymmetrical wall thickening or polypoid intraluminal masses may be indistinguishable from primary gallbladder cancer (Fig. 39).[104] Malignant melanoma is the most common source of gallbladder metastases which may be asymptomatic or simulate acute cholecystitis.[105]

Worms

Certain worms which parasitise man may find their way into the gallbladder and/or bile ducts and may be recognised on ultrasound.

Ascariasis Infestation by the *Ascaris lumbricoides* roundworm is endemic in the Far East, CIS, Latin America and Africa, and world-wide is probably second only to gallstones as a cause of acute biliary symptoms. The

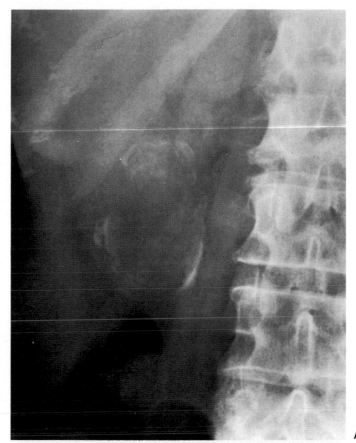

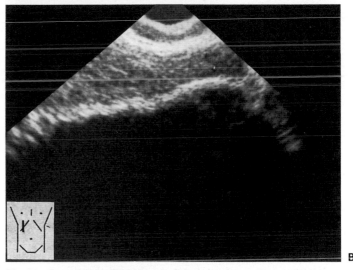

Fig. 38 Porcelain gallbladder. A: X-ray showing typical gallbladder wall calcification. **B:** Scan of gallbladder area showing total reflection of sound at the gallbladder wall. Figure courtesy of Dr A. E. A. Joseph.

adult worm is 15 to 50 cm long and some 5 mm thick, and lives mainly in the jejunum. It has a propensity to migrate up into the common bile duct from where it may enter the gallbladder or intrahepatic bile ducts. It may then cause biliary colic or acute cholecystitis. Ultrasound scans will

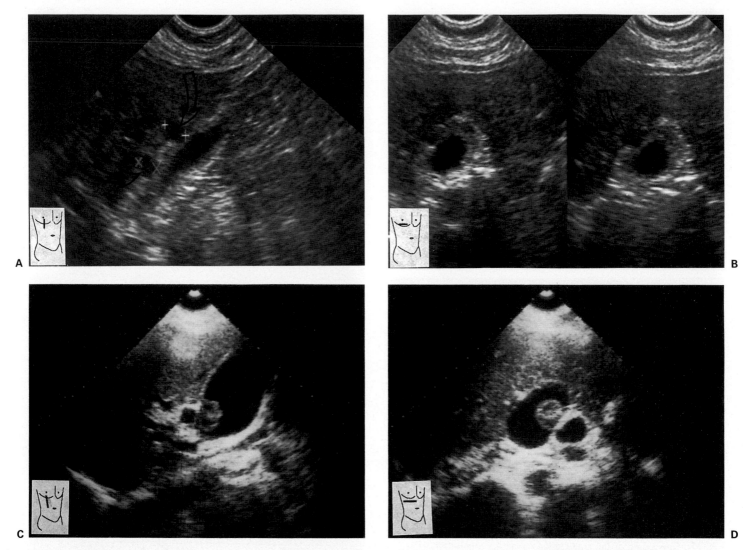

Fig. 39 Metastatic deposits (arrows) from an anaplastic lung primary are seen in the gallbladder wall as echo-poor nodules. **A:** Longitudinal scan. **B:** Transverse scans. **C:** Metastases from malignant melanoma giving rise to a clearly defined, slightly heterogeneous soft tissue lesion arising from the gallbladder wall, oblique scan and **D:** transverse scan.

demonstrate the worms in the common duct or gallbladder as single strips, multiple strips, coils, or as amorphous fragments (Fig. 40).[106] The writhing movements of the living worm are striking on real time scanning.

Clonorchiasis Man ingests the *Clonorchis sinensis* liver fluke by eating raw freshwater fish and the disease is endemic in the Far East. The adult worms are some 5 mm in length and reside in the medium or small intrahepatic bile ducts and occasionally also in the extrahepatic ducts and gallbladder. Intrahepatic duct dilatation and cholangitis are the main features of the disease, and form the bulk of the ultrasound findings, but the parasites can be demonstrated in the gallbladder, where they cause floating or dependent, discrete, non-shadowing, intraluminal reflective foci, which are fusiform in shape and measure 3 to 6 mm. Spontaneous movements of these structures have been observed on ultrasound, representing movement of

living worms. Thickening of the gallbladder wall has also been noted.[107]

Liver flukes Adult *fasciola* worms have recently been observed within the gallbladder on ultrasound as irregular, linear reflective structures 20 to 30 mm long,[108] and similar findings are documented in the gallbladder of a patient with *Opisthorchis viverrinii*.[109]

Hydrops

Enlargement of the gallbladder is a subjective judgement as the range of normal variation precludes precise ranges for the normal dimensions. The long axis measurement should not exceed 10 cm and the short axis 5 cm, but these figures are only a rough guide as many abnormally distended gallbladders will be smaller than these sizes, and some normal gallbladders will be larger.

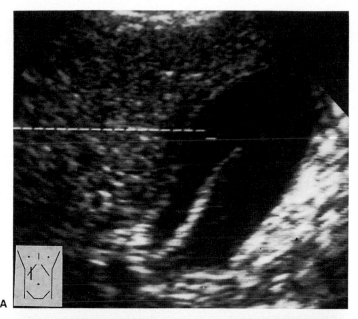

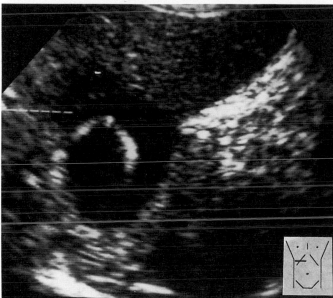

Fig. 40 Worms in gallbladder. A: Longitudinal and **B:** transverse scan showing curved worm in the gallbladder lumen.

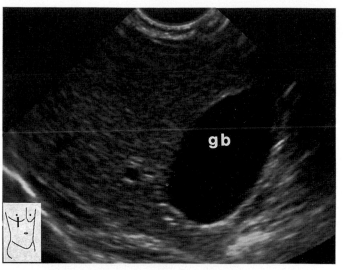

Fig. 41 Hydrops of the gallbladder due to mucocutaneous lymph node (Kawasaki) syndrome in a child aged 3 months.

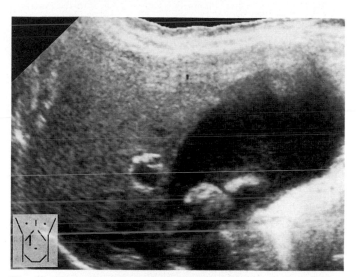

Fig. 42 Mucocele of the gallbladder. The gallbladder is distended, thin walled and contains stones.

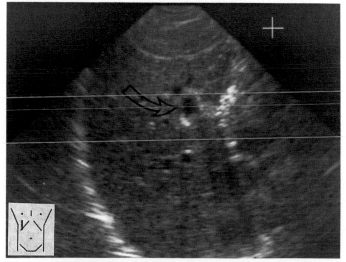

Fig. 43 Microgallbladder (arrow) in a fasted patient with cystic fibrosis.

There are several conditions in which the gallbladder enlarges (e.g. diabetes, pregnancy,[110] and in response to narcotic and anticholinergic drugs),[111] but the term 'hydrops' is probably best reserved for gallbladders which are distended due to blockage of the cystic duct, and these will give a more rounded and tense appearance due to the raised intraluminal pressure (Fig. 41).

Acute dilatation of the gallbladder may develop in children with typhoid, leptospirosis or other systemic infections.[112] It has also been reported in mucocutaneous lymph node (Kawasaki) syndrome,[113,114] Sjogren's disease,[115] and in systemic sclerosis.[116] Chronic dilatation may be due to stones in Hartman's pouch or the cystic duct giving rise to a mucocele of the gallbladder (Fig. 42).

Microgallbladder

If the gallbladder measures less than 3 cm × 1 cm in the fasting state it is classified as a microgallbladder and this occurs in approximately 30% of patients with cystic fibrosis.[117] The gallbladder usually contains colourless viscid mucus – 'white bile' – and the cystic duct may be atrophic or occluded with mucus. There is an increased incidence of gallstones in cystic fibrosis due to a combination of factors which include loss of bile salts because of malabsorption, increased biliary lipid composition and bile stasis, while thickening of the gallbladder wall may develop if secondary cholecystitis occurs (Fig. 43).[118]

REFERENCES

1 Health and Policy Committee, American College of Physicians. How to study the gallbladder. Ann Int Med 1988; 109: 752–754

2 Bush W H. Renal cell carcinoma discovered incidentally during gallbladder ultrasonography. AJR 1990; 154: 196

3 Bartrum R J Jr, Crow H C, Foote S R. Ultrasonic and radiographic cholecystography. N Engl J Med 1977; 296: 538–541

4 Crade M, Taylor K J W, Rosenfield A T, de Graaf C S, Minihan P. Surgical and pathologic correlation of cholecystosonography and cholecystography. AJR 1978; 131: 227–229

5 Cooperberg P L, Burhenne H J. Real time ultrasonography: diagnostic technique of choice in calculous gallbladder disease. N Eng J Med 1980; 302: 1277–1279

6 Cooperberg P L, Gibney R G. Imaging of the gallbladder, 1987. Radiology 1987; 163: 605–613

7 Marton K I, Doubilet P. How to image the gallbladder in suspected cholecystitis. Ann Int Med 1988; 109: 722–729

8 Simeone J F, Mueller P R, Ferrucci J T. Non-surgical therapy of gallstones: implications for imaging. AJR 1989; 152: 11–17

9 Lees W R, Kellett M J. Gallbladder stones: new roles for the radiologist. Clin Radiol 1989; 40: 561–563

10 Bellamy P R, Hicks A. Assessment of gallbladder function by ultrasound: implications for dissolution therapy. Clin Radiol 1988; 39: 511–512

11 Mathieson J R, So C B, Malone D E, Becker C D, Burhenne H J. Accuracy of sonography for determining the number and size of gallbladder stones before and after lithotripsy. AJR 1989; 153: 977–980

12 Birnholz J C. Population survey: ultrasonic cholecystography. Gastrointest Radiol 1982; 7: 165–167

13 Barbara L. Epidemiology of gallstone disease: the 'Sirmione Study'. In: Capocaccia L, Ricci G, Angelico F, Angelico M, Attili A F. eds. Epidemiology and prevention of gallstone disease. Lancaster: MTP Press. 1984: p 23–25

14 GREPCO. Prevalence of gallstone disease in an Italian adult female population. Am J Epidemiol 1984; 119: 796–805

15 Gracie W A, Ransohoff D F. The natural history of silent gallstones: the innocent gallstone is not a myth. N Engl J Med 1982; 307: 798–800

16 Dowling R H. Epidemiology and medical treatment of cholesterol gallstones: recurrence, post-dissolution management and the future. In: Capocaccia L, Ricci G, Angelico F, Angelico M, Attili A F. eds. Epidemiology and prevention of gallstone disease. Lancaster: MTP Press. 1984: p 116–128

17 Filly R A, Allen B, Minton M J, Bernhoft R, Way L W. In vitro investigation of the origin of echoes within biliary sludge. JCU 1980; 8: 193–200

18 Sommer F G, Taylor K J W. Differentiation of acoustic shadowing due to calculi and gas collections. Radiology 1980; 135: 399

19 Carroll B A. Gallstones: in vitro comparison of physical, radiographic and ultrasonic characteristics. AJR 1978; 131: 223–226

20 Filly R A, Moss A A, Way L W. In vitro investigation of gallstone shadowing with ultrasonic tomography. JCU 1979; 7: 255

21 Jaffe C C, Taylor K J W. The clinical impact of ultrasonic beam focussing patterns. Radiology 1979; 131: 469–472

22 Taylor K J W, Jacobson P, Jaffe C C. Lack of an acoustic shadow on scans of gallstones: a possible artefact. Radiology 1979; 131: 463–464

23 Harbin W P, Ferucci J T, Wittenberg J, Kirkpatrick R H. Non-visualised gallbadder by cholecystosonography. AJR 1979; 132: 727–728

24 Callen P W, Filly R A. Ultrasonographic localisation of the gallbladder. Radiology 1979; 133: 693–698

25 Conrad M R, Leonard J, Landay M J. Left lateral decubitus sonography of gallstones in the contracted gallbladder. AJR 1980; 134: 141–144

26 MacDonald F R, Cooperberg P L, Cohen M M. The WES triad – A specific sign of gallstones in the contracted gallbladder. Gastrointest Radiol 1981; 6: 39–41

27 Ratpopoulos V, D'Orsi C, Smith E, Reuter K, Moss L, Kleinman P. Dynamic cholecystosonography of the contracted gallbladder: The double-arc-shadow sign. AJR 1982; 138: 275–278

28 Kane R A, Jacobs R, Katz J, Costello P. Porcelain gallbladder: ultrasound and CT appearance. Radiology 1984; 152: 137–141

29 Crow H C, Bartrum R J, Foote S R. Expanded criteria for the ultrasonic diagnosis of gallstones. JCU 1976; 4: 289

30 Scheske G A, Cooperberg P L, Cohen M M, Burhenne H J. Floating gallstones: the role of contrast material. JCU 1980; 8: 22–27

31 Love M B. Sonographic features of milk of calcium bile. J Ultrasound Med 1982; 1: 325–327

32 Chun G H, Deutsch A L, Scheible W. Sonographic findings in milk of calcium bile. Gastrointest Radiol 1982; 7: 371–373

33 Conrad M R, Janes J O, Dietchy J. Significance of low level echoes within the gallbladder. AJR 1979; 132: 967–972

34 Simeone J F, Mueller P R, Ferrucci J T, Harbin W P, Wittenberg J. Significance of non-shadowing focal opacities at cholecystosonography. Radiology 1980; 137: 181–185

35 Messing B, Bories C, Kunstlinger F, Bernier J J. Does total parenteral nutrition induce gallbladder sludge formation and lithiasis? Gastroenterology 1983; 84: 1012–1019

36 Bolondi L, et al. Early detection of biliary sludge and gallstones after surgery of the G. I. tract. In: Barbara L, Dowling R H, Hofman A F, Roda E. eds. Recent advances in bile acid research. New York: Raven Press. 1985: p 281–285

37 Goldstein A, Madrazo B L. Slice thickness artefacts in gray scale ultrasound. JCU 1981; 9: 365–375

38 Anastasi B, Sutherland G R. Biliary sludge ultrasonic appearance simulating neoplasm. Br J Radiol 1981; 54: 679–681

39 Fakhry J. Sonography of tumefactive biliary sludge. AJR 1982; 139: 717–719

40 Britten J S, Golding R H, Cooperberg P L. Sludge balls to gallstones. J Ultrasound Med 1984; 3: 81–82

41 Engel J M, Deitch E A, Sikkema W. Gallbladder wall thickness: sonographic accuracy and relation to disease. AJR 1979; 134: 907–909

42 Finberg H J, Birnholtz J. Ultrasound evaluation of the gallbladder wall. Radiology 1979; 133: 693–698

43 Marchal G, Van de Voorde P, Van Dooren W, Ponette E, Baert A. Ultrasonic appearance of the filled and contracted normal gallbladder. JCU 1980; 8: 439–442

44 Lewandowski B J, Winsberg F. Gallbladder wall thickness distortion by ascites. AJR 1981; 137: 519–521

45 Sanders R C. The significance of sonographic gallbladder wall thickening. JCU 1980; 8: 143–146

46 Fiske C E, Laing F C, Brown T W. Ultrasonographic evidence of gallbladder wall thickening in association with hypoalbuminemia. Radiology 1980; 135: 713–716

47 Ralls P W, Quinn M F, Juttner H U, Halls J M, Boswell W D. Gallbladder wall thickening: patients without intrinsic gallbladder disease. AJR 1981; 137: 65–68

48 Saverymuttu S H, Grammatopoulos A, Meanock C I, Maxwell J D, Joseph A E A. Gallbladder wall thickening (congestive cholecystopathy) in chronic liver disease: a sign of portal hypertension. Br J Radiol 1990; In press

49 Shlaer W J, Leopold G R, Scheible F W. Sonography of thickened gallbladder wall: a non-specific finding. AJR 1981; 136: 337–339

50 Maudgal D P, WansboroughJones M H, Joseph A E A. Gallbladder abnormalities in acute infectious hepatitis. Dig Dis Sci 1984; 29: 257–260

51 Juttner H-U, Ralls P W, Quinn M F, Jenney J M. Thickening of gallbladder wall in acute hepatitis: ultrasound demonstration. Radiology 1982; 142: 465–466

52 Brandt D J, MacCarty R L, Charbonneau J W, LaRusso N F, Wiesner R H, Ludwig J. Gallbladder disease in patients with primary sclerosing cholangitis. AJR 150: 571–574

53 Romano A J, vanSonnenberg E, Casola G, et al. Gallbladder and bile duct abnormalities in AIDS: sonographic findings in eight patients. AJR 1988; 150: 123–127

54 McClure J, Banerjee S S, Schofield P S. Crohn's disease of the gallbladder. J Clin Pathol 1984; 37: 516–518

55 Carroll B A. Gallbladder wall thickening secondary to focal lymphatic obstruction. J Ultrasound Med 1983; 2: 89–91

56 Laudanna A A, Ferreyra N P, Cerri G G, Bettarello A. Thickening of the gallbladder wall in alcoholic hepatitis verified by ultrasonographic examination. Scand J Gastroenterol 1987; 22: 521–524

57 Cerri G G, Alves V, Magalhaes A. Sonography in hepatobiliary schistosomiasis. Radiology 1984; 153: 777

58 Bouchier I A D. New drugs: gallstones. BMJ 1990; 300: 592–597

59 Laing F C, Federle M P, Jeffrey R B, Brown T W. Ultrasonic evaluation of patients with acute right upper quadrant pain. Radiology 1981; 190: 449–455

60 Handler S J. Ultrasound of gallbladder wall thickening and its relation to cholecystitis. AJR 1979; 132: 581–585

61 Marchal G J F, Casaer M, Baert A L, Goddeeris P G, Kerremans R, Fevery J. Gallbladder wall sonolucency in acute cholecystitis. Radiology 1979; 133: 429–433

62 Kane R A. The Biliary system. In: Kurtz A B, Goldberg B B. eds. Gastrointestinal ultrasonography. New York: Churchill Livingstone. 1988: p 75–137

63 Sherman M, Ralls P W, Quinn M, Halls J, Keats J B. Intravenous cholangiography and sonography in acute cholecystitis: prospective evaluation. AJR 1980; 135: 311–313

64 Clain A. Hamilton Bailey's Physical Sign in Clinical Surgery. 14th ed. Bristol: Wright. 1967

65 Ralls P W, Halls J, Lapin S A, Quinn M F, Morris U L, Boswell W. Prospective evaluation of the sonographic Murphy sign in suspected acute cholecystitis. JCU 1982; 10: 113–115

66 Ralls P W, Colletti P M, Lapin S M, et al. Real time sonography in suspected acute cholecystitis. Radiology 1985; 155: 767

67 Jeffrey R B, Laing F C, Wong W, Callen P W. Gangrenous cholecystitis: diagnosis by ultrasound. Radiology 1983; 148: 219–221

68 Kane R A. Ultrasonographic diagnosis of gangrenous cholecystitis and empyema of the gallbladder. Radiology 1980; 134: 191–194

69 Jenkins M, Golding R H, Cooperberg P L. Sonography and computed tomography of haemorrhagic cholecystitis. AJR 1983; 140: 1197–1198

70 Wales L R. Desquamated gallbladder mucosa: unusual sign of cholecystitis. AJR 1982; 139: 810–811

71 Simeone J F, Brink J A, Mueller P R, et al. The sonographic diagnosis of acute gangrenous cholecystitis: importance of the Murphy sign. AJR 1989; 152: 289–290

72 Bergman A B, Neiman H L, Kraut B. Ultrasonographic evaluation of pericholecystic abscesses. AJR 1979; 132: 201–203

73 Madrazo B L, Francis I, Hricak H, Sandler M A, Hudak S, Gitschlag K. Sonographic findings in perforation of the gallbladder. AJR 1982; 139: 491–496

74 Hunter N D, Macintosh P K. Acute emphysematous cholecystitis: an ultrasonic diagnosis. AJR 1980; 134: 592–593

75 Blaquiere R M, Dewbury K C. The ultrasound diagnosis of emphysematous cholecystitis. Br J Radiol 1982; 55: 114–116

76 Parulekar S G. Sonographic findings in acute emphysematous cholecystitis. Radiology 1982; 145: 117–119

77 Bloom R A, Fisher A, Pode D, Asaf Y. Shifting intramural gas: a new ultrasound sign of emphysematous cholecystitis. JCU 1984; 12: 40–42

78 Nemcek A A, Gore R M, Vogelzang R L, Grant M. The effervescent gallbladder: a sonographic sign of emphysematous cholecystitis. AJR 1988; 150: 575–577

79 Bloom R A, Libson E, Lebensart P D, et al. The ultrasound spectrum of emphysematous cholecystitis. JCU 1989; 17: 251–256

80 Deitch E A, Engel J M. Acute acalculous cholecystitis: an ultrasonic diagnosis. Am J Surg 1981; 142: 290–292

81 Shuman W P, Rogers J V, Ruydd T G, Mack L A, Plumley T, Larson E B. Low sensitivity of sonography and cholescintigraphy in acalculous cholecystitis. AJR 1984; 142: 531–534

82 Mirvis S E, Vainright J R, Nelson A W, et al. The diagnosis of acute acalculous cholecystitis: A comparison of sonography, scintigraphy, and CT. AJR 1986; 147: 1171–1175

83 McGahan J P, Walter J R. Diagnostic percutaneous aspiration of the gallbladder. Radiology 1985; 155: 619–622

84 McGahan J P, Lindfors K K. Acute cholecystitis: diagnostic accuracy of percutaneous aspiration of the gallbladder. Radiology 1988; 167: 669–671

85 Berk R N, van der Vegt J H, Lichtenstein J E. The hyperplastic cholecytoses: cholesterolosis and adenomyomatosis. Radiology 1983; 146: 595–601

86 Raghavendra B N, Subramanyam B R, Balthazar E J, Horii S C, Megibow A J, Hilton S. Sonography of adenomyomatosis of the gallbladder: radiologic-pathologic correlation. Radiology 1983; 146: 747–752

87 Fowler R C, Reid W A. Ultrasound diagnosis of adenomyomatosis of the gallbladder: ultrasonic and pathological correlation. Clin Radiol 1988; 39: 402–406

88 Price R J, Stewart E T, Foley W D, Dodds W J. Sonography of polypoid cholesterolosis. AJR 1982; 139: 1197

89 Jacyna M R, Bouchier I A D. Cholesterolosis: a physical cause of 'functional' disorder. BMJ 1987; 295: 619–620

90 Carter S J, Rutledge J, Hirsch J H. Papillary adenoma of the gallbladder: ultrasonic demonstration. JCU 1978; 6: 433

91 Foster D R, Foster D B E. Gallbladder polyps in Peutz-Jeghers syndrome. Postgrad Med J 1980; 56: 373–376

92 Niv Y, Kosakov K, Shcolnik B. Fragile papilloma (papillary adenoma) of the gallbladder. A cause of recurrent biliary colic. Gastroenterology 1986; 91: 999–1001

93 Kozuka S, Kurashina M, Tsubone M, Hachisuka K, Yasui A. Significance of intestinal metaplasia for the evolution of cancer in the biliary tract. Cancer 1984; 54: 2277–2285

94 Williamson R C N. Acalculous disease of the gallbladder. Gut 1988; 29: 860–872

95 Majeski J A. Polyps of the gallbladder. J Surg Oncol 1986; 32: 16–18

96 Olken S M, Bledsoe R, Newmark H. The ultrasonic diagnosis of primary carcinoma of the gallbladder. Radiology 1978; 129: 481–482

97 Crade M, Taylor K J W, Rosenfield A T, et al. The varied ultrasonic character of gallbladder tumour. JAMA 1979; 241: 2195–2196

98 Yeh H-C. Ultrasonography and computed tomography of carcinoma of the gallbladder. Radiology 1979; 133: 167–173

99 Dalla Palma L, Rizzatto G, Pozzi-Mucelli R S, Bazzocchi M. Grey scale ultrasonography in the evaluation of carcinoma of the gallbladder. Br J Radiol 1980; 53: 662–667

100 Yum H Y, Fink A H. Sonographic findings in primary carcinoma of the gallbladder. Radiology 1980; 134: 693–696

101 Ruiz R, Teyssou H, Fernandez N, et al. Ultrasonic diagnosis of primary carcinoma of the gallbladder: a review of 16 cases. JCU 1980; 8: 489–495

102 Koga A, Yamauchi S, Izumi Y, Hamanaka N. Ultrasonographic detection of early and curable carcinoma of the gallbladder. Br J Surg 1985; 72: 728–730

103 Diehl A K, Beral V. Cholecystectomy and changing mortality from gallbladder cancer. Lancet 1981; ii: 187–189

104 Phillips G, Pochaczevsky R, Goodman J, et al. Ultrasound patterns of metastatic tumours in the gallbladder. JCU 1982; 10: 379

105 Bundy A L, Richie W G M. Ultrasonic diagnosis of metastatic melanoma presenting as acute cholecystitis. JCU 1982; 10: 285

106 Schulman A, Loxton A J, Heydenrych J J, Abdurahman K E. Sonographic diagnosis of biliary ascariasis. AJR 1982; 139: 485–489

107 Lim J H, Ko Y T, Lee D H, Kim S Y. Clonorchiasis: sonographic findings in 59 proved cases. AJR 1989; 152: 761–764

108 Bassily S, Iskander M, Youssef F G, El-Masry N, Bawden M. Sonography in diagnosis of Fascioliasis. Lancet 1989; 1: 1270–1271

109 Wong R K, Peura D A, Mutter M L, Heit H A, Birns M T, Johnson L F. Hemobilia and liver flukes in a patient from Thailand. Gastroenerology 1985; 88: 1958–1963

110 Braverman D Z, Johnson M L, Kern F Jr. Effects of pregnancy and contraceptive steroids on gallbladder function. N Engl J Med 1980; 302: 362

111 Kane R A. Ultrasonographic evaluation of the gallbladder. Crit Rev Diagn Imaging 1982; 17: 107

112 Cohen E K, Stringer D A, Smith C R, Daneman A. Hydrops of the gallbladder in typhoid fever as demonstrated by sonography. JCU 1986; 14: 633–635

113 Slovis T L, Hight D W, Philippart A I, Dubois R S. Sonography in the diagnosis and management of hydrops of the gallbladder in children with mucocutaneous lymph node syndrome. Pediatrics 1980; 65: 789–794

114 Koss J C, Coleman B G, Mulhern C B et al. Mucocutaneous lymph node syndrome with hydrops of the gallbladder diagnosed by ultrasound. JCU 1981; 9: 477–479

115 Tanaka K, Shimada M, Hattori M, Utsunomiya T, Oya N. Sjogren's syndrome with abnormal manifestations of the gallbladder and central nervous system. J Pediatr Gastroenterol Nutr 1985; 4: 148–151

116 Copeman P W M, Medd W E. Diffuse systemic sclerosis with abnormal liver and gallbladder. BMJ 1967; 3: 353–354

117 Wilson-Sharp R C, Irving H C, Brown R C, Chalmers D M, Littlewood J M. Ultrasonography of the pancreas, liver, and biliary system in cystic fibrosis. Arch Dis Child 1984; 59: 923–926

118 Wilson-Sharp R C, Irving H C. Abdominal ultrasonography in cystic fibrosis. Le Journal Francais d'Echographie 1985; 3: 191–200

Bile duct pathology

Henry C. Irving

Jaundice

Jaundice is due to an increase in the serum bilirubin level above the normal range of 1 to 15 mg/l (1.7 to 25 μmol/l). When the increase is mild its presence may only be detected on biochemical analysis of the blood, but when the bilirubin level rises sufficiently there is clinically detectable yellow discoloration of the skin, sclerae and mucous membranes.

The pathological mechanisms that give rise to jaundice can be classified into three main groups: haemolytic (or prehepatic), hepatocellular (or hepatic), and obstructive.

The haemolytic nature of jaundice is readily apparent from haematological and biochemical blood tests, and imaging has little part to play in diagnosis or management.

There are many causes of hepatocellular jaundice, most of which will be diagnosed on biochemical, serological or histological examinations of the blood or liver, but some will cause structural changes in the liver which may be detectable on ultrasound scans. The ultrasonographic features of parenchymal liver diseases such as the various types of hepatitis and cirrhosis, of primary and secondary malignant disease of the liver, and of inflammatory processes such as pyogenic liver abscesses, are discussed in Chapters 16 and 18. Ultrasound may suggest the cause of hepatocellular jaundice and it can be used to guide a needle for a diagnostic aspiration or biopsy (see Ch. 6).

Obstructive jaundice is strictly defined as due to a block in the pathway between the site of conjugation of bile in the liver cells and the entry of bile into the duodenum through the ampulla. The block may be intrahepatic, at the biochemical, cellular, or canalicular level, or extrahepatic in the bile ducts. It is this latter group of causes of extrahepatic obstructions that are referred to as SURGICAL jaundice, to simplify their distinction from all other causes of jaundice which are then referred to as MEDICAL.

Although the cause can often be diagnosed on the basis of a careful history and examination, the differing managements of medical and surgical jaundice make early differential diagnosis essential. Conventional blood testing will usually confirm the present of cholestasis (obstruction), but they provide little or even misleading information about the site of obstruction and its cause. A variety of techniques for visualising the biliary tree is now available and, because some are expensive and some involve risks, it is important that patients be subjected only to a sensible and rational programme of investigation.[1] Ultrasound scores highly on grounds of safety, simplicity, cost and accuracy, and has therefore come to be universally regarded as the best initial imaging procedure.[2]

Ultrasound has been shown to be highly accurate in diagnosing surgical jaundice, detecting dilatation of the intrahepatic or extrahepatic biliary tree in 85% to 95% of patients with proven obstruction,[3–9] and has a high positive predictive value for obstruction with an incidence of false positive findings of less than 5%. Ultrasound is also highly accurate at defining the level of obstruction, although the actual cause may be diagnosed in only about a third of patients.

Obstruction may occur without duct dilatation (see below) and thus there is a false negative rate of up to 25% in patients with gallstone jaundice in most of the early published series,[10] although, more recently, the reported sensitivity for the detection of choledocholithiasis has increased to over 80%.[11,12] These results are attributable to improvements in equipment and meticulous scanning technique.

As in all areas of medicine, undue reliance must not be placed upon a single test (in this case ultrasound), and where clinical suspicion continues, a negative ultrasound scan must not preclude the option of proceeding to direct cholangiography.

Bile duct dilatation

The ultrasound diagnosis of obstructive or surgical jaundice depends upon the detection of bile duct dilatation.

Within the liver, the normal non-dilated small bile ducts are not visualised on ultrasound. The larger main right and left bile ducts can be identified as tubular structures running anterior to and parallel with the right and left branches of the portal vein and measure up to 2 mm in diameter in the non-dilated system (Fig. 1).[13,14] The diameter of the normal common duct at the porta hepatis should be less than 5 mm,[15,16] increasing slightly (less than 6 mm) as the duct runs caudally in the free edge of the lesser omentum[17] and within the head of the pancreas. The diameter of the non-obstructed duct does increase with age

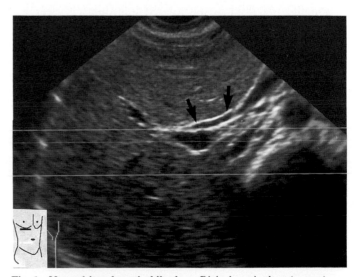

Fig. 1 Normal intrahepatic bile duct. Right hepatic duct (arrows) seen running anterior to right branch of portal vein.

(see Ch. 11),[18] after cholecystectomy[19-21] or if there has been previous obstruction.[22]

Dilatation of the intrahepatic bile ducts will result in one or more of the following ultrasound findings:

Parallel channel sign
Double-barrel shot-gun sign
Stilette sign
'Too many tubes' in the liver
Stellate pattern near porta
Enhancement distal to ducts.

The 'parallel channel'[23] and 'double-barrelled shot-gun'[24] signs depend upon the bile ducts dilating to become equal to or greater than the diameter of the adjacent portal vein branch. When scanned along their long axes, these structures are seen as two parallel channels, while in cross-section the appearance is apparently reminiscent of looking into a double-barrelled shot-gun (Fig. 2)! When the parallel channels occur in a fatty liver, the outer walls may be masked by the high reflectivity of the liver parenchyma. In this case all that is seen is the interface between the vein and duct giving rise to the 'stilette' sign (Fig. 2C).[25]

When scanning a patient with dilated intrahepatic ducts, there is an immediate overall impression of 'too many tubes' in the liver, and when the scans are analysed carefully, it can be seen that these tubes do not correspond to hepatic arteries, veins or portal veins, and must be bile ducts (Fig. 3).[26]

The nature of the branching pattern of the intrahepatic bile duct system is such that when dilated, the ducts are seen to converge together giving a characteristic 'stellate pattern'. This is in contradistinction to the branching pattern of the portal veins which have a more orderly arrangement whereby the peripheral branches all take origin from the main right and left branches (Fig. 4).[27]

Finally, the fluid in the dilated bile ducts is clear bile and ultrasound is transmitted without attenuation – unlike blood which attenuates the ultrasound beam at about the same rate as the liver. When, as is usual, the time-gain compensation (swept gain) is set to compensate for the liver's attenuation, there will be increased through transmission of sound (enhancement) beyond dilated ducts but not beyond the intrahepatic blood vessels (Fig. 5). Although this sign is useful when distinguishing dilated ducts from blood vessels, it is often disadvantageous in the clinical situation when the patchy enhancement beyond the dilated bile ducts so disturbs the normally uniform echo pattern of the liver parenchyma that it becomes impossible to diagnose small metastatic lesions with confidence.

Obstruction without dilatation Unfortunately, complete reliance upon the ultrasound detection of duct dilatation to detect obstruction will lead to a false negative diagnosis in some cases since it has been well-documented that obstruction may occur without dilatation.[28-31]

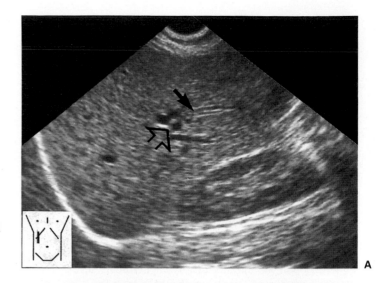

A

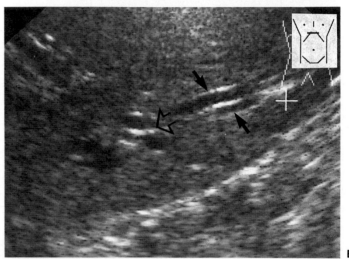

B

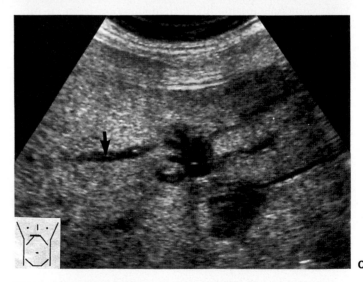

C

Fig. 2 Dilated intrahepatic bile duct. 'Parallel channel' (arrows), and 'double-barrelled shot-gun' (open arrows) signs. **A**: Longitudinal scan. **B**: Transverse scan (magnified). **C**: Stilette sign; the linear echoes (arrow) represent the interface between the dilated bile duct and the adjacent portal vein.

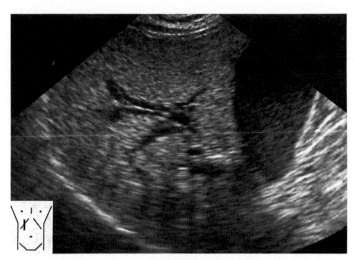

Fig. 3   **Dilated intrahepatic bile ducts** – 'too many tubes' within the liver. Note the distended gallbladder with echogenic bile.

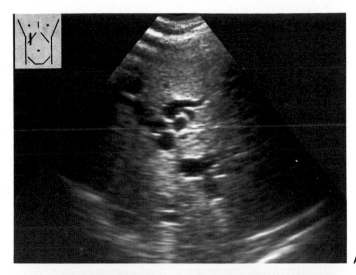

A

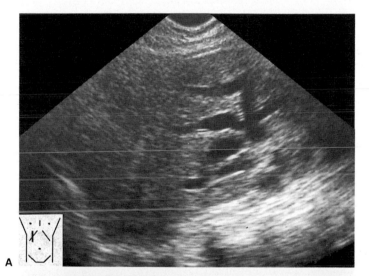

A

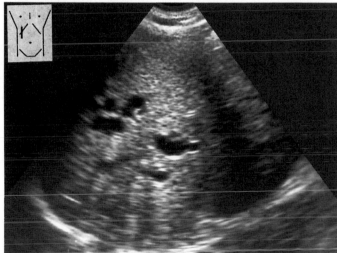

B

Fig. 5   **Dilated intrahepatic bile ducts**. **A**: 'Enhancement beyond dilated ducts'. **B**: Results in patchy echo texture within liver.

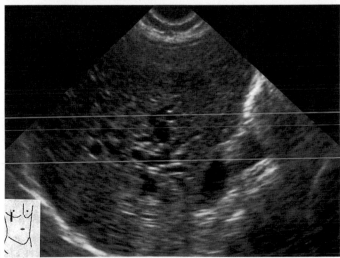

B

Fig. 4   **Dilated intrahepatic bile ducts** – 'stellate branching pattern'.
A: Patient supine. **B**: Patient in right anterior oblique position.

If the obstruction is of recent onset, the ducts may not have had time to dilate despite the onset of jaundice.[32] Rescanning after an interval of a couple of days may well detect these cases, and is recommended if the ultrasound findings do not fit with the clinical impression.

It is possible to detect stones in non-dilated ducts on ultrasound, but a negative scan in suspicious clinical circumstances should lead to further investigations such as CT scanning or direct cholangiography via the percutaneous transhepatic or endoscopic retrograde routes.[1,12]

Other causes of obstruction without dilatation are encasement of the common duct by tumour[30] or fibrosis of the duct wall as in sclerosing cholangitis,[4,33] and in cases of chronic hepatitis or cirrhosis dilatation of intrahepatic ducts may be impossible due to rigidity of the surrounding liver parenchyma.

Whilst   direct   cholangiography   remains   the   'gold standard' for the exclusion of biliary obstruction, adjuncts to ultrasound scanning such as fatty meal sonography,[34-37] and endosonography[38] offer improved accuracy and significantly lessen the false negative rate for ultrasound (see Ch. 11).

Dilatation without jaundice Ultrasound detection of biliary dilatation may precede the onset of clinically detectable jaundice.[39-41] This situation may occur in several different clinical settings: a) when segments of the intrahepatic biliary tree are obstructed by tumour while other parts remain unobstructed; b) when there are stones in the common duct causing a ball-valve effect, the intermittent relief of obstruction allows clearance of the bile so that jaundice may not develop; c) in chronic incomplete or slowly progressive obstruction such as may be caused by tumour in the head of pancreas or chronic pancreatitis, the wider extrahepatic portions of the biliary tree dilate more, in keeping with Laplace's law. These pathological conditions must be differentiated from the non-pathological dilatation of the common duct with increasing age[18] and from post-cholecystectomy dilatation;[18-20] fatty meal sonography may again prove helpful in a number of these cases.[34-37] However, it should also be noted that while the serum bilirubin may not be elevated, so that the patient remains anicteric, the serum level of alkaline phosphatase is more sensitive and will almost always be raised if the duct dilatation is pathological, and this finding should aid the decision to proceed to CT scan or direct cholangiography.[41]

Rapid changes in duct diameter The diameter of the common duct may respond rapidly to both physiological and pathological changes in intraduct pressure[42-44] and thus the ultrasound measurement of duct calibre at any one moment of time may not convey the entire picture. The walls of the extrahepatic ducts are composed mainly of elastic fibres and connective tissue with little or no smooth muscle.[45] The stretch potential of the elastic fibres permits duct dilatation while the elastic recoil of the fibres is responsible for return of the duct to normal size after relief of an obstruction.

An increase in the volume of bile within the biliary system will result in increased intraductal pressure and the common duct will dilate.[46] The bile volume is controlled by the balance between bile production (choleresis) and bile outflow, which is itself controlled in health by the tone of the sphincter of Oddi and the reservoir function of the gallbladder.

After cholecystectomy, a choleresis may so stress the capacity of the common duct that marked dilatation may result. This would be particularly liable to occur in 'floppy' ducts which have been subject to previous obstruction and dilatation.

Furthermore, it is apparent that an abrupt increase in bile duct volume caused by the direct injection of contrast medium into the bile duct at cholangiography may result

in an assessment of duct diameter that is significantly discrepant from the preceding ultrasound scan.[44,47]

Gallbladder distension Courvoisier's law states that, 'if in a jaundiced patient the gallbladder is enlarged, it is not a case of stone impacted in the common duct, for previous cholecystitis which existed when the stone was in the gallbladder, must have rendered the gallbladder fibrotic and incapable of dilatation'.[48] We now know that, as with all rules in medicine, there are exceptions to this law. Stones can form de novo in the common duct leaving the gallbladder wall in pristine condition, there may be double impaction of stones when the stone in the cystic duct causes a distended gallbladder and the stone in the common duct causes jaundice (Fig. 6), or there may be a pancreatic calculus impacted at the ampulla obstructing both bile and pancreatic ducts.

However, whenever duct dilatation is encountered, it is useful to assess the degree of distension of the gallbladder as this may offer a clue to the level of the obstructing lesion. A distended gallbladder suggests a low common duct obstruction, while a contracted gallbladder is consistent with obstruction above the level of the cystic duct insertion. But the possibility of dual pathology must always be considered, and the gallbladder findings must be regarded as supportive rather than of primary importance.

Choledocholithiasis

Initial euphoria in the late 1970's for the value of ultrasound in assessing the biliary tract was followed in the early 1980's by deep depression at the poor results for the ultrasound detection of stones in the common duct,[49-52] with sensitivity rates of less than 33%. One report[51] did indicate that the results in the last 16 months of their 40 month study period were significantly better than in the first 24 months, due to improved scanning techniques and developments in high resolution real time equipment. These same authors have published further results[11,53] confirming that the sensitivities for diagnosing stones in the common duct may be as high as 75% to 80%, and other workers have confirmed these findings.[12,54]

Scale of the problem Choledocholithiasis occurs in approximately 15% of patients with stones in the gallbladder,[55] but may also occur in the absence of cholelithiasis, and may be found in as many as 4% of post-cholecystectomy cases,[56] many of whom will present with abdominal symptoms without jaundice.[22]

The classical clinical presentations of choledocholithiasis include biliary colic, jaundice, and fluctuating fever – Charcot's triad. However, one or more of these components is often absent, the clinical features depending upon the varying degrees of bile duct obstruction, inflammation and infection present in any individual case.

Causes of the problem There are several explanations

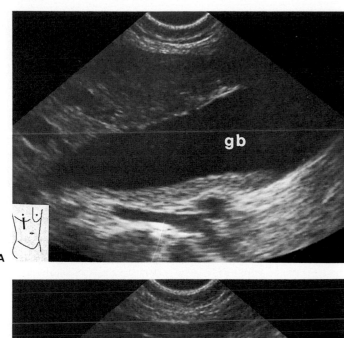

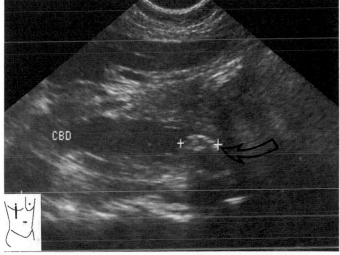

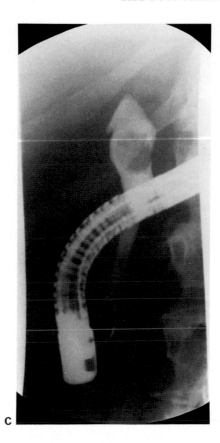

Fig. 6 Choledocholithiasis. A: Distended gallbladder (gb) due to **B:** a stone (arrow) obstructing the common duct (CBD). **C:** Confirmed on ERCP.

for the low sensitivity of ultrasound in the diagnosis of choledocholithiasis:

a) Gas in the first and second parts of the duodenum interferes with the ultrasound demonstration of the common duct, which accounts for the finding that stones in the proximal portion of the duct are very much more often detected than stones in the distal portion (Fig. 7).[11,53]

b) Lack of dilatation of common ducts that contain stones, even in the presence of obstruction is now well-recognised[30,31] and may occur in as many as 25% of acutely obstructed ducts (Fig. 8).[50,51] Explanations for this phenomenon include the so-called 'ball-valve effect'[50] whereby the intermittent nature of the obstruction prevents the intraduct pressure from rising sufficiently to cause duct dilatation, and the 'temporal lag' between onset of obstruction and onset of dilatation.[32]

c) The absence of a bile pool around stones in the duct

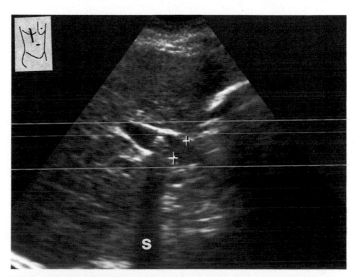

Fig. 7 Choledocholithiasis. Stone in the dilated common duct casting acoustic shadow (s).

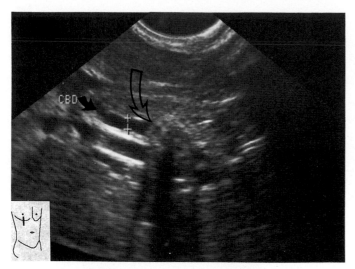

Fig. 8 **Stone in non-dilated duct**. Stone (open arrow) within a normal calibre common duct (CBD, solid arrow) (4 mm).

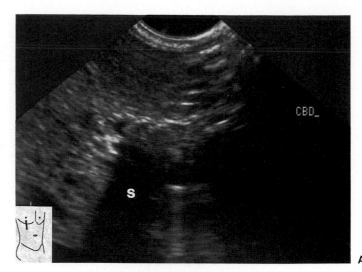

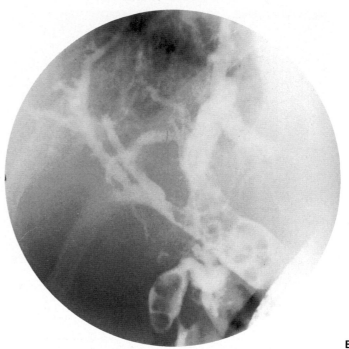

Fig. 9 **Stones filling the lumen of the common duct**.
A: Longitudinal scan with patient in right anterior oblique position (s – shadow). B: ERCP shows duct full of stones.

impairs the ability of the ultrasonographer to spot the stones. The contrast between the reflectivity of solid stone and the echo-free nature of fluid bile that is so useful in the diagnosis of stones in the gallbladder, is often not present since the stones are in direct contact with the highly reflective walls of the duct and the adjacent gas-containing bowel. A particularly embarrassing situation can arise when the duct is absolutely full of stones giving rise to a highly reflective structure with distal acoustic shadowing which is misdiagnosed as bowel gas (Fig. 9).

d) As many as 10% of common duct stones may lack a distal acoustic shadow,[52,57,58] especially when the stones are at the lower end of the duct (Fig. 10). This phenomenon may be due to the differing composition of common duct stones (as compared to gallbladder stones), and indeed some are merely conglomerations of soft sludge, or to technical factors such as gain settings, transducer frequency and focusing, and reflection/refraction of sound by the curved walls of the duct. Non-shadowing stones in the duct cannot be distinguished from other intraluminal pathology such as blood clot, tumour or parasitic infection.

e) Gas in the bile duct may give ultrasound appearances identical to those of stones i.e. high reflectivity and acoustic shadowing emanating from within the duct lumen (Fig. 11), and will thus obscure the presence of stones from the sonographer. The gas is usually widely distributed throughout the intrahepatic biliary ducts and thus the nature of the problem should be apparent to the sonographer. However, the increasing incidence of endoscopic sphincterotomy severely restricts the usefulness of ultrasound in searching for retained stones after surgical or endoscopic procedures.

Solutions to the problem Developments in equipment and transducer technology now permit the demonstration of small stones within minimally dilated, or even normal calibre ducts, as long as meticulous scanning technique is employed (see Ch. 11). It is important to scan the common duct in both longitudinal and transverse scan planes (Fig. 12), to be prepared to move the patient into both right and left anterior oblique (Fig. 13), as well as upright and semi-upright positions, and to use water in the stomach and duodenum, all in an effort to demonstrate pathology in the common duct. An important clue to a calculous aetiology of biliary obstruction is the disproportionate dilatation of the extrahepatic biliary tree in comparison to the intra-

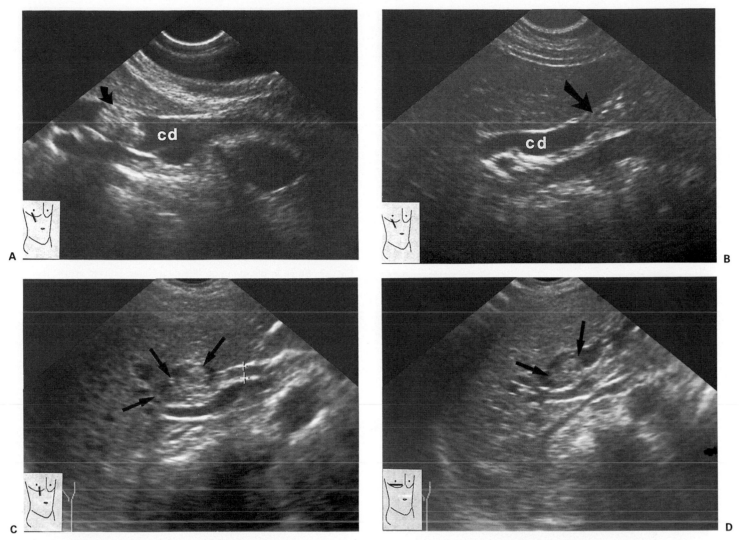

Fig. 10   No shadowing from stones within the common duct. A: Stone (arrow) in mid-duct. **B:** Stone (arrow) at lower end of duct (cd – common duct). **C** and **D:** Longitudinal and transverse scans in another patient. The calculus is producing a mass effect in the common duct.

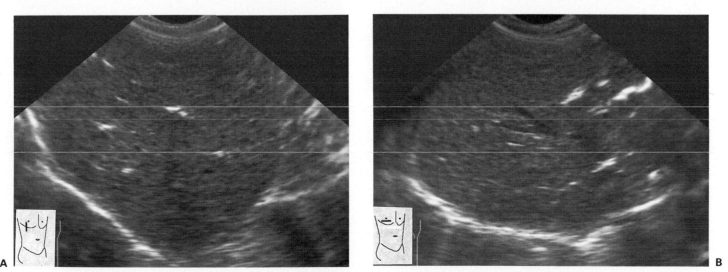

Fig. 11   Gas in the bile ducts. A: Longitudinal and **B:** transverse scans showing gas in intrahepatic bile ducts.

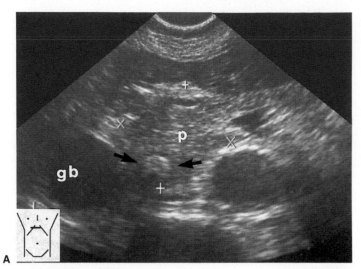

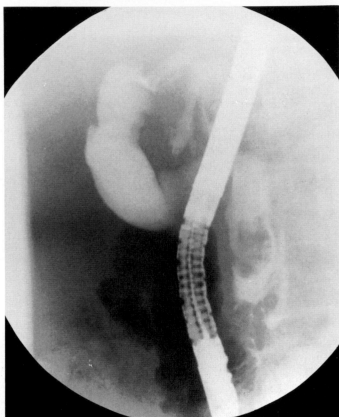

Fig. 12 Stone in the lower end of the common bile duct. A: Stone (arrows) identified within the lower end of common duct in a swollen head of pancreas (p) on transverse scan (gb – gallbladder). **B:** Confirmed on ERCP.

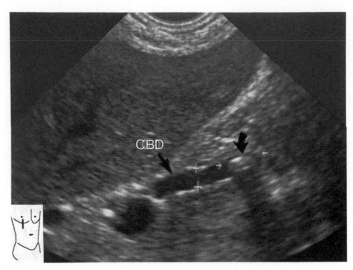

Fig. 13 Stone in the common bile duct. Stone (curved arrow) seen in common duct (CBD) only on the right anterior oblique view.

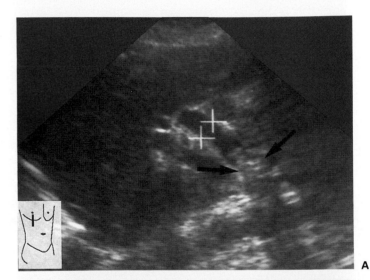

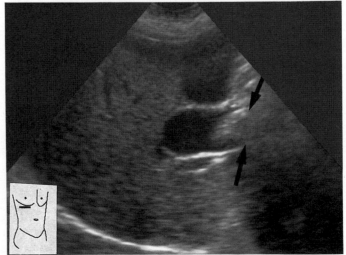

Fig. 14 Stone in the common bile duct. Stones (arrows) impacted within the lower end of the common duct. **A:** Longitudinal scan. **B:** Transverse scan in a different patient.

hepatic ducts. When this is noted, the search for a calculus should be even more diligent. However, despite all these efforts, approximately 30% of common duct stones will be missed – mainly due to impaction in the lower end of the common duct where they are hidden by the duodenum (Fig. 14). Endosonography and fatty meal sonography have already been referred to as offering opportunities for further improvement in this application of ultrasound (see Ch. 11).

Bile duct neoplasms

Tumours of the bile ducts may be benign, but these are all extremely rare, and include papillomas, adenomas, cystadenomas and granular cell myoblastomas.[57,59-62] Papillomas and solid adenomas appear as solid, non-shadowing intraluminal masses, while cystadenomas are multiloculated cystic masses which usually occur in young females. These latter originate from the bile duct epithelium but usually do not communicate with the biliary tree. The differential diagnosis includes echinococcal cysts, cystic metastases, abscesses, partially liquefied haematomas and hepatic artery aneurysms.

Primary malignant tumours of the bile ducts – cholangiocarcinomas – although rare, are much more common than benign tumours and their incidence is thought to be increasing. They may develop at any level within the biliary tree, and when they involve the confluence of the left and right hepatic ducts at the porta hepatis they are referred to as Klatskin tumours, following his original description in 1965.[63]

The ultrasound features of cholangiocarcinomas have been well-documented,[64-70] although the frequency with which these signs are detected varies greatly depending upon the site and size of the tumour.

Dilatation of the biliary tree can be followed down to the point of obstruction where it may be possible to detect a solid poorly reflective mass, which, if large enough, can be seen to have a heterogeneous internal echo pattern and ill-defined margins (Fig. 15). Occasionally an intraluminal

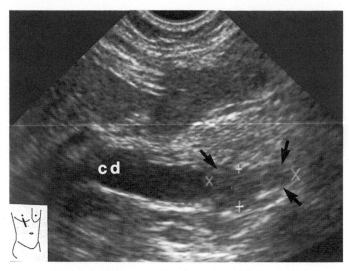

Fig. 16 Cholangiocarcinoma – intraluminal mass (arrows) (cd – common duct).

mass is detected (Fig. 16), while in other cases thickening of the walls of the bile duct may be the only evidence of a tumour (Fig. 17). These ultrasound signs are a direct representation of the gross pathology since these tumours can vary from large solid masses to lesions that infiltrate the submucosa with a thickness of only a few millimetres, when they may be undetectable to both palpation by the surgeon and naked eye inspection by the pathologist. It is this latter form of cholangiocarcinoma that presents on ultrasound as biliary dilatation without a detectable mass, possibly with some increased reflectivity and thickening of the duct wall, and is thus extremely difficult to diagnose.

The ultrasound visibility of these tumours may increase after a biliary stent has been inserted (percutaneous or en-

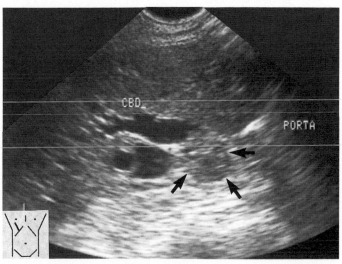

Fig. 15 Klatskin tumour (arrows) obstructing the common duct.

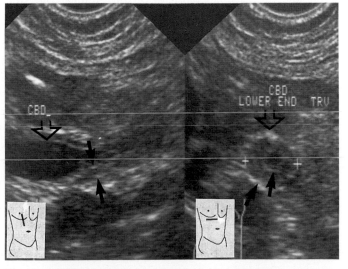

Fig. 17 Cholangiocarcinoma – thickening of walls (solid arrows) of common duct seen on both longitudinal and transverse scans.

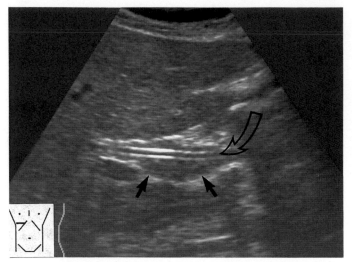

Fig. 18   Cholangiocarcinoma (solid arrows) has become visible after insertion of a stent (open arrow).

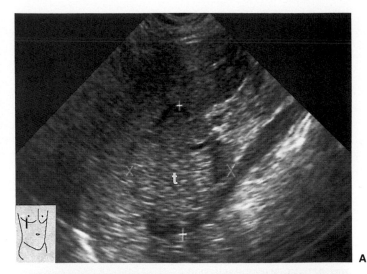

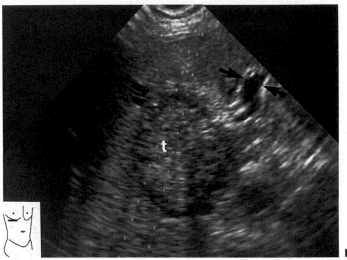

Fig. 19   Cholangiocarcinoma (t) invading liver and occluding portal vein (arrows). **A**: Longitudinal scan. **B**: Transverse scan with biopsy lines in place.

doscopic) (Fig. 18), and it is often then possible to visualise the lesion sufficiently well to permit ultrasound guided biopsy. However, cholangiocarcinomas have a fibrous nature making it difficult to obtain samples adequate for cytological confirmation via fine needle aspiration, so that a cutting biopsy for a histological sample is often necessary.

The role of ultrasound extends beyond the diagnosis of cholangiocarcinomas to assessment of operability by demonstrating evidence of spread of the tumour. Direct invasion to involve surrounding structures such as the portal vein, hepatic artery and liver substance, as well as metastatic spread to regional lymph nodes, are all demonstrable on ultrasound (Fig. 19) which has been shown to be more accurate than CT scanning in this respect.[68]

As well as metastasising to the liver, cholangiocarcinomas may be multifocal and may be indistinguishable from hepatic metastatic disease on ultrasound, and from sclerosing cholangitis on cholangiography due to the multiple strictures in the biliary tree.

Other tumours obstructing the bile ducts

The bile ducts may be obstructed by intrahepatic tumour, enlarged lymph nodes at the porta hepatis, carcinoma of the head of the pancreas and ampullary tumours.

The lymph nodes at the porta hepatis are not demonstrable on ultrasound scans unless pathologically enlarged. By virtue of their proximity to the confluence of the right and left hepatic ducts and their distribution along the length of the common duct, lymphomatous or metastatic disease in the nodes may compress and obstruct the bile ducts. The nodal nature of a mass at the porta hepatis is usually obvious on ultrasound by carefully observing the interfaces that indicate that the tumour is composed of several discrete individual masses and, whilst it is true that

lymphoma usually results in large nodes that are particularly poorly reflective, biopsy is required for accurate distinction between lymphoma and metastases (most frequently from colon, stomach, pancreas and breast) (Fig. 20).

Enlargement of the head of the pancreas, whether due to inflammation or malignancy, may compress the lower end of the common duct as it traverses the gland prior to entering the duodenal papilla. Acute pancreatitis may cause transient extrahepatic duct dilatation but usually does not result in intrahepatic duct dilatation (Fig. 21), whereas the fibrous stricturing of the common duct of chronic pancreatitis may be indistinguishable from malignant disease both on ultrasound and at surgery. Carcinomas of the head of the pancreas are characteristically echo-poor solid masses into which the dilated common duct can be followed (Fig. 22) (see Ch. 10). Detection of coexistent pancreatic duct

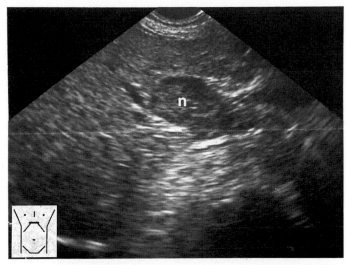

Fig. 20   **Lymph node mass** (n) at porta hepatis (Hodgkin's disease).

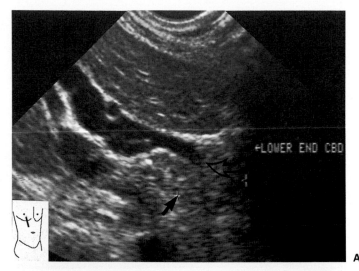

A

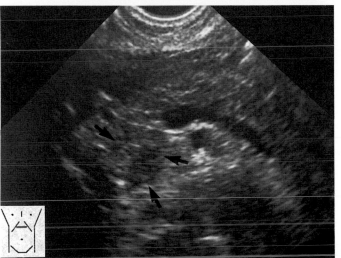

B

Fig. 22   **Dilated common duct due to pancreatic carcinoma** (solid arrows). **A**: Longitudinal scan. **B**: Transverse scan.

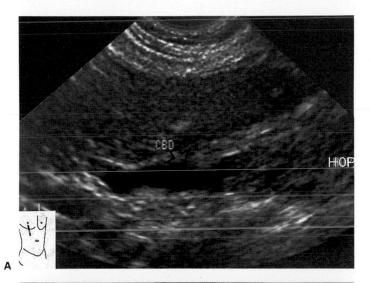

A

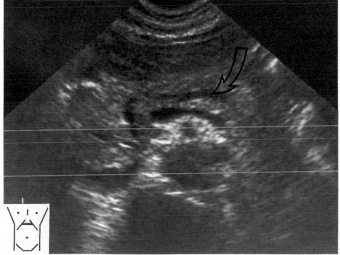

B

Fig. 21   **Dilated common duct due to acute pancreatitis.**
A: Longitudinal scan. **B**: Transverse scan showing dilated pancreatic duct (curved arrow) (HOP – head of pancreas).

dilatation provides useful confirmatory evidence of pancreatic pathology and 'ultrasonic double duct dilatation' may be caused by chronic pancreatitis, impacted pancreatic and biliary calculi, and ampullary carcinoma, as well as by pancreatic carcinoma. Ultrasound is highly sensitive for duct dilatation but has less specificity than the ERCP sign of 'double duct obstruction' which is almost invariably due to pancreatic carcinoma (Fig. 23).

Ampullary carcinoma is difficult to identify on ultrasound. The findings of dilatation of the common duct with a normal head of pancreas should raise the suspicion of this tumour, especially if pancreatic duct dilatation is also detected. The diagnosis must be made endoscopically, and it is important that it is not overlooked, since these tumours often present early with jaundice (due to their strategic location) and radical surgery may offer a good chance of cure.

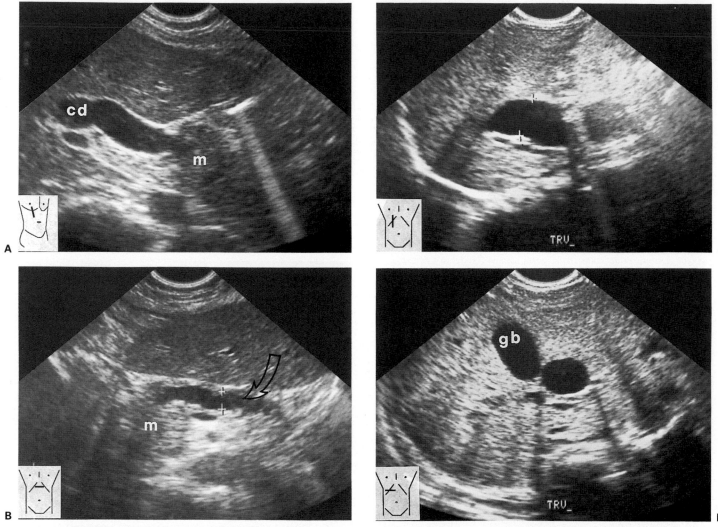

Fig. 23 Double duct obstruction due to pancreatic carcinoma (m). **A:** Longitudinal scan (cd – common duct). **B:** Transverse scan (arrow – pancreatic duct).

Fig. 24 Choledochal cyst. A: Longitudinal scan. **B:** Transverse scan showing aneurysmally dilated common duct in a young child.

Choledochal cysts

Choledochal cysts usually present in children or young adults, and are discussed more fully in Chapter 26. The ultrasound appearances are usually of massive cystic dilatation of the extrahepatic common duct, although the main intrahepatic ducts may be affected.[71–74] The underlying anomaly is thought to be an abnormal insertion of the common duct into the distal pancreatic duct, resulting in reflux of pancreatic secretions into the common duct that cause fibrotic stricturing and obstruction to the biliary tree.[75,76] The condition is more common in females and Orientals and presents with jaundice, fever and pain (due to cholangitis) with a palpable right upper quadrant mass (Fig. 24). As well as recurrent cholangitis, complications include stone formation with progression to biliary cirrhosis and portal hypertension and an increased incidence of

cholangiocarcinoma. The differential diagnosis includes other fluid-filled masses such as hepatic cyst, pancreatic pseudocyst, enteric duplication, hepatic artery aneurysm[77] and echinococcal disease (Fig. 25). Confirmation of the diagnosis may be obtained from ^{99m}Tc-HIDA scintigraphy when excretion of radioactivity into the cyst will confirm its continuity with the biliary system.

Caroli's disease

Caroli's disease – congenital dilatation of the intrahepatic bile ducts,[78] otherwise known as communicating cavernous ectasia of the intrahepatic ducts[79] – is an autosomal recessive disorder in which ultrasound scanning reveals multiple cyst-like spaces throughout the liver substance (Fig. 26).[80,81] These 'cysts' are seen on cholangiography to com-

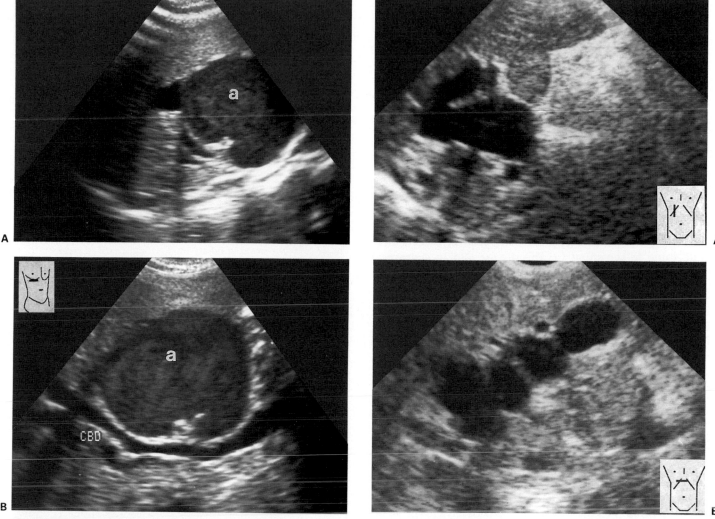

Fig. 25   Hepatic artery aneurysm (a) obstructing the common duct. **A**: Longitudinal scan. **B**: Transverse scan. Note the low level echoes within the aneurysm due to blood clot in this case.

Fig. 26   Caroli's disease. A and **B**: Cystic dilatation of the biliary tree in a child, subsequently shown to be Caroli's disease.

municate with the dilated intrahepatic biliary tree, whilst the extrahepatic bile ducts are usually unaffected. Stones may form within the cysts or dilated ducts, giving rise to attacks of cholangitis which may progress to the formation of pyogenic liver abscesses. There may be an association with renal tubular ectasia or other forms of cystic disease of the kidney, and there is a rather uncertain relationship to congenital hepatic fibrosis in which there is bile duct proliferation and multiple strictures with proximal cystic dilatation[82] – also in association with renal cystic disease, usually of the infantile polycystic type. Caroli himself classified the condition into two types: the pure form without hepatic fibrosis or portal hypertension, and a second type associated with congenital hepatic fibrosis.[83]

The differential diagnosis includes severe biliary dilatation due to any of the other causes of biliary obstruction, polycystic disease of the liver (in which the cysts do not communicate with the bile ducts or each other) and congenital hepatic fibrosis. Other non-invasive imaging tests, such as ^{99m}Tc-HIDA scanning, may help in diagnosis,[84] but, as alluded to above, it has been speculated that Caroli's disease, polycystic disease and congenital hepatic fibrosis are all parts of the same spectrum,[79] and hence cholangiography and even liver biopsy may be needed for a specific diagnosis.

Oriental cholangiohepatitis

Recurrent pyogenic cholangitis, also known as oriental cholangiohepatitis, is endemic in south east Asia, and is characterised by recurrent attacks of cholangitis. It is due to peribiliary fibrosis which causes biliary duct strictures, and is caused by the adult worms of the *Chlonorchis sinensis* liver fluke which are ingested by man in raw freshwater fish. However, the parasites are not found in all patients with the clinical condition, and some authorities question the causal relationship.

The ultrasound features consist of massively dilated bile ducts with multiple strictures, the common duct being most frequently involved, followed by left, then right hepatic ducts. The parasites may be identified within the ducts[85] and also within the gallbladder.[86] There are often bilirubinate stones within the ducts; these are often soft and sludge-like. In most patients there is secondary bacterial infection with *E. coli* in the bile. Gas-forming organisms may result in pneumobilia and there is an increased incidence of cholangiocarcinoma – presumably as a result of chronic irritation leading to dysplasia. All these pathological processes result in a complex ultrasonographic picture,[85–88] and although ultrasound may be of considerable value in screening for the disease and in suggesting the diagnosis, cholangiography will be needed for full evaluation.

Biliary ascariasis

As described in Chapter 12, the *Ascaris lumbricoides* roundworm is an extremely common cause of biliary pathology world-wide. The worms infest the small bowel but can migrate up the common bile duct and may enter the gallbladder and the intrahepatic ducts. Biliary colic is common, while jaundice, ascending cholangitis and parasitic liver abscesses occur occasionally.

The worm may be seen as a non-shadowing reflective linear structure within the lumen of the common duct, and multiple worms may produce a spaghetti-like appearance. The digestive tract of the worm may be visualised as an echo-free tubular structure within the worm and as a bull's eye appearance on transverse scan,[89] and movements of the worms in the common duct and gallbladder may be observed using real time ultrasound (Fig. 27).[90] The diagnosis is confirmed by isolating the worms or their eggs from the stool, and medical treatment is usually effective in eradicating the infestation.

Sclerosing cholangitis

Sclerosing cholangitis predominantly affects young men and it may be idiopathic or associated with inflammatory bowel disease. Histologically there is non-specific inflammation of bile duct walls, and the ultrasound findings are

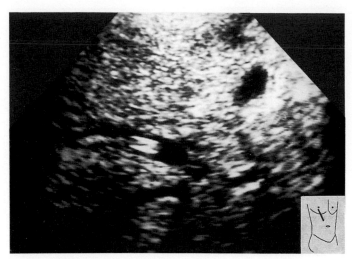

Fig. 27 *Ascaris* **worm in biliary tract.** Oblique view of common hepatic duct showing the typical 'tramline' appearance of *Ascaris* in the duct.

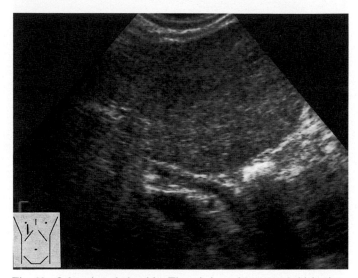

Fig. 28 Sclerosing cholangitis. There is irregular mucosal thickening in the common duct.

of dilatation of the intrahepatic bile ducts which may be confined to one or more segments or lobes, depending upon the anatomical location of the strictures.[91] Thickening of the wall of the common duct has been reported (Fig. 28),[33] but the findings are not specific and the differential diagnosis includes cholangiocarcinoma and other causes of ascending cholangitis.

REFERENCES

1 Scharsschmidt B F, Goldberg H I, Schmid R. Approach to the patient with cholestatic jaundice. N Engl J Med 1983; 308: 1515–1519

2 Lunderquist A. The radiology of jaundice. Clin Gastroenterol 1989; 3: 387–406

3 Taylor K J W, Rosenfield A T. Grey scale ultrasonography in the differential diagnosis of jaundice. Arch Surg 1977; 112: 820–825

4 Sample W F, Sarti D A, Goldstein L I, Weiner M, Kadell B M. Gray-scale ultrasonography of the jaundiced patient. Radiology 1978; 128: 719–725

5 Vallon A G, Lees W R, Cotton P B. Gray-scale ultrasonography in obstructive jaundice. Gut 1979; 20: 51–54

6 Koenigsberg M, Wiener Sn, Walzer A. Accuracy of sonography in the differential diagnosis of obstructive jaundice: a comparison with cholangiography. Radiology 1979; 133: 157–165

7 Dewbury K C, Joseph A E A, Hayes S, Murray C. Ultrasound in the evaluation and diagnosis of jaundice. Br J Radiol 1979; 52: 276–280

8 Wild S R, Cruikshank J G, Fraser G G M, Copland W A, Grieve D C. Grey-scale ultrasonography and percutaneous transhepatic cholangiography in biliary tract disease. BMJ 1980; 281: 1524–1526

9 Haubek A, Pedersen J H, Buscharth F, Gammelgaard J, Hancke S, Willumsen L. Dynamic sonography in the evaluation of jaundice. AJR 1981; 136: 1071–1074

10 Ruddell W S J. Ultrasound in biliary tract disease. BMJ 1981; 282: 311

11 Laing F C, Jeffrey R B, Wing V W, Nyberg D A. Biliary dilatation: defining the level and cause by real time ultrasound. Radiology 1986; 160: 39–42

12 Lindsell D R M. Ultrasound imaging of pancreas and biliary tract. Lancet 1990; 335: 390–393

13 Dewbury K C. Visualisation of normal biliary ducts with ultrasound. Br J Radiol 1980; 53: 774–780

14 Bressler E L, Rubin J M, McCracken S. Sonographic parallel channel sign: a reappraisal. Radiology 1987; 164: 343–346

15 Cooperberg P L. High resolution real time ultrasound in the evaluation of the normal and obstructed biliary tract. Radiology 1978; 129: 477–480

16 Cooperberg P L, Li D, Wong P, Cohen M M, Burhenne H J. Accuracy of common hepatic duct size in the evaluation of extrahepatic biliary obstruction. Radiology 1980; 135: 141–144

17 Parulekar S G. Evaluation of common bile duct size. Radiology 1979; 133: 703–707

18 Wu C-C, Ho Y-H, Chen C-Y. Effect of aging on common bile duct diameter: a real time sonographic study. JCU 1984; 12: 473

19 Graham M F, Cooperberg P L, Cohen M M, et al. The size of normal common hepatic duct following cholecystectomy: an ultrasonic study. Radiology 1980; 135: 137

20 Mueller P R, Ferrucci J T Jr, Simeone J F, et al. Postcholecystectomy bile duct dilatation: myth or reality? AJR 1981; 136: 355

21 Wedmann B, Borsch G, Coenen C, Paassen A. Effect of cholecystectomy on common bile duct diameters; a longitudinal prospective ultrasonographic study. JCU 1988; 16: 619–624

22 Ruddell W S J, Ashton M G, Lintott D J, Axon A T R. Endoscopic retrograde cholangiography and pancreatography in investigation of post-cholecystectomy patients. Lancet 1980; i: 444–447

23 Weill F, Eisencher A, Zeltner F. Ultrasonic study of the normal and dilated biliary tree: 'shot-gun sign'. Radiology 1978; 127: 221

24 Conrad M R, Landay M J, Janes J O. Sonographic 'parallel channel' sign of biliary tree enlargement in mild to moderate obstructive jaundice. AJR 1978; 130: 279

25 Ingram C, Joseph A E A. The stilette sign: the appearance of dilated ducts in the fatty liver. Clin Radiol 1989; 40: 257–258

26 Laing F C, London L A, Filly R A. Ultrasonographic identification of dilated intrahepatic bile ducts and their differentiation from portal venous structures. JCU 1978; 6: 90

27 Taylor K J W, Rosenfield A T, De Graaff C S. Anatomy and pathology of the biliary tree as demonstrated by ultrasound. In: Taylor K J W. ed. Diagnostic ultrasound in gastrointestinal disease. Clinics in Diagnostic Ultrasound. Edinburgh: Churchill Livingstone. 1979: pp 103–121

28 Muhletaler C A, Gerlock A J, Fleischer A C, James A E. Diagnosis of obstructive jaundice with non-dilated bile ducts. AJR 1980; 134: 1149–1152

29 Thomas J L, Zornoza J. Obstructive jaundice in the absence of sonographic biliary dilatation. Gastrointest Radiol 1980; 5: 357–360

30 Beinart C, Efremidis S, Cohen B, Mitty H A. Obstruction without dilatation. JAMA 1981; 245: 353–356

31 Greenwald R A, Pereiras R, Morris S J, Schiff E R. Jaundice, choledocholithiasis, and a non-dilated common duct. JAMA 1978; 240: 1983–1984

32 Fried A M, Bell R M, Bivins B A. Biliary obstruction in a canine model: sequential study of the sonographic threshold. Invest Radiol 1981; 16: 317–319

33 Carroll B A, Oppenheimer D A. Sclerosing cholangitis: sonographic demonstration of bile duct wall thickening. AJR 1982; 139: 1016

34 Simeone J F, Mueller P R, Ferrucci J T, et al. Sonography of the bile ducts after a fatty meal: an aid in detection of obstruction. Radiology 1982; 143: 211–215

35 Simeone J F, Butch R J, Mueller P R, et al. The bile ducts after a fatty meal: furthur sonographic observations. Radiology 1985; 154: 763–768

36 Wilson S A, Gosink B R, vanSonnenberg E. Unchanged size of a dilated common bile duct after a fatty meal; results and significance. Radiology 1986; 160: 29–31

37 Darweesh R M A, Dodds W J, Hogan W J, et al. Fatty meal sonography for evaluating patients with suspected partial common duct obstruction. AJR 1988; 151: 63–68

38 Amouyal P, Palazzo L, Amouyal G, et al. Endosonography: promising method for diagnosis of extrahepatic cholestasis. Lancet 1989; ii: 1195–1198

39 Weinstein D P, Weinstein B J, Brodmerkel G J. Ultrasonography of biliary tract dilatation without jaundice. AJR 1979; 132: 729–734

40 Weinstein B J, Weinstein D P. Biliary tract dilatation in the non-jaundiced patient. AJR 1980; 134: 899

41 Zeman R, Taylor K J W, Burrell M I, et al. Ultrasonic demonstration of anicteric dilatation of the biliary tree. Radiology 1980; 134: 689

42 Glazer G M, Filly R A, Laing F C. Rapid change in calibre of the non-obstructed common duct. Radiology 1980; 140: 161–162

43 Scheske G A, Cooperberg P L, Cohen M M, et al. Dynamic changes in the caliber of the major bile ducts, related to obstruction. Radiology 1980; 135: 215–216

44 Mueller P R, Ferrucci J T Jr, Simeone J F. Observations on the distensibility of the common bile duct. Radiology 1982; 142: 467–472

45 Mahour G H, Wakim K G, Soule E H, et al. Structure of the common bile duct in man. Ann Surg 1967; 166: 91–94

46 Schein C F, Beneventano T C. Choledochal dynamics in man. Surg Gynecol Obstet 1968; 126: 591–596

47 Sauerbrei E E, Cooperberg P L, Gordon P, Li D, Cohen M M, Burhenne HJ. The discrepancy between radiographic and sonographic bile duct measurements. Radiology 1980; 137: 751–755

48 Clain A. Hamilton Bailey's physical signs in clinical surgery. 14th ed. Bristol: Wright. 1967

49 Gross B H, Harter L P, Gore R M, et al. Ultrasonic evaluation of common bile duct stones; prospective comparison with endoscopic retrograde cholangiopancreatography. Radiology 1983; 146: 471–474

50 Cronan J J, Mueller P R, Simeone J F, et al. Prospective diagnosis of choledocholithiasis. Radiology 1983; 146: 467–469

51 Laing F C, Jeffrey R B. Choledocholithiasis and cystic duct obstruction: difficult ultrasonographic diagnosis. Radiology 1983; 146: 475–479

52 Einstein D M, Lapin S A, Ralls P W, Halls J M. The insensitivity of sonography in the detection of choledocholithiasis. AJR 1984; 142: 725–728

53 Laing F C, Jeffrey R B, Wing V W. Improved visualisation of choledocholithiasis by sonography. AJR 1984; 143: 949–952

54 Dong B, Chen M. Improved sonographic visualisation of choledocholithiasis. JCU 1987; 15: 185–190

55 Way L W, Sleisenger M H. Biliary obstruction, cholangitis, and choledocholithiasis. In: Sleisenger M H, Fordtran J S. eds. Gastrointestinal disease. Philadelphia: W B Saunders. 1983: p 1389–1403

56 Glenn F. Postcholecystectomy choledocholithiasis. Surg Gynecol Obstet 1972; 134: 249–252

57 Kane R A. The biliary system. In: Kurtz A B, Goldberg B B. eds. Gastrointestinal ultrasonography. Clinics in Diagnostic Ultrasound. Edinburgh: Churchill Livingstone. 1988: p 75–137

58 Dewbury K C, Smith C L. The misdiagnosis of common bile duct stones with ultrasound. Br J Radiol 1983; 56: 625–630

59 Carroll B A. Biliary cystadenoma and cystadenocarcinoma: gray scale ultrasound appearance. JCU 1978; 6: 337–340

60 Bondstam S, Kivilaakse E O, Standetskjold-Nordenstam C-G M, Holmstrom T, Hastebaeka J. Sonographic diagnosis of a bile duct polyp. AJR 1980; 135: 610–611

61 Stanley J, Vujic I, Schabel S I, Gobien R P, Reines H D. Evaluation of biliary cystadenoma and cystadenocarcinoma. Gastrointest Radiol 1983; 8: 245–258

62 Marchal G, Gelin J, Van Steenbergen W V, et al. Sonographic diagnosis of intraluminal bile duct neoplasm; a report of 3 cases. Gastrointest Radiol 1984; 9: 329–333

63 Klatskin G. Adenocarcinoma of the hepatic duct at its bifurcation within the porta hepatis. Am J Med 1965; 38: 241–256

64 Dillon E, Peel A L G, Parkin G J S. The diagnosis of primary bile duct carcinoma (cholangiocarcinoma) in the jaundiced patient. Clin Radiol 1981; 32: 311–317

65 Meyer D G, Weinstein B J. Klatskin tumors of the bile ducts: sonographic appearance. Radiology 1983; 148: 803–804

66 Subramanyam B R, Raghavendra B N, Balthazar E J, et al. Ultrasonic features of cholangiocarcinoma. J Ultrasound Med 1984; 3: 405

67 Marchan L, Muller N L, Cooperberg P L. Sonographic diagnosis of Klatskin tumors. AJR 1986; 147: 509

68 Gibson R N, Yeung E, Thompson J N, et al. Bile duct obstruction; radiologic evaluation of level, cause and tumour resectability. Radiology 1986; 160: 43–47

69 Karstrup S. Ultrasound diagnosis of cholangiocarcinoma at the confluence of the hepatic ducts (Klatskin tumours). Br J Radiol 1988; 61: 987–990

70 Yeung E Y C, McCarthy P, Gompertz R H, Benjamin I S, Gibson R N, Dawson P. The ultrasonographic appearances of hilar cholangiocarcinoma (Klatskin tumours). Br J Radiol 1988; 61: 991–995

71 Filly R A, Carlsen E N. Choledochal cyst: report of a case with specific ultrasonographic findings. JCU 1979; 4: 7–10

72 Reuter K, Raptopoulos V D, Cantelmo N, Fitzpatrick G, Hawes H L E. The diagnosis of a choledochal cyst by ultrasound. Radiology 1980; 136: 437–438

73 Han B K, Babcock D S, Gelfand M H. Choledochal cyst with bile duct dilatation; sonography and ^{99m}Tc IDA cholescintigraphy. AJR 1981; 136: 1075–1079

74 Kangarloo H, Sarti D A, Sample W F, et al. Ultrasonographic spectrum of choledochal cysts in children. Pediatr Radiol 1980; 9: 15

75 Kimura K, Ohto M, Ono T, et al. Congenital cystic dilatation of the common bile duct: relationship to anomalous pancreaticobiliary ductal union. AJR 1977; 128: 571–577

76 Jona J Z, Babitt D P, Starshak R J, Laporta A J, Glicklich M, Cohen R D. Anatomic observations and etiologic and surgical considerations in choledochal cyst. J Pediatr Surg 1979; 14: 315–320

77 Filly R A, Freimanis A K. Thrombosed hepatic artery aneurysm – report of a case diagnosed echographically. Radiology 1970; 97: 629–630

78 Caroli J, Spoupaut R, Kossakowski J, Plocker L, Paradowska M. La dilatation polykistique congenitale des voies biliaires interhepatiques: essai de classification. Seminars Hospital Paris 1958; 34: 488–495

79 Mujahed Z, Glenn F, Evans J. Communicating cavernous ectasia of the intrahepatic bile ducts (Caroli's disease). AJR 1971; 113: 21–26

80 Bass E M, Funston M R, Shaff M I. Caroli's disease: an ultrasound diagnosis. Br J Radiol 1977; 50: 366–369

81 Mittelstaedt C A, Volberg F M, Fischer G J, et al. Caroli's disease: sonographic findings. AJR 1980; 134: 585–587

82 Rosenfield A T, Siegel N J, Kappelman N B, Taylor K J W. Gray scale ultrasonography in medullary cystic disease of the kidney and congenital hepatic fibrosis with tubular ectasia: new observations. AJR 1977; 129: 297–303

83 Caroli J. Diseases of intrahepatic bile ducts. Isr J Med Sci 1968; 4: 213–215

84 Imai Y, Watanabe M D, Kondo Y, Nakanishi M D. Caroli's disease: its diagnosis with non-invasive methods. Br J Radiol 1981; 54: 526–528

85 Morikawa P, Ishida H, Niizawa M, Komatsu M, Arakawa H, Masamune O. Sonographic features of biliary clonorchiasis. JCU 1988; 16: 655–658

86 Lim J H, Ko Y T, Lee D H, Kim S Y. Clonorchiasis: sonographic findings in 59 proved cases. AJR 1989; 152: 761–764

87 Ralls P W, Colletti P M, Quinn M F, et al. Sonography in recurrent oriental pyogenic cholangitis. AJR 1981; 136: 1010

88 Federle M P, Cello J P, Laing F C, Jeffrey R B. Recurrent pyogenic cholangitis in Asian immigrants. Radiology 1982; 143: 151

89 Schulman A, Loxton A J, Heydenrych J J, Abdurahman K E. Sonographic diagnosis of biliary ascariasis. AJR 1982; 139: 485–489

90 Cerri G C, Leite G J, Simoes J B, et al. Ultrasonographic evaluation of ascaris in the biliary tract. Radiology 1983; 146: 753–754

91 Doyle T C A, Roberts-Thomson I C. Radiological features of sclerosing cholangitis. Australas Radiol 1983; 27: 163

14

Liver anatomy

Anatomy
Ultrasound appearances
Variations
Assessment of liver size

David O. Cosgrove

Anatomy

The liver, the largest abdominal organ weighing 1.5 kg, lies in the upper abdomen, predominantly on the right side (Fig. 1).[1-3] It has an overall wedge-shape, tapering from right to left with a domed upper surface that fits under the cupola of the right hemidiaphragm. The flatter inferior surface is actually tilted quite markedly so that it faces posteriorly and to the left – thus it is more informatively described as the visceral surface.

The superior surface is relatively featureless but, by contrast, the visceral surface is complex because it contains the liver hilum (the porta hepatis) and also is indented by the shallow fossae that accommodate the organs that are in direct contact with the liver. These are the stomach on the left and, moving to the right, the duodenum and gall bladder, the inferior vena cava and the right kidney. In addition, the visceral surface is marked by fissures that separate some of the liver segments (vide infra). Posteriorly the superior and visceral surfaces continue smoothly into each other, while the infero-anterior border is sharp and is indented by the ligamentum teres and the gallbladder.

The porta lies approximately transversely; through it pass the portal vein, the hepatic artery and the bile duct (Fig. 2). The portal vein usually divides into left and right branches before actually penetrating the liver substance though, like so many anatomical features of the liver vasculature, this is subject to some variation. However the vein always lies posterior to the artery and duct, with the duct lying laterally and deviating further to the right as it passes inferiorly to enter the duodenum. The medial position of the hepatic artery can be remembered from the fact that it originates in the midline from the coeliac axis; it retains this relatively medial position throughout its course.

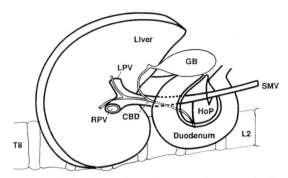

Fig. 2 The hepatic pedicle. The relations of the vessels in the hepatic pedicle are illustrated in this cutaway diagram in which the porta is viewed from the right. Those portions of the bile duct that are overlain by duodenum are shown dotted to indicate the difficulty of imaging these parts with ultrasound. CBD – common bile duct, GB – gallbladder, HoP – head of pancreas, LPV – left portal vein, RPV – right portal vein, SMV – superior mesenteric vein.

The right branch of the portal vein passes transversely within the liver substance for a few centimetres before dividing into anterior and posterior branches, while the left branch curves anteriorly, giving branches to the parts of the liver it traverses. The hepatic arterial branches follow the same pattern.

The overall arrangement of the bile ducts is similar, the smaller ducts joining to form right and left ducts which generally lie anterior to the associated portal vein branches. As it passes infero-medially to the porta, the right hepatic duct crosses over the right portal vein with the right hepatic artery lying between them (though the artery is more variable and lies anterior to the duct in some 10% of subjects). The right and left hepatic ducts emerge from the liver substance before joining to form the common hepatic duct which passes down antero-lateral to the main portal

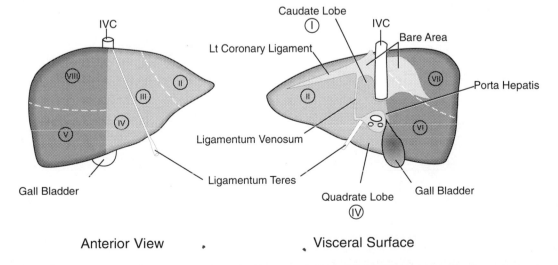

Anterior View • • Visceral Surface

Fig. 1 Anatomy of the liver. Two views of the liver are shown in diagrammatic form. The diaphragmatic surface is much simpler than the visceral surface which contains the porta hepatis. Note that in vivo the visceral surface is tilted to face infero-medially. Coinaud's segmental numbering system is indicated.

vein, posterior to the duodenum (first part) and across the posterior surface of the pancreas before turning laterally (to the right) to enter the second part of the duodenum at the papilla (ampulla) of Vater. At some point along this course, most often in the porta itself, the common hepatic duct is joined by the cystic duct; below this it is referred to as the common bile duct. The overall lie of the bile duct is infero-lateral, approximately at right angles to the costal margin, but this also is variable, depending mainly on the level of the pancreas, so in some subjects the common bile duct may run almost transversely while in others it lies in the sagittal plane.

Three main hepatic veins drain the liver; they empty into the upper part of the inferior vena cava. The right hepatic vein lies in the coronal plane and empties separately into the inferior vena cava. The middle passes from the position of the gallbladder fossa and joins the left to form a short common trunk of a centimetre or so in length, so that both empty together into the anterior aspect of the inferior vena cava. The left hepatic vein commonly lies in the mid-sagittal plane but may lie to one or other side. In addition, a series of smaller, short hepatic veins drain the portions of the liver which are in direct contact with the inferior vena cava, i.e. the supero-medial part of the right lobe and the caudate lobe; these are known as the inferior group of hepatic veins (vide infra).

The liver is divided into segments based on the arterial and portal supply (Fig. 3). The separation between the right and left lobes is along a line joining the gallbladder fossa inferiorly with the fossa for the inferior vena cava superiorly; it passes through the porta and demarcates the parts of the liver supplied by the right and left bile ducts. The middle hepatic vein lies in this plane, but the line of demarcation is not obvious on the surface of the liver (this is why, despite its significance, this major division was not recognised until the importance of the vascularisation of the liver emerged with the increase in hepatic surgery). The two lobes are approximately equal in size and so their veins, arteries and bile ducts are of similar diameters. While generally their designations are appropriate to their position in the upper abdomen, the plane separating them is usually tilted to face anteriorly and to the left, so that the portions of the left lobe near the porta overlie the medial portions of the right lobe. Each lobe is further subdivided: the right into anterior and posterior portions more or less along the coronal plane, corresponding to the line of the right hepatic vein, the left into medial and lateral segments by the ligamentum teres and the falciform ligament (Fig. 4). The lateral segment is one of the most variable, in some subjects being rudimentary, in others being large and extending far inferiorly on the left. The square shape of the medial segment with the gallbladder fossa postero-laterally and the ligamentum teres medially gives it its alternative title, the quadrate lobe.

An important though small additional segment of the liver is the caudate lobe which may be considered as a finger-like extension from the upper posterior part of the right lobe.[4,5] It passes to the left across the subdiaphragmatic portion of the inferior vena cava and then expands into a variable sized lobe that commonly extends inferiorly. Here it lies immediately posterior to the lateral segment of the left lobe, the two being separated by a fissure in which the ligamentum venosum is buried.

A numbering system for the liver segments developed by Coinaud[6] has become widely accepted;[7] it is useful when a precise description of the position of a lesion is required

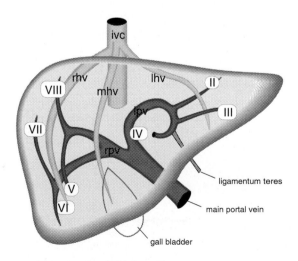

Fig. 3 Blood vessels of the liver. The main branches of the portal vein and the way they interdigitate with the three main hepatic veins are illustrated. The segmental divisions are indicated in Roman numerals. ivc – inferior vena cava, lhv – left hepatic vein, lpv – left portal vein, mhv – middle hepatic vein, rhv – right hepatic vein, rpv – right portal vein.

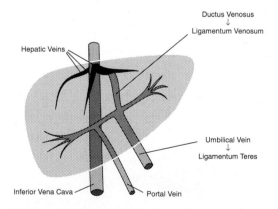

Fig. 4 Fetal circulation through the liver. The venous bypass in the fetus takes blood returning from the placenta via the umbilical vein to the left portal vein and thence directly to the left hepatic vein and on into the inferior vena cava. The temporary vessels which carry this blood (the umbilical vein and the ductus venosus) undergo vasospasm at birth and they subsequently thrombose to form the ligamentum teres and ligamentum venosum respectively. If the spasm extends into the left portal vein itself, lateral parts of the left lobe of the liver become ischaemic. This may account for the marked variability in size of this segment.

for example for planning liver surgery. In this system the segments are numbered clockwise, starting with the caudate as Segment I, Segments II and III being the left and right portions of the lateral segment of the left lobe and Segment IV the quadrate lobe. Segments V and VI are the posterior and anterior portions of the right lobe inferiorly while VII and VIII are the corresponding portions of the superior part of the right lobe (Fig. 3).

The liver is almost entirely covered by peritoneum which is folded in a rather complex way, especially around the porta and the caudate lobe (Fig. 1). Over the superior (diaphragmatic) surface the peritoneum is drawn into transverse folds, triangular in shape with their apices laterally where the visceral layer (on the liver capsule) folds over to continue as the parietal layer on the inferior surface of the diaphragm. These triangular folds leave an unperitonealised 'bare' area where the liver is in direct contact with the diaphragm (mainly its central tendinous portion). Anteriorly the peritoneal folds continue into the falciform ligament that forms a crescentic double fold that passes toward the free edge of the left lobe. Here it folds over the ligamentum teres which lies in its free edge. Posteriorly the peritoneal folds continue into the fissure for the ligamentum venosum.

The complexity of the peritoneum of the visceral surface results from the layers that form the lesser sac of the omentum.[8] Its anterior wall consists of the lesser omentum, a double peritoneal layer that extends as a sheet from the lesser curve of the stomach to the liver and thus also known as the hepato-gastric ligament. It attaches in the depths of the fissure for the ligamentum venosum and from there folds back on itself to continue as the peritoneal layer covering the liver itself. At the oesophago-gastric region the anterior layer continues over the diaphragm as the parietal peritoneum while the posterior layer is reflected over the posterior abdominal wall (mainly covering the body and tail regions of the pancreas) as the posterior wall of the lesser sac. On the right the two layers separate to enfold the hepatic pedicle (comprising the portal vein, the hepatic artery and the bile duct), fusing lateral to them to form a free border that stretches up from the first part of the duodenum to the lateral part of the porta hepatis where the layers again continue into the peritoneum covering the liver. Thus a foramen is formed immediately posterior to the porta hepatis where the general peritoneum communicates with the recess (the lesser sac); it is known as the 'foramen of Winslow' or the 'additus to the lesser sac' and its posterior margin overlies the inferior vena cava. The other walls of the lesser sac are formed by the posterior wall of the stomach and the peritoneum over the upper retroperitoneal structures so that part of the pancreas lies immediately posterior to it (this is why pseudocysts so commonly collect in the lesser sac). On the left it extends up to the splenic hilum. Most of the caudate lobe lies within it.

The triangular (or coronary) ligaments over the diaphragmatic surface of the liver divide the subphrenic peritoneal space into anterior and posterior portions which are more completely separated on the right where the ligament is more extensive. The posterior subphrenic space continues into the hepato-renal space ('Morrison's pouch'). These spaces delimit regions in which ascitic fluid and infective collections tend to form.

Ultrasound appearances

In longitudinal sections through the left lobe, the liver has a triangular shape with a rounded upper surface and a sharp inferior border; its margins are clearly defined by the reflective capsular line (Fig. 5). The parenchymal echoes are a mid-grey and consist of a uniform, sponge-like pattern interrupted only by the vessels. Tomograms to the right show the same basic shape but the liver here is larger, especially the upper portion, while the various impressions produced by the contiguous organs are apparent (Fig. 6). In transverse sections the wedge shape of the liver is seen, tapering to the left (Fig. 7). The caudate lobe (Fig. 8) is seen as an extension of the right lobe in transverse sections and as an almond-shaped structure posterior to the left lobe in longitudinal views. The position of the ligamentum teres is marked by an intensely reflective focus in transverse sections (Fig. 9).

The appearance of the complex of vessels at the porta depends on their orientation in the slices viewed; two main projections need to be considered. When the tomogram runs along the line of the hepatic pedicle, the portal vein is cut lengthways (Fig. 10); tomograms slightly laterally also cut the bile duct which is seen as a smaller tubular

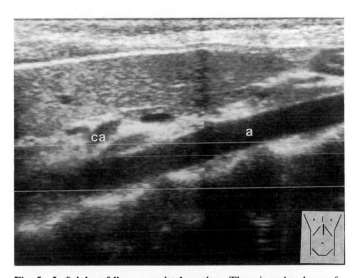

Fig. 5 Left lobe of liver – sagittal section. The triangular shape of the left lobe is somewhat exaggerated in this aesthenic subject in whom the liver is thinned antero-posteriorly. It overlies the aorta with its midline branches. a – aorta, ca – coeliac axis.

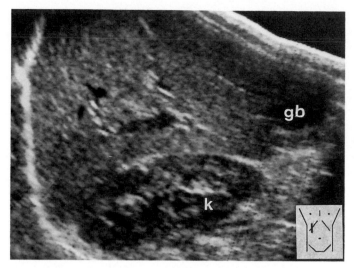

Fig. 6 Right lobe of liver – sagittal section. The bright bow of the diaphragm outlines the upper surface of the liver while posteriorly it overlies the right kidney. Its parenchyma is interrupted by spaces for the veins. k – kidney, gb – gallbladder.

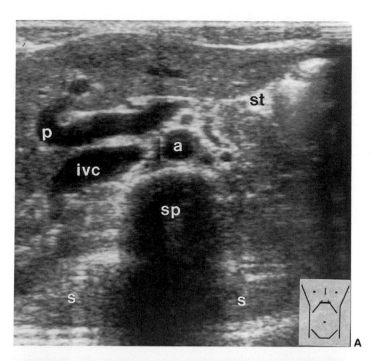

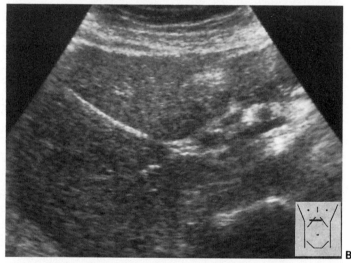

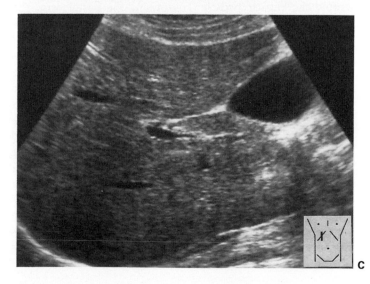

structure running parallel to the portal vein and lying anterior to it. Often the duct is only apparent from the mid-position of the porta and below because above this level (i.e. above the point of fusion of the left and right ducts) they are seen as small rings cut in cross section, lying to the left and right of the portal vein respectively and so are difficult to recognise. Sections along the hepatic pedicle and slightly medially image the hepatic artery immediately anterior to the portal vein; usually the artery divides somewhat lower than the level of junction of the hepatic ducts and so the right branch is more often imaged as a ring passing across to the right and lying between the portal vein and the bile duct (either the right hepatic or the common duct). As a normal variant the artery lies anterior to the duct but the position of both these anterior to the portal vein is practically inviolable. Seen in transverse section (Fig. 11) the portal vein appears as a ring with the duct and artery anterior to it in the same relative positions as in the longitudinal sections.

The portal vein branches can be traced from the porta, the right passing more or less transversely for a few centimetres before dividing into its main anterior and posterior branches (Fig. 12). The left portal vein curves anteriorly

Fig. 7 The liver in transverse section. A: In transverse section the liver has a wedge shape, narrowing to the left. This means that the visceral surface is tilted to the left and also inferiorly, though this can only be appreciated on a sagittal section. This tomogram has passed through the porta hepatis. a – aorta, ivc – inferior vena cava, p – portal vein, s – sacro-spinalis muscle, sp – spine, st – stomach. **B:** Transverse image showing the main interlobar fissure separating the left and right lobes. **C:** Longitudinal scan showing the fissure lying between the porta hepatis and the gallbladder fossa.

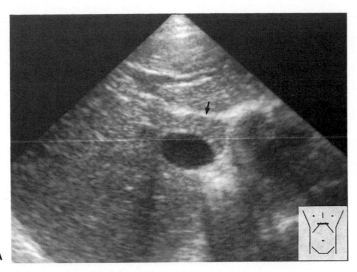
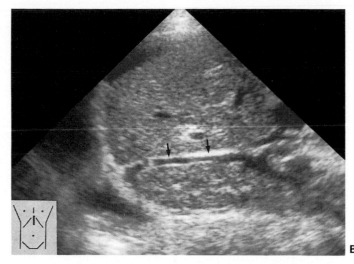

A B

Fig. 8 **The caudate lobe. A:** In transverse section the caudate lobe is seen as an extension medially of the right lobe. It lies immediately anterior to the inferior vena cava. **B:** In longitudinal section it is seen as an oval or almond-shaped portion of liver tissue posterior to the left lobe from which it is separated by the fissure for the ligamentum venosum (arrows). In this case a trace of ascites surrounds the caudate lobe, indicating its position within the lesser sac.

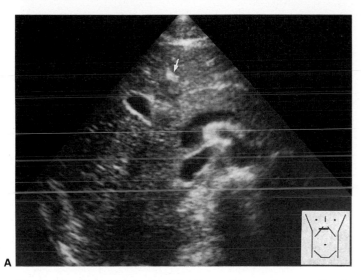
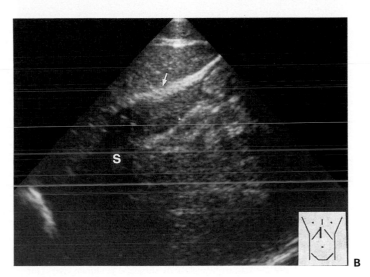

A B

Fig. 9 **The ligamentum teres.** The fibrous tissue and surrounding fat give the ligamentum teres strong echoes. **A:** Cut in cross-section (arrow) it appears as a spot while **B:** cut lengthways a band is seen; it often casts a marked shadow (s) which interferes with imaging of structures immediately deep to it.

as well as crossing to the left (reflecting the generally more anterior position of the left lobe of the liver) before giving off superior and inferior branches to the various segments it traverses. One notable branch passes inferiorly towards the ligamentum teres; usually it thins to a fine thread as it enters the ligamentum itself, often being too small to be resolved here. It is an important vein because, as the remnant of the left umbilical vein (Fig. 4), it represents one of the potential sites of portosystemic anastomosis which can open up and become very prominent in portal hypertension (see Ch. 19).

Sections high in the liver show the larger hepatic veins as they converge towards the upper cava (Fig. 13). Their relations are best shown in cross-sections: the right hepatic vein generally lies in the coronal plane and curves medially to enter the cava a centimetre or so below the diaphragm. The middle hepatic vein can be traced from the general position of the gallbladder curving superiorly and posteriorly to enter the anterior part of the cava immediately below the diaphragm. Commonly the left vein joins it so that these two empty together, the left hepatic vein having curved from left to right. The smaller inferior group

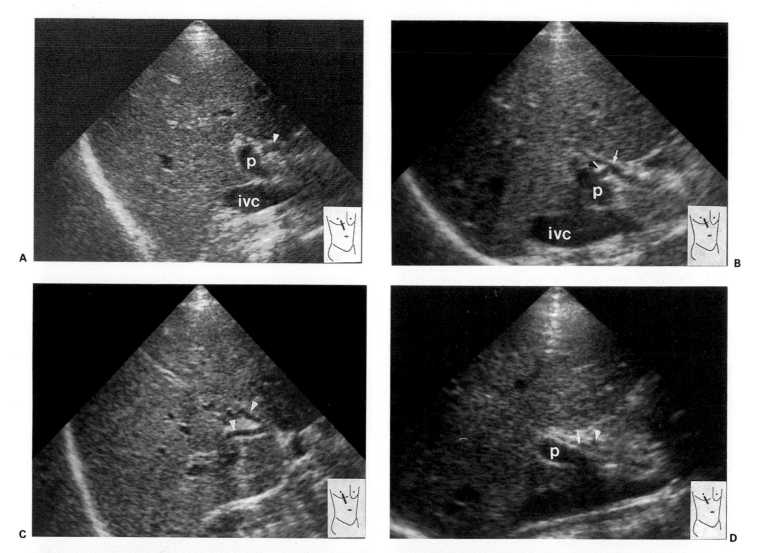

Fig. 10 The porta hepatis cut lengthways. Oblique cuts through the porta medially show **A:** the hepatic artery (arrowhead) lying anterior to the portal vein (p) while **B:** slightly further laterally the common bile duct (arrow) overlies the vein in a characteristic configuration with the hepatic artery (arrowhead) in between. **C:** In this subject a cut further laterally still reveals the hepatic artery dividing into two branches (arrowheads) – presumably these represent the right and left main branches. If this is the correct interpretation, this depicts a relatively uncommon anomaly of the hepatic artery in which the main division occurs further laterally than usual. **D:** A much commoner anomaly, where the artery (arrowhead) lies anterior to the bile duct (arrow) (10% of subjects) is shown. ivc – inferior vena cava.

of hepatic veins may sometimes be demonstrated as short vessels passing directly from the caudate lobe and the medial portion of the right lobe where the cava is in direct contact with the liver (Fig. 14).

The two sets of veins tend to have distinctive appearances on ultrasound, the portal veins having thicker, reflective walls while the hepatic veins appearing merely as defects in the liver parenchyma. This corresponds to their anatomical structures since the hepatic veins are essentially large sinusoids whose walls are thin or absent while the portal veins have fibromuscular walls and in addition are accompanied by smaller hepatic arterial branches and by small radicles of the biliary tree. However, as always in ultrasound imaging, the actual appearances depend as

much on the angle of interrogation as on the anatomy so that a portal vein cut at a more oblique angle may have inapparent walls while sometimes an hepatic vein which has been cut so that its walls lie at 90° to the ultrasound beam has strongly reflective walls. The overall anatomy also helps in their distinction and they may be traced towards the porta or the inferior vena cava where a definite designation is required. Doppler (Plate 1), provides a direct means of demonstrating the flow direction[9] (though it must be remembered that flow in the portal veins may be reversed in extreme portal hypertension (see Ch. 19)).

Within the liver parenchyma the normal bile ducts are too small to be demonstrated except under good imaging conditions (Fig. 15). However, the left and right main

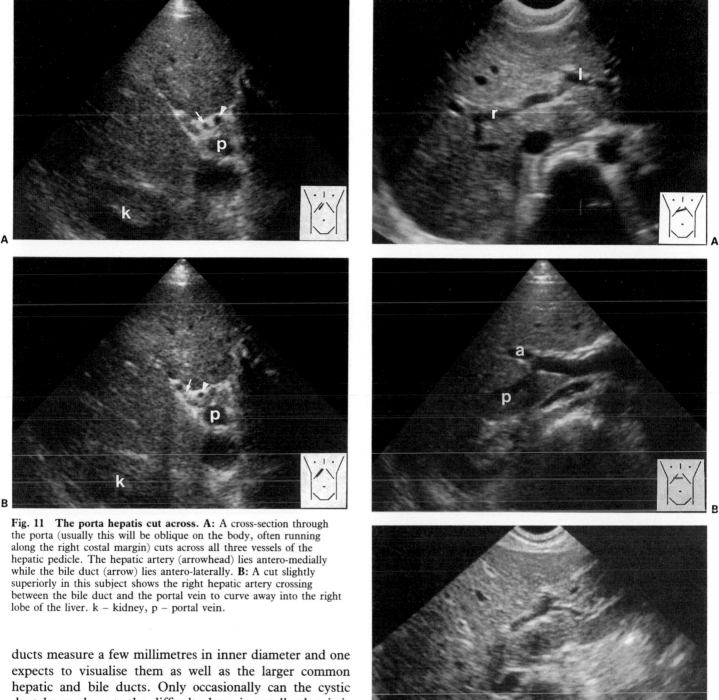

Fig. 11 The porta hepatis cut across. A: A cross-section through the porta (usually this will be oblique on the body, often running along the right costal margin) cuts across all three vessels of the hepatic pedicle. The hepatic artery (arrowhead) lies antero-medially while the bile duct (arrow) lies antero-laterally. **B:** A cut slightly superiorly in this subject shows the right hepatic artery crossing between the bile duct and the portal vein to curve away into the right lobe of the liver. k – kidney, p – portal vein.

ducts measure a few millimetres in inner diameter and one expects to visualise them as well as the larger common hepatic and bile ducts. Only occasionally can the cystic duct be made out; the difficulty here is usually that it is extremely tortuous (Fig. 16). The diameter of the lumen of the bile duct is considered by many to increase slightly with age, though this is still somewhat controversial, as is the case also with the pancreatic duct (see Ch. 8). The conventional position to measure the bile duct lumen is within the porta at the level of the right portal vein where the duct is cut across (Fig. 17); at this level the hepatic artery can usually also be demonstrated, probably actually the right hepatic artery. A convenient and easily remembered formula is 1 mm per decade of life; this allows for the

Fig. 12 The portal veins. The main portal vein divides into the main right and left branches within the porta. **A:** A cut just superior to this shows the main branches with the right branch (r) passing transversely and the left (l) passing antero-medially. **B:** A cut through the right branch shows its division into anterior (a) and posterior (p) segmental branches. **C:** Similarly on the left the two main segmental divisions of the portal vein are shown.

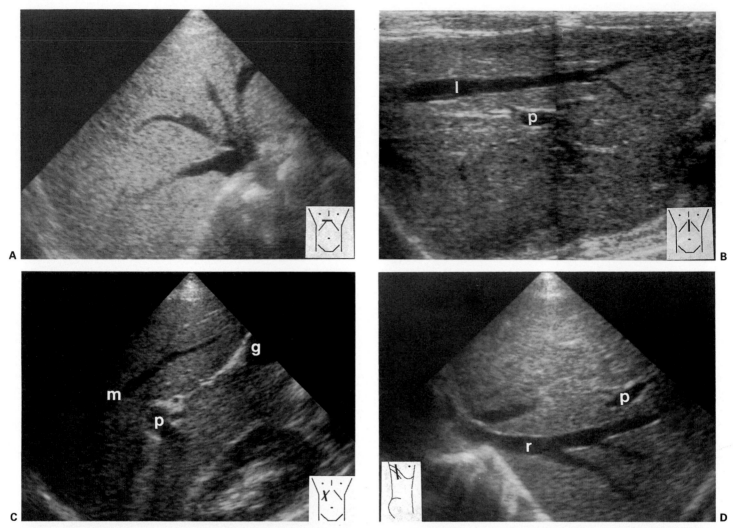

Fig. 13 Main hepatic veins. A: In a high transverse section inclined upwards the main hepatic veins are well-seen as they converge on the inferior vena cava. **B** and **C:** Longitudinal sections in the sagittal plane show the path of the left and middle hepatic veins (l and m) lying approximately in the midline and in the right mid-clavicular lines respectively. **D:** The right hepatic vein (r) is best demonstrated in a coronal section through the lower intercostal spaces. g – gallbladder, p – portal vein.

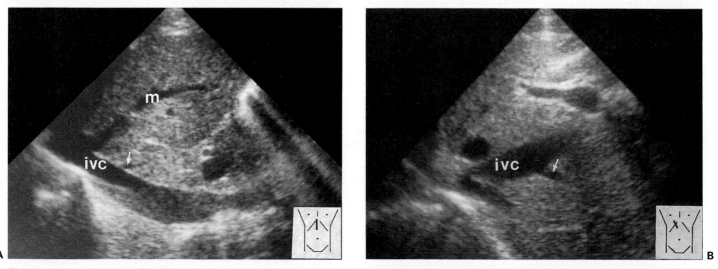

Fig. 14 Inferior hepatic veins. The main hepatic veins are supplemented by a small set of veins, the inferior group (arrows), which drain those parts of **A:** the caudate and **B:** right lobes that are in direct contact with the cava. ivc – inferior vena cava, m – middle hepatic vein.

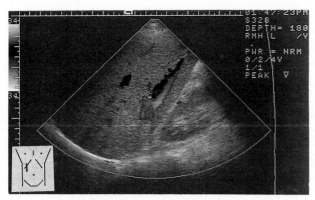

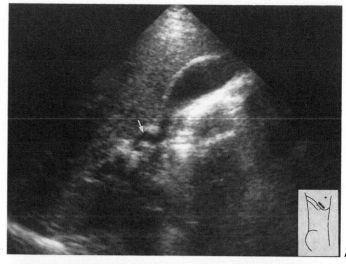

Plate 1 Colour Doppler of the right lobe of the liver. The flow in the main portal vein is shown as a red colour because it runs towards the transducer; whereas the flow in the hepatic vein is coded as blue because it is away from the transducer. This figure is reproduced in colour in the colour plate section at the front of this volume.

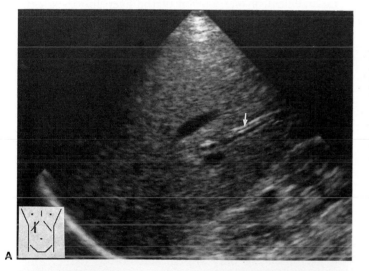

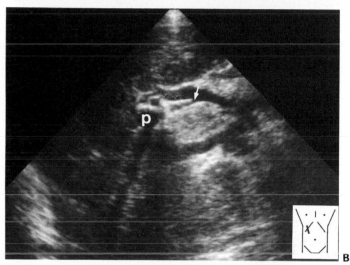

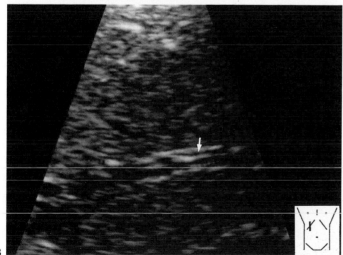

Fig. 15 Intrahepatic bile ducts. A: Under good imaging conditions with a high resolution scanner normal intrahepatic bile ducts (arrow) can sometimes be detected lying close to the larger portal vein branches. Provided these are less than 1 mm in calibre, they can be accepted as normal. Colour Doppler demonstrates that some of these vessels accompanying the portal veins are arterial branches; the anatomical relationship of these three vessels is more variable than at the porta hepatis. **B:** A magnification of the relevant portion of A.

Fig. 16 Cystic duct. A: The cystic duct is often visualised at the point where it leaves the gallbladder (arrow) but **B:** the point of junction with the common duct (arrow) is rarely demonstrated. p – right portal vein.

smaller duct calibre in the paediatric age group and for progressive enlargement with age, while for the average adult the value of 4 to 5 mm corresponds with the commonly quoted measurements. The duct expands as it descends and receives the cystic duct, so if only the more inferior (extrahepatic) portions can be accessed, an additional few millimetres must be allowed.

When compared with the duct diameter measured during a cholecystogram or a cholangiogram (either percutaneous or retrograde endoscopic) the ultrasound sizes seem too small. This discrepancy caused much debate before the complex of factors that explain it was understood and the measurements could be reconciled. Ultrasound tends to underestimate the calibre of ducts in general because of infilling due to the beam width artefact that causes the reflective walls to appear thickened and to spread into the lumen. On the other hand, on X-ray the tube-film distance magnifies the image and this is added

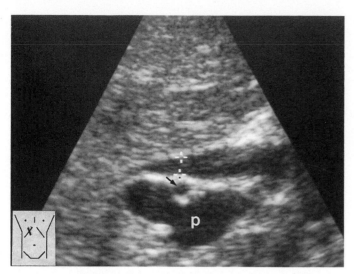

Fig. 17   Measurement of the common duct. The recommended position for measuring the calibre of the common duct is at the point where it crosses the hepatic artery (caliper crosses). In this patient the duct is at the upper limit of normal (4.1 mm). arrow – hepatic artery, p – portal vein.

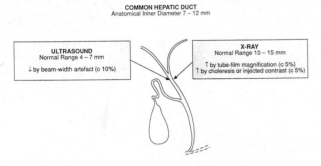

Fig. 18 Discrepancy between X-ray and ultrasound normal ranges for the bile duct. While the ultrasound measurement of the diameter of the bile duct is underestimated because of infilling due to beam spreading, the cholangiographic measurement is exaggerated because of magnification effects. In addition the contrast-induced choleresis ensures that the duct is filled during the X-ray measurement. When the duct has an oval cross-section, the X-ray measurement is of the long axis while the ultrasound measurement is of the short axis. These factors account well for the discrepancy.

to the fact that the duct is distended either by injected contrast or by the choleresis induced by the biliary contrast agent. These factors combine to account well for the discrepancy (Fig. 18).

Variations

True variants of the liver may be divided into cases of failure of development of a lobe or segment and cases where abnormal development has occurred.[10] The commonest examples of failure affect the left lobe, especially its lateral segments (II and III), and are often compensated by hypertrophy of the right and quadrate lobes. The small left lobe may result from a developmental failure (i.e. true

hypoplasia) but an alternative mechanism concerning the fetal bypass system seems probable in many cases. At birth the umbilical vein and sinus venosus are occluded by vasospasm thus closing the placento-splenic liver bypass; the ligamentum teres and ligamentum venosum are formed by the fibrosed remnants of these vessels (Fig. 4). The left portal vein branch is closely attached to these fetal blood vessels; if the spasm extends abnormally, the lateral portion of the left lobe may become ischaemic. Though difficult to establish with certainty, the frequency with which a small lateral segment of the left lobe is replaced by a fibrous band is suggestive of this aetiology. Generally this anomaly is of no clinical significance, though occasionally it is associated with defective development of the diaphragm. Absence of the right lobe is much rarer; again a diaphragmatic hernia may coexist.

Enlargement of one portion of the liver also most commonly affects the left lobe which may stretch across to the left costal margin. Here it lies superior to the spleen giving a confusing appearance that is easily mistaken for a subphrenic collection. Alternatively the enlargement may form a thin sheet of liver in the epigastrium that extends well below the costal margin. These two variants probably should be considered as changes in shape rather than as anomalies where a true additional lobe is found. Usually these more severe developmental anomalies form as sessile lobes consisting of marked enlargements of a liver segment; the Reidel's lobe, a 'linguiform prolongation of the right lobe', is very common. It may appear simply as a long right lobe or may have a modest narrowing overlying the right kidney so that it is almost pedunculated (Fig. 19). True pedunculated accessory lobes are rarer; the stalk may contain liver tissue or only vessels and fibrous tissue. Since they may be found in any position in the abdomen, they

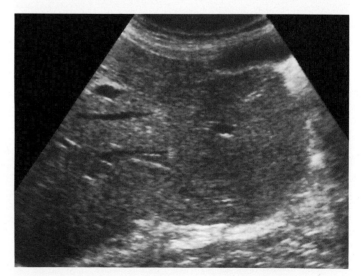

Fig. 19   Reidel's lobe. Reidel's lobe is an inferior extension of the right lobe which often overlies the kidney. Because it lies very superficially, it is obvious on palpation and thus raises the suspicion of hepatomegaly.

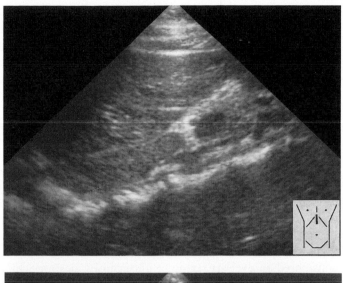

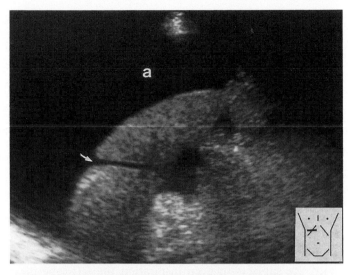

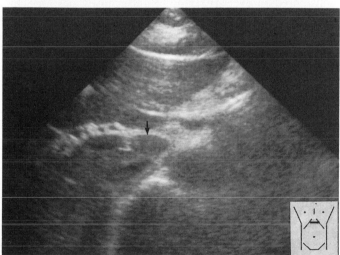

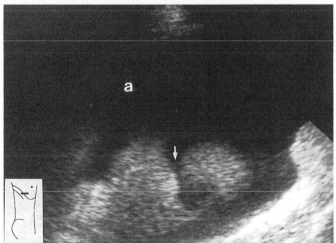

Fig. 20 Long caudate lobe. The caudate lobe is very variable in size. **A:** When it extends far inferiorly, as in this subject.
B: Transverse cuts through its tip may suggest the presence of a pre-aortic mass (arrow) that is separate from the liver, such as an enlarged lymph node but cuts further superiorly demonstrate its continuity with the liver.

Fig. 21 Accessory fissure in the liver. Under normal conditions accessory fissures are difficult to detect on ultrasound because the surfaces are apposed; in this patient ascitic fluid (a) separating the surfaces reveals the fissure (arrow) extending deep into the right lobe from its lateral surface.

are particularly confusing especially when affected by pathology such as masses or torsion.

Marked variability of the caudate lobe has been mentioned: it may be very small or may extend inferiorly as a tongue below the level of the free border of the left lobe (Fig. 20). Seen in transverse section, the tip seems to be separate from the liver and at first might suggest a pancreatic mass or lymphadenopathy.

Indentations on the liver surface from adjacent structures can be quite marked and masses often impress themselves on the liver parenchyma as it is soft and yielding. The same effect often produces grooves on the diaphragmatic surface where prominent leaflets indent it producing furrows. True accessory fissures are sometimes encountered on this surface forming deep peritoneal folds in the liver substance that are fixed in position (Fig. 21).

Assessment of liver size

The wide normal variation in the configuration of the liver makes assessment of its size difficult, whatever means are employed. The bulk of the liver may lie mainly on the right, perhaps with a Reidel's lobe and a correspondingly small left lobe, or there may be a small right lobe with a large left lobe that extends across to lie under the left hemidiaphragm above the spleen. In the midline such a large left lobe may cover the upper epigastric organs.

Clinical evaluation is notoriously unreliable,[11,12] a Reidel's lobe, for example, easily being mistaken for hepatomegaly. Tomographic techniques are difficult to use because each image represents only one projection of the anatomy so that the full series of slices must be evaluated before the true dimensions of the liver can be appreciated.

This is difficult to perform automatically and can only be approximated by eye. Because it is non-tomographic, isotope scintigraphy is in some respects the most reliable method for size evaluation since the whole outline of the liver is demonstrated.[13] Again the problem of projections, here those of the liver surfaces rather than of slices, is difficult to overcome. An additional problem with isotope methods is the variable image magnification. Though this can be calibrated by the use of a scale applied to the patient's body, this adds another stage to the scan and has not proved routinely practical.

With tomographic techniques such as ultrasound, the simplest approach to evaluate liver size is from linear measurements in standard positions. In a series of 1000 normal subjects anteroposterior (AP) longitudinal diameters were measured in the midline and at the mid-clavicular line.[14] With the subjects in deep inspiration the left lobe measurements were straightforward but on the right overlying lung usually prevented access to the uppermost part of the liver, so the level of the lung was taken as the limit (Fig. 22). The results (Table 1) of the linear measurements were not improved upon by working out areas and the longitudinal and AP measurements were closely enough correlated for most subjects so that use of the longitudinal

value alone was accurate enough for routine purposes, except in very thin or very obese subjects. This is because the liver tends to be elongated in thin subjects, so that the longitudinal measurement on its own gives an overestimation, while the reverse is true of obese subjects, whose livers tend to be short and deep.

Quite similar figures were proposed in another study[15] in which linear measurements were compared with autopsy measurements of liver size. The span (supero-inferior distance) of the right lobe was measured in the scan plane half-way between the midline and the lateral extent of the right lobe (in practice this is very close to the mid-clavicular line). When this measurement was correlated with autopsy measurements 93% of those livers with a span less than 13 cm were normal while 75% of those larger than 15 cm were abnormal. The 13 to 15 cm group was considered an overlap region of uncertainty, despite which this type of linear measurement is useful for assessment of changes in liver size, for example when following the response of liver metastases to chemotherapy.

In a slight elaboration of this method, longitudinal measurements of the left lobe in the midline and of the right lobe in the mid-clavicular line have been extensively assessed and provide a surprisingly good correlation with other physical measurements such as body weight and surface area.[14] In this study of almost one thousand healthy subjects, the normal values on the left were 8.3 ($\pm$ 1.7), and on the right 10.5 ($\pm$ 1.5) cm. Only in very heavy and very light subjects was it important to add AP measurements; in these somatotypes the horizontal and vertical lie of the liver respectively leads to an under- and overestimation of liver size when only longitudinal measurements are used.

Table 1 Dimensions of the normal liver[14]

		Diameter (cm) (mean $\pm$ SD)	95th Percentile (cm)
Mid-clavicular	longitudinal	10.5 $\pm$ 1.5	12.6
	AP	8.1 $\pm$ 1.9	11.3
Midline	longitudinal	8.3 $\pm$ 1.7	10.9
	AP	5.7 $\pm$ 1.5	8.2

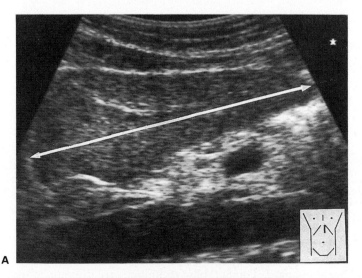
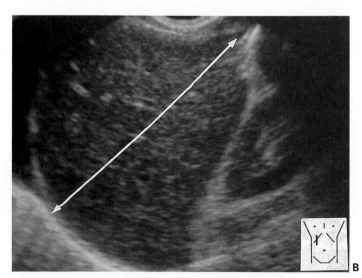

A   B

Fig. 22 Linear measurements of the liver. The size of the liver can be assessed by **A**: taking the span in the midline and **B**: in the mid-clavicular line; the former averages 8 cm and the latter 10 cm. Only in very thin or very heavily built patients is it necessary also to take the antero-posterior measurements to compensate for their different liver shapes.

A slightly more complex method, in which the height, breadth and thickness of the liver are combined, mathematically also gives good correlations.[16] In one method, the product of these three (in centimetres) is divided by 27 (3^3) to give an index of liver volume which is nominally 100%. The standard deviation is between 95% and 140% (75 subjects). Another way to incorporate the data is to plot the values graphically and derive an equation for the best linear fit. The liver volume (LV) in ml is approximated by the equation:

$$LV = 133.2 + 0.422 \ (h \times b \times l) \ cm$$

Since both these methods require the transverse span of the liver to be measured, they are not readily applicable to real time scanners; possibly this is the reason for their failure to gain routine acceptance.

A more elaborate method to estimate the liver volume involves measuring the area of each of a spaced series of tomograms.[17] If the slices are all in the same plane (usually either transverse or sagittal sections) and are spaced 1 cm apart, simply summing the areas (in cm^2) gives the liver volume (in ml) and this equals the weight, assuming that the liver's density is one. A slight refinement can be incorporated to allow for the difficulty in measuring the areas of the topmost and lowermost slices whose outlines tend to be blurred because of the partial volume effect. If other sets of slices, such as radial, are chosen, more complex formulae must be used, but the same results can be obtained. Using a static scanner, accuracies of 5% have been obtained in vivo and this represents a great improvement on clinical or simple linear ultrasound measurements. However, the technique is time consuming and necessitates the use of a static scanner (the field of view of real time systems being too small to accommodate the whole area of the central tomograms through the liver). In addition, in many subjects, the complete set of slices cannot be obtained, gas or bone preventing access for some parts of the liver. For most departments therefore, this type of evaluation is too tedious and cumbersome for routine use; the same method is much more easily applied to CT scans.

In practice therefore, the ultrasound evaluation of liver size is a subjective affair; the experienced sonologist can gain a useful impression of liver size from tomographic views in different directions covering both lobes with due allowance for the patient's size. For example, if both left and right lobes project below the costal margin, suspicion of hepatomegaly is raised and can often be confirmed by noting that the free edge of the liver has lost its normal sharp configuration and become rounded, a non-specific feature of hepatomegaly of any cause. Though crude, this form of subjective evaluation is often useful, especially in refuting a clinical impression of hepatomegaly which is often readily explained by the presence of a Reidel's lobe (especially if it overlies a high right kidney) or perhaps by a flat right hemidiaphragm.

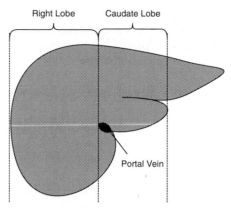

Transverse Section

Fig. 23 Measurement of the caudate lobe. The position for measurement of the caudate lobe in the transverse plane is shown. The normal caudate is less than two thirds the transverse diameter of the right lobe.

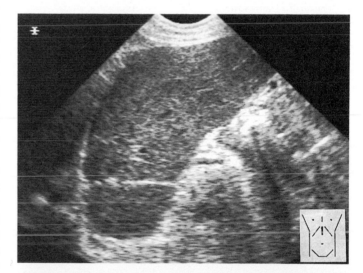

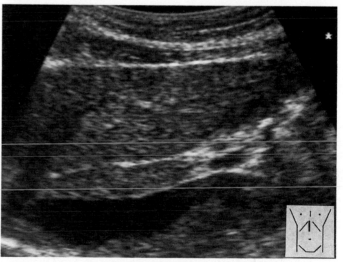

Fig. 24 AP measurement of the caudate lobe. The AP measurement of the caudate lobe should be no more than one third of the AP measurement of the overlying left lobe. These two patients show that the rule applies even in wide variations of liver shape.

One lobe of the liver whose size can be assessed on a linear measurement is the caudate lobe which is often particularly enlarged in cirrhosis and in hepatic vein occlusion (the Budd-Chiari syndrome). Again a subjective evaluation is often sufficient, especially to exclude enlargement, but when there is doubt or when a baseline measurement is required, its transverse diameter at the level of the porta may be measured and compared with the transverse diameter of the right lobe (Fig. 23). The normal caudate lobe is less than two thirds of the right lobe and there is only a small overlap with normal.[18] A more practical alternative is to compare the AP thickness of the caudate with the left lobe immediately anterior to it; the caudate should be less than half the thickness of the left lobe (Fig. 24).

REFERENCES

1 Valleix D, Sautereau D, Pouget X, et al. Ultrasonographic anatomy of the liver. Surg Radiol Anat 1987; 9: 123–134
2 Gelfand D W. Anatomy of the liver. Radiol Clin North Am 1980; 18: 187–194
3 Marks W M, Filly R A, Callen P W. Ultrasonic anatomy of the liver: a review with new applications. JCU 1979; 7: 137–146
4 Brown B M, Filly R A, Callen P W. Ultrasonographic anatomy of the caudate lobe. J Ultrasound Med 1982; 1: 189–192
5 Heloury Y, Leborgne J, Le Neel JC, Malvy P, Barbin J Y, Hureau J. The caudate lobe of the liver. Anatomical study. Surgical applications. J Chir (Paris) 1987; 124: 651–657
6 Couinaud C. Le Foie; études anatomique et chirurgicales. Paris: Masson. 1957
7 Mukai J K, Stack C M, Turner D A, et al. Imaging of surgically relevant hepatic vascular and segmental anatomy. Part 1. Normal anatomy. AJR 1987; 149: 287–292
8 Balfe D M, Mauro M A, Koehler R E, et al. Gastrohepatic ligament: normal and pathologic CT anatomy. Radiology 1984; 150: 485–490
9 Berland L L, Lawson T L, Foley W D. Porta hepatis: sonographic discrimination of bile ducts from arteries with pulsed Doppler with new anatomic criteria. AJR 1982; 138: 833–840
10 Champetier J, Yver R, Letoublon C, Vigneau B. A general review of anomalies of hepatic morphology and their clinical implications. Anat Clin 1985; 7: 285–299
11 Naftalis J, Leevy C M. Clinical estimation of liver size. Am J Dig Dis 1963; 8: 236–243
12 Sullivan S, Krasner N, Williams R. The clinical estimation of liver size. BMJ 1976; 2: 1042–1043
13 Peternel W W, Schaefer J W, Schiff L. Clinical evaluation of liver size and hepatic scintiscan. Am J Dig Dis 1966; 11: 346–350
14 Niederau C, Sonnenberg A, Müller J E, Erchenbrecht J F, Scholten T, Fritsch W P. Sonographic measurements of the normal liver, spleen, pancreas and portal vein. Radiology 1983; 149: 537–540
15 Gosink B B, Leymaster C F. Ultrasonic estimation of hepatomegaly. JCU 1981; 9: 37–41
16 Kardel T, Holm H H, Rasmusen S N, Mordensen T. Ultrasonic determination of liver and spleen volumes. Scand J Clin Lab Invest 1971; 27: 123–128
17 Rasmussen S N. Liver volume determination by ultrasonic scanning. Dan Med Bull 1978; 25: 1–46
18 Harbin W P, Robert N J, Ferrucci J T. Diagnosis of cirrhosis based on regional changes in hepatic morphology: a radiological and pathological analysis. Radiology 1980; 135: 273–283

15

Intra-operative ultrasound

Graham R. Plant

243

INTRODUCTION

Where it is important to depict anatomy that cannot be viewed directly during surgery, ultrasound offers several advantages over conventional X-ray methods. These include lack of radiation, cheapness, high resolution display of anatomy and pathology and an interactive, real time approach that appeals to the surgeon.

Conventional ultrasound scans through the skin and body wall provide excellent tissue visualisation in slim patients but have limitations in obese or very muscular subjects. Intra-operative ultrasound, in which there are no intervening body structures, gives excellent imaging on all patients. Surgeons and radiologists have used ultrasound in a wide variety of operative procedures and the increasing availability of the equipment and expertise in operating theatres have resulted in ever greater utilisation of the technique. Initially a number of problems presented themselves but the development of new machines, better understanding of the ultrasound anatomy and abilities of the technique, and improved training have resulted in rapid growth in the use of intra-operative ultrasound.

This chapter will discuss the equipment and techniques, present the body areas in which intra-operative ultrasound is presently used and define the uses of particular interest.

Equipment

If ultrasound examinations are to be performed within the operative field the equipment used must fulfil certain requirements:

> the risks of infection must be eliminated;
> the transducer may need to be used in areas where there is only limited room to manoeuvre;
> the equipment as a whole will be used in atmospheres possibly containing flammable anaesthetic gases;
> the transducer will be in direct contact with the patient's viscera and hence electrical safety must be assured.

The only components that need significant change from standard equipment are the transducers. As in conventional ultrasound, transducers are available as linear array and sector types. These may be used as end or side viewing, depending on the application required.

There are a number of commercially available portable ultrasound machines that support intra-operative transducers. These machines are attractive by reason of their portability and simplicity and also because they are relatively inexpensive. Although they offer the ability to perform intra-operative ultrasound, reservations have to be expressed about their overall image quality and ability to detect very small or ill-defined masses. Hence their true usefulness may be limited.

Transducers

Linear arrays Linear array transducers are the main type used in intra-abdominal and vascular work. This is because they can in general be used in sites where the space for access is limited. It is possible to save space in the transducer head itself by mounting some of the electrical components at the proximal end of the transducer cable and therefore have the smallest possible working head whilst still maintaining a useful footprint size. A side viewing transducer is particularly useful as it can be slipped alongside the organ in question. An end viewing system is often too cumbersome to fit into tight spaces (e.g. between the right lobe of the liver and the body wall) as it would need to be turned inwards for the active surface to make contact with the liver. The end viewing systems are, however, eminently suitable for examining the exposed pancreas.

I-shaped or T-shaped transducers are also available, dependent on the position of insertion of the cable. The latter are in general easier to hold with the fingertips in confined spaces. For intra-abdominal work transducers operating between 3 and 7.5 MHz are available. The usual trade-off between the depth of field and image quality applies so that a 5 MHz transducer gives the best overall results for upper abdominal work. If only shallow structures need to be examined, a 7.5 MHz transducer gives better resolution.

Sector scanners Whilst it is quite possible to use sector scanners on easily accessible areas, their larger size is limiting. It is worth remembering, however, that it is quite possible to use a conventional surface scanning transducer in situations when the limited range of a dedicated probe is inadequate, as may occur with large liver tumours. Since

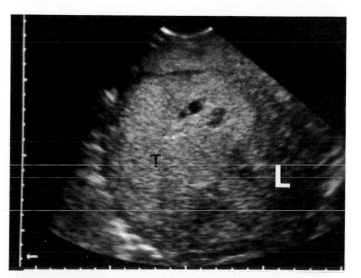

Fig. 1 Large hepatic tumour (T) demonstrated by the use of a conventional end viewing 5 MHz sector transducer using a sheath for sterility when the sterilisable intra-operative transducer did not have sufficient depth of penetration. L – liver.

these transducers are not generally sterilisable, they need to be covered with a sterile sheath (Fig. 1). In areas where only direct surface contact to an easily accessible area is required, they may be very useful.

Techniques

In general no major changes to conventional techniques are necessary, though contact gel is not usually required as the operative field is usually wetted by body fluids. It is often helpful to dim the surgical lights and this will also reduce drying due to the heat from them.

As with extra-corporeal scanning, lesions close to the transducer may be poorly seen even though they may be palpable. Depending on circumstance the area may be immersed in saline, a small stand-off device such as a saline bag may be used or the organ may be visualised from its contralateral surface.

Wherever appropriate it is advantageous for the surgeon to expose the whole of the area or organ that is being investigated. This allows the best visualisation of internal structures to be obtained.

Transducer sterilisation

The important requirement of sterility for intra-operative scanning can be met either by sterilising the transducer itself or by enclosing it in a sterile sheath.

The transducer may be sterilised in ethylene chloride gas; however, the facilities for this may not always be instantly available and so it may be necessary to have more than one transducer. Alternatively the transducer may be immersed in glutaraldehyde 2% (Cidex®); 10 minutes' immersion will kill most pathogens including *Pseudomonas*, HIV and HBV, 1 hour's immersion kills *Mycobacterium tuberculosis* while 3 hours are necessary to kill all spores of the *Clostridia* strains. Before use the probe must be rinsed with sterile water to remove traces of the glutaraldehyde which is tissue toxic. Although theoretically less effective against some pathogens, this system is quick and readily performed and has not been shown to have significant drawbacks. The electrical connectors at the scanner end of the transducer cable are not waterproof and therefore cannot be immersed; prolonged immersion of the transducer and cable in glutaraldehyde may damage the plastic casing of some transducers.

Whichever system is used, scrupulous cleaning of the transducer is mandatory after each study and before sterilisation to remove any dried blood or debris on the casing.

The sterile sheath method is applicable to all transducers but is somewhat cumbersome. It may also degrade the image due to the extra layers through which the sound passes and because of the possibility of air bubbles being

trapped between the scanning head and sheath. A little contact gel is necessary between transducer and sheath.

Body areas

Liver

Liver surgery is the area in which intra-operative ultrasound is most extensively used.[1]

Intra-operative ultrasound is of use in five ways:

a) It is very accurate at identifying lesions within the liver. Whilst conventional pre-operative imaging has a detection rate in the liver of between 60% and 90%,[2–4] intra-operative ultrasound has been shown to detect more lesions than the best pre-operative technique.[4,5] Patients coming to surgery for liver tumours will have had intensive liver imaging. Despite this it is not uncommon for intra-operative ultrasound to detect further small tumours that determine the resectability and prognosis (Fig. 2). Where there has been a delay between the imaging and the resection, intra-operative ultrasound can check that no further change has occurred.

b) Modern liver resection relies on the concepts of segmental anatomy described by Couinaud.[6,7] Intra-operative ultrasound helps delineate the liver into its eight segments by allowing identification of the vascular elements that supply and drain the segments of the liver.[8]

Visualising the vessels and especially the hepatic venous drainage is also of extreme importance to the surgeon. If a tumour involves all three hepatic veins (usually because it lies close to their insertion into the vena cava) then resection is impossible. This information may be difficult to obtain pre-operatively as metastases, particularly from

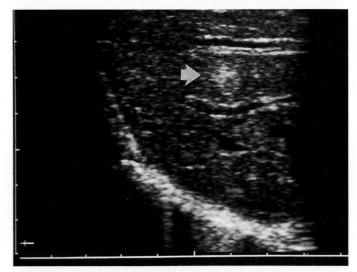

Fig. 2 Small hepatic metastasis (arrow) sandwiched between two vascular bundles. Identified by intra-operative ultrasound, it was impalpable and not visualised on pre-operative imaging.

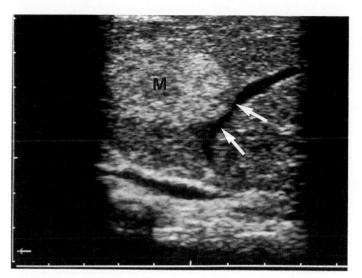

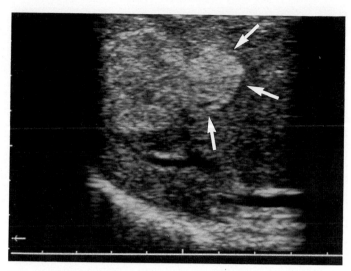

Fig. 3 **Hepatic metastasis** from a colonic carcinoma (M) impinging on the middle hepatic vein (arrows). As is common with this type of tumour, the wall of the vessel was not involved.

Fig. 4 **Hepatic metastasis** from a colonic carcinoma showing a bilobed appearance. The main lesion was palpable, the nodule (arrows) was not.

colorectal tumours (probably the commonest tumour resected from the liver), often abut the hepatic veins without necessarily involving them (Fig. 3).

Occasionally an accessory vein will provide venous drainage of segments 5 and 6 directly into the vena cava. This allows preservation of these segments when the rest of the right lobe is resected. This vein is usually visible at operation but occasionally intra-operative ultrasound may help in its detection.

c) Intra-operative ultrasound allows the surgeon to inspect the proposed resection plane. It renders the liver 'transparent' and hence occasionally it will allow the plane of the resection to be slightly adjusted to encompass a nodule of tumour that is impalpable while retaining a margin of uninvolved tissue around the tumour (Fig. 4).

d) When there are multiple lesions on imaging or at laparotomy, intra-operative ultrasound is invaluable in defining the lesions, particularly if small benign cysts are present since they may be missed on pre-operative imaging or masquerade as small tumour deposits. Intra-operative ultrasound will rapidly dismiss these lesions from consideration, but if doubt remains guided biopsy can be performed accurately.[9]

e) Some surgical teams, notably that of Bismuth in Paris,[10] also use the visualisation provided by intra-operative ultrasound to cannulate the hepatic vasculature either to control bleeding or to delineate the segments to be resected by injection of coloured dye.

It should be emphasised that, whilst intra-operative ultrasound has high sensitivity, the specificity as to the type of lesion is not significantly better than conventional ultrasound. However, biopsy of lesions under ultrasound

control for histology is easily performed as part of the intra-operative study.

It is well-known from conventional ultrasound that lesions of histologically similar types may give rise to different ultrasound appearances. Similarly, on intra-operative ultrasound colorectal metastases may appear of either increased or decreased reflectivity (Fig. 5). Usually this does not pose a problem with intra-operative ultrasound but, in common with pre-operative imaging, haemangiomas are difficult to differentiate from malignant lesions. One lesion that is often possible to differentiate is

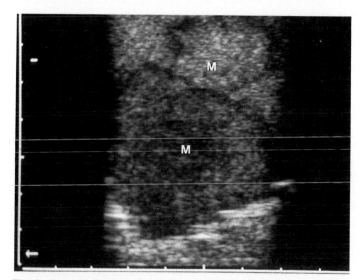

Fig. 5 **Hepatic metastases** (M) from a colonic carcinoma demonstrating that both reflective and echo-poor appearances may be produced by the same histological type.

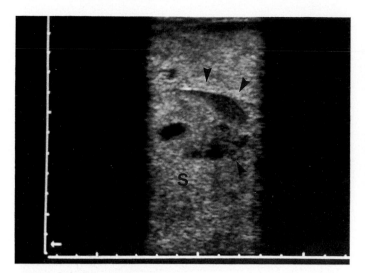

Fig. 6 Hepatic sarcoma (S) showing some of the characteristic fluid spaces (arrowheads) which honeycomb part of this large tumour.

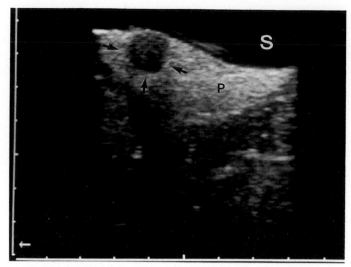

Fig. 7 Pancreatic insulinoma (arrows) visualised as a well-defined, poorly reflective mass in the body of the pancreas (P). Scanning has been performed using a stand-off device (a saline bag) (S) to improve near field visualisation.

the sarcoma which often has characteristic fluid spaces within it (Fig. 6).

Equally importantly there are a few lesions that are not easily visualised on ultrasound. Some will have been detected on pre-operative imaging while others are palpable; in these cases the false negative ultrasound is not serious. Some lesions may be detected by virtue of a halo of tissue around them or because of subtle alterations in the parenchymal pattern. This applies particularly to hepatocellular carcinomas, especially when they occur on a background of cirrhosis, but is sometimes also a problem with metastases from colorectal and breast carcinomas.

Though the main application of intra-operative ultrasound is in malignancy, it can also be useful for other types of lesion where localisation within the liver is important. For example, abscesses may honeycomb the liver making both percutaneous drainage and conventional surgical treatment difficult. In these cases the use of intra-operative ultrasound allows accurate puncture of the multiple loculi to be performed with minimal hepatic damage.

Pancreas

Intra-operative ultrasound is very useful in detecting small tumours such as insulinomas that may not be visualised pre-operatively, and which are not always palpable at operation.[11–13] The availability of intra-operative ultrasound in patients coming to surgery with a provisional diagnosis of insulinoma but in whom the lesion has not been visualised can be very reassuring.

Insulinomas appear as well-defined, poorly reflective areas within the pancreatic parenchyma (Fig. 7). As they may be multiple it is very important to examine the whole pancreas once it has been surgically exposed. Ultrasound

also helps resolve questions as to the significance of palpable lesions. Echo-poor lesions on the surface of the gland are usually lymph nodes; they may be removed for histological diagnosis.

In the surgery of pancreatic pseudocysts, intra-operative ultrasound allows identification of the exact site of the cyst and its relationship to gastrointestinal structures. This is helpful prior to drainage of a pseudocyst into the gut, and can be performed before extensive dissection has been carried out. The stomach may be outlined by fluid instilled via a nasogastric tube.

The ability of intra-operative ultrasound to visualise intraparenchymal structures also enables location of an impalpable pancreatic duct; multiloculated abscesses can be identified and drained.

Biliary surgery

Intra-operative ultrasound is useful to detect calculi in the gallbladder, biliary tree and, most importantly, in the distal common bile duct. In the gallbladder it is more accurate than palpation in the detection of small calculi.[14]

Intra-operative ultrasound has been compared to intra-operative cholangiography in the detection of distal common bile duct calculi,[14] with a reported sensitivity of 92% as opposed to 85% for cholangiography. However, it is a technically demanding examination and it may be prudent for both tests to be carried out especially when experience with intra-operative ultrasound is limited.

When the surgeon needs to dissect regions where the anatomy is complex or variable (e.g. the porta hepatis) and especially when distortion or scarring make the dissection hazardous, the ability to locate critical structures such as the hepatic artery or bile duct by intra-operative ultrasound is reassuring and probably speeds the procedure.

Renal surgery

Intra-operative ultrasound is useful during pyelolithotomy to localise calculi (especially when they are mobile), to guide a marker to them and to check for complete clearance following the procedure. This use of ultrasound may limit the extent and duration of surgery and decrease the number of nephrectomies performed.

Although this technique remains useful, it has to some extent been overtaken by the newer procedures of lithotripsy and percutaneous nephrolithotomy.

Vascular surgery

During vascular reconstruction intra-operative ultrasound can quantify the amount of atheroma in a vessel. It has also been shown to be accurate in assessing a vessel wall for the presence of intimal flaps, strictures and thrombi.

Neurosurgery

Precise localisation is of major importance in neurosurgery, both for the biopsy of lesions and for surgery. While stereotactic biopsy is the usual technique employed, intra-operative ultrasound allows the surgeon to visualise masses accurately with their relationship to surrounding vital structures. In common with the experience using ultrasound elsewhere, the capacity for characterisation of tissue is limited.

The procedure is usually performed with an end viewing transducer and here the small footprint of the sector probe is an advantage. A multifrequency transducer optimises visualisation in the relatively shallow depth range usually encountered. The use of attachable needle guides for easy accurate biopsy is helpful. The ability to confirm the position of the needle tip in real time gives greater confidence and therefore fewer biopsy passes are required. If haemorrhage occurs following the biopsy this can be recognised rapidly and treated.

Personnel and training

The question of who should perform intra-operative ultrasound examinations is difficult. Surgeons view it as an extension of their practice while radiologists feel that it falls in their provenance as an imaging technique. Both are valid points of view. In terms of controlling the scanner and familiarity with the ultrasound appearances, the radiologist has an undoubted advantage and can learn the relevant anatomy while the surgeon may equally become experienced in the use of ultrasound.

To inspect a proposed resection plane, the surgeon needs to hold the transducer during scanning in order to understand fully the exact relationships of the structures imaged. The organisational difficulties in scheduling a radiologist for the operating theatre without prolonging the anaesthetic unduly or wasting too much of his time should not be underestimated.

Ideally the answer lies in a team approach, especially for the more complicated procedures, with the radiologist being heavily involved with the pre-, intra- and post-operative imaging. If this can be achieved with mutual respect and understanding then most of the logistic and territorial problems disappear.

Our experience indicates that if the radiologist scans to ascertain the presence and sites of pathology and the surgeon reviews the surgically relevant anatomy then an ideal balance develops. This is a field in which enthusiasm and inventiveness have a large part to play and will result in maximal benefit to the patient.

Conclusion

Intra-operative ultrasound has become routine in some important areas, notably in checking the liver for metastases before radical colectomy and in planning liver segmentectomy. Once an intra-operative scanner becomes available, applications in new problems can be explored; although thus far no formal study has been reported demonstrating savings in time or efficiency, the information provided improves confidence and thus presumably, patient care.

REFERENCES

1 Seltzer S E, Holman B L. Imaging hepatic metastases from colorectal carcinoma: identification of candidates for partial hepatectomy. AJR 1989; 152: 917–923

2 Hayashi N, Yamamoto K, Tamaki N, et al. Metastatic nodules of hepatocellular carcinoma: detection with angiography, CT and US. Radiology 1987; 165: 61–63

3 Heiken J, Weyman P J, Lee J K T, et al. Detection of focal hepatic masses: prospective evaluation with delayed CT, CT during arterial portography, and MR imaging. Radiology 1989; 171: 47–51

4 Clouse M E. Current diagnostic imaging modalities of the liver. Surg Clin North Am 1989; 69: 193–234

5 Machi J, Isomoto H, Yamashita Y, et al. Intraoperative ultrasonography in screening for liver metastases from colorectal cancer: comparative accuracy with traditional procedures. Surgery 1987; 101.6: 678–684

6 Couinaud C. Le Foie. Etudes anatomiques et chirurgicales. Paris: Masson. 1957

7 Bismuth H. Surgical anatomy and anatomical surgery of the liver. World J Surg 1982; 6: 3–9

8 Kane R A, Clarke M, Hamilton E S, et al. Prospective comparison of pre-operative imaging and intra-operative ultrasound in the detection of liver tumours. Radiology 1987; 165[P] (suppl): 286–287

9 Rifkin N D, Rosato F E, Branch M, et al. Intraoperative ultrasound of the liver: an important adjunctive tool for decision making in the operating room. Ann Surg 1987; 205: 466–471

10 Bismuth H, Castaing D. Operative ultrasound of the liver and bilary ducts. Paris: Springer-Verlag

11 Shawker T H, Doppman J L. Intra-operative US. Radiology 1988; 166: 568–569

12 Galiber A K, Reading C C, Charboneau J W, et al. Localisation of pancreatic insulinoma: comparison of pre- and intra-operative US with CT and angiography. Radiology 1988; 166: 405–408

13 Sigel B, Machi J, Ramos J R, et al. The role of imaging ultrasound during pancreatic surgery. Ann Surg 1984: 200; 486–493

14 Sigel B. ed. Operative ultrasonography, 2nd edition. New York: Raven Press. 1988

FURTHER READING

Deixonne B, Lopez F-M. eds. Operative ultrasonography during hepatobiliary and pancreatic surgery. Berlin: Springer-Verlag. 1988.

Makuuchi M. ed. Abdominal intraoperative ultrasonography. Tokyo: Igaku-Shoin. 1987.

Mukai J K, Stack C M, Turner D A, et al. Imaging of surgically relevant hepatic vascular and segmental anatomy. Part 2. Extent and resectability of hepatic neoplasms. AJR 1987; 149: 293–297.

Benign focal liver lesions

Keith C. Dewbury

INTRODUCTION

A focal liver lesion is, by definition, a discrete abnormality arising within the liver. Clearly, to some degree the distinction between focal and diffuse abnormalities is artificial and the two merge together. Difficulty in separating an intra- from an extrahepatic mass is sometimes a problem. Identification of the exact organ involved is essential in the diagnostic process as well as in treatment and prognostication. Ultrasonic features suggesting an intrahepatic origin include movement of the mass with the liver in respiration, bulging of the liver capsule, displacement and distortion of the portal and hepatic vessels and posterior displacement of the inferior vena cava. The larger the lesion, the more difficult the distinction may be. Masses of less than 10 cm are usually more accurately assessed. It is appropriate for

CT to be used to complement ultrasound when difficulties remain. The advantages of demonstration of all tissues including gas and bone may be invaluable. The limitless multiplanar scanning to delineate boundaries between contiguous viscera and the real time capabilities remain important contributions for ultrasound.

Simple cyst

Ultrasound is highly accurate in the demonstration of cystic lesions in any organ and this applies particularly in the liver.[1] Fine detail is well-shown and a careful evaluation of cyst wall smoothness and regularity, septa, fluid levels and internal echoes should be made in addition to the posterior acoustic enhancement. This fine internal detail may be better evaluated with ultrasound than with CT.[2] Fine

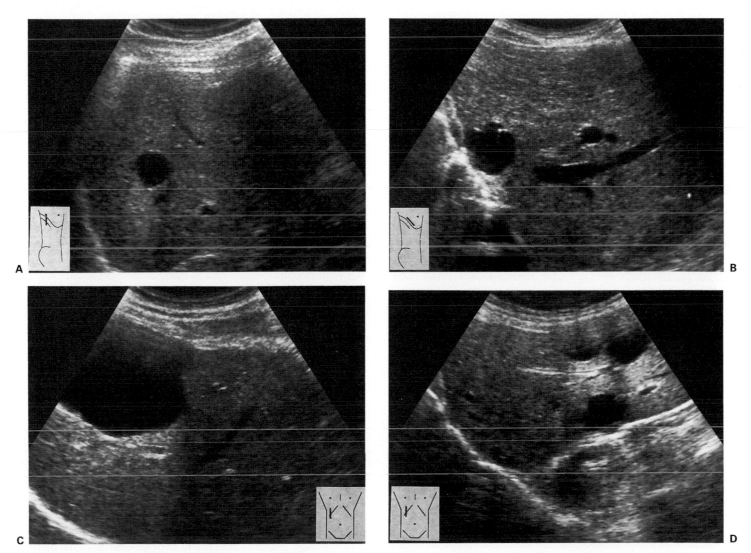

Fig. 1 Liver cyst. A: Small, simple liver cyst in the right lobe of the liver showing a clear well-defined wall and distal acoustic enhancement. **B:** Longitudinal scan showing a simple liver cyst with partial septation anteriorly. Distal acoustic enhancement is poorly appreciated due to the lesion's location adjacent to the diaphragm. **C:** Large simple liver cyst. Note the prominence of the distal acoustic enhancement. **D:** Three simple cysts in the right lobe of the liver.

septations are not uncommonly seen and should not be cause for concern. Simple hepatic cysts may be primary or secondary. Primary liver cysts are congenital and arise from developmental defects in the formation of bile ducts.[3] They are relatively uncommon, tend to be superficial and are lined with cuboidal epithelium. They usually do not cause liver enlargement and are rarely palpable. The right lobe of the liver is affected more often than the left (Fig. 1). The incidence is said to be one in 600 at laparotomy.[4] Occasionally simple cysts may present with pain, as a right upper quadrant mass or with symptoms secondary to haemorrhage or infection (Fig. 2).[5] The average cyst size is 3 cm.

Acquired cysts are usually secondary to trauma, inflammation or parasitic infection and are essentially indistinguishable from primary cysts on ultrasound. The

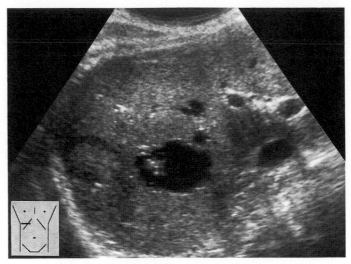

Fig. 3 **Liver cyst and metastasis**. Transverse scan of the right lobe of the liver showing a solid metastasis and adjacent to this a cystic metastasis which may be mistaken for a simple liver cyst. The irregularity of its wall should arouse suspicion.

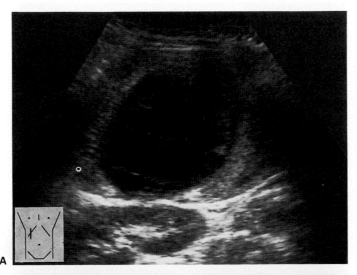

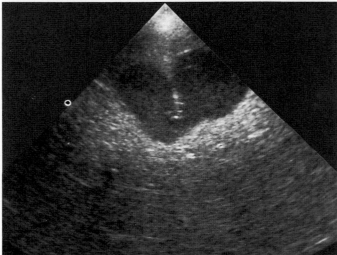

Fig. 2 **Liver cyst. A:** A large simple cyst in the right lobe of the liver showing stranding due to haemorrhage. **B:** Placement of a needle for diagnostic aspiration of a simple cyst into which haemorrhage has occurred.

diagnostic accuracy of ultrasound in the diagnosis of simple liver cysts approaches 100%. The differential diagnosis will include a necrotic metastasis, hydatid cyst, hepatic cyst-adenocarcinoma, haematoma or abscess (Fig. 3). If there is any concern about the diagnosis or the patient is symptomatic, guided percutaneous aspiration may be performed with cytological analysis.[5] In common with cysts in other organs most simple cysts recur following aspiration.[6] Occasionally, an intrahepatic gall bladder may simulate a solitary intrahepatic cyst.[7] Biliary cystadenoma is usually quite distinctive with multiple septations and papillary projections. The choledochal cyst with its continuation with the extrahepatic biliary tree is also usually quite characteristic (see Chs 13 and 26).[8] Occasionally, a choledochal cyst may be rather localised and intrahepatic in site causing diagnostic confusion (Fig. 4).[8] Radioactive excretion studies with Technetium HIDA will establish the correct diagnosis in this instance.

Polycystic liver disease

Multiple cysts in the liver occasionally occur as an isolated phenomenon; however, they are most commonly seen in patients with underlying polycystic disease. The majority of patients with polycystic liver disease have renal cysts (Fig. 5).[9] Polycystic renal disease is a relatively common congenital condition affecting one in 500. It has an autosomal dominant mode of inheritance. Approximately one third of patients with polycystic kidney disease are found to have liver cysts.[3,4] Polycystic liver disease is more likely to be symptomatic than single cysts, the most common presentation being with hepatomegaly. As with single cysts, haemorrhage or infection in any of the cysts may cause

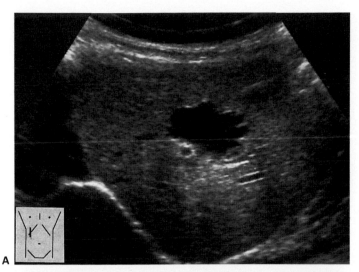

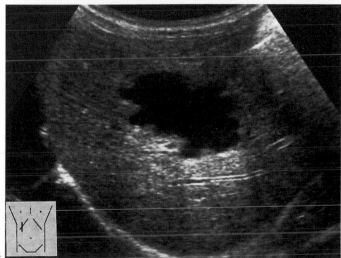

Fig. 4 Cyst with irregular margins. A and **B:** Longitudinal scans taken in an infant at 1 and at 4 months of age. They show a unilocular cyst with a crenated margin within the right lobe of the liver. This lies centrally and has enlarged during the period of observation. The lobulated margin raises the possibility of a biliary origin.

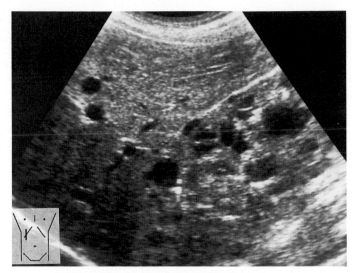

Fig. 5 Polycystic disease. Longitudinal scan showing the enlarged right kidney of a patient with adult polycystic renal disease with small cysts. Two or three small cysts are also noted in the liver.

pain. The presence of multiple cysts in the liver may distort the normal liver architecture considerably. Acoustic enhancement beyond each cyst may produce the impression of an abnormal liver pattern in addition to the cysts (Fig. 6). A similar appearance may also be seen with marked intrahepatic biliary duct dilatation and in Caroli's disease.

Echinococcal cyst (hydatid disease)

The liver is the organ most frequently involved by hydatid disease where more than half the cysts are found.[10] Other sites of involvement in decreasing order of frequency include the lungs, the bones, the brain and the peritoneal cavity.[3] The parasite is endemic in certain areas, particu-

larly where sheep and cattle grazing are common. The Middle East has a high incidence. The eggs of the worm (*Echinococcus granulosus*) are excreted in the faeces of infected dogs. Cattle, sheep, goats and humans serve as the intermediate host. The eggs hatch in the upper intestine and the embryos permeate the intestinal mucosa to enter the blood stream. The larvae lodge in an organ and cause an inflammatory reaction. Some larvae encyst and slowly grow at up to 1 cm per year. Enclosing the fluid within the cyst is an inner nucleated germinal layer which gives rise to the brood capsules and an outer opaque non-nucleated layer. The outer layer is quite distinctive with numerous delicate laminations like tissue paper. Outside this is an inflammatory reaction. Daughter cysts may develop from the inner germinal layer.

A variety of ultrasound appearances may be demonstrated by hydatid cysts.[11]

Solitary cyst A single cyst may vary in size from 1 to 20 cm and may be quite indistinguishable from a simple congenital liver cyst. In endemic regions, all liver cysts are considered to be hydatid until proven otherwise (Fig. 7). The distinction between simple and hydatid cysts may be aided by noting the following features:

a) wall calcification may occur many years after the initial infection. Simple liver cysts rarely, if ever, calcify. The presence of a complete rind of calcification suggests an inactive lesion (Fig. 8);[12]

b) debris consisting of sand or scolices may be present within hydatid cysts. This can be accentuated by moving the patient during the examination;[13]

c) it may be possible to discern the two layers of the wall of a hydatid cyst.

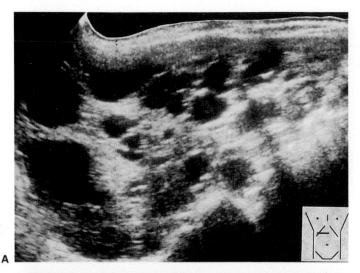

A

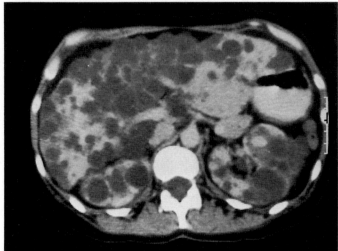

B

Fig. 6 Polycystic disease. Transverse ultrasound scan with a corresponding CT slice in a patient with marked polycystic liver disease associated with adult polycystic kidneys. Note that in the ultrasound scan the distortion of the parenchyma by the multiple cysts and the irregular distal enhancement beyond them produces a very abnormal liver textural pattern.

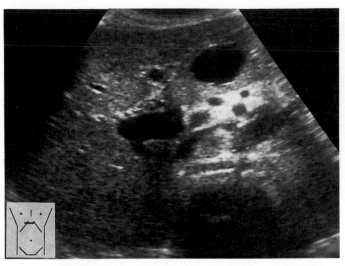

Fig. 7 Hydatid disease – simple type. Transverse scan through the liver showing a single simple cyst in the left lobe in a patient from the Middle East. A complement fixation test suggested the presence of hydatid disease.

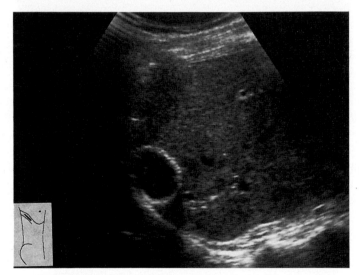

Fig. 8 Calcified hydatid. Oblique scan through the right lobe of the liver showing a single calcified hydatid cyst.

Separation of the membrane Separation of the membrane producing an 'ultrasound water lily sign' results from detachment and collapse of the inner germinal layer from the exocyst. This produces a pathognomonic appearance for hydatid disease. The collapsed germinal layer is seen as an undulating linear collection of echoes either floating in the cyst or lying in the most dependent portion (Fig. 9).[14]

Daughter cysts The development of daughter cysts from the lining germinal membrane produces a characteristic appearance of cysts enclosed within a cyst. This appearance is extremely characteristic, producing what

may be described as a cartwheel or honeycomb cyst (Fig. 10).[15]

Multiple cysts With heavy or continued infestation multiple primary parent cysts may develop within the liver. This will often produce hepatomegaly. Normal liver tissue is demonstrated between the individual cysts. In the absence of membrane separation or daughter cyst formation the diagnosis of hydatid disease may be difficult. The differential diagnosis should include necrotic hepatic metastases, chronic haematomas, abscess, simple cysts, polycystic disease and bile duct cysts.[10] Uncomplicated

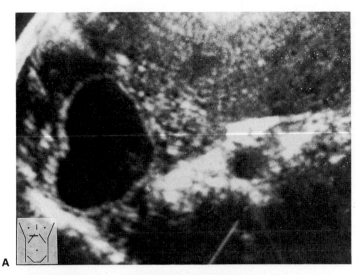

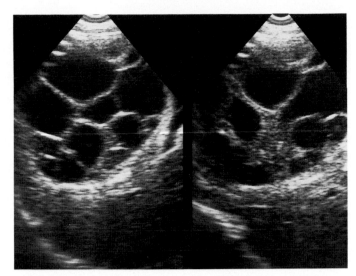

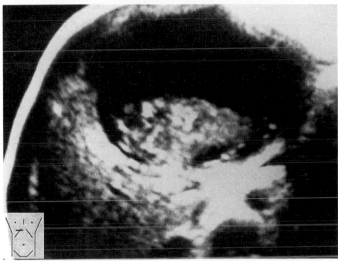

Fig. 9   Hydatid cysts. A: Transverse scan of the liver showing an hydatid cyst appearing as a flattened sphere. Note the early detachment of the capsule laterally. **B:** Hydatid cyst in which the membranes have become completely detached producing the 'floating membranes sign'. (Figure courtesy of Professor Sawat Hussein, Karachi).

percutaneous aspiration of hydatid cysts has been reported.[16] Anaphylaxis is a well-recorded risk of fluid leakage and skin tests or complement fixation tests should be performed if there is a suspicion of the diagnosis of hydatid disease.[5] When hydatid cysts become secondarily infected a different pattern may be seen with filling of the cyst with echoes (Fig. 11). The membrane may separate, producing a bizarre appearance. As cysts grow they may compress vascular structures or the biliary tree. In practice, significant biliary obstruction may mean that there is communication of the cyst with the biliary tree.[17] Cysts arising in the upper portion of the liver may communicate with the bronchi by a trans-diaphragmatic pathway.

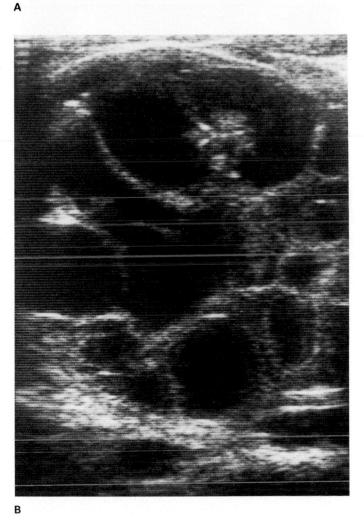

Fig. 10   Classical hydatid cysts. A: and **B:** Examples of the pathognomonic appearance of hydatid cysts in which daughter cysts have developed from the lining germinal membrane producing the characteristic cartwheel or honeycomb pattern. (Figure courtesy of Professor Sawat Hussein, Karachi.)

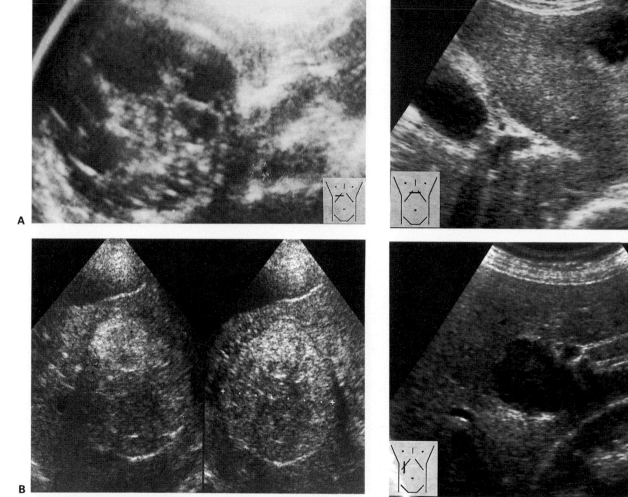

Fig. 11   Complicated hydatid cysts. A: Transverse scan showing an infected hydatid cyst. Many of the daughter cysts are filled with debris and the margins of the cyst have become rather indistinct. **B:** Infected hydatid cyst where the whole cyst has become more highly reflective than adjacent liver and the increased reflectivity within the cyst has almost totally obscured the margins of the daughter cysts. (Figure courtesy of Professor Sawat Hussein, Karachi.)

Fig. 12   Pyogenic abscess. A: Typical small pyogenic abscess in the left lobe of the liver. The wall is slightly thickened and irregular. A few low level echoes are present within the abscess cavity and acoustic enhancement is noted beyond the abscess. **B:** A more clearly defined abscess in the right lobe of the liver but showing similar features with a little debris within the abscess and distal enhancement beyond. In this patient a second lesion is just visible adjacent to the hemidiaphragm. Multiplicity of pyogenic abscesses is common and should be excluded by a systematic search.

Abscess

Pyogenic abscess Intrahepatic abscesses most frequently arise as a complication of an intra-abdominal infection with direct portal venous spread to the liver.[18,19] Common aetiological sites of infection include the biliary tract, colonic diverticulitis and appendiceal abscess. Abscesses may also result from prior abdominal surgery, trauma, neoplasm or bacteraemia in an immuno-compromised patient. Frequently, the source of infection is not found. The agent is most commonly *Escherichia coli*, but anaerobic bacteria such as *Clostridia* and *Bacteroides* are also

found.[20] Rapid diagnosis and prompt appropriate treatment are important since the morbidity and mortality from untreated abscess is high.[21,22] The clinical presentation may be variable but fever, pain, pleurisy, nausea and vomiting are all common. There is usually a leukocytosis with abnormal liver function tests and anaemia. Ultrasound will typically show a spherical, oval or slightly irregular echopoor lesion with distal enhancement (Fig. 12). This is a pattern present in three quarters of cases.[23] Great variability is, however, common and will to a large extent depend upon both the age of the abscess and the causative organism. In the genesis of an abscess inflammatory destruction of liver parenchyma is followed by pyogenic exudation within the cavity formed. The reflectivity of the contents and the marginal definition will change in a dynamic way with time (Fig. 13). A significant number of abscesses can be higher in reflectivity than adjacent normal liver. This may be related to air or microbubbles within the fluid or to a mixture of differing content producing strong acoustic interfaces.[24,25] Larger amounts of gas within an abscess will produce the typical ultrasound appearances associated with parenchymal gas.[26,27] In a chronic abscess a wall of variable thickness may be present. The differential diagnosis of an abscess includes complicated hepatic cysts and necrotic tu-

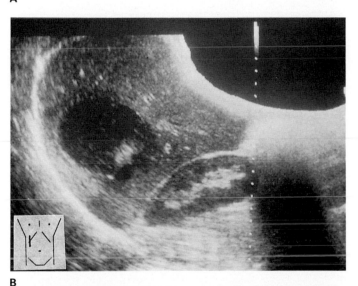

A

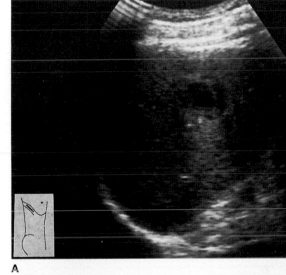

A

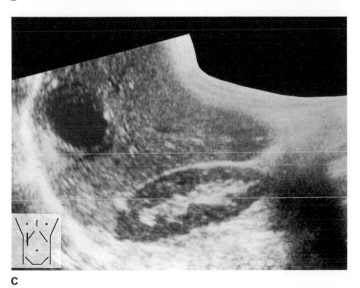

C

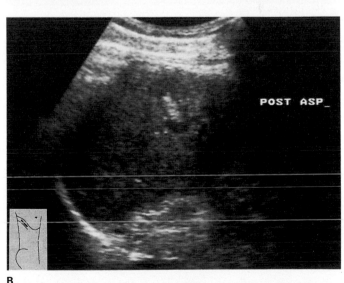

POST ASP

B

Fig. 13 Abscess – serial studies. Longitudinal scans through the right lobe of the liver taken at monthly intervals showing the change in size and appearance of an abscess on treatment.

Fig. 14 Abscess – pre- and post-aspiration. A: Oblique scan through the right lobe of the liver showing a small echo-poor focal lesion with distal enhancement, suspicious of an abscess. **B:** Post-aspiration appearances after 20 ml of thick pus had been removed.

mours. A diagnostic fine needle aspiration is invaluable and should be readily performed (Fig. 14) (see Ch. 6).

Amoebic abscess *Entamoeba histolytica* primarily infects the colon. The disease is contracted by ingesting the cysts in contaminated food and water. The walls of the cysts dissolve in the alkaline contents of the small bowel and the trophozoites emerge to colonise and ulcerate the colon. The right half of the colon is most commonly involved.[20] Patients may be asymptomatic. Invasion of the colonic mucosa allows the amoebae to be carried in the portal venous system to the liver. Hepatic abscess formation occurs in 25% of patients infected and is the most common non-enteric complication.[28] An amoebic abscess may be indistinguishable from a pyogenic abscess. Characteristically there is:

a) lack of a significant wall echo so that they appear to be punched out lesions;
b) symmetrical oval or round configuration;
c) lower reflectivity than liver with a rather homogeneous pattern of internal echoes;
d) distal acoustic enhancement;
e) subcapsular location (Fig. 15).[28–32]

When the infection has been established there is liquefaction necrosis of the hepatocytes with little leukocytic response or fibrotic reaction, producing the classical 'anchovy sauce' contents. Pathologically, the walls of this abscess have a shaggy fibrin lining surrounded by scant fibrovascular response. Aspiration is rarely indicated as the diagnosis can be confirmed by haemoglutination titres and

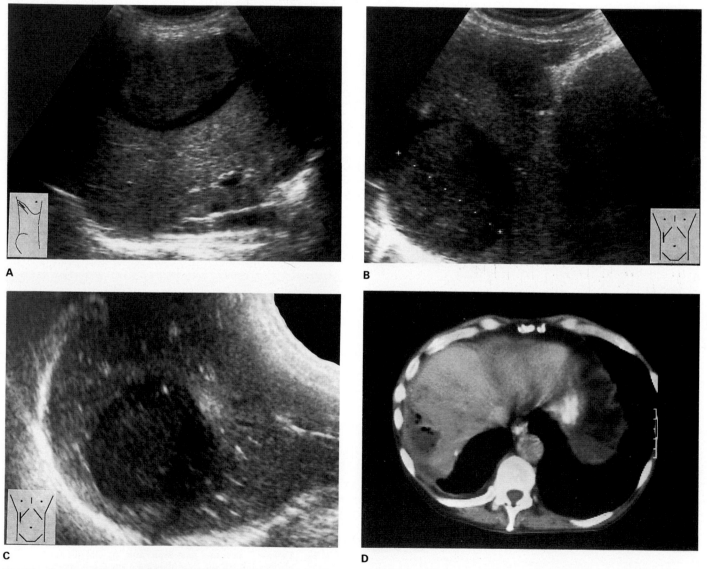

A   **B**   **C**   **D**

Fig. 15 Amoebic abscess. A and **B:** Large amoebic abscesses showing typical features of lack of a significant wall echo, an oval configuration, low, uniform reflectivity of internal echoes and distal acoustic enhancement. Both abscesses also show a typical peripheral location. **C:** Ultrasound and **D:** CT images of an amoebic abscess in which there is a small amount of gas present, shown by high reflectivity on ultrasound and low density on CT.

response to metronidazole therapy. Serial follow up after therapy shows a decrease in the size of the lesion and a decrease in its reflectivity. At this stage the lesion has the characteristics of fluid on ultrasound but in fact the contents are semi-solid and cannot easily be aspirated. Complete resolution can be expected eventually although this may take as long as 2 years.[33] Occasionally a cystic focal area may persist indistinguishable from a simple liver cyst.

Candidiasis Hepatic candidiasis is uncommon and usually follows haematogenous spread of infection to the liver in an immunologically compromised patient. The typical ultrasound appearances are of a target lesion with a small highly reflective centre and a poorly reflective halo. This outer halo is often a little irregular and lobular in outline (Fig. 16). Multiple lesions are characteristic. The outer rim is assumed to be necrotic and inflammatory debris and the central reflectivity either fungal mycelia or the collagen vascular bundle. Lymphoma and leukaemia are the important differential diagnoses, although target lesions are unusual in these conditions.[34,35] Fine needle aspiration is necessary for definitive diagnosis.

Cavernous haemangioma Benign hepatic neoplasms are rare with the exception of the cavernous haemangioma. This is the most common benign tumour of the liver and is reported in up to 7% of patients at autopsy.[36] The tumour is composed of a network of vascular endothelial lined spaces filled with blood. The majority are entirely asymptomatic and require no treatment.[37,38] Their importance lies in positive differentiation from lesions that do require therapy or may change patient management.

The spectrum of appearances on ultrasound is variable. However, the majority have a very distinctive pattern. This is of a sharply defined, highly reflective round tumour usu-

ally less than 2 cm in diameter and with a homogeneous echo pattern. Lesions may be single or multiple.[36,37,39,40] The high reflectivity is most likely due to the multiple interfaces between the vascular spaces. Lesions may occur anywhere within the liver but are more common in the right lobe. There is a tendency towards a peripheral location. Those occurring centrally usually lie close to the main hepatic veins (Fig. 17).[41]

Larger tumours may develop a lobular margin (Fig. 18). Haemangiomas larger than 2.5 cm in diameter are reported to show posterior acoustic enhancement (Fig. 19). This is an unusual feature although not unique in highly reflective masses and probably relates to the vascularity.[42] As the haemangioma undergoes degeneration and fibrous replacement the reflectivity becomes more heterogeneous. This is

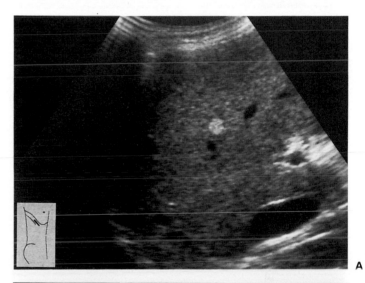

A

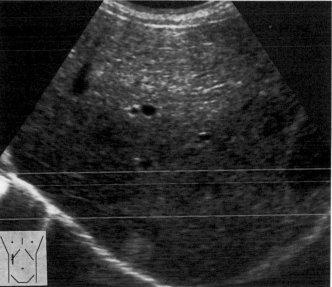

B

Fig. 17 Haemangiomas. A: Typical example of a tiny highly reflective cavernous haemangioma. **B:** Haemangioma of slightly lower reflectivity; detail and contrast resolution are reduced because the lesion lies beyond the focal zone.

Fig. 16 Fungal abscess. Transverse scan through the liver in a patient with disseminated candidiasis. The lesions show the typical pattern of multiple slightly echo-poor lesions with a reflective nidus.

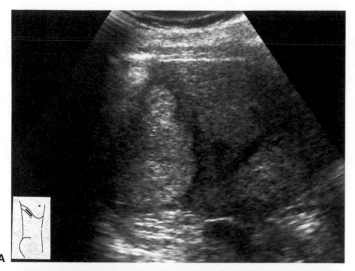

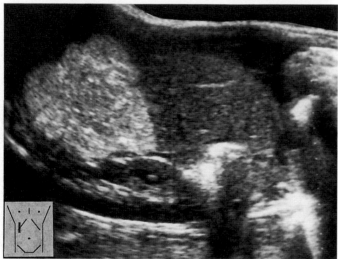

Fig. 18 Large haemangioma. A: Large lesion of high reflectivity with a lobular margin. **B:** Large lesions may be confusing and need either additional imaging or histology for full evaluation.

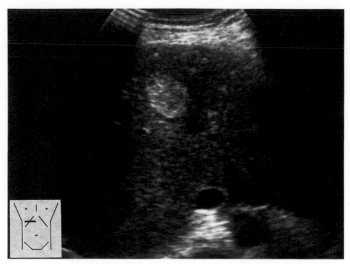

Fig. 19 Haemangioma with enhancement. Typical 3 cm haemangioma showing the unusual finding of slight distal accentuation.

more frequently seen with larger lesions. Atypical appearances make distinction from other focal hepatic lesions difficult or impossible.

In asymptomatic patients with no known history of malignancy it is safe to consider these classical appearances as diagnostic of haemangioma. Where there is an unusual ultrasound appearance or clinical concern a dynamic CT should be done. A characteristic enhancement pattern is then typically shown (Fig. 20). Lesions smaller than 1 to 1.5 cm in diameter may be difficult to evaluate accurately with dynamic CT. However, these small haemangiomas are usually extremely typical on ultrasound.[43] Magnetic resonance imaging (MRI) has been reported to be more sensitive than dynamic CT or ultrasound for detection of haemangiomas.[44] If this is not available and any doubt persists, biopsy of these lesions can safely be performed with

a fine needle particularly if a long liver path is chosen (see Ch. 6).[45]

A rare but interesting group of haemangiomatous tumours is seen in the liver during infancy.[46] Again, often multiple, massive shunting can occur resulting in their occasional presentation with cardiac failure. There is hepatomegaly and there may be associated cutaneous haemangiomas. Although well-defined, these do not generally have the appearance of adult haemangiomas on ultrasound but rather have a non-homogeneous, irregular appearance with mixed reflectivity. In addition, large draining veins may be seen and there may be some enlargement of the proximal abdominal aorta due to shunting through the hepatic artery. Serial ultrasound scans are useful since the natural history of these lesions is to decrease in size over 6 months until they are no longer visible (Fig. 21).

Focal nodular hyperplasia Focal nodular hyperplasia is a rare benign tumour of the liver often discovered by chance. Typically, it is discovered in women of 20 to 40 years of age but occurs in both sexes and in all age groups.[47] Most patients are asymptomatic but up to a third may have pain or hepatomegaly. Focal nodular hyperplasia is generally a solid lesion in a subcapsular location. It is well-circumscribed but non-encapsulated. The mass is composed of normal hepatocytes, Kupffer cells, bile duct elements and fibrous connective tissue. Multiple nodules are separated by bands of fibrous tissue often radiating from a central stellate scar or a linear fibrous scar.[48] The ultrasound features are variable. The lesions are usually homogeneous with a slightly differing reflectivity to the normal liver which may be higher or lower (Fig. 22). An echo complex corresponding to the central fibrous scar, although classical, is infrequently demonstrated.[49] Because the lesions contain Kupffer cells they may concentrate

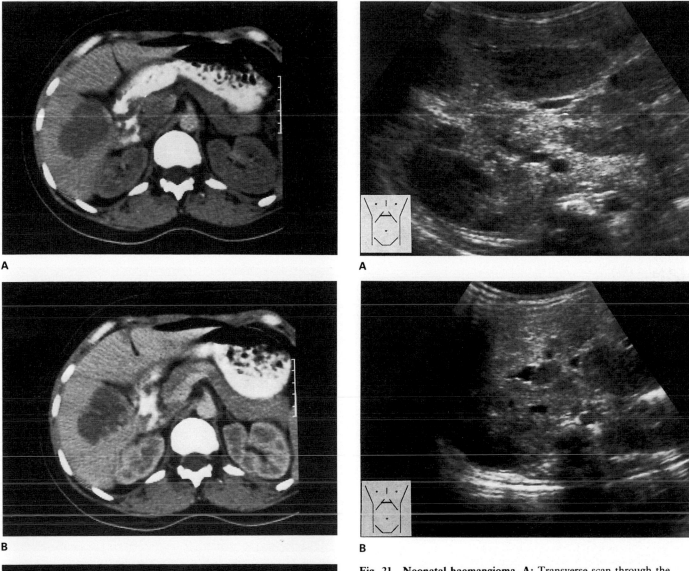

A

B

C

Fig. 20 Haemangioma – dynamic CT scan. A, B and **C**: Part of a dynamic CT scan following contrast, showing the typical filling-in of the lesion during the course of the examination. Delayed slices over several minutes may be required to demonstrate the infilling.

A

B

Fig. 21 Neonatal haemangioma. A: Transverse scan through the liver of a neonate who had a congenital cardiac anomaly and multiple visible haemangiomas on the skin. The patient was developing heart failure. The liver is full of large relatively well-defined echo-poor focal lesions. Arteriography of the liver at the time of cardiac catheterisation confirmed that these were haemangiomas. **B:** Follow up scan 3 months later, although done at different magnification, shows a dramatic spontaneous reduction in size of the focal liver lesions; this is a typical finding in multiple haemangiomatous tumours of the liver in infancy.

radio-colloids. This combination of a lesion larger than 2 cm diameter on ultrasound (or CT) without a cold area on the isotope scan is almost diagnostic of focal nodular hyperplasia.[48,50]

Liver cell adenoma Liver cell adenoma consists of normal or slightly atypical hepatocytes containing areas of bile stasis and focal haemorrhage or necrosis but, unlike focal nodular hyperplasia, not containing bile ducts or Kupffer cells.[50] They are usually manifest as smooth solitary masses that are well-marginated and completely or

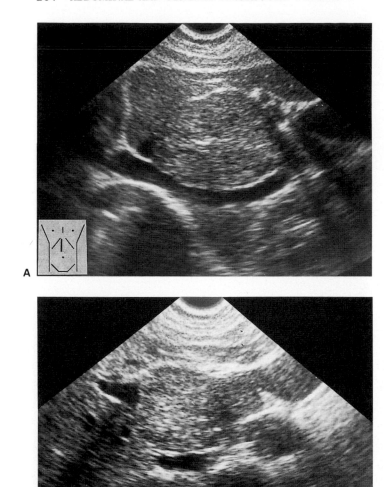

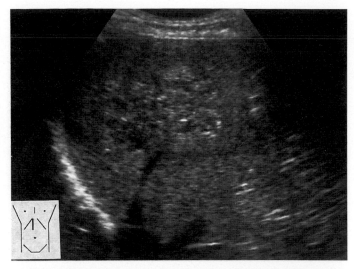

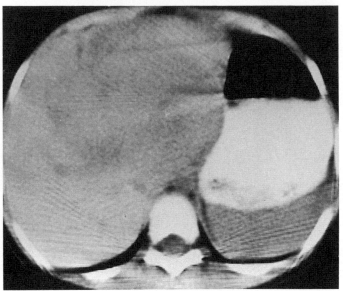

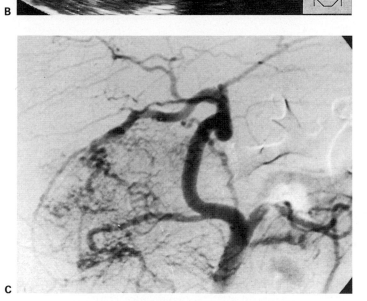

Fig. 23 Adenoma. A: Ultrasound and **B:** CT images showing a large rather poorly defined focal mass in the left lobe of the liver. Obvious necrotic clefts are shown on the ultrasound scan. Both ultrasound and CT suggested this was a malignant tumour but at biopsy it turned out to be a liver cell adenoma.

Fig. 22 Focal nodular hyperplasia. A: Longitudinal and **B:** transverse scans of the liver showing a well-defined focal lesion expanding the caudate lobe of the liver. Its texture is little different from adjacent liver tissue. **C:** Selective arteriogram showing a uniform vascularity of this lesion which, at biopsy, was proven to be focal nodular hyperplasia.

partially encapsulated. There is a close association with the use of oral contraceptives and it is much commoner in women.[20,51,52] Up to 60% of patients with hepatic adenoma have areas of haemorrhage and necrosis compared with 6% in focal nodular hyperplasia (Fig. 23). The mass is usually symptomatic with presentations including a palpable mass, right upper quadrant pain and haemorrhage. This may be into the tumour or from rupture into the peritoneum. There are no definitive ultrasound features that distinguish hepatic adenoma from focal nodular hyperplasia.[50] The clinical presentation should be helpful. Distinction is important as focal nodular hyperplasia may be followed conservatively whilst surgery is the treatment of choice for hepatic adenoma. Hepatic adenomas may regress following cessation of the contraceptive pill.

The precise ultrasound pattern is very variable depending on the amount of bleeding that has occurred and the timing of the scan in relation to the episode of bleeding.

Hepatic adenomas also occur in association with glycogen storage disease where there is an 8% incidence (see Ch. 27). In type I disease the incidence is reportedly as high as 40%.[53,54] In Von Geirke's disease the overall liver texture is abnormal with an increase in size and reflectivity due to fatty and glycogen infiltration. Against this background adenomas stand out with a variable appearance ranging from low to high reflectivity.

Lipomas and focal fatty change   Lipomas are rare primary benign tumours arising from mesenchymal elements. They are non-encapsulated and in continuity with the normal liver parenchyma. They show the typical high reflectivity of fatty tumours (Fig. 24).[55]

Fatty infiltration of the liver is a common occurrence resulting from increased deposition of triglyceride in hepatocytes. This arises from a variety of nutritional disturbances or toxic insults to the liver.[56,57] These include obesity, nutritional deficiencies, diabetes mellitus, pregnancy, steroids, hepatotoxic drugs and alcoholism.[58] The development of fatty infiltration is a dynamic process and changes may be seen within a few weeks of an insult and may regress within days.[57,59] Most characteristically, the fatty involvement is uniform or geographic in distribution. However, occasionally it may be nodular or multifocal when it can be indistinguishable from other focal hepatic lesions.[60] Features suggesting the true nature of the process are sharp angular boundaries to the lesions and no evidence of displacement or effacement of venous structures (Fig. 25).

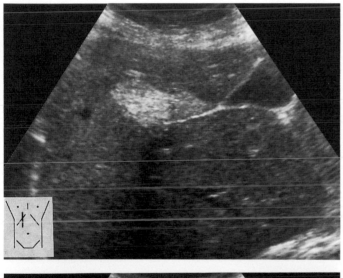

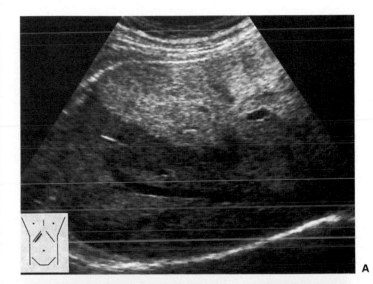

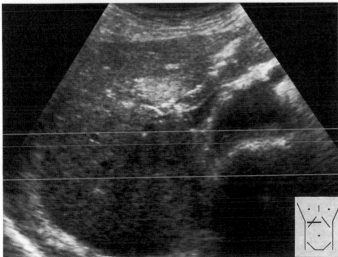

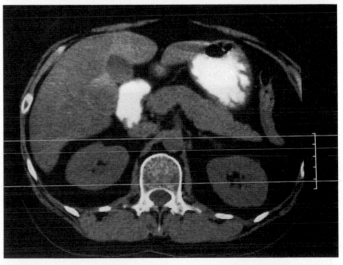

Fig. 24   Fatty lesion. A and **B:** A fairly well-defined reflective focal lesion lying just above the hepatic interlobar fissure. Guided biopsy of this lesion revealed fatty tissue; the differential diagnosis is between focal fatty change and lipoma.

Fig. 25   Focal fatty change. A: Transverse scan through the right lobe of the liver showing the typical geographic distribution of focal fatty infiltration, in this example most marked anteriorly with sparing posteriorly. There is no disturbance of the normal vascular architecture. **B:** CT scan in another case showing similar features.

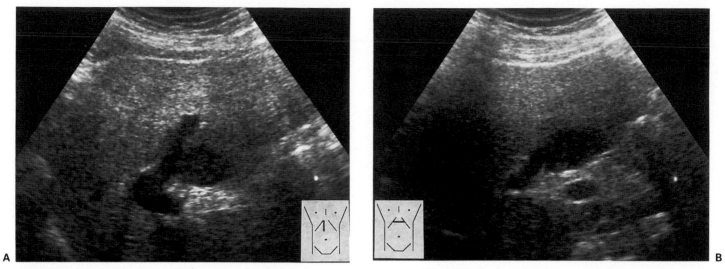

Fig. 26 Focal fatty sparing. A and **B:** The typical oval area of focal sparing from a more generalised fatty infiltration of the liver is shown.

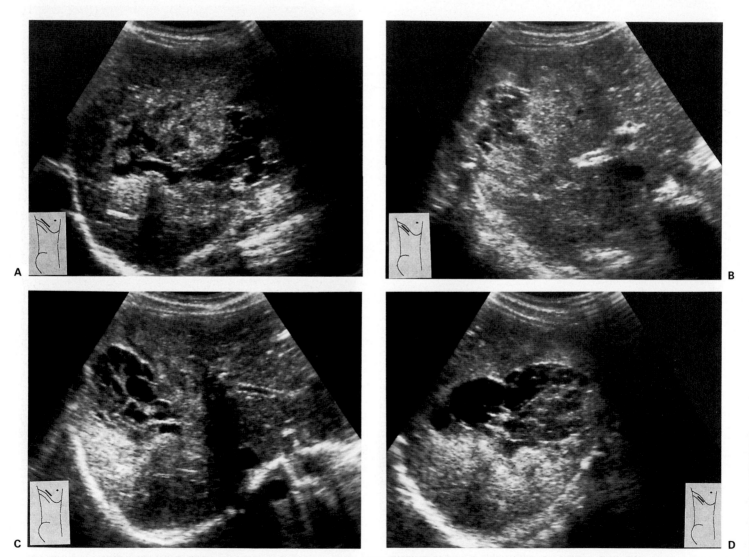

Fig. 27 Liver trauma. A and **B:** Oblique intercostal liver images of a child who suffered liver trauma following a fall from a horse. Note the irregular patchy high reflectivity involving much of the right lobe of the liver. **C** and **D:** Follow up scans 4 days later showing some decrease in reflectivity corresponding to liquefaction of the clot.

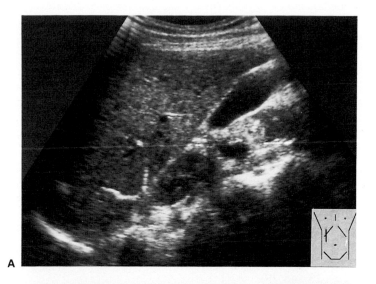

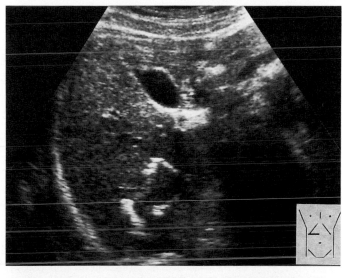

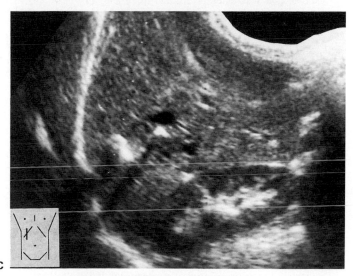

Another well-recognised variant is focal sparing of small areas of normal liver in a more generalised fatty infiltration. The spared area appears as an echo-poor focal mass. A characteristic location for the spared area is the quadrate lobe anterior to the portal vein bifurcation or related to the gallbladder bed.[59-61] The shape of the spared area or pseudomass is typically ovoid. Its location has led to the suggestion that the sparing relates to alteration of blood flow in this area (Fig. 26).[61]

Liver haematoma The aetiology of a liver haematoma may be blunt abdominal trauma or rupture of a neoplasm such as a hepatic adenoma or cavernous haemangioma. In children blunt abdominal trauma causing liver trauma is a common problem. This may be attributed to the greater flexibility of the rib cage and the lack of surrounding fat.[62-64]

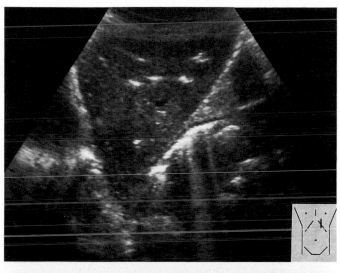

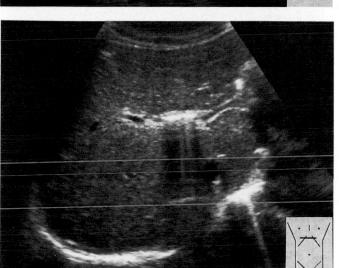

Fig. 28 Calcification in the liver. A: Longitudinal and **B:** oblique scans showing curvilinear calcification, presumably related to previous abscess formation or trauma to the right lobe of the liver.
C: Calcifications with marked acoustic shadowing beyond.

Fig. 29 Pneumobilia. A: Longitudinal and **B:** transverse scans showing small focal areas of high reflectivity with distal shadowing and reverberation artefacts. This is due to gas within the biliary tree and is to be compared with Figure 28.

There are three major categories of liver trauma:

a) rupture of the liver and its capsule. This is the most serious injury. The patient may be too ill for any imaging to be undertaken. This type of injury will usually be most fully demonstrated with CT;

b) subcapsular haematoma;

c) central haematoma. In the acute situation a central haematoma tends to be highly reflective due to fibrin and erythrocytes forming multiple acoustic interfaces. With time the clot undergoes liquefaction which corresponds with decreasing reflectivity and an apparent increase in the size of the haematoma (Fig. 27). This increase in size is due to fluid absorption into the lesion as a result of increased osmotic pressure secondary to blood breakdown in the devitalised tissues. Over a period of months the haematoma may become cystic and develop internal stranding. This eventually resolves with regeneration of liver tissue, but residual fibrous scar or a small cystic space may persist in the long-term.

Subcapsular haematomas, if small, will go through a similar sequence of changes but if larger they may initially appear to be poorly reflective due to the larger amount of fluid blood present within them.

In addition to evaluating the liver, ultrasound is helpful in evaluating other abdominal viscera and assessing the presence of free blood. Liver rupture will often require surgical intervention but the large majority of patients with liver haematomas require minimal or no surgical intervention. Serial follow up is of value and interest to monitor progressive resolution.

Calcification   Liver calcification is not a disease process but is seen as the end result of a number of infections and infestations including tuberculosis, syphilis and parasitic diseases.[65] Liver abscesses and haematomas may also develop dystrophic calcification in the long-term. In these situations the calcification can be regarded as the 'tomb stones' of the disease in question. As with calcification elsewhere, the appearances are typical with a focus of very high reflectivity and clear cut distal acoustic shadowing (Figs 28 and 29).

Paediatric liver tumours

Benign tumours of the liver in children include haemangioendothelioma, mesenchymal hamartoma, multiple haemangiomas, adenoma, and cystic hepatoblastoma. These will all be discussed in more detail in Chapter 27.

REFERENCES

1 Federle M P, Filly R A, Moss A A. Cystic hepatic neoplasms: complimentary roles of CT and sonography. AJR 1981; 136: 345

2 Brick S H, Hill M C, Lande I M. The mistaken or indeterminate CT diagnosis of hepatic metastases: the value of sonography. AJR 1987; 148: 723

3 O'Brien M J, Gottlieb L S. The liver and biliary tract. In: Robins S L, Cotran R S. eds. Pathologic basis of disease. Philadelphia: W B Saunders. 1979: p 1009

4 Taylor K J W, Viscomi G N. Ultrasound diagnosis of cystic disease of the liver. J Clin Gastroenterol 1980; 2: 197

5 Roemer C E, Ferruci J T Jnr, Mueller P R, et al. Hepatic cysts: diagnosis and therapy by sonographic needle aspiration. AJR 1981; 136: 1065

6 Saini S, Mueller P R, Ferruci J T Jnr, et al. Percutaneous aspiration of hepatic cysts does not provide definitive therapy. AJR 1983; 141: 559

7 Spiegel R M, King D L, Green W M. Ultrasonography of primary cysts of the liver. AJR 1978; 131: 235

8 Austin R M, Sussman S, McArdle C R, et al. Computed tomographic and ultrasound appearances of a solitary intrahepatic choledochal cyst. Clin Radiol 1986; 37: 149

9 Kuni C C, Johnson N L, Holmes J H. Polycystic liver disease. JCU 1978; 6: 332

10 Choliz J D, Olaverri F J L, Casas T F, Zubieta S O. Computed tomography in hepatic echinococcosis. AJR 1982; 139: 699

11 Hadidi A. Ultrasound findings in liver hydatid disease. JCU 1979; 7: 365

12 Itzchuk Y, Rubinstein Z, Shilo R. Ultrasound in tropical diseases. In Sanders R C, Hill M C. eds. Ultrasound Annual. New York: Raven Press. 1983: p 69

13 Lewell D B, McCorkell S J. Hepatic echinococcal cysts: sonographic appearance and classification. Radiology 1985; 155: 773

14 Niron E A, Ozer H. Ultrasound appearances of liver hydatid disease. Br J Radiol 1981; 54: 335

15 Babcock D S, Kaufman L, Cosnow I. Ultrasound diagnosis of hydatid disease (echinococcosis) in two cases. AJR 1978; 131: 895

16 Mueller P R, Dawson S L, Ferucci J T Jnr, Nardi G L. Hepatic echinococcal cyst: successful percutaneous drainage. Radiology 1985; 155: 627

17 Gharbi H A, Hassine W, Brauner M W, Dupuch K. Ultrasound examination of the hydatic liver. Radiology 1981; 139: 459

18 Kuligowska E, Connors S K, Shapiro J H. Liver abscess: sonography in diagnosis and treatment. AJR 1982; 138: 253

19 Silver S, Weinstein A, Cooperman A. Changes in the pathogenesis and detection of intrahepatic abscess. Am J Surg 1979; 137: 608

20 Wright R, Milward-Sadler G H, Alberti K G M M, Karran S. In: Liver and biliary disease, 2nd edition. Eastbourne: Balliere Tindall. 1985: p 1077

21 Freeny P C. Acute pyogenic hepatitis: sonographic and angiographic findings. AJR 1980; 135: 388

22 Kuligowska E, Noble J. Sonography of hepatic abscess. In: Raymond H W, Zwiebel W J. eds. Seminars in ultrasound, vol 4: 2. New York: Grunne and Stratton. 1983: p 102

23 Terrier F, Becker C D, Triller J K. Morphologic aspects of hepatic abscesses at computed tomography and ultrasound. Acta Radiol Diag 1983; 24: 129

24 Subramanyan B R, Balthazer E J, Raghavendra B N, et al. Ultrasound analysis of solid appearing abscesses. Radiology 1983; 146: 487

25 Powers T A, Jones T B, Carl J H. Echogenic hepatic abscess without radiographic evidence of gas. AJR 1981; 137: 159

26 Jones M, Kovak A, Geshner J. Acoustic shadowing by gas producing abscesses. South Med J 1981; 74: 247

27 Burt T B, Knochel J Q, Lee T G. Gas as a contrast agent and diagnostic aid in abdominal sonography. J Ultrasound Med 1; 1982: 179

28 Ralls P W, Colletti P M, Quinn M F, Halls J. Sonographic findings in hepatic amoebic abscess. Radiology 1982; 145: 123

29 Boultbee J E, Simjee A E, Rooknoodeen F, Engelbrecht H E. Experiences with grey scale ultrasonography in hepatic amoebiasis. Clin Radiol 1979; 30: 683

30 Dalrymple R B, Fataar S, Goodman A, et al. Hyperechoic amoebic

liver abscess: an unusual ultrasonic appearance. Clin Radiol 1982; 33: 541

31 Sukov R J, Cohen L J, Sample W F. Sonography of hepatic amoebic abscess. AJR 1980; 134: 911

32 Abul-Khair M H, Kenawi M M, Korasky E E, Arafa N M. Ultrasonography and amoebic liver abscesses. Ann Surg 1981; 193: 221

33 Ralls P W, Quinn M F, Boswell W D Jnr, Colletti P M, et al. Patterns of resolution in successfully treated hepatic amoebic abscess: sonographic evaluation. Radiology 1983; 149: 541

34 Ho B, Cooperberg P L, Li D K B, et al. Ultrasonography and computed tomography of hepatic candidiasis in immunosuppressed patients. J Ultrasound Med 1982; 1: 157

35 Miller J H, Greenfield L D, Wald B R. Candidiasis of the liver and spleen in childhood. Radiology 1982; 142: 375

36 Onodera H, Ohta K, Oikawa M, et al. Correlation of the real time sonographic appearance of hepatic haemangiomas with angiography. JCU 1983; 11: 421

37 Wiener S N, Paruleker S G. Scintigraphy and ultrasonography of hepatic haemangioma. Radiology 1979; 132: 149

38 Park W C, Phillips R. The role of radiation therapy in the management of haemangiomas of the liver. JAMA 1970; 212: 1496

39 Mirk P, Rubaltelli L, Bazzocchi M, et al. Ultrasonographic patterns in hepatic haemangiomas. JCU 1982; 10: 373

40 Freeny P C, Vimont T R, Barnett D C. Cavernous transformation of the liver: ultrasonography, arteriography and computed tomography. Radiology 1979; 132: 143

41 Bruneton J N, Drouillard J, Fenart D, et al. Ultrasonography of hepatic cavernous haemangioma. Br J Radiol 1983; 56: 791

42 Taboury J, Porcel A, Tubiana J-M, Monnier J-P. Cavernous haemangiomas of the liver studied by ultrasound. Radiology 1983; 149: 781

43 Itai Y, Ohtomo K, Araki T, et al. Computed tomography and sonography of cavernous hemangiomas of the liver. AJR 1983; 141: 315

44 Glazer G M, Aisen A M, Francis I R, et al. Hepatic cavernous haemangioma: magnetic resonance imaging. Radiology 1985; 155: 417

45 Solbiati L, Livraghi T, De Pra L, et al. Fine needle biopsy of hepatic hemangioma with sonographic guidance. AJR 1985; 144: 471

46 Stanley P, Gates G F, Eto R, Miller S W. Hepatic cavernous hemangiomas and hemangioendotheliomas in infancy. AJR 1977; 129: 317

47 Scatarige J C, Fishman E K, Sanders R C. The sonographic 'star sign' in focal nodular hyperplasia of the liver. J Ultrasound Med 1982; 1: 275

48 Rogers J V, Mack L A, Freeny P C, et al. Hepatic focal nodular hyperplasia: angiography, CT, sonography and scintigraphy. AJR 1981; 137: 983

49 Welch T J, Sheedy P F, Johnson C M, et al. Focal nodular hyperplasia and hepatic adenoma: comparison of angiography, CT, ultrasound and scintigraphy. Radiology 1985; 156: 593

50 Sandler M A, Petrocelli R D, Marks D S, Lopez R. Ultrasonic features and radionuclide correlation in liver cell adenoma and focal nodular hyperplasia. Radiology 1980; 135: 393

51 Klatstein G. Hepatic tumours: possible relationship to use of oral contraceptives. Gastroenterology 1977; 73: 386

52 Quinn S K, Hanks J, Shaffer H. Sonographic diagnosis of a liver cell adenoma. South Med J 1986; 79: 372

53 Bowerman R A, Samuels B I, Silver T N. Ultrasonographic features of hepatic adenomas in type I glycogen storage disease. J Ultrasound Med 1983; 2: 51

54 Brunelle F, Tammam S, Odievre M, Chaumont P. Liver adenomas in glycogen storage disease in children. Ultrasound and angiographic studies. Pediatr Radiology 1984; 14: 94

55 Kurdziel J C, Itines J, Parache R M, Chaulieu C. Adenolipoma of the liver: a unique case with ultrasound and CT pattern. Eur J Radiol 1984; 4: 45

56 Foster K J, Dewbury K, Griffith A, Wright R. The accuracy of ultrasound in the detection of fatty infiltration of the liver. Br J Radiol 1980; 53: 440

57 Quinn S F, Gosink B B. Characteristic sonographic signs of hepatic infiltration. AJR 1985; 145: 753

58 Saverymutto S H, Joseph A E A, Maxwell J D. Ultrasound scanning in the detection of hepatic fibrosis and steatosis. BMJ 1986; 292: 13

59 Bashist B, Hecht H L, Harley W D. Computed tomographic demonstration of rapid changes of fatty infiltration of the liver. Radiology 1982; 142: 691

60 Yates C K, Streight R A. Focal fatty infiltration of the liver simulating metastatic disease. Radiology 1986; 159: 83

61 Kawashima A, Suehiro S, Murayama S, Russell W J. Focal fatty infiltration of the liver mimicking a tumour: sonographic and CT features. J Comput Assist Tomogr 1986; 10: 329

62 Lam A H, Shulman'L. Ultrasonography in the management of liver trauma in children. J Ultrasound Med 1984; 3: 199

63 VanSonnenberg E, Simeone J F, Mueller P R, et al. Sonographic appearance of haematomas in the liver, spleen and kidney: A clinical, pathologic and animal study. Radiology 1983; 147: 507

64 Moon K L Jnr, Federle M P. Computed tomography in hepatic trauma. AJR 1983; 141: 309

65 Weeks L E, McCune B R, Martin J F, O'Brien T F. Differential diagnosis of intrahepatic shadowing on ultrasound examination. JCU 1978; 6: 399

Malignant liver disease

David O. Cosgrove and Luigi Bolondi

General ultrasound features

Ultrasound detects liver tumours, whether primary or secondary, by demonstrating the lesion itself together with changes due to its expanding or invasive nature. As with other applications, the detection of liver lesions depends on a combination of resolution and contrast, so that smaller masses can be detected when there is a marked difference in reflectivity (and sometimes of texture) from the background, while low contrast lesions must be larger to be demonstrable. For such lesions, the masking produced by the random speckled structure of the basic ultrasound image has a serious detrimental effect (see Ch. 2). Liver tumours may be more or less strongly reflective than the liver parenchyma; subjectively strongly reflective lesions seem to be easier to detect at a given contrast ratio, though this has not been subjected to scientific scrutiny.

As tumours expand, they distort the nearby architecture. Recognition of this may provide useful clues in drawing attention to the abnormality. Enlargement of the liver, the most fundamental, is often difficult to detect until gross because of the wide range of normal variations (see Ch. 14), but rounding of the free edge of the liver is sometimes very obvious (Fig. 1) – like other signs of expansion, this is non-specific and can also be produced by many infective and degenerative processes (e.g. granulomata, early cirrhosis or hepatic storage diseases). Care must be taken when there is a Riedel's lobe for these often have a bulbous shape with a rounded margin, even when normal (Fig. 2). Focal mass effects may be seen as local humps on the liver surface (Fig. 3) or as deviations of the normal straight or gently curved course of the liver veins (Fig. 4). As with cirrhotic nodules malignant humps are more obvious when the liver is surrounded by ascites, but if looked for carefully they can often be demonstrated in its absence. Since much of the liver surface lies close to the skin a transducer with good near field resolution is required. The diaphragmatic surface of the liver is often indented by prominent or hypertrophic leaflets of the diaphragmatic muscle; viewed from below, these simulate humps on tomographic views though they are actually ridges of liver tissue protruding between the muscular bands (Fig. 5). Careful observation of their shape in two dimensions should avoid this diagnostic error. In addition as the diaphragm moves with respiration, the position of the 'humps' moves as the diaphragm slides over the liver – observation of the relative movement of the liver and diaphragm may provide additional important clues on the position and nature of both real and apparent abnormalities.

The invasive properties of tumours may be confirmed by the demonstration of vascular involvement (Fig. 6). Both the portal and the hepatic veins may be invaded, often

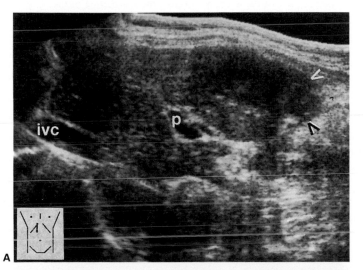

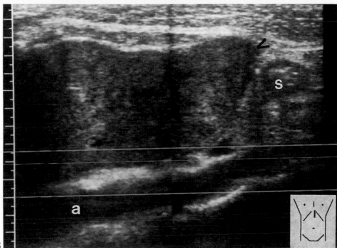

Fig. 1 Rounded free edge of liver. The free margin of the liver is normally sharply angled. Rounding (arrowheads) results from any disease process causing hepatomegaly and thus forms a useful but non-specific indicator of liver pathology. a – aorta, p – portal vein, s – stomach, ivc – inferior vena cava.

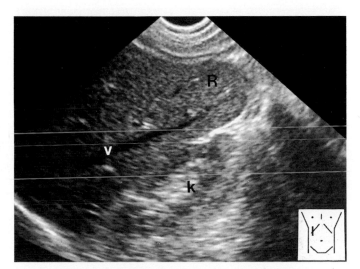

Fig. 2 Riedel's lobe. While the free margin of the liver is normally sharp, in the case of a Riedel's lobe (R) it may be rounded without signifying underlying pathology. k – kidney, v – hepatic vein.

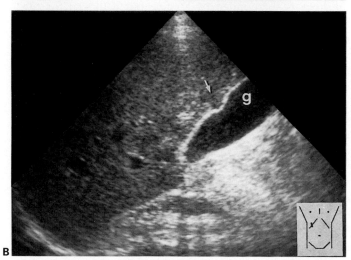

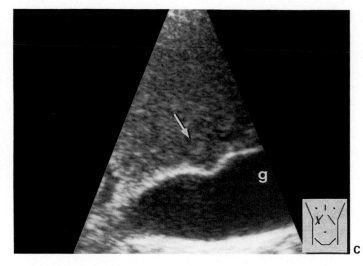

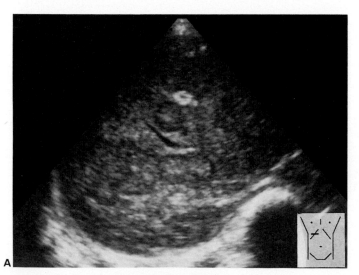

Fig. 3 Surface humps in liver malignancy. Subcapsular masses may cause nodularity of the liver contour. **A:** This is easier to detect when the deeper parts of the liver are affected, the indentation of the adjacent organs indicating their position. k – kidney, p – portal vein. **B** and **C:** Note that the 'hump' (arrow) may be obvious though the echo-contrast is minimal ('isoechoic' lesion). Superficial 'humps' are more difficult to detect because they are obscured by reverberation and lie close to the transducer, where resolution is poor. g – gallbladder.

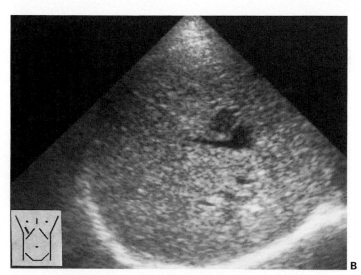

Fig. 4 Deviation of liver veins in malignancy. Masses may distort the normally gently curving paths of nearby blood vessels. In these examples the offending tumours (a 'target' lesion in (A)) are easily seen, but sometimes this feature can draw attention to an otherwise subtle lesion.

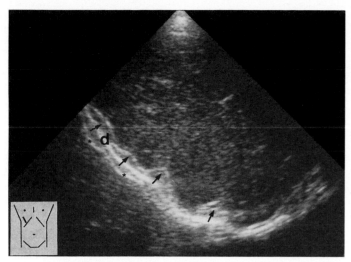

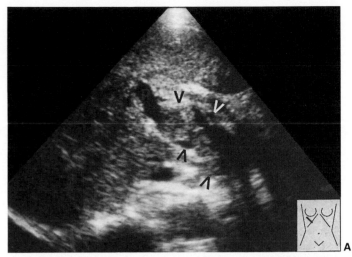

Fig. 5 Diaphragmatic 'humps'. Whereas the liver surface is normally smooth, because the muscle of the diaphragm may form into thickened bundles that indent the surface of the liver, 'nodularity' or 'humps' on this surface do not carry the same implications and should be ignored. This example shows marked indentations (arrowheads) of the upper surface of the liver in a patient with chronic airways obstruction. Note the mirror-image artefact (★) which gives a double outline to the hypertrophied muscular layer of the diaphragm (d) (see Ch. 4).

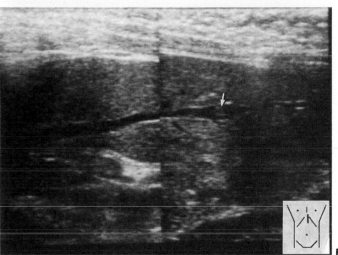

leading to occlusion and, in the latter case, extension to the cava may be observed. The intravascular tumour may be visualised as reflective material within the vessel but, if the tumour is poorly reflective, it may not be distinguishable from the echoes in blood and only the expansion of the vessel may be apparent, depending on the size of the mass. Secondary signs of occlusion such as splenomegaly in the case of portal vein or compensatory dilatation of still-patent hepatic veins in a partial Budd-Chiari syndrome may be helpful, but the most direct way to make the diagnosis is using Doppler to evaluate the flow. Some form of duplex Doppler is obligatory because the deep position of the ves-

Fig. 6 Vascular invasion in liver malignancy. More aggressive tumours may invade the liver's blood vessels. **A:** A metastatic ovarian carcinoma has invaded the portal vein (arrowheads). **B:** A malignant melanoma has invaded the middle hepatic vein (arrow). In both cases the veins are expanded, a typical feature of tumour involvement that is not seen with simple thrombosis.

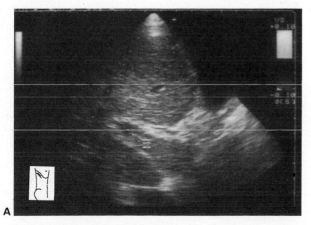

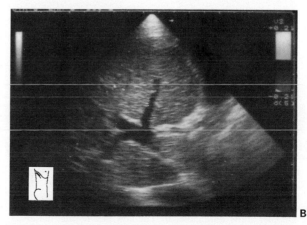

Plate 1 Tumour involvement of the portal vein. A: Though solid tissue completely fills the vessel's lumen, colour flow mapping displays a little hepatopetal flow. **B:** A portal vein branch shows reversed flow. This figure is reproduced in colour in the colour plate section at the front of this volume.

sels necessitates correlation of the flow position with the anatomy; pulsed Doppler is effective (Fig. 7) but colour Doppler gives a dramatic overall display of the vascular anatomy and allows a more confident diagnosis of absence of flow (Plate 1). Any type of liver tumour may invade vessels but it is observed more frequently in the more aggressive types and is especially common in primary hepatocellular carcinoma.

Bile ducts may also be invaded and occluded, producing the classic features of intrahepatic duct dilatation (see Ch. 13) with the parallel channel and double-barrel shotgun signs (Fig. 8). Bile duct invasion is a particular feature of cholangiocarcinoma (see Ch. 13) but may also be en-

countered in any other primary or secondary tumour. Obstructive jaundice does not usually result because the liver's reserve for bile excretion is well able to compensate for the loss of one segment. Jaundice, when it develops in liver malignancy, is more likely to be due to very extensive replacement of the liver volume by tumour – in the lymphomas the para-neoplastic syndrome of obstructive jaundice at the cannalicular level should also be considered.

Precise localisation of the segmental position of a lesion may be important, for example when a segmental resection is planned. The segmental numbering system described by Coinaud is used (see Ch. 14) and it is often possible to define precisely in which segment a lesion lies by noting its position with respect to internal landmarks. The primary distinction is the main left-right lobe division which corresponds with the lie of the middle hepatic vein and runs from the gall bladder fossa upwards to the IVC. The left lobe is then divided at the position of the ligamentum teres into medial and lateral segments while the right lobe is divided by the position of the right hepatic vein (usually this lies in the coronal plane) into anterior and posterior segments. Further subdivisions into superior and inferior segments are not as easily defined on ultrasound though they roughly correspond with the level of the main portal vein trunks. It may be straightforward to decide that a mass lies clearly within one segment or that it is confined to one lobe but, when the position is marginal or the lesion's margins are ill-defined, these decisions may not be possible with ultrasound. Angiography and CT may be useful alternatives.

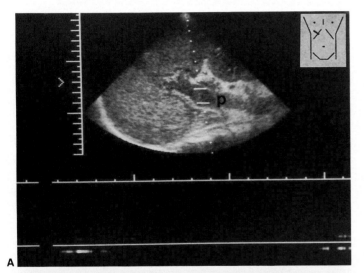

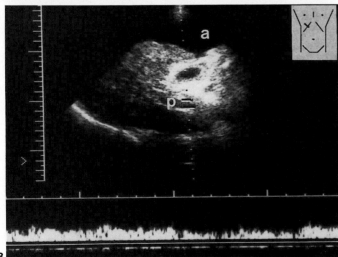

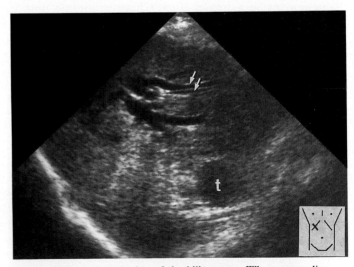

Fig. 7 **Doppler study of portal vein invasion. A:** A pulsed Doppler study of an occluded portal vein shows no signal, indicated by the flat spectral trace in the lower part of the figure. Although in many anatomical situations in the abdomen, geometric constraints make a negative Doppler study unreliable. **B:** The flow in a normal portal vein is so readily obtained that failure to demonstrate it is significant. The liver in (B) is heavily replaced by metastatic disease and surrounded by ascites (a). p – portal vein.

Fig. 8 **Malignant occlusion of the biliary tree.** When a mass lies close to the biliary tree, the duct may be occluded, giving rise to the same 'parallel channel sign' (arrows) of intrahepatic biliary tree dilatation as occurs in obstruction to the main duct, but in this case confined to the affected segment. In this patient with lymphoma, the offending mass is not seen in this tomogram, though another, subcapsular lesion is demonstrated (t).

Hepatocellular carcinoma

Clinical background

Primary liver cancer is one of the major malignancies in many countries throughout the world, particularly in sub-Saharan Africa and in the Far East;[1,2] it has been increasing in incidence in many countries in recent years but at the same time it is probably decreasing in a few others, including the USA.[3]

Primary liver cancer consists of two major histopathological types: hepatocellular carcinoma (HCC) and cholangiocarcinoma. The ratio of hepatocellular carcinoma to cholangiocarcinoma varies from five to one to nearly 40 to one, depending upon the frequency of hepatocellular carcinoma, which varies widely around the world.[4] Both are very rare in infancy where another type of cancer predominates: the hepatoblastoma. Since the prevalence of hepatocellular carcinoma is so much higher than that of other forms of primary liver cancer, the large majority of studies in the literature, particularly in recent years, is devoted to this type of tumour. Its aetiology, epidemiology and pathology are now well-understood.

A close association between hepatocellular carcinoma and cirrhosis, particularly the post-hepatitic or macronodular variety, was demonstrated many years ago.[5] The development of hepatocellular carcinoma in cirrhotic livers is particularly frequent in the Far East and in the West where 80% of patients with hepatocellular carcinoma have cirrhosis,[6,7] whereas this association is less frequent in South Africa (40% of cases). The carcinogenic properties of the hepatitis B virus (HBV) provides an explanation. Evidence supporting the aetiological role of HBV can be summarised as follows:[8]

a) parallelism between the prevalence of hepatocellular carcinoma and the frequency of HBsAg carriers;
b) familial clustering of hepatocellular carcinoma, cirrhosis and carriers;
c) high rate of positive HBV markers in patients with hepatocellular carcinoma;
d) presence of HBsAg positive patients with hepatocellular carcinoma;
e) production of HBsAg by cell lines derived from human hepatocellular carcinoma;
f) integration of HBV DNA in liver cancer cell DNA;
g) development of hepatocellular carcinoma in animal species infected by Hepa-DNA virus.

The importance of chronic non-A non-B liver disease in the development of hepatocellular carcinoma has also been recognised, since these infections are a direct cause of macronodular cirrhosis. The role of hepatitis virus C infection, which is responsible for the large majority of non-A, non-B chronic liver disease, has been emphasised recently in the development of hepatocellular carcinoma.[9] The liver in alcoholic cirrhosis, which is more common in Western

countries, has a reduced regenerative capacity compared to macronodular cirrhosis. Chemical carcinogens, such as aflatoxin, seem to play an important role in South African hepatocellular carcinoma.

Grossly, hepatocellular carcinomas can be classified into four types.[10]

a) infiltrative: these neoplastic lesions are not clearly demarcated and tumour thrombi are frequently found in the portal venous system;
b) expansive: a single nodule of hepatocellular carcinoma or many nodules in the same liver can display this pattern. In these cases the lesion is sharply demarcated from the surrounding parenchyma. Tumour invasion of portal vein branches is usually absent;
c) mixed infiltrative and expansive: when an infiltrative pattern, such as disruption of the capsule, is seen in nodules of the expansive type;
d) diffuse: this pattern consists of numerous small nodules (5 to 10 mm diameter) scattered throughout a cirrhotic liver.

The most important serological marker of hepatocellular carcinoma is the alpha-fetoprotein (AFP). Normal values in healthy humans are lower than 20 ng/ml. A rise in serum levels generally occurs in chronic liver disease and so the discriminant value for a specific diagnosis of hepatocellular carcinoma is 400 ng/ml. It has been recognised that the serum AFP is not always elevated to a diagnostic level, particularly in small hepatocellular carcinomas where its sensitivity is about 40%;[11,12] the sensitivity seems to be even lower in Western series of hepatocellular carcinoma.

The advent of real time ultrasonography, particularly the development of convex array transducers, has increased the accuracy of the diagnosis of focal lesions in the liver and significantly contributed to improve the detection of early hepatocellular carcinoma (HCC) thus defining the true incidence and natural history of this disease. Since the beginning of the 1980s, screening and follow up programmes in patients with chronic liver disease have been undertaken in the Far East using a combination of real time ultrasound and serum AFP.[13] These studies lead to the detection of a large number of asymptomatic small hepatocellular carcinomas, opening up new therapeutic options. From these investigations it is now clear that real time ultrasound plays the most important role in the diagnosis and follow up of hepatocellular carcinoma in this patient group.

Ultrasound appearances

Before the early 1980s only advanced cases of hepatocellular carcinoma were diagnosed and the sonographic appearances of the small hepatocellular carcinomas had not been described. Though most cases are still only detected when advanced, early lesions are seen in population surveys

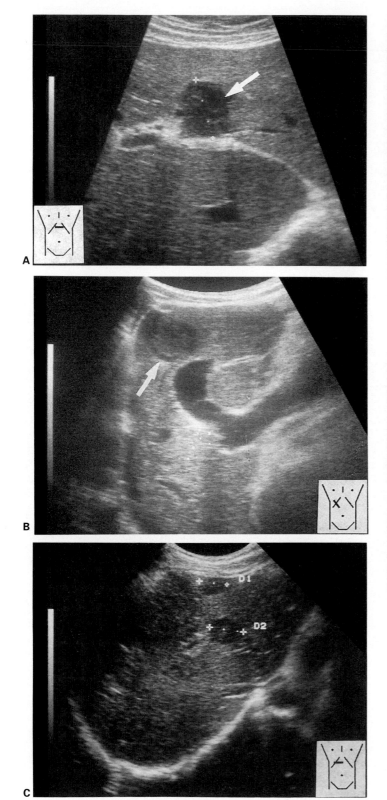

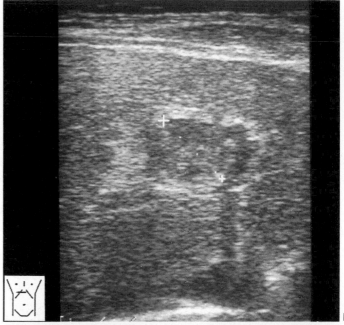

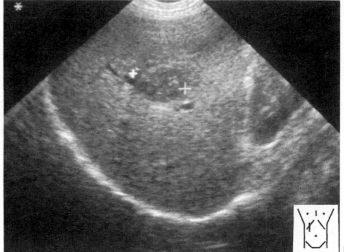

Fig. 9 Small hepatocellular carcinomas – echo-poor. A: The 2.8 cm nodule (arrow) is located proximal to the portal bifurcation. **B:** A tumour nodule (arrow) with a thin echo-poor rim, located close to the left branch of the portal vein. **C:** Two small echo-poor nodules (2.4 and 1.9 cm) are visible in the same patient. **D** and **E:** Larger hepatocellular carcinomas (> 3 cm) tend to be more reflective than the smaller lesions.

and in patients with cirrhosis who are under surveillance; their ultrasound appearances depend on their stage.

The shape of the tumour depends on its size and the invasiveness; three patterns have been described:[14]

a) nodular, when the contour of the tumour is regular and the boundary with the parenchyma is well-defined (Figs 9 to 11); the nodules may be single or multiple;

b) massive, when the tumour is large (> 5 cm) and the boundary with the liver parenchyma is difficult to recognise (Fig. 12);

c) diffuse, when the mass is indistinct and large portions of liver parenchyma are involved by tumour (Fig. 13).

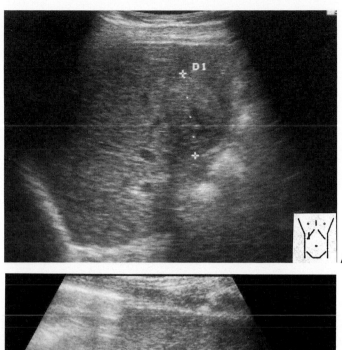

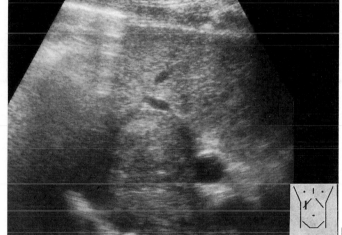

Fig. 11 Hepatocellular carcinoma – subtle. When the reflectivity of the tumour matches that of the surrounding liver, lesions are difficult to detect. In these examples the echo-poor halo draws attention to their presence.

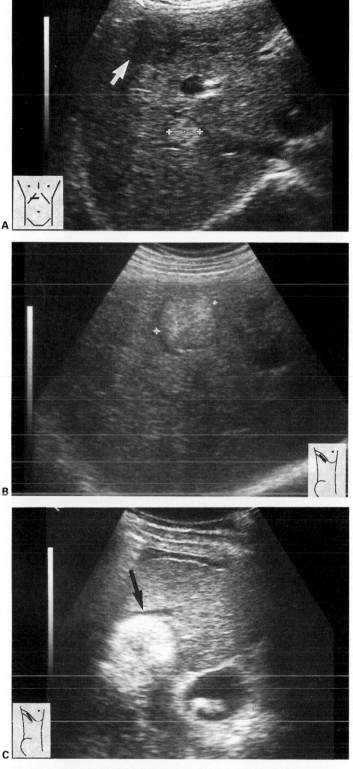

Fig. 10 Hepatocellular carcinomas – highly reflective. A: Small (2 cm) HCC with highly reflective pattern (between markers). A larger echo-poor nodule (arrow) is visible near to the liver surface. **B:** The nodule of HCC shows a highly reflective pattern with an echo-poor rim. **C:** HCC (4.5 cm) with intensely reflective pattern (arrow). A small quantity of ascitic fluid is visible around the liver and the gallbladder contains calculi.

Various degrees of reflectivity are found in hepatocellular carcinomas depending on their size and duration (Fig. 14) and on their pathological characteristics. The mass may show reflectivity less than, equal to, or greater than that of the normal liver (Figs 10 and 11). In other instances a mixed echo pattern, with areas of both increased and reduced reflectivity, is found. An echo-poor nodule may occasionally be found within a large mass, representing differentiation of cell lines within a pre-existing tumour, the 'tumour in tumour phenomenon' (Fig. 15). An echo-poor ring is frequently visualised around small nodules of hepatocellular carcinomas (Fig. 11). This ring is generally not visible when the nodule is smaller than 2 cm, while edge shadows are seen with lesions larger than 3 cm.

The influence of tissue characteristics on the reflectivity of the neoplasm has been investigated;[15] there is a close

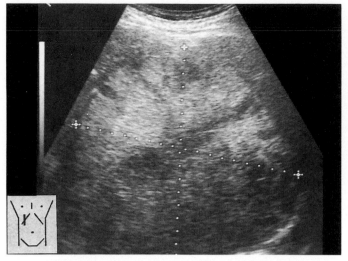

Fig. 12   Large hepatocellular carcinoma. Massive tumours tend to have heterogeneous internal structure.

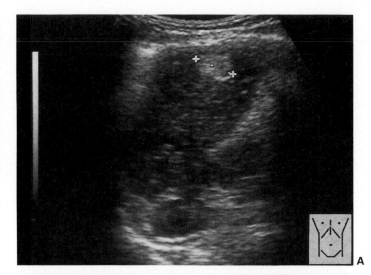

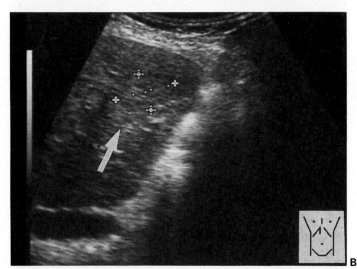

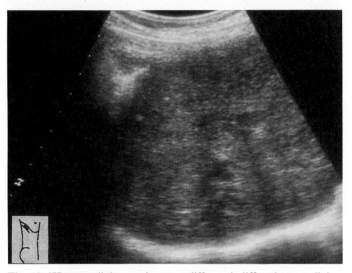

Fig. 13   Hepatocellular carcinoma – diffuse. A diffuse hepatocellular carcinoma involving large portions of liver parenchyma without a clear line of demarcation from the non-neoplastic tissue is shown. The echo pattern is highly heterogeneous with areas of both high and low reflectivity.

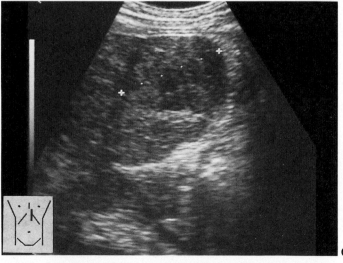

relationship between increasing reflectivity and the presence of necrosis and haemorrhage within the tumour. The highly reflective pattern is the most frequent, being found in about half of all cases.[16,17] However, small hepatocellular carcinomas (< 3 cm diameter) tend to be poorly reflective (77.4% of cases) (Table 1).[18] In a study on the natural history of small hepatocellular carcinomas (< 3 cm diameter), Ebara et al correlated the ultrasound pattern of the nodules with their size,[19] and demonstrated a tendency for them to develop from generally echo-poor lesions to a pattern with an echo-poor periphery and a more reflective centre and finally to large lesions with high

Fig. 14   Changing reflectivity of hepatocellular carcinomas during growth. A: At the time of the initial scan this 2 cm lesion was highly reflective. **B:** 6 months later (3.4 cm) it displayed an isoechoic pattern and was difficult to visualise (arrow). **C:** After a further 3 months (4.9 cm) it displayed a poorly reflective pattern.

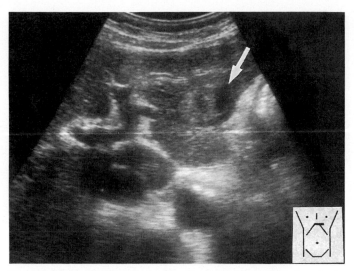

Fig. 15 Hepatocellular carcinoma – iso-echoic. The majority of this lesion is difficult to detect because it has the same reflectivity as the surrounding liver. However a small echo-poor nodule (arrow) is visible within this lesion ('tumour in tumour phenomenon').

Table 1 Ultrasound patterns of small hepatocellular carcinoma

Tumour size (cm)	No of tumours (%) Reflectivity of liver			
	Low	Equal	High	Total
1–2	15 (83.3%)	1 (5.6%)	2 (11.1%)	18 (100%)
2–3	9 (69.2%)	1 (7.7%)	3 (23.1%)	13 (100%)
Total	24 (77.4%)	2 (6.4%)	5 (16.1%)	31 (100%)

Sheu, Radiology 1984[18]

level echoes in advanced disease. The increase in reflectivity occasionally noted in small hepatocellular carcinomas is probably related to diffuse fatty change within the malignant tissue.[14,20] These lesions can be differentiated from haemangiomas if the peripheral echo-poor ring characteristic of carcinomas can be demonstrated.

Fibrolamellar hepatocellular carcinomas usually have a particular appearance with surface lobulations and a central scar.[21]

Growth pattern Some characteristics of the shape and reflectivity of hepatocellular carcinomas depend on the pattern and speed of growth of the tumour. It has been suggested that the presence of an echo-poor ring and a regular contour with sharp delimitation from the liver parenchyma represents a growth pattern of the expansive type. Partial or complete lack of these characteristics indicates an infiltrative growth pattern that produces a diffuse tumour which is difficult to recognise on ultrasound, because it may be similar in appearance to some cases of advanced cirrhosis. However, the ability of ultrasound to differentiate these growth patterns reliably is not fully established.

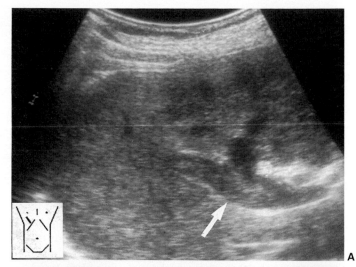

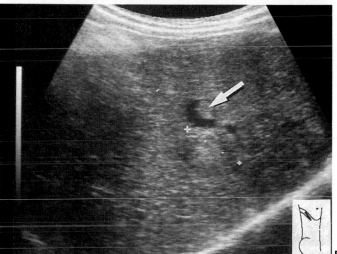

Fig. 16 Tumour involvement of the portal venous system.
A: Echogenic material in the main and right portal veins. Material is seen within the vessel lumen (arrow). **B:** Partial occlusion of a branch of the right portal vein (arrow). The nodule of hepatocellular carcinoma (2.9 cm) is located proximal to the vessel.

The ultrasound pattern has also been related to the growth rate of the tumour, particularly for small hepatocellular carcinomas found in the Japanese surveys. Here small echo-poor tumours tend to grow slowly whereas those with an echo-poor ring tend to grow faster.[19] This behaviour has not yet been confirmed in Western populations.

Vascular involvement Hepatocellular carcinoma has a strong tendency to invade the portal venous system. The hepatic veins[22,23] and the inferior vena cava may also be involved less frequently. Vascular invasion is recognisable as a mass within a major portal branch or even in the portal trunk (Fig. 16). Portal vein involvement is more frequently detected by ultrasound than by CT or angiography (71.4%, 28.6% and 14.5% respectively). However, tumour spread within peripheral portal branches, typical of the infiltrative type of growth, is not easily visualised by ultrasound or by any other technique.

Doppler features Pulsed and colour Doppler investigations have opened up new possibilities for characterising hepatocellular carcinomas and especially the blood vessel invasion that is so typical of this tumour.[24–26] The complex origins of the Doppler vascular signals from tumour masses have been clarified by recent studies.[27] It is well-accepted that tumour growth depends on its blood supply and most of this neovascularisation is concentrated in a ring at the periphery of the tumour. Though these arterioles are too small to be visualised by non-invasive imaging techniques, Doppler signals may be detected from them. Arterio-venous shunts are characteristic of some hepatocellular carcinomas and they too may be detectable.

Even in small hepatocellular carcinomas, abnormal signals are characterised by high peak Doppler shift frequencies, often over 4 KHz, due to the high pressure gradient in arterio-portal shunting.[24,25,28] These high peak signals may be associated with broadening of the spectrum due to marked flow disturbances (Fig. 17). Another pulsed Doppler feature consistent with hepatocellular carcinoma is high diastolic flow probably through large intratumoural vascular lakes with low impedance (Fig. 18). Colour Doppler mapping facilitates and speeds the search for these signals.

In a large series,[29] low impedance signals were detected in 87% of 55 hepatocellular carcinomas, in 28% of 25 metastatic cancers and in only 13% of 30 haemangiomas. In another series[26] arterial signals were found within and at the periphery of the tumour in 76% of small hepatocellular carcinomas (< 3 cm in diameter) and in all hepatocellular carcinomas larger than 3 cm diameter. This method also proved quite sensitive (83%) in the diagnosis of hepatocellular carcinoma, but its specificity seems to be low, because similar signals can be found also in liver metastasis, in cholangiocarcinomas and in some benign lesions such as focal nodular hyperplasia. It has not yet been established if the presence and the pattern of these vascular signals is related to the growth rate of the tumour or whether it predicts a tendency to vascular invasion.

Differential diagnosis

Solid focal lesions are quite frequently detected within the liver, this often raises problems of interpretation. An overall clinical assessment is fundamental to interpreting the ultrasound finding of a mass and to assessing the probability of its being malignant. In a patient with cirrhosis, every solid nodule found in the liver must be suspected of being a hepatocellular carcinoma until proved otherwise by guided biopsy or some other technique (such as angiography).

There are however, some characteristic echo patterns, which can help in the differential diagnosis:

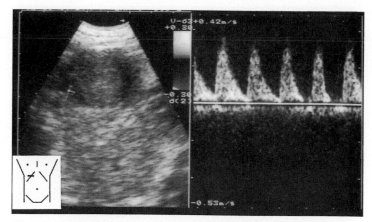

Fig. 17 Doppler analysis of hepatocellular carcinoma. A high peak arterial signal is detected at the periphery of the tumour.

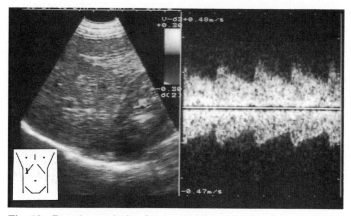

Fig. 18 Doppler analysis of a small highly reflective hepatocellular carcinoma. Low impedance arterial signals within the tumour.

a) small (1 to 3 cm) highly reflective nodules, single or multiple, often incidental findings in healthy subjects, are generally haemangiomas;

b) an echo-poor ring or a 'target lesion' pattern suggests malignancy.

c) an anechoic area seen within a reflective lesion generally corresponds to necrosis in the centre of a metastatic deposit.

There are also other non-neoplastic lesions which sometimes require differentiation from benign and malignant tumours: for example focal fatty infiltration and hydatid cysts,[30] which sometimes display a solid pattern (see Ch. 16).

Diagnostic accuracy

Comparative studies on the sensitivity of various imaging modalities in the diagnosis of hepatocellular carcinoma in Japan indicate that real time ultrasound has a higher detection rate than CT, angiography or scintigraphy, particularly where the nodules are smaller than 2 to 3 cm in diameter. The reported detection rates were 94% for ultrasound, 84% for CT, 76% for angiography and 12% for scintigraphy.

Real time ultrasound also proved superior to abdominal angiography and CT in the diagnosis of neoplastic involvement of portal branches.[31] Contrast CT (after Lipiodol injection though the hepatic artery) and magnetic resonance evaluation have been introduced but their accuracy in comparison with other techniques, and particularly with ultrasound, has not yet been definitely established.

Metastatic tumours

Clinical background

Terminal metastatic involvement of the liver is the rule in all but central nervous system malignancies (Table 2)[32] and as such is taken as a grave prognostic sign which underlies the importance of liver assessment in tumour staging. However the liver may be involved early in some tumour types, particularly those arising in the splanchnic bed whose venous drainage passes directly to the liver, so that the liver may be the sole metastatic site. Colo-rectal carcinomas are an example in which the metastasis may be resected if this is surgically feasible (solitary lesion restricted to one segment or lobe). The route of tumour spread to the liver is more likely to be haematogenous rather than lymphatic since, for the most part, the liver's lymphatics are hepatofugal. An exception is the lymph drainage of the gall bladder, the early and extensive involvement of the porta hepatis region that is characteristic of this tumour, though no doubt partly due to direct contiguous invasion, may be partly lymphatic.

Whether the vascular route is arterial or via the portal venous system depends on the site of the primary.[33] Systemic lesions, such as carcinomas of the lung and breast, can only reach the liver via the arterial system (having first traversed the lung bed) whereas tumours arising in the gastrointestinal tract might spread by either route – the slight predilection for gastrointestinal tumours to involve the portion of the liver that corresponds to the distribution of the portal vein blood draining them is evidence in favour of a predominantly venous route. (Caecal and ascending colonic tumours, for example, tending to metastasise to the right lobe while those arising in the descending colon and the rectum, which drain via the inferior mesenteric vein, preferentially affecting the left lobe.[34]) Regardless of the vascular route involved in the metastatic process, liver metastases take most of their blood supply from the hepatic artery rather than the portal vein.[35] In general they are not particularly vascular lesions, though there are exceptions to this.

Animal experiments, supported by observations in humans, show that single cells shed from a malignant tumour are not capable of growth when they embolise into the capillary bed of a potential metastatic site. Larger clumps of a few hundred cells are the smallest capable of taking root. To survive the tumour nidus must establish its own blood supply, because diffusion can only supply oxygen and nutriments to lesions smaller than about 1 mm diameter.[36,37] Neovascularisation depends on the tumour secreting a protein 'hormone', the tumour angiogenesis factor which promotes the development and ingrowth of buds from nearby capillaries. The smallest viable metastasis measures only a fraction of a millimetre in diameter: such a lesion is several orders of magnitude smaller than the smallest detectable on ultrasound or any imaging technique either currently available or realistically envisaged. Potentially the lesion grows exponentially, doubling the number of cells every week for a highly aggressive tumour such as Burkitt's lymphoma at one extreme, to doubling every 6 months for a slow growing tumour. A tumour of 1 mm diameter, the earliest that detection is possible even by the most sophisticated means under optimum circumstances, represents a tumour that has already undergone some 20 doublings – at 40 doublings a tumour might weigh as much as 1 kg and at this size is usually lethal (Fig. 19).[38] Thus it is apparent that most of the growth cycle of a metastasis has already occurred by the stage at which it can be detected by imaging methods; the goal of detecting 'early' deposits is far from realised. The same depressing considerations apply to primary malignant tumours.

Table 2 Frequency of liver metastases (adapted from[2])

Tumour type	Frequency of metastases (%) At presentation	At post-mortem
Carcinomas		
Bladder	> 5	30–50
Breast	1	45–60
Bronchus (oat)	10	30
Cervix	< 1	15–35
Colo-rectal	25	70
Kidney	15	35–40
Melanoma	6	70
Nephroblastoma	3–10	40
Neuroblastoma	25	70
Ovary	< 5	10–15
Pancreas	NA	50–70
Prostate	1	15
Stomach	NA	35–50
Testis	< 1	s 50, t 80
Thyroid	4	60
Uterus	< 1	15–30
Sarcomas		
Osteosarcoma	< 5	< 5
Rhabdomyosarcoma	10	45
Lympho-reticular		
Hodgkin's	8	60
Non-Hodgkin's	1–16	50

(s – seminoma, t – teratoma, NA – information not available)

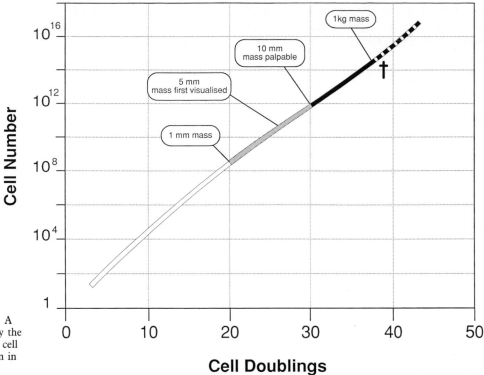

Fig. 19 Time scale of tumour cell division. A typical tumour has enlarged to a lethal size by the time it has undergone some 40 generations of cell division. At 20 doublings it has reached 1 mm in diameter.

Liver metastases are characteristically multiple and show a range of sizes with a uniform distribution. This suggests that they have seeded on a continual basis over long periods of time, probably since the primary has grown large enough to invade its vascular system. The alternative hypothesis, that seeding is a sporadic affair, tumour clumps being shed in intermittent showers, would be expected to produce clustering of the size of metastases corresponding to their several ages, unless variable growth rates are assumed to occur.

Ultrasound appearances

A bewildering range of appearances is encountered in liver metastatic disease (Table 3) and their overlap with non-malignant disorders inevitably results in lack of specificity.[39,40] Focal lesions are commonest but the malignancy may also infiltrate widely. The commonest focal pattern is of echo-poor masses (Fig. 20) whose texture differs

Table 3 Ultrasonic patterns of metastases

Poorly reflective	Any type (typical of lymphomas)
Highly reflective	Typically gastro-intestinal and uro-genital tract 1°
Cystic	Mucin secreting 1°
	Necrosis in any type
Calcified	Typical of colo-rectal 1°
Confluent	Any extensive 1° or 2° tumour
Diffuse	Lymphoma and leukaemia

little from the surrounding liver.[41] The difference in reflectivity may be sufficient that the lesions are very obvious and they may even be virtually echo-free. This is particularly often the case for lymphomas and sarcomas, presumably because these tumours have a very uniform cellular architecture with little stromal reaction so that few ultrasound interfaces are produced. Not uncommonly however, the contrast in reflectivity is slight, so that the lesions are difficult to demonstrate except by the mass effects and invasive features discussed above. Echo-poor lesions may be produced by any type of primary tumour; they are typical of many of the commonest malignancies such as carcinoma of the breast and bronchus. Usually the attenuation in the lesion is the same as the liver itself so that neither distal shadowing nor enhancement are present and the surrounding liver is unremarkable. A special case occurs when metastases develop in a fatty liver: the TGC is set to be correct for the increased attenuation of the fatty liver, but this is inappropriate for the lesion, so that enhancement is produced (Fig. 21). This combination of pathologies is not rare because fatty change can be produced by anorexia and by anticancer drugs. The resulting appearance is easily confused with simple liver cysts.

When the deposit is more reflective than the liver, the lesion is easier to detect, tending to catch the eye as the beam is swept across it in the real time search (Fig. 22). Again a range of contrasts in intensity is seen, from those that are obvious, to subtle lesions that are difficult to detect, and enhancement or shadowing are not generally

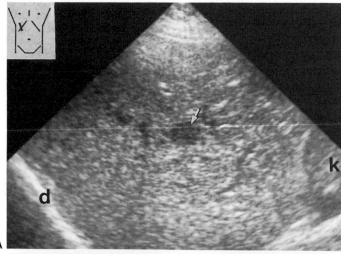

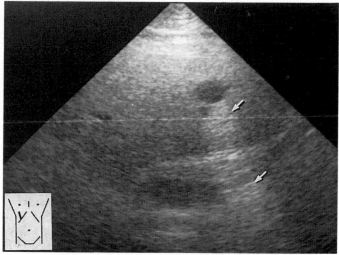

Fig. 21 Pseudo-enhancement of metastasis in a fatty liver. This lymphomatous lesion in the liver shows marked distal enhancement (arrows), most obviously interpreted as being due to a cystic lesion. In fact, the lesion is solid but with a lower attenuation than the fatty liver that surrounds it. Since the TGC has been adjusted to compensate for the abnormally high attenuation of the fatty liver, it pulls up the distal echoes, falsely suggesting that the lesion is cystic.

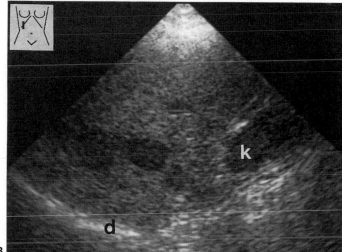

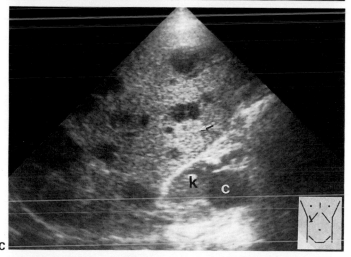

Fig. 20 Echo-poor metastases. Lesions with slightly lower intensity echoes than the surrounding liver are the commonest type of metastasis. **A:** The solitary deposit (arrow) was metastatic from a bronchial carcinoma. **B** and **C:** The multiple lesions were from breast and non-Hodgkin's lymphoma respectively. The kidney in (C) contains a simple cyst. Note the apparent enhancement deep to some of the lesions in (C) (arrow); this is attributable to the relatively lower attenuation within the lesion compared to the surrounding liver (compare with Fig. 21). c – cyst, d – diaphragm, k – kidney.

produced. However, highly reflective lesions may be surrounded by an echo-poor band which may be merely a fine line (known as a halo) or be obvious as a border several millimetres thick. This type is known as the target or 'bull's eye' pattern (Fig. 23) and is more often encountered with larger lesions, perhaps representing the effects of haemorrhage or necrosis. Highly reflective and target lesions are typical of tumours originating in the gastrointestinal and urogenital tracts, being common for example in colo-rectal carcinomas and in carcinoma of the ovary, pancreas and kidney. However, it is important to note that a proportion of such tumours may also produce echo-poor deposits and the different types may be mixed within the same liver (Fig. 24).

The reasons for these different appearances on ultrasound are not clear. The low level echoes of the common type may correspond with lesions that have a high water content: in general with ultrasound high water levels are associated with low reflectivity, the clearest example being the echo-poor appearance of oedematous tissue, e.g. acute pancreatitis. For the highly reflective variety a correlation with vascularity has been suggested[42] as is the case with haemangiomas,[43] but it is by no means a strong link and other factors such as stromal collagen content turn out to be equally important.[44–46] Tumour necrosis, fatty replacement[47] and calcification may also play a part. The nature of the echo-poor halo surrounding highly reflective deposits remains a controversy. Some authors claim that it represents increase in fluid at the tumour margin whilst others suggest that it results from pressure-atrophy of the hepatocytes in response to the enlargement of the tumour

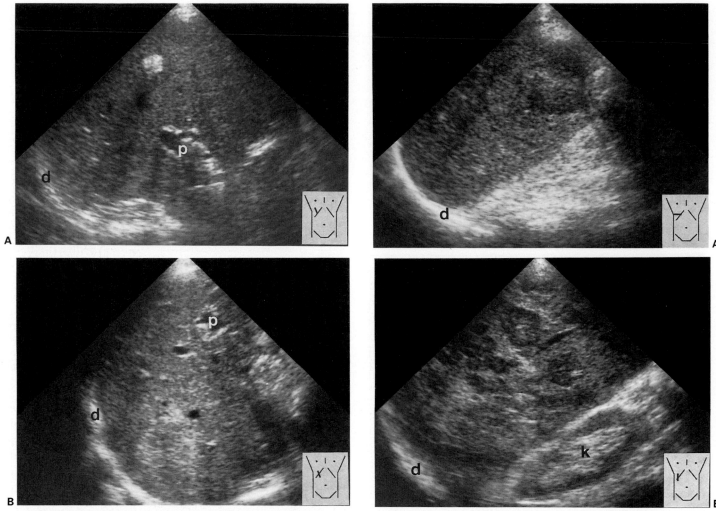

Fig. 22 Highly reflective metastases. Deposits with high amplitude echoes are commonly due to metastases from the gastrointestinal and urogenital tracts. These typical solitary lesions were metastases from colonic and rectal primaries respectively. p – portal vein, d – diaphragm.

Fig. 23 Target lesions. A and **B:** The concentric ringed pattern of the 'target' or 'bull's eye' lesion is shown in these two cases. This pattern is more often seen with larger lesions. d – diaphragm, k – kidney.

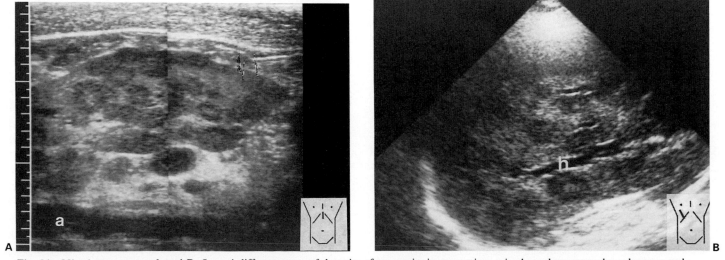

Fig. 24 Mixed metastases. A and **B:** Several different types of deposits often coexist in one patient – in these three examples echo-poor and target lesions are intermixed. a – aorta, h – hepatic vein.

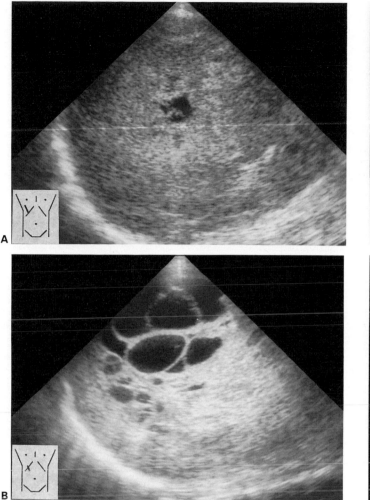

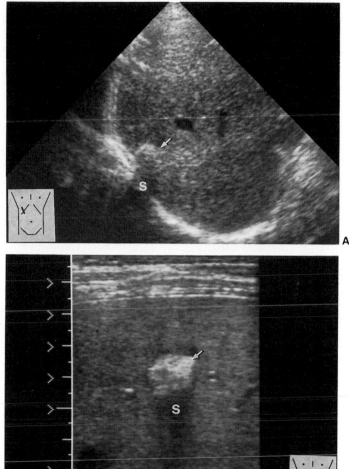

Fig. 25 Cystic metastases. The two varieties of cystic metastasis are illustrated. **A:** The shaggy wall of the fluid space suggests that it has resulted from necrosis in the centre of a tumour, presumably because of ischaemia. The irregularity of the surrounding tissue represents the viable portion of the metastasis. This pattern simulates an abscess cavity. **B:** When the cyst results from mucin secretion the walls of the cavity are smooth suggesting a benign lesion; this multicystic lesion might be misdiagnosed as polycystic liver disease or as biliary cysts. If only a single cyst were present it would probably be considered to be a simple cyst. Only growth over serial observations provides the clue to their malignant nature. The commonest source of this type is the ovary, but any tissue capable of secreting mucin can be responsible – this patient had a testicular teratoma.

Fig. 26 Calcified metastases. Metastases from the gastrointestinal tract are prone to calcify. The typical ultrasound features are of a highly reflective lesion (arrows) with shadowing (s).

leaving the sinusoidal blood vessels as the halo.[48] However it is by no means clear that such vessels would be echo-poor, the increased number of interfaces between the blood and the vessel walls produces high level echoes in other situations such as in haemangiomas.[43]

For the less common types of liver metastasis the correspondence between pathology and ultrasonic appearance is more readily understood. Fluid filled lesions, recognised by their distal enhancement, are an example (Fig. 25); they are echo-free when they contain clear fluid, as may be produced by mucin-secreting lesions (e.g. carcinoma of the

ovary, pancreas, etc.) but contain debris when the fluid represents tumour necrosis.[49,50] This type tend to have a shaggy wall and so are not likely to be confused with simple cysts, but the mucin-secreting types are indistinguishable except for their progressive enlargement when studied sequentially over a period of months.

Calcified lesions have very intense echoes and may show shadowing if the foci of calcium are sufficiently large (Fig. 26). Calcification commonly occurs in secondaries from colo-rectal and gastric carcinomas as well as in neuroblastomas.

One of the more difficult differential diagnoses is from haemangiomas which also have a variety of appearances but are most commonly highly reflective (Fig. 27) (see Ch. 16).[51] While an absolutely definite differential diagnosis is not possible with ultrasound, haemangiomas are typically situated in a subcapsular or perivascular position, are usually solitary, measure a few centimetres in diameter

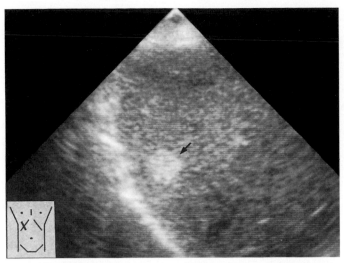

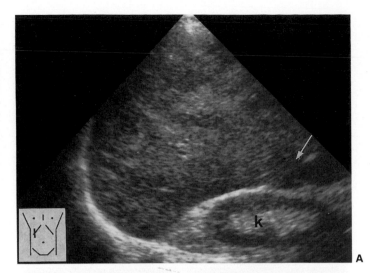

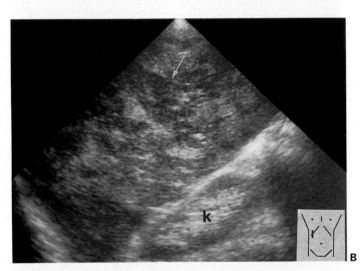

Fig. 27 Haemangioma. A solitary well-defined highly reflective focus (arrow) is the typical appearance of a haemangioma, but this finding in a patient undergoing a staging scan always raises doubt. The lack of any changes in the surrounding liver (halo, distortion) and the position under the capsule are helpful features suggesting a benign lesion.

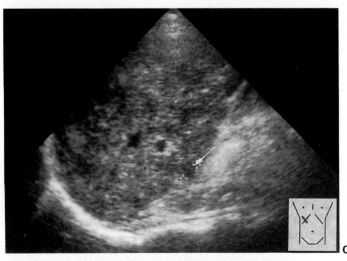

and have uniform, high amplitude echoes. There are no mass effects nor evidence of invasion and they lack the echo-poor halo that may be seen around highly reflective metastases. Occasionally large haemangiomas may show distal enhancement, a feature not described with highly reflective metastases. In children haemangiomas are echo-poor and sometimes present a disorganised appearance that may suggest metastatic disease; their vascular nature is obvious on colour Doppler (see Ch. 27). Doppler studies on adult haemangiomas are unfortunately unhelpful, generally being negative (as also in metastases[52,53]) probably because the flow through the meshwork of tortuous vessels is too slow for detection with current equipment. Biopsy is safe provided the lesion is approached via surrounding liver (so that any bleeding is confined) but interpretation of a cytological sample may be difficult,[54] a definitive diagnosis can usually be made on histology of a cutting needle specimen. Angiography (often performed with CT) is usually definitive[55,56] though rare examples of metastases showing the delayed filling from the periphery that typifies haemangiomas have been reported.[57]

Metastases (and primary hepatocellular carcinomas) may become diffuse by confluent growth of initially separate foci (Fig. 28). The resultant appearance is of an irregular pattern throughout the affected portion (commonly this is the entire liver) with ill-defined patchiness consisting of geographic echo-poor areas. These textural changes are often very subtle and easily missed altogether or confused with the irregular texture of diffuse infiltrative or degenerative diseases such as focal fatty infiltration and cirrhosis.[58] Liver enlargement, together with the absence of the typical

Fig. 28 Diffuse metastases. When metastatic disease becomes extensive the individual lesions may coalesce so that their margins are lost. The resulting pattern is of a grossly distorted texture whose malignant origin may not be obvious. Usually, as in these examples (arrows), some definable masses can be detected amongst the overall texture disturbance. k – kidney.

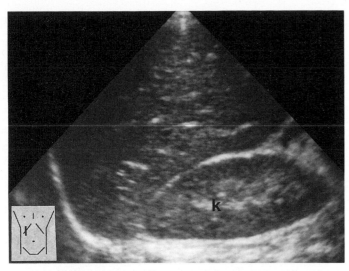

Fig. 29 Dark liver – lymphoma. The liver's echoes are normally higher than those of the renal cortex (evaluated at the same depth in the scan). Some acute diffuse processes cause a reduction in the liver's echo intensity (the so-called 'dark liver'); these include lymphomatous and leukaemic infiltration. Since identical changes are sometimes produced by reactive infiltration in the same patients, the findings are non-specific and biopsy confirmation is required. In this patient diffuse lymphoma was found. k – kidney.

ancillary features of cirrhosis, may be suggestive of metastatic disease. In most cases a careful search will reveal at least a few focal abnormalities which indicate the true diagnosis.

Diffuse involvement is also a feature of the lymphomas and leukaemias, though in the former there may also be focal involvement.[59] The liver is enlarged and shows reduced reflectivity (the 'dark liver pattern') identical to that produced by conditions such as acute hepatitis and acute cardiac failure (Fig. 29) (see Ch. 18). Unfortunately, in lymphoma and leukaemia the liver is commonly affected by reactive cellular infiltration (round-cell inflammatory changes) which produces exactly the same ultrasonic appearance, therefore this finding is of little diagnostic value.

In general the differential diagnostic considerations for focal liver lesions include all the benign focal processes, but often the clinical picture will make some so unlikely (or probable) as to shorten the list of possible causes considerably. A pyogenic or amoebic abscess, for example, can simulate a metastasis exactly but the liver is usually locally tender and the story of fever is suggestive. Likewise, trauma will usually be suspected from the patient's history. Hepatic (oestrogen) adenomas and focal nodular hyperplasia (FNH) pose difficult diagnostic problems: they cannot reliably be distinguished from metastases with present imaging techniques though the Kupffer cells usually present in FNH take up colloids, producing a normal isotope scan, which is very reassuring.[60,61]

Focal fatty change is also a difficult diagnostic problem (see Ch. 16); the fatty tissue appears as regions of increased reflectivity which can be misdiagnosed as highly reflective masses.[62] Features that should be looked for are the typical distribution of focal fatty change as triangular or polygonal regions that project onto one of the liver surfaces (perhaps a fissure or the porta) and the uniform echoes with no disturbance of the adjacent liver architecture (no halo, no mass or invasive effects). In addition, the foci tend to progress or regress rather rapidly, so that a study a week or so later may reveal complete clearing or wide extension. Confirmation can be obtained from a liver scintigram (using S-colloid) which shows no loss of function in the affected region. The counterpart, where all but a small portion of the liver has become infiltrated with fat, leaving an apparently dark segment, is even more difficult to distinguish from a deposit.[63] Again the process develops on a segmental basis, so the spared region is seen as a wedge projecting onto a liver surface; this is especially common close to the gall bladder. As with focal fatty change, there are no mass or invasive effects. The predilection for the portions of the liver near the gallbladder (especially the quadrate lobe) is interesting for this region has an unusual portal blood supply. In some subjects it is supplied by portal veins passing directly from the gallbladder, in others the cystic veins first empty into one of the main portal vein branches before passing into the liver sinusoids. Possibly the cystic blood does not contain the toxic substance that causes fatty change in the main part of the liver, accounting for the focal sparing (or vice versa, toxins being present in

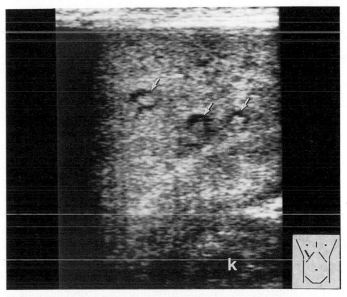

Fig. 30 Candida micro-abscess. Multiple small lesions of a target pattern (arrows) are seen in patients with fungal septicaemia and liver (or spleen) involvement. The central punctum may represent the arteriole in which the septic embolus lodged. This patient, who was recovering from a bone marrow transplant, developed monilial infection of the upper gastrointestinal tract and subsequently a fever. Typical lesions were seen on the scan and confirmed by the demonstration of hyphae on fine needle biopsy. k – kidney.

the cystic veins in the case of focal fatty change occurring here). CT is sometimes helpful in this problem, showing a low density in the fatty segments, but ultrasound seems to be more sensitive than CT since in many cases CT is negative when the ultrasound changes are obvious. If focal fatty change (or sparing) is considered before a biopsy, then it is prudent to take samples both from the apparent abnormality and from the surrounding liver – the seemingly normal liver may actually turn out to be the abnormality!

In oncology departments patients who are severely immunocompromised may occasionally develop widespread multifocal fungal abscesses which, if present in the liver, may be difficult to distinguish from malignancy (Fig. 30) (see Ch. 16).[64]

Accuracy of ultrasound in liver malignancy

In comparison with other non-invasive techniques for imaging the liver, ultrasound has the advantage of availability, cost effectiveness and simplicity for the patient. The earliest of the methods in this group was isotope scanning (currently performed using ^{99m}Tc labelled colloids of sulphur) which provides a map of Kupffer cell activity.[65–67] Most lesions appear as regions of reduced uptake and so are easily masked by overlying tissue of normal function. Because of this and the inherently limited spatial resolution of the gamma camera, isotope techniques cannot offer a sensitivity comparable to ultrasound. However, the ability to demonstrate function is valuable in some differential diagnostic problems, notably the distinction of focal fatty change and focal nodular hyperplasia,[68] both of which show normal function, from other focal lesions, both benign and malignant (see Ch. 16). Developments in isotope techniques may extend its role: improved resolution is available both from positron cameras and from the new generation of single photon tomographic gamma cameras (high resolution SPECT),[69] and new radio-pharmaceuticals will continue to be developed.[70]

CT (computed tomographic X-ray) scanners, when used with contrast,[71] offer similar resolution to ultrasound with the benefits that all of the liver can be imaged in almost every patient, CT not being limited by the patient's body habitus or by the presence of gas. Some parts of the liver are less easily studied, especially the upper portions at the dome of both right and left lobes where movement and partial volume effects make smaller lesions undetectable. The lack of sagittal and coronal projections and the need to use contrast for optimum results are further limitations. Comparing ultrasound and CT for liver tumours is difficult because there is no 'gold standard' but several studies have shown a marginally higher sensitivity for CT,[72,73] while both lack specificity in the sense that the precise nature of focal lesions is often indeterminate. CT fares somewhat better than ultrasound in this respect, mainly because it

can distinguish most cases of haemangioma using haemodynamic criteria.

The most striking finding to emerge from these studies is the overall poor sensitivity of either technique to small metastatic lesions. For example, when post-mortem liver specimens are scanned, many or even most of the deposits that can be seen by naked-eye on the cut surfaces are not demonstrated by CT or ultrasound either in vivo or in vitro.[74,75] Similarly, when pre-operative ultrasound staging studies are compared with the findings of intra-operative scans, a marked increase in the number of lesions detected is noted.[76,77]

The accuracy of these techniques is usually quoted as in the high 80% to 90% range[78,79] (Table 4) but this refers to the ability to stage a patient correctly as having metastatic disease or not, rather than the ability to detect each lesion correctly. In clinical practice, both ultrasound and CT are successful because of the fact that in most patients metastatic disease is multiple with at least some of the lesions being large enough and with sufficient contrast to be detected, rather than because of their intrinsic sensitivity.

In practice most investigators use ultrasound as the initial method to study the liver;[80] a positive result is usually adequate for management decisions, supplemented if necessary by ultrasound guided biopsy.[81,82] The significance of a negative result has to be weighed in the clinical context. For example, if a crucial management decision is to be based on demonstrating that the liver (or part of it, when a segmental resection is planned) is unaffected, then a negative ultrasound should be followed up by a contrast CT study and, if this is negative, possibly by angiography or nuclear magnetic resonance imaging (MRI), though the number of additional lesions demonstrated by additional tests diminishes progressively so that multiple tests are not cost effective in routine staging.[83] MRI of the liver, especially when gadolinium contrast enhancement is used, offers higher sensitivity than either ultrasound or CT scanning;[84] it is probably the most sensitive method for the detection of liver tumours but its expense and time consuming nature will probably restrict its use to special problems.

Table 4 Table of reported accuracy of ultrasound in liver metastases

1° Tumour Type	Sens	Spec	Acc	Cases	Reference
mixed	54	92	–	137	59
lymphoma	85	72	–	51	59
GI tract	84	90	–	100 prospective laparoscopy	72
mixed	73	94	84	108 retrospective	67
colon & breast	82	85	–	122 prospective	72
GI tract	–	–	88	50 prospective, op correlation	79
mainly GI tract	61	94	80	80 prospective, op correlation	74

Special techniques

a) Intra-operative ultrasound

Using small, high frequency linear array transducers applied directly onto the liver surface after laparotomy produces very high resolution images which allow the detection of metastases missed on conventional studies.[85,86] Any abnormality demonstrated can be biopsied under ultrasound guidance. More accurate staging, for example in colo-rectal carcinoma, allows more appropriate surgical management: a segmental resection can be added when a solitary lesion is found, or a planned radical procedure limited to simple resection of the primary if multiple metastases are demonstrated.[87,88]

b) Biopsy guidance

Using ultrasound to guide placement of fine or cutting biopsy needles improves tissue sampling and so reduces false negative and indeterminate results.[81,82] It also reduces risk because vulnerable structures such as the gall bladder can be avoided. Ultrasound guidance should be used for any focal lesion unless it is massive and obviously palpable.

c) Ultrasound contrast enhancement

A variety of contrast agents has been used experimentally to enhance contrast for ultrasound. Particulate materials[89] have the disadvantage of potential toxicity, while perfluorohydrocarbons,[90] because they have to be taken up by liver cells, must be injected several hours before scanning but are effective at increasing contrast between tumours and the liver background. Perhaps the most promising are encapsulated gas bubbles, either in sugar particles or more recently, in human serum albumen (Albunex).[91,92] These particles can be made small enough to cross the pulmonary capillary bed and so increase the reflectivity of the vascular bed. The vascular contrast lasts several hours after an intravenous injection and they appear to be safe. The effect on real time images is dramatic, a flush of intense echoes appearing in the larger vessels and then filling the vascular parts of the organ as smaller vessels become filled. On Doppler a marked increase in signal strength is observed, both on spectral traces and on colour images enabling smaller vessels to be evaluated. In experimental animals liver tumours can be imaged more readily and the tumour vessels detected on colour Doppler.

REFERENCES

1 Kew M C, Geddes E W. Hepatocellular carcinoma in rural Southern African blacks. Medicine 1982; 61: 98–108

2 Yu S Z. Epidemiology of primary liver cancer. In: Tang Z Y. ed. Subclinical hepatocellular carcinoma. Beijing, China: China Academic Publisher, 1985: 189–211

3 Saracci R, Repetto F. Time trends of primary liver cancer: Indication of increased incidence in selected cancer registry populations. J Natl Cancer Inst 1980; 65: 241–247

4 Okuda K, Kubo Y, Okazaki N, et al. Clinical aspects of intrahepatic bile duct carcinoma including hilar carcinoma. A study of 57 autopsy-proven cases. Cancer 1977; 39: 232–246

5 Edmondson H A, Steiner P E. Primary carcinoma of the liver. A study of 100 cases among 48 900 necropsies. Cancer 1954; 7: 462–503

6 Shikata T. Primary liver carcinoma and liver cirrhosis. In: Okuda K, Peters R L. eds. Hepatocellular carcinoma. New York: Wiley. 1976: p 53–72

7 Peters R L. Pathology of hepatocellular carcinoma. In: Okuda K, Peters R L. eds. Hepatocellular carcinoma. New York: Wiley. 1976: p 107–168

8 Okuda K. Primary liver cancer. Dig Dis Sci 1986; 31: 133–146

9 Colombo M, Donato M F, Rumi M G, et al. Prospective study of primary liver carcinoma in patients with cirrhosis and hepatitis C virus infection. Hepatology 1989; 10: 645A

10 Kojiro M, Nakashima T. Pathology of hepatocellular carcinoma. In: Okuda-Ishak. eds. Neoplasms of the liver. Tokyo: Springer Verlag. 1987: p 81–104

11 Chen D S, Sung J L, Sheu J C, et al. Serum alpha feto protein in the early stage of human hepatocellular carcinoma. Gastroenterology 1984; 86: 1404–1409

12 Bolondi L, Benzi G, Santi V, et al. Relationship between Alphafeto protein serum levels, tumor volume and growth rate of hepatocellular carcinoma in a European series. Ital J Gastroenterol, 1990 in press

13 Shinagawa T, Ohto M, Kimura K, et al. Diagnosis and clinical features of small hepatocellular carcinoma with emphasis on the utility of real time ultrasonography. A study in 51 patients. Gastroenterology 1984; 86: 495–502

14 Ohto M, Ebara M, Okuda K. Ultrasonography in the diagnosis of hepatic tumor. In: Okuda-Ishak. ed. Neoplasms of the Liver. Tokyo: Springer Verlag. 1987: p 251–258

15 Itoh K, Yasuda Y, Ueno E, Kasahara K, Zhao L. Studies on the relationships between acoustic patterns produced by liver carcinoma in ultrasonography and in scanning acoustic microscopy. Asian Med J 1983; 26: 585–597

16 Cottone M, Marcenò M P, Maringhini A, et al. Ultrasound in the diagnosis of hepatocellular carcinoma associated with cirrhosis. Radiology 1983; 147: 517–519

17 Zhi-zhang Xu. Real time B-Mode ultrasonography in localization of subclinical carcinoma. In: Tang Zhao-you. eds. Subclinical hepatocellular carcinoma. Berlin: Springer Verlag. 1985: 36–53

18 Sheu J C, Sung J L, Chen D S, et al. Ultrasonography of small hepatic tumors using high-resolution linear-array real time instruments. Radiology 1984; 150: 797–802

19 Ebara M, Ohto M, Shinagawa T, et al. Natural history of minute hepatocellular carcinoma smaller than three centimeters complicating cirrhosis. A study in 22 patients. Gastroenterology 1986; 90: 289–298

20 Yoshikawa J, Matsui O, Takashima T. Fatty metamorphosis in hepatocellular carcinoma: radiological features in 10 cases. AJR 1988; 151: 717–720

21 Brandt D J, Johnson C D, Stephens D H, Weiland L H. Imaging of fibrolamellar hepatocellular carcinoma. AJR 1988; 151: 295–299

22 Mathieu D, Guinet C, Bouklia-Hassane A, Vasile N. Hepatic vein involvement in hepatocellular carcinoma. Gastrointest Radiol 1988; 13: 55–60

23 Sugiura N, Ohto M, Kimura K, Ebara M, Okuda K. Imaging diagnosis of portal vein tumour thrombosis and its pathophysiology in hepatocellular carcinoma. Jpn J Gastroenterol 1986; 83: 2151–2160

24 Taylor K J W, Ramos I, Morse SS, Fortune K L, Hammers L, Taylor C R. Focal liver masses: differential diagnosis with pulsed Doppler US. Radiology 1987; 164: 643–647

25 Bolondi L, Gaiani S, Li Bassi S, et al. Colour Doppler and duplex investigation of vascular signals arising from hepatocellular carcinoma (HCC). Gastroenterol Int 1989; 2: 30–32

26 Ohnishi K, Nomura F. Ultrasonic Doppler studies of hepatocellular carcinoma and comparison with other hepatic focal lesions. Gastroenterology 1989; 97: 1489–1497

27 Taylor K J W, Ramos I, Carter D, Morse S S, Snower D, Fortune K L. Correlation of Doppler US tumor signals with neovascular morphologic features. Radiology 1988; 166: 57–62

28 Taylor C R, Taylor K J W. Diagnostic imaging of hepatocellular carcinoma: progress in non invasive tissue characterization. J Clin Gastroenterol 1988; 10: 452–457

29 Yasuhara K, Kimura K, Ohto M, et al. Pulsed Doppler in the diagnosis of small liver tumors. Br J Radiol 1988; 61: 898–902.

30 Lewall D B, McCorkell S J. Hepatic echinococcal cyst: sonographic appearance and classification. Radiology 1985; 155–775

31 Igawa S, Sakai K, Kinoshite H, Hirohashi K. Intraoperative sonography: clinical usefulness in liver surgery. Radiology 1985; 156: 473–478

32 Gilbert H A, Kagan A R. Liver Metastases. In: Weiss L. ed. Fundamental Aspects of Metastases. Amsterdam: Elsevier. 1976: Ch. 26

33 Wilson M A. Metastatic Disease of the Liver. In: Wilson M A, Ruzicka F F. eds. Modern Imaging of the Liver. New York: Dekker. 1989: Ch. 17

34 Desai A G, Bennet R, Sheriff S. Streaming in the portal vein: its effect on the spread of metastases to the liver. Clin Nucl Med 10: 1985: 556–559

35 Ackerman N B. The blood supply of experimental liver metastases. Surgery 1974; 75: 589–596

36 Schor A M, Schor S L. Tumour angiogenesis. J Pathol 1983; 141: 385–413

37 Folkman J, Merler E, Abernathy C, Williams G. Isolation of a tumour factor responsible for angiogenesis. J Exp Med 1971; 33: 275

38 DeVita V. Single agent vs combination chemotherapy. CA 1975; 25: 152

39 Green B, Bree R L, Goldstein H M, Stanley C. Gray scale evaluation of hepatic neoplasms: patterns and correlations. Radiology 1977; 124: 203–208

40 Scheible W, Gosink B B, Leopold G R. Gray scale echographic patterns of hepatic metastatic disease. AJR 1977; 129: 983–987

41 Koischwitz D. Sonomorphologie primäre und secondäre Leberneoplasmen. Fortschr Rontgenstr 1980; 133: 372–378

42 Rubaltelli L, Del Maschio A, Candiani F. The role of vascularisation in the formation of echographic patterns of hepatic metastases. Br J Radiol 1980; 53: 1166–1168

43 Marchal G, Baert A L, Favery J. Ultrasonography of liver haemangioma. Fortschr Rontgenstr 1983; 138: 201–207

44 Marchal G, Tshibwabwa-Tumba E, Verbeken E, Baert A, Lauweryns J. Influence of tumoral and peritumoral vascularization on the sonographic appearance of liver metastases. In: Ferrucci J T, Mathieu D G. eds. Advances in hepatic radiology. St Louis: Mosby. 1990: p 109–128

45 Marchal G J, Pylyser K, Tshibwabwa-Tumba E A, et al. Anechoic halo in solid liver tumors: sonographic, microangiographic, and histologic correlation. Radiology 1985; 156: 479–483

46 Marchal G, Tshibwabwa-Tumba E, Oyen R, Pylyser K, Goddeeris R. Correlation of sonographic patterns with histology and microangiography. Invest Radiol 1985; 20: 79–84

47 Tanaka S, Kitamura T, Imaoka S. Hepatocellular carcinoma: sonographic and histological correlation. AJR 1983; 140: 701–707

48 Schonland M M, Milward-Sadler G H, Wright D H, Wright R. Hepatic tumours. In: Wright R, Alberti K G, Karran S, Milward-Sadler G H. Liver and biliary diseases. London: Saunders. 1979: p 919

49 Federle M P, Filly R A, Moss A A. Cystic hepatic neoplasms: complementary roles of CT and ultrasonography. AJR 1981; 136: 345–348

50 Schlauri H, Hacki W H, von Schulthess G K, Stamm B. Liver apudoma simulating cystic liver. Dtsch Med Wochenschr 1987; 112: 1986–1989

51 Reading N G, Forbes A, Nunnerley H B, Williams R. Hepatic haemangioma: a critical review of diagnosis and management. Q J Med 1988; 67: 431–445

52 Yasuhara K, Kimura K, Ohto M, et al. Pulsed Doppler in the

53 Taylor K J, Ramos I, Morse S S, Fortune K L, Hammers L, Taylor C R. Focal liver masses: differential diagnosis with pulsed Doppler US. Radiology 1987; 164: 643–647

54 Brambs H J, Spamer C, Volk B, Wimmer B, Koch H. Histological diagnosis of liver hemangiomas using ultrasound-guided fine needle biopsy. Hepatogastroenterology 1985; 32: 284–287

55 Freeny P C, Marks W M. Patterns of contrast enhancement of benign and malignant hepatic neoplasms during bolus dynamic and delayed CT. Radiology 1986; 160: 613–618

56 Suramo I, Lahde S. Computed tomography of small asymptomatic haemangiomas of the liver. Acta Radiol Diagn 1982; 23: 577–583

57 Brick S H, Hill M C, Lande I M. The mistaken or indeterminate CT diagnosis of hepatic metastases: the value of sonography. AJR 1987; 148: 723–726

58 Chafetz N, Taylor A, Alazraki N P, Gosink B B. The heterogeneous liver scan: ultrasound correlation. Radiology 1979; 130: 201–213

59 Scholmerich J, Volk B A, Gerok W. Value and limitations of abdominal ultrasound in tumour staging – liver metastases and lymphoma. Eur J Radiol 1987; 7: 243–245

60 Sandler M A, Petrocelli R D, Marks D S, Lopez R U. Ultrasonic features and radionuclide correlation in liver cell adenoma and focal nodular hyperplasia. Radiology 1980; 135: 393–397

61 Kerlin P, Davis G L, McGill D B, Weil L H, Adson M A, Sheedy P F. Hepatic adenoma and focal nodular hyperplasia: clinical, pathologic, and radiologic features. Gastroenterology 1983; 84: 994–1002

62 Kawashima A, Suehiro S, Murayama S, Russell W J. Focal fatty infiltration of the liver mimicking a tumor: sonographic and CT features. J Comput Assist Tomogr 1986; 10: 329–331

63 Kissin C M, Bellamy E A, Cosgrove D O, Slack N, Husband J E. Focal sparing in fatty infiltration of the liver. Br J Radiol 1986; 59: 25–28

64 Maxwell A J, Mamtora H. Fungal liver abscesses in acute leukaemia – a report of two cases. Clin Radiol 1988; 39: 197–201

65 Tanascescu D E, Waxman A D, Drickman M V, et al. Liver scanning in colon carcinoma. Radiology 1982; 145: 453–455

66 Ostfield D A, Meyer J A. Liver scanning in cancer patients with short interval autopsy correlation. Radiology 1981; 138: 671–673

67 McGarrity T J, Samuels T, Wilson F A. An analysis of imaging studies and liver function tests to detect hepatic neoplasia. Dig Dis Sci 1987; 32: 1113–1117

68 Rogers J V, Mack L A, Freeny P C, Johnson M L, Sones P J. Hepatic focal nodular hyperplasia: angiography, CT, sonography and scintigraphy. AJR 1981; 137: 983–990

69 Khan O, Ell P J, Jarrit P H, Cullum I D, Williams E D. Comparison between emission and transmission computed tomography of the liver. BMJ 1981; 283: 1212–1214

70 Moldofsky P J, Powe J, Mulhern C B Jnr, et al. Metastatic colon carcinoma detected with radiolabeled F(ab')2 monoclonal antibody fragments. Radiology 1983; 149: 549–555

71 Foley W D, Berland L L, Lawson T L, Smith D F, Thorsen M K. Contrast enhancement for dynamic hepatic computed tomographic scanning. Radiology 1983; 147: 797–803

72 Alderson P O, Adams D F, McNeil B J, et al. Computed tomography, ultrasound and scintigraphy of the liver in patients with colon or breast carcinoma: a prospective study. Radiology 1983; 149: 225–230

73 Flowerdew A D, Taylor I. Pre-operative scanning of the liver for colorectal liver metastases. Scand J Gastroenterol Suppl 1988; 149: 62–80

74 Smith T J, Kemeny M M, Sugarbaker P H, et al. A prospective study of hepatic imaging in the detection of metastatic disease. Ann Surg 1982; 195: 486–491

75 Finlay I G, Meek D R, Gray H W, Duncan J G, McArdle C S. Incidence and detection of occult hepatic metastases in colorectal carcinoma. BMJ 1982; 284: 803–805

76 Parker G A, Lawrence W Jnr, Horsley J S 3d, et al. Intraoperative ultrasound of the liver affects operative decision making. Ann Surg 1989; 209: 569–576

77 Igawa S, Sakai K, Kinoshita H, Hirohashi K. Intraoperative

sonography: clinical usefulness in liver surgery. Radiology 1985;
156: 473–478

78 Cilizza S, Lupatelli R, De Fazio S, Preziosi P, Karakachi F,
Cucchiara G. Combined ultrasound and CEA in the preoperative
assessment of hepatic metastases from gastrointestinal malignancies.
J Surg Oncol 1985; 28: 161–164

79 Cave-Bigley D J, Lamb G H. The value of pre-operative
ultrasound of the liver in colonic and gastric neoplasia. Br J Radiol
1985; 58: 13–14

80 Silberstein E B, Gilbert L A, Pu M Y. Comparative efficacy of
radionuclide, ultrasound and computed tomography for hepatic
metastases. Concepts Diagn Nucl Med 1985; 2: 3–12

81 Huber K, Heuhold N. Rapid diagnosis of liver cancer by
ultrasound-guided fine-needle aspiration biopsy. Cancer Detect
Prev 1987; 10: 383–387

82 Limberg B, Hopker W W, Kommerell B. Histological differential
diagnosis of focal liver lesions by ultrasonically guided fine needle
biopsy. Gut 1987; 28: 237–241

83 Schreiber M H. Wilson's law of diminishing returns (Editorial).
AJR 1982; 138: 786–788

84 Curati W L, Halevy A, Gibson R N, Carr D H, Blumgart L H,
Steiner R E. Ultrasound, CT, and MRI: comparison in primary
and secondary tumors of the liver. Gastrointest Radiol 1988;
13: 123–128

85 Gozzetti G, Mazziotti A, Bolondi L, et al. Intraoperative
ultrasonography in surgery for liver tumors. Surgery 1986;
99: 523–530

86 Simeone J T. Intraoperative ultrasonography of liver tumours. In:
Ferrucci J T, Mathieu D G. eds. Advances in hepatobiliary
radiology. New York: Mosby. 1990: p 229–238

87 Castaing D, Garden O J, Bismuth H. Segmental liver resection
using ultrasound-guided selective portal venous occlusion. Ann
Surg 1989; 210: 20–23

88 Machi J, Isomoto H, Kurohiji T, et al. Detection of unrecognized
liver metastases from colorectal cancers by routine use of operative
ultrasonography. Dis Colon Rectum 1986; 29: 405–409

89 Parker K J, Tuthill T A, Lerner R M, Violante M R. A
particulate contrast agent with potential for ultrasound imaging of
liver. Ultrasound Med Biol 1987; 13: 555–566

90 Mattrey R F, Strich G, Shelton R E, et al. Perfluorochemicals as
US contrast agents for tumor imaging and hepatosplenography:
preliminary clinical results. Radiology 1987; 163: 339–343

91 Matsuda Y, Yabuuchi I. Hepatic tumors: ultrasound contrast
enhancement with CO_2 microbubbles. Radiology 1986; 161: 701–705

92 Hilpert P L, Mattrey R F, Mitten R M, Peterson T A D. IV
injection of air-filled human albumin microspheres to enhance
arterial Doppler signals: a preliminary study in rabbits. AJR 1989;
153: 613–616

Diffuse liver disease

Henry C. Irving

INTRODUCTION

The assessment of the echoes from the liver parenchyma forms part of virtually every upper abdominal ultrasound examination, and yet the information derived from these ultrasound reflections is one of the least well-utilised facets of ultrasound scanning.

The normal liver parenchyma returns a homogeneous background of low level echoes within which the normal hepatic and portal venous structures can be identified. Various pathological processes may result in either increase or decrease in echo amplitude, disturbances in echo pattern, and alterations in the size of the liver. All these ultrasound features need to be evaluated whenever the liver is examined.

Echo amplitude

The echo amplitude of the liver parenchyma can be assessed by comparing it with the reflectivity of the renal parenchyma and the portal vein walls.

The amplitude of the parenchymal liver echoes is slightly higher than those returned from the renal cortex at the same depth in the image (Fig. 1A). It is important that the comparison is between echoes at similar depths in order to avoid errors introduced by the application of swept gain (time-gain compensation). Obviously, the comparison is only valid if the renal parenchyma is itself normal; many intrinsic renal diseases affect the reflectivity of the renal parenchyma and may lead to false diagnoses of liver disease if this is not recognised (Fig. 1B).

The echoes from the walls of the portal venous radicles should be of higher amplitude than the adjacent liver parenchyma, so that these vessel walls can be resolved as clear white lines (Fig. 2A). Loss of this clarity of the portal vein wall echoes is a reliable indicator of increased reflectivity of the liver parenchyma (Fig. 2B).[1] Conversely, the portal vein wall echoes may become unduly prominent signifying reduced reflectivity of the liver parenchyma – the so-called 'dark liver'.

Attenuation

Loss in amplitude with depth is attenuation, and attempts to measure attenuation are a logical extension of the visual assessment of liver parenchymal reflectivity described above. Normal liver parenchyma attenuates the ultrasound beam at around 0.5 dB/MHz/cm of path length (or 1 dB/MHz/cm of depth) and it has been shown that abnormal liver parenchyma does show either increased or decreased attenuation.[2] Attenuation may be measured using the reflected signal amplitude or alternatively by using frequency shift (based on the principle that higher frequencies are attenuated more rapidly than lower, resulting in a shift in spectral content towards the lower

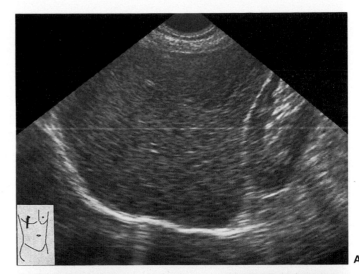

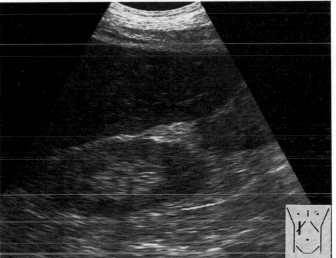

Fig. 1 Relationship between renal and hepatic echoes. A: Scan to show relationship between echo amplitude of normal liver and normal renal parenchyma. B: Scan to show abnormal kidney with increased parenchymal echoes giving false diagnosis of 'dark' liver.

frequencies). Many studies have been performed to evaluate the different methods of measuring liver attenuation and to correlate the changes in attenuation with pathological processes[2-6] and, whilst some encouraging results have been published, the techniques have not yet been adopted for general clinical use (see Vol. 2, Ch. 57).

Echo pattern

The other component of echo texture that can be assessed visually is echo pattern. Normal liver parenchyma consists of interleaving linear echoes that are uniform in size and shape, forming a homogeneous network. These echoes may become finer and more closely packed (Fig. 3A), coarser and more loosely arranged (Fig. 3B), or irregular and non-

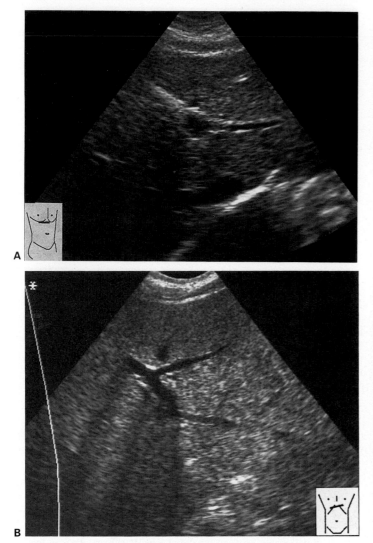

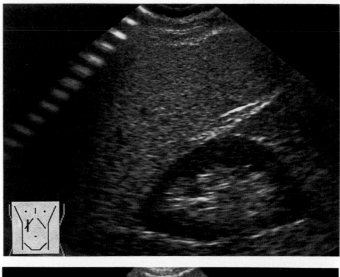

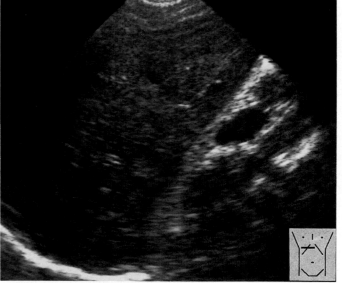

Fig. 2   Periportal echoes. A: Scan to show normal portal vein wall echoes standing out from adjacent liver parenchyma. **B:** Loss of portal vein wall echo indicating 'bright' liver.

Fig. 3   Abnormal echo patterns in 'bright' liver. A: Fine, closely packed echoes. **B:** Coarse, loosely arranged echoes.

uniform in size, shape and pattern – according to the nature of the pathology. However, it must be realised that the apparent 'texture' of the liver is at least as dependent on technical factors in the ultrasound scanner as on liver architecture. There is not a one-to-one correlation between small scale liver anatomy and the ultrasound echo pattern.

Liver size

Estimation of liver size has long been one of the key components of a general physical examination and ultrasound imaging offers a scientific approach to this assessment (see Ch. 14). Because of the complex shape of the liver, accurate volume estimation of the organ is tedious and time consuming,[7,8] and investigators have shown that unidimensional longitudinal measurements,[9,10] or bi-dimensional longitudinal and transverse measurements[11] can quantitate hepatomegaly accurately. A useful single measurement is the longitudinal mid-clavicular diameter, which is less than 13 cm in over 95% of normals.[10] However, most ultrasonographers find that a subjective assessment of liver size, using reference organs such as the kidneys and observations of shape and surface contours, is sufficiently accurate for clinical purposes, and measurements tend to be reserved for therapeutic trials when serial estimation of liver size is required.

Accuracy

Using the ultrasound criteria described above, questions arise as to the reliability of ultrasound in predicting the presence of diffuse parenchymal liver disease, its accuracy in suggesting the correct histological diagnosis and the possibility of replacing the invasive liver biopsy. While many workers agree that ultrasound is a sensitive technique for distinguishing normal from abnormal liver,[10,12–20] there has been much less confidence over the ability of ultrasound to specify individual pathological processes such as steatosis and fibrosis[13,14,17–22] and the consensus is that liver biopsy for histological diagnosis remains the 'gold standard', although ultrasound has much to offer in detecting and monitoring liver disease and its complications.

Fatty infiltration

The accumulation of fatty droplets within hepatocytes occurs in response to a variety of injuries to the liver that interfere with normal metabolism, deficiency of lipotropic factors or transportation of abnormally large amounts of fat to the liver cells. The more important causes encompass a long list including alcohol, diabetes mellitus, obesity, pregnancy, drugs (especially corticosteroids) and toxic substances, malnutrition due to dietary deficiency or wasting diseases, parenteral hyperalimentation and inborn errors of metabolism.[23,24] Fatty infiltration is a dynamic process: its severity may alter rapidly, over weeks or even days,[25,26] and is usually completely reversible.[16,27]

Ultrasound appearances

Fat causes increased reflectivity,[28] presumably due to the interfaces produced by the multiple fat droplets producing increased echo amplitude of the liver parenchyma, giving the typical appearances of a 'bright liver'.[14,19,21,23] The echo pattern is usually that of fine, closely packed echoes (Fig. 4),[22,23] and there is often hepatomegaly (75% of cases[23]) which is a helpful distinguishing feature from cirrhosis, when the liver is normal in size or shrunken.[29]

It is the fat which is predominantly responsible for the increased attenuation of the ultrasound beam that is seen in some 'bright livers', and this feature may also be used to distinguish fatty infiltration from other causes of this ultrasound appearance.[2,6,18,30] It is important that as high a frequency transducer as possible (e.g. 5 MHz) be used in order to optimise the detection of increased attenuation if mild degrees of fatty infiltration are not to be missed.[20,22]

However, whilst ultrasound is highly sensitive for the detection of fatty infiltration (sensitivity 86% for mild and almost 100% for moderate and severe degrees[22]) the specificity is lower, probably due to the fact that fatty infiltration may develop concurrently with other pathological changes such as fibrosis in many of the conditions listed above.

Focal fatty infiltration

Fatty infiltration is commonly a generalised process, affect-

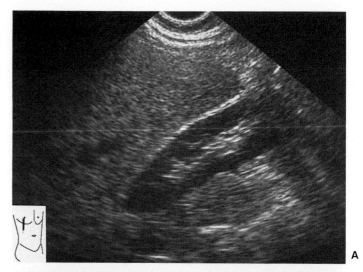

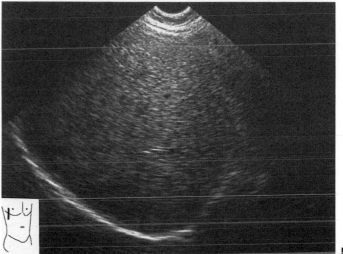

Fig. 4 Fatty liver. A and **B:** Longitudinal sections to show the increased reflectivity of the 'bright' liver. Note that the liver is enlarged with increased attenuation so that the deeper parts of the liver are not imaged.

ing the entire liver volume in a uniform fashion and causing a diffuse abnormality. However, this is not always the case: fatty infiltration may be patchy, i.e. lobar, segmental or sub-segmental in distribution, when it is known as focal fatty infiltration (or focal steatosis).[31,32]

In these situations, regions of increased reflectivity form adjacent to regions of normal liver echo texture. The boundaries are often angulated or geometric in shape or there may be characteristic interdigitating margins.[33] Regions of fatty infiltration have no mass effect and normal vessels can be seen to pass through the affected portions of liver without displacement.[34] These features usually allow a confident ultrasonographic diagnosis to be made – but the differentiation from highly reflective metastatic deposits may be difficult when the fatty infiltration results in single or multiple discrete areas of increased reflectivity (Fig. 5).[27,35–37]

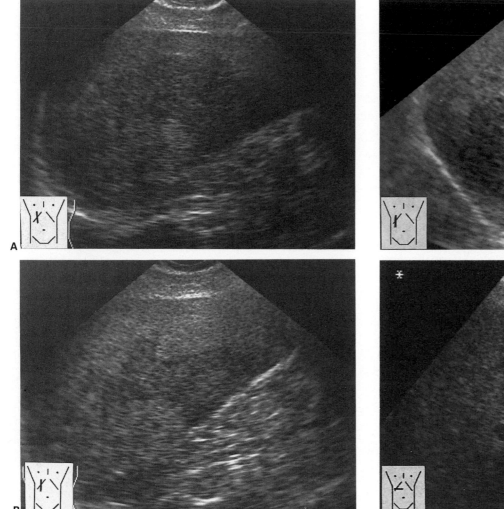

Fig. 5 Focal fatty infiltration. A and **B:** Two longitudinal sections showing the geographic areas of increased reflectivity typical of irregular fatty infiltration.

Fig. 6 Focal fatty sparing. A: Geographic echo-poor area in the posterior portion of the right lobe and **B:** similar region in a typical position close to the gallbladder. Both are due to focal sparing in extensive but incomplete fatty change.

Fatty infiltration with focal areas of sparing

Similar diagnostic dilemmas may be encountered when the fatty infiltration is almost totally uniform but there are single or multiple islands of liver which are spared. These regions of normal liver echo texture appear reduced in echo amplitude in comparison to the surrounding 'bright liver' and may be misinterpreted as echo-poor lesions (Fig. 6).[38]

Typical sites of focal fatty sparing are the quadrate lobe anterior to the portal vein bifurcation, areas adjacent to the gallbladder fossa, and subsegmental subcapsular regions.[39–41] The location of these spared areas has led to speculation that there is a vascular factor associated with the aetiology of this phenomenon,[42] such as the presence of portosystemic venous collaterals permitting shunting which may act as protection from the fatty infiltration.[39]

Cirrhosis

The pathological features of cirrhosis of the liver are parenchymal destruction with nodular regeneration and fibrosis resulting in architectural distortion. It is an end result of a wide variety of causes which may be classified on either an aetiological or morphological basis, or using a combination of both systems.

Ultrasound appearances

The ultrasound appearances are not specific for any particular type of cirrhosis and, whilst some cirrhotic livers may appear normal on ultrasound scans, abnormalities can be recognised in approximately two thirds of cases.[21,12] The essential ultrasonographic features are increased reflectivity

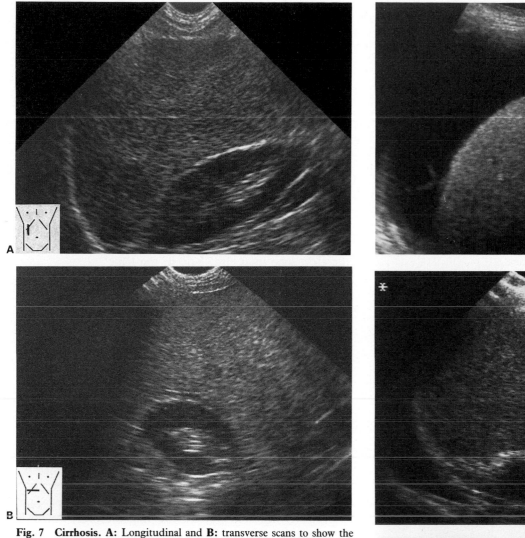

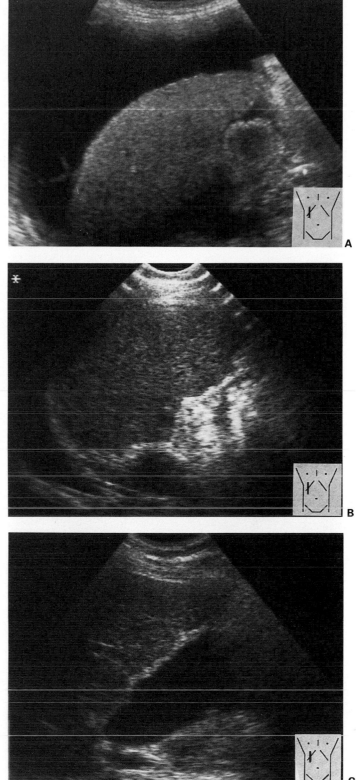

Fig. 7 Cirrhosis. A: Longitudinal and **B:** transverse scans to show the increased echo amplitude and irregular echo pattern without increase in attenuation typical of cirrhosis without additional fatty change.

of the fibrous tissue and a concomitant loss of definition of portal vein walls[16,18,19,21] but no significant increase in attenuation,[2,5,6] disturbance of echo pattern, which is usually coarse and irregular,[15] although the echoes can be fine and even[12] and a generalised heterogeneity of texture partly corresponding to the disorganisation of structure seen pathologically (Fig. 7).[16]

The lack of attenuation of the ultrasound beam by fibrosis is useful in distinguishing fibrosis from fatty infiltration[2,5,6] but, especially in alcoholic disease, the two pathologies often coexist, causing confusion.[16] However, some workers have been able to identify the coarse echo pattern of fibrosis in the background of the fine echo pattern of fatty infiltration and have suggested that the mixed pattern of pathologies is recognisable on ultrasound.[22]

Regenerative nodules may give a generalised granularity to the liver echo texture in forms of micronodular cirrhosis,

Fig. 8 Nodular liver surface. A: Nodularity of the liver surface is most easily seen when there is ascites. **B:** In the absence of ascites the nodularity may be apparent on the inferior liver surface. Note the right pleural effusion. **C:** A distended gallbladder facilitates assessment of the inferior surface of the liver, revealing mild nodularity in this case.

while the larger nodules of macronodular disease may give an ultrasonically recognisable surface nodularity. Surface nodularity is most easily detected in the presence of ascites; otherwise it can be identified by careful examination of the inferior surface of the liver, especially in relation to the gallbladder and right kidney (Fig. 8). Larger nodules may mimic tumour masses[43] – an awkward differential diagnosis since cirrhosis is a risk factor for hepatoma and ultrasound is used to screen for this complication (Fig. 9) (see Ch. 17).[44] Since most hepatomas are vascular while regenerating nodules are not, Doppler studies are helpful in this problem (see Ch. 17).

The morphology of the liver may assist in the ultrasound diagnosis of cirrhosis. Although a cirrhotic liver may be normal in size, the liver tends to shrink as the disease progresses. Furthermore, the right lobe of the liver may shrink while the caudate lobe occupies a relatively larger proportion of the liver volume.[45] A ratio of caudate lobe to right lobe can be derived from a transverse scan of the liver immediately below the portal vein bifurcation: this is less than 0.6 in normals (see Ch. 14), it is greater than 0.65 in cirrhosis with 100% specificity but sensitivities of 84% and 43% in two different series.[45,46] Similar results have been obtained for right lobe to left lobe longitudinal diameter ratios,[29] and the two later studies found that the sensitivity rates were higher in post-necrotic (post-hepatitic) cirrhosis than in the alcohol related disease.

Shrinkage of the right lobe with sparing or hypertrophy of the caudate and/or left lobes is thought to be related to the vascular anatomy – probably the arrangement of venous drainage which leads to more extensive fibrosis and relatively less compensatory hypertrophy and regeneration in the right lobe than elsewhere in the liver.

Other ultrasound findings in cirrhosis are related to the complications associated with hepatocellular failure and portal hypertension; these include ascites, splenomegaly, the development of collateral venous channels and other abnormalities of the portal venous system, all of which are discussed in detail in Chapter 19.

Hepatitis

Acute viral hepatitis

The main value of ultrasound in acute viral hepatitis is in excluding an obstructive (surgical) cause of jaundice (see Ch. 13) but, once bile duct dilatation has been excluded, the ultrasonographer may be able to suggest hepatitis as the underlying aetiology of the hepatocellular (medical) jaundice.

The so-called 'dark liver' of ultrasound refers to an appearance in which the portal vein walls appear of higher echo amplitude than usual in comparison to the surrounding liver parenchyma, which appears less reflective than normal (Fig. 10). This appearance has also been termed the 'centrilobular pattern'[19,47] and is thought to be caused by the cellular swelling and oedema in the centrilobular portion of the liver lobules with sparing of the portal tracts. However, although in the original description, the centrilobular pattern was seen in 13 of 16 patients with acute hepatitis,[47] a later study which include 791 patients with acute hepatitis failed to show a significant increase in the incidence of this pattern in the hepatitis patients over a control group (32% and 31% respectively).[48] Another often striking feature of acute hepatitis is marked thickening of the gallbladder wall (see Ch. 12). This may also be seen, to a lesser extent, in patients with a wide variety of chronic liver diseases.

The 'dark liver' appearance has also been observed in leukaemic infiltration,[47] toxic shock syndrome,[49] congestive cardiac failure, AIDS,[50] and radiation injury,[51] as well

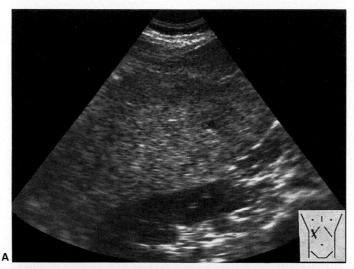

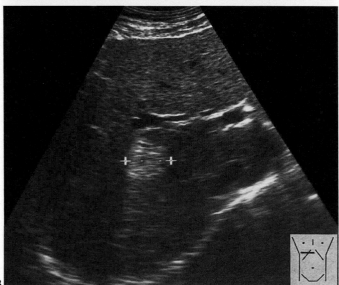

Fig. 9 Cirrhosis. A: The nodular echo pattern is shown in this case with advanced cirrhosis. **B:** The mass of increased reflectivity represents a hepatoma.

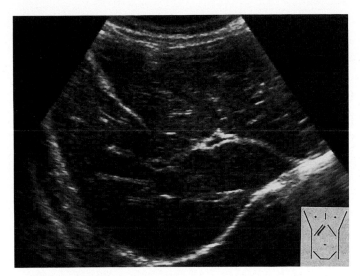

Fig. 10 'Dark' liver (centrilobular) pattern.

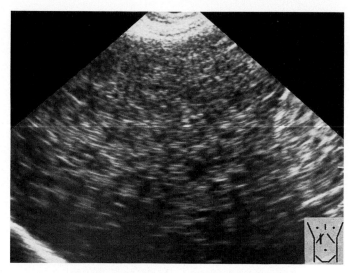

Fig. 11 **Granulomatous hepatitis** – 'target lesion' representing a granuloma. (Figure courtesy of Dr A. Joseph.)

as in normals,[42] so caution must be advised in the clinical application of this ultrasound sign.

Acute alcoholic hepatitis

Acute alcoholic hepatitis can vary from a mild anicteric illness to fulminant hepatic failure. It may be completely reversible but may progress to frank cirrhosis. The liver is almost always enlarged, there is increased reflectivity and attenuation.[16,52]

These appearances of an enlarged 'bright' liver are indistinguishable from other causes of fatty infiltration and the ultrasound appearances must be correlated with the clinical history.

Chronic hepatitis

The classification of chronic hepatitis is complex but the underlying pathological changes that give rise to abnormal ultrasound findings are diffuse inflammation with varying degrees and distributions of necrosis, fatty change and fibrosis.

The ultrasound findings are of increased parenchymal reflectivity and altered echo patterns. Increased attenuation is not a marked feature of chronic hepatitis but sometimes occurs, depending upon the amount of fatty infiltration and necrosis as compared to fibrosis.[13,47]

Granulomatous hepatitis

Some chronic inflammatory diseases characteristically form granulomata. In these, epithelioid macrophages and tissue histiocytes aggregate and become surrounded by small lymphocytes while multinucleated giant cells may be formed by the coalescence of epithelioid cells. In tuber-culosis the granulomata often undergo central necrosis (caseation) and subsequent fibrosis and calcification.

Granulomatous liver diseases may produce a 'bright liver' indistinguishable from other causes[50,53] but it has been reported that the granulomata can be recognised as small, moderately reflective lesions 3 to 5 mm in diameter surrounded by an echo-poor halo (Fig. 11).[53] These granulomata have been seen in tuberculosis, sarcoidosis and brucellosis, and echo-poor nodules in tuberculous hepatitis have been confused with metastatic disease.[54,55]

Infestations

Infestations of the liver are well-described as causes of focal lesions on ultrasound scans (see Ch. 16). However, on a world-wide basis, the single most common infestation of the liver is by the blood fluke *Schistosoma mansoni* which causes a form of cirrhosis that eventually results in portal hypertension.

Marked fibrosis occurs around the portal tracts throughout the liver in response to a granulomatous re-action caused by the parasite implanting along portal vein branches. This is referred to pathologically as 'pipe-stem fibrosis' and is seen on ultrasound as increased reflectivity and thickening of portal vein walls. This ultrasound pattern of periportal fibrosis is typical of schistosomiasis.[56–58] Although splenomegaly usually coexists, in endemic areas the ultrasound appearance of the liver may be the only clue to the diagnosis of hepatosplenic schistosomiasis[56,59] and ultrasound has been used to assess the success of a large scale chemotherapy programme.[60]

Cystic fibrosis

Liver disease in cystic fibrosis becomes commoner with

age, and is thus seen more frequently as patients survive the respiratory complications of the disease and live longer. Fatty infiltration may occur, giving the typical ultrasound features, but it is of little clinical consequence. Of more importance is a distinctive type of focal biliary cirrhosis with eosinophilic concretions; in approximately 5% of cases this progresses to a multilobular biliary cirrhosis, eventually giving rise to portal hypertension.

The clinical diagnosis of liver involvement is difficult because overinflation of the lungs makes assessment of liver and spleen size unreliable and biochemical liver function tests are unhelpful because of the focal nature of the disease.

Ultrasound of the liver may show diffuse or patchy increase in reflectivity[61] and accentuation of the periportal echoes has also been described,[62,63] as has an irregularity of the liver edge[64] – presumably indicating surface nodularity (Fig. 12).

While these appearances are not specific, their detection will alert the clinician to the development of liver disease and serial scans may be useful in monitoring progress.

Biliary cirrhosis

Biliary cirrhosis is divided into primary and secondary depending on the aetiology.

Primary biliary cirrhosis

The aetiology of primary biliary cirrhosis remains obscure but autoimmune factors are implicated; the disease is far more common in females. It typically presents with pruritis in middle aged women and progresses slowly giving rise to jaundice after an interval of several years. Ultrasound imaging is disappointing, the size and appearances of the

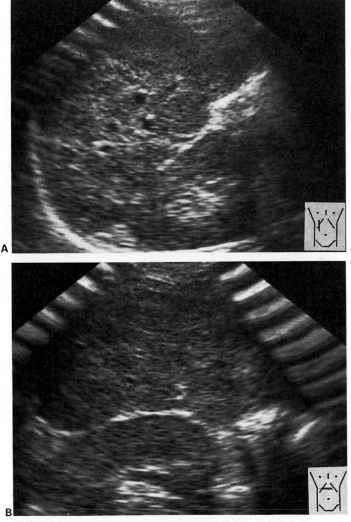

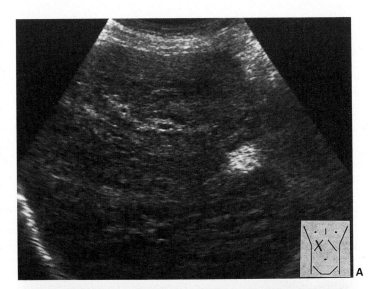

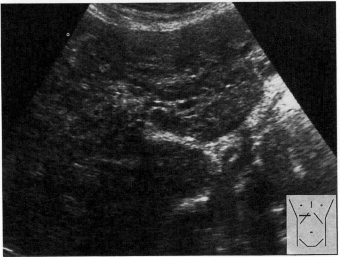

Fig. 12 Cystic fibrosis. A: Longitudinal and **B:** transverse scans to show diffuse changes and patchy (periportal) changes.

Fig. 13 Primary biliary cirrhosis. A: Longitudinal and **B:** transverse scans. Note the prominent periportal reflectivity and coarse, slightly irregular texture of the liver.

liver being normal.[13] There is, however, usually evidence of portal hypertension and splenomegaly is invariably present. In a minority of advanced cases textural changes are shown consisting of coarse nodularity and accentuation of the portal tracts (Fig. 13). Very rarely the liver may be small in size with a nodular surface. There is a significant increase in the incidence of gallstones in primary biliary cirrhosis, many patients having required cholecystectomy prior to diagnosis.

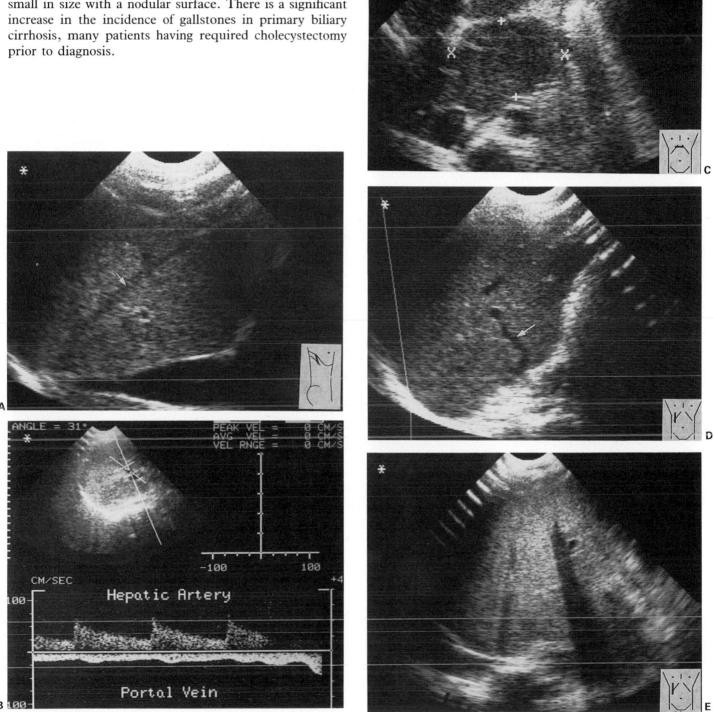

Fig. 14 Budd Chiari syndrome. A: Thrombus (arrow) within a major hepatic vein. **B:** Reverse flow in the portal vein with a compensatory increase in hepatic arterial flow. **C:** In this well-established case, the caudate lobe (+X) shows marked enlargement. **D:** Serpiginous dilated peripheral segment of an hepatic vein (arrow). **E:** Focal areas of attenuation with acoustic shadowing.

Secondary biliary cirrhosis

Secondary biliary cirrhosis arises as a result of long-standing bile duct obstruction. The dilated ducts may be apparent but often are remarkably minor. There are no characteristic ultrasound findings apart from those relating to the initiating cause (e.g. Caroli's disease, choledochal cyst, bile duct stricture).

Budd Chiari syndrome

This syndrome is caused by partial or complete obstruction of the hepatic venous outflow. The obstruction may be central or peripheral and is occasionally a result of inferior vena caval web but is more frequently associated with hypercoagulable states. If the venous obstruction is complete and of rapid onset, patients usually die of acute liver failure. Those that present for imaging investigations usually have a disease of slow onset and sparing of one or more of the major hepatic veins.

The ultrasound features in the acute phase are of hepatomegaly and ascites and relatively normal spleen size. Thrombus may be seen within the major hepatic veins (Fig. 14A) and there is often reverse flow in the portal vein (Fig. 14B). As the disease progresses there is compensatory hypertrophy of the caudate lobe (Fig. 14C), often with the detection of dilated serpiginous veins (Fig. 14D) and there is progressive splenomegaly. In long-standing Budd Chiari syndrome the liver texture is abnormal, often with small focal areas of high attenuation giving rise to acoustic shadowing (Fig. 14E).

Conclusions

Ultrasound can provide a great deal of useful information about the nature and extent of diffuse liver disease, although the differential diagnosis usually remains wide (Tables 1 and 2), and liver biopsy for histological diagnosis remains the final arbiter.[65] Even in this context, ultrasound has a role to play in guiding biopsy needles in order to maximise diagnostic accuracy and safety. It should also be noted that ultrasound can be used for guiding 'plugged' biopsies, so enabling tissue cores to be obtained from patients in whom the liver disease has rendered conventional biopsy unsafe due to impaired blood coagulation.[66,67]

Table 1 Causes of the 'bright' liver

Fatty infiltration[14,21]
Cirrhosis[12,13]
Chronic hepatitis[13,47]
Alcoholic hepatitis[16,52]
Granulomatous hepatitis[53]
Chronic congestive cardiac failure[13]
Portal fibrosis[13]
Schistosomiasis[56,58]
Cystic fibrosis[61,62]
Glycogen storage (Gaucher's) disease[6]
Niemann-Pick disease[6]

Table 2 Causes of the 'dark' liver

Acute viral hepatitis[47,48]
Congestive cardiac failure
Leukaemic infiltration[47]
Toxic shock syndrome[49]
AIDS[50]
Radiation injury[51]
Normal[48]

REFERENCES

1 Kurtz A B, Dubbins P A, Rubin C S. Echogenicity: analysis, significance, and masking. AJR 1981; 137: 471

2 Taylor K J W, Riely C A, Flax S, Weltin G, Kuc R, Barwick K W. Quantitative US attenuation in normal liver and in patients with diffuse liver disease: importance of fat. Radiology 1986; 160: 65–71

3 Ralls P W, Johnson M B, Kanel G, et al. FM sonography in diffuse liver disease: prospective assessment and blinded analysis. Radiology 1986; 161: 451–454

4 Aufrichtig D, Lottenberg S, Hoefs J, et al. Frequency-demodulated US: evaluation in the liver. Radiology 1986; 160: 59–64

5 Kuni C C, Johnson T K, Crass J R, Snover D C. Correlation of Fourier spectral shift-determined hepatic acoustic attenuation coefficients with liver biopsy findings. J Ultrasound Med 1989; 8: 631–634

6 Garra B S, Insana M F, Shawker T H, Russell M A. Quantitative estimation of liver attenuation and echogenicity: normal state versus diffuse liver disease. Radiology 1987; 162: 61–67

7 Rasmussen S N. Liver volume determination by ultrasonic scanning. Br J Radiol 1972; 45: 579–585

8 VanThiel D H, Hagler N G, Scade R R, et al. In vivo hepatic volume determination using sonography and computed tomography. Gastroenterology 1985; 88: 1812

9 Gosink B B, Laymaster C E. Ultrasonic determination of hepatomegaly. JCU 1981; 9: 37

10 Niederau C, Sonnenberg A. Liver size evaluated by ultrasound: ROC curves for hepatitis and alcoholism. Radiology 1984; 153: 503

11 Niederau C, Sonnenberg A, Muller J E, Erckenbrecht J F, Scholten T, Fritsch W P. Sonographic measurements of the normal liver, spleen, pancreas, and portal vein. Radiology 1983; 149: 537–540

12 Dewbury K C, Clark B. The accuracy of ultrasound in the detection of cirrhosis of the liver. Br J Radiol 1979; 52: 945–948

13 Joseph A E, Dewbury K C, McGuire P G. Ultrasound in the detection of chronic liver disease (the 'bright' liver). Br J Radiol 1979; 52: 184–188

14 Foster K J, Dewbury K C, Griffith A H, Wright R. The accuracy of ultrasound in the detection of fatty infiltration of the liver. Br J Radiol 1980; 53: 440–442

15 Debongie J C, Pauls C, Fievez, Wibin E. Prospective evaluation of the diagnostic accuracy of liver ultrasonography. Gut 1981; 22: 130

16 Taylor K J W, Gorelick F S, Rosenfield A T, Riely C A. Ultrasonography of alcoholic liver disease with histological correlation. Radiology 1981; 141: 157–161

17 Meek D R, Mills P R, Gray H W, Duncan J G, Russel R I, McKillop J H. A comparison of computed tomography, ultrasound

and scintigraphy in the diagnosis of alcoholic liver disease. Br J Radiol 1984; 57: 23–27

18 Sanford N L, Walsh P, Matis C, Baddeley H, Powell L W. Is ultrasonography useful in the assessment of diffuse parenchymal liver disease? Gastroenterology 1985; 89: 186–191

19 Needleman L, Kurtz A B, Rifkin M D, Cooper H S, Pasto M E, Goldberg B B. Sonography of diffuse benign liver disease: accuracy of pattern recognition and grading. AJR 1986; 146: 1011–1015

20 Saverymuttu S H, Joseph A E, Maxwell J D. Ultrasound scanning in the detection of hepatic fibrosis and steatosis. BMJ 1986; 292: 13–15

21 Gosink B B, Lemon S K, Scheible W, Leopold G R. Accuracy of ultrasonography in diagnosis of hepatocellular disease. AJR 1979; 133: 19–23

22 Joseph A E A, Saverymuttu S H, Al-Sam S, Cook M G, Maxwell J D. Comparison of liver histology with ultrasonography in assessing diffuse parenchymal liver disease. Clin Radiol 1991; 43: 26–31

23 Scatarige J C, Scott W W, Donovan P J, Seigelman S S, Sanders R C. Fatty infiltration of the liver: ultrasonographic and computed tomographic correlation. J Ultrasound Med 1984; 3: 9–14

24 Campillo B, Bernuau J, Witz M O, et al. Ultrasonogrphy in acute fatty liver of pregnancy. Ann Intern Med 1986; 105: 383–384

25 Bashist B, Hecht H L, Harley W D. Computed tomographic demonstration of rapid changes in fatty infiltration of the liver. Radiology 1982; 142: 691

26 Clain J E, Stephens D H, Charboneau J W. Ultrasonography and computed tomography in focal fatty liver. Report of two cases with special emphasis on changing appearances over time. Gastroenterology 1984; 87: 948

27 Swobodnik W, Wechsler J G, Manne W, Ditschuneit H. Multiple regular circumscript fatty infiltrations of the liver. JCU 1985; 13: 577–580

28 Behan M, Kazam E. The echographic characteristics of fatty tissues and tumors. Radiology 1978; 129: 143–151

29 Goyal A K, Pokharna D S, Sharma S K. Ultrasonic diagnosis of cirrhosis: reference to quantitative measurements of hepatic dimensions. Gastrointest Radiol 1990; 15: 32–34

30 Lin T, Ophir J, Potter G. Correlation of ultrasonic attenuation with pathologic fat and fibrosis in liver disease. Ultrasound Med Biol 1988; 14: 729–734

31 Scott W W Jnr, Sanders R C, Siegelman S S. Irregular fatty infiltration of the liver: diagnostic dilemmas. AJR 1980; 135: 67–71

32 Mulhern C B, Arger P H, Coleman B G, Stein G N. Nonuniform attenuation in computed tomography study of the cirrhotic liver. Radiology 1979; 132: 399

33 Quinn S F, Gosink B B. Characteristic sonographic signs of hepatic fatty infiltration. AJR 1985; 145: 753–755

34 Halvorsen R A, Korobkin M, Ram P C, Thompson W M. CT appearances of focal fatty infiltration of the liver. AJR 1982; 139: 277–281

35 Middleton W D. Sonography case of the day: focal hepatic fatty infiltration adjacent to falciform ligament. AJR 1989; 152: 1326–1327

36 Yoshikawa J, Matsui O, Takashima T, et al. Focal fatty change of the liver adjacent to the falciform ligament: CT and sonographic findings in five surgically confirmed cases. AJR 1987; 149: 491–494

37 Kawashima A, Suehiro S, Murayama S, Russell W J. Case report: focal fatty infiltration of the liver mimicking a tumour: sonographic and CT findings. J Comput Assist Tomogr 1986; 182: 239

38 Kissin C M, Bellamy E A, Cosgrove D O, Slack N, Husband J E. Focal sparing in fatty infiltration of the liver. Br J Radiol 1986; 59: 25–28

39 Marchal G, Tshibwabwa-Tumba E, Verbeken E, et al. 'Skip areas' in hepatic steatosis: a sonographic-angiographic correlation. Gastrointest Radiol 1986; 11: 151–157

40 Sauerbrei E E, Lopez M. Pseudotumor of the quadrate lobe in hepatic sonography: a sign of generalised fatty infiltration. AJR 1986; 147: 923–927

41 White E M, Simeone J F, Mueller P R, Grant E G, Choyke P L, Zeman R K. Focal periportal sparing in hepatic fatty infiltration: a cause of hepatic pseudomass on US. Radiology 1987; 162: 57–59

42 Arai K, Matsui O, Takashima T, Ida M, Nishida Y. Focal spared areas in fatty liver caused by regional decreased portal flow. AJR 1988; 151: 300–302

43 Okazaki N, Yoshida T, Yoshino M, Matue H. Screening of patients with chronic liver disease for hepatocellular carcinoma by ultrasonography. Clin Onc 1984; 10: 241

44 Cottone M, Marceno M P, Maringhini A, et al. Ultrasound in the diagnosis of hepatocellular carcinoma associated with cirrhosis. Radiology 1983; 147: 517–519

45 Harbin W P, Rabert N J, Ferrucci J T Jnr. Diagnosis of cirrhosis based on regional changes in hepatic morphology. A radiological and pathological analysis. Radiology 1980; 135: 273

46 Giorgio A, Amoroso P, Lettieri G, et al. Cirrhosis: value of caudate to right lobe ratio in diagnosis with US. Radiology 1986; 161: 443

47 Kurta A B, Rubin C S, Cooper H S, et al. Ultrasound findings in hepatitis. Radiology 1980; 136: 717–723

48 Giorgio A, Amoroso P, Fico P, et al. Ultrasound evaluation of uncomplicated and complicated acute viral hepatitis. JCU 1986; 14: 675–679

49 Lieberman J M, Bryan P J, Cohen A M. Toxic shock syndrome: sonographic appearances of the liver. AJR 1981; 137: 606

50 Grumbach K, Coleman B G, Gal A A, et al. Hepatic and biliary tract abnormalities in patients with AIDS. Sonographic-pathologic correlation. J Ultrasound Med 1989; 8: 247–254

51 Garra B S, Shawker T H, Chang R, Kaplan K, White R D. The ultrasound appearance of radiation-induced hepatic injury. Correlation with computed tomography and magnetic resonance imaging. J Ultrasound Med 1988; 7: 605–609

52 Shepherd D F C, Dewbury K C. Sequential imaging of the process of acute alcoholic hepatitis with ultrasound and isotopes. Br J Radiol 1980; 53: 163–165

53 Mills P, Saverymuttu S, Fallowfield D, Nussey S, Joseph A E. Ultrasound in the diagnosis of granulomatous liver disease. Clin Radiol 1990; 41: 113–115

54 Blangy S, Cornud F, Sibert A, Vissuzaine C, Saraux J L, Benacerraf R. Hepatitis tuberculosis presenting as tumoral disease on ultrasonography. Gastrointest Radiol 1988; 13: 52–54

55 Ferandes J D, Nebesar R A, Wall S G, Minihan P T. Report of tuberculous hepatitis presenting as metastatic disease. Clin Nucl Med 1984; 9: 245–247

56 Hussain S, Hawass N D, Zaidi A J. Ultrasonographic diagnosis of schistosomal periportal fibrosis. J Ultrasound Med 1984; 3: 449–452

57 Abdel-Wahab M F, Esmat G, Milad M, Abdel-Razek S, Strickland G T. Characteristic sonographic pattern of schistosomal hepatic fibrosis. Am J Trop Med Hyg 1989; 40: 72–76

58 Cerri G G, Alves V A F, Magalhaes A. Hepatosplenic schistosomiasis mansoni: ultrasound manifestations. Radiology 1984; 153: 777

59 Homeida M, Ahmed S, Dafalla A, et al. Morbidity associated with Schistosoma mansoni infection as determined by ultrasound: a study in Gezira, Sudan. Am J Trop Med Hyg 1988; 39: 196–201

60 Homeida M A, Fenwick A, DeFalla A A, et al. Effect of antischistosomal chemotherapy on prevalence of Symmers' periportal fibrosis in Sudanese villages. Lancet 1988; 2: 437–440

61 Wilson-Sharpe R C, Irving H C, Brown R C, Chalmers D M, Littlewood J M. Ultrasonography of the pancreas, liver and biliary system in cystic fibrosis. Arch Dis Child 1984; 59: 923–926

62 Willi U V, Reddish J M, Littlewood Teele R. Cystic fibrosis: its characteristic appearance on abdominal ultrasonography. AJR 1980; 134: 1005–1010

63 Graham N, Manhire A R, Stead R J, Lees W R, Hodson M E, Batten J C. Cystic fibrosis; ultrasonographic findings in the pancreas and hepatobiliary system correlated with clinical data and pathology. Clin Radiol 1985; 36: 199–203

64 McHugo J M, McKeown C, Brown M T, Weller P, Shah K J. Ultrasound findings in children with cystic fibrosis. Br J Radiol 1987; 60: 137–141

65 Celle G, Savarino V, Picciotto A, Magnolia M R, Scalabrini P, Dodero M. Is hepatic ultrasonography a valid alternative tool to liver biopsy? Report on 507 cases studied with both techniques. Dig Dis Sci 1988; 33: 467–471

66 Riley S A, Ellis W R, Irving H C, Lintott D J, Axon A T R, Losowsky M S. Percutaneous liver biopsy with plugging of the needle track: a safe method for use in patients with impaired coagulation. Lancet 1984; 2: 436

67 Irving H C. Sheath needle for liver biopsy. Radiology 1988; 168: 879

The portal venous system

Luigi Bolondi, Stefano Gaiani and Luigi Barbara

Sonographic findings in portal hypertension

Portal hypertension develops when increased resistance to portal flow ('backward flow theory') and/or increased portal blood flow ('forward flow theory') occur; recent evidence suggests that both mechanisms are involved in the maintenance of chronic portal hypertension.[1,2] The consequence of these mechanisms may be the enlargement of the extrahepatic portal vessels and the development of spontaneous portosystemic collaterals. Sonographic examination of the upper abdomen demonstrates some of the collateral pathways and changes in the main vessels of the portal venous system.

Changes of the calibre of the portal vessels

The portal vessels have been measured both in normal subjects and in patients with portal hypertension,[3-23] but there are wide discrepancies in the quoted upper normal values of the diameter of the portal vein (Table 1).[5,24-30] It is known that many factors, such as respiration,[29] posture changes[31] and absorptive state,[32,33] influence the calibre of the portal vein. Measurements should therefore be taken in basal conditions (quiet respiration, supine and fasting).

In our experience the upper normal limit of the portal vein diameter is 13 mm (Fig. 1A).[3,27] Dilatation of the portal vein occurred in 56% (73 out of 129 cases) of patients with portal hypertension due to liver cirrhosis. Among these 73 cases the calibre was over 15 mm in 46, and between 13 and 15 mm in the remaining 27 cases. In attempts to identify patients with high risk for variceal bleeding some authors[25,28] have compared the dilatation of the portal vein with the presence of oesophageal varices, demonstrating that the latter is correlated with a significant calibre increase of the portal vein and that a calibre over 17 mm is 100% predictive for large varices.[25] A normal calibre of the portal vein cannot however exclude portal hypertension. In some cases with alcoholic liver cirrhosis we found a portal vein with a calibre of 11 to 12 mm (Fig. 1B) even in the presence of large varices. The main intrahepatic portal branches are usually also dilated in portal hypertension, whereas the peripheral intrahepatic branches appear nar-

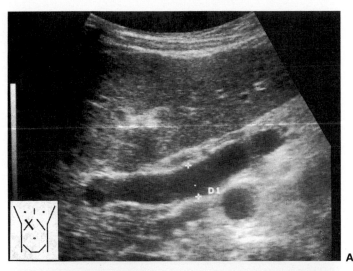

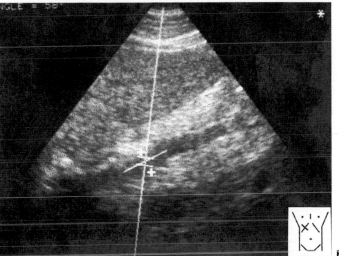

Fig. 1 **A: Dilated portal vein** (over 15 mm) in patient with post-hepatitic liver cirrhosis and portal hypertension. **B:** Portal hypertension due to alcoholic cirrhosis. In these patients the calibre of the portal vein may sometimes be normal such as in the example (11.4 mm).

rowed and tortuous, presumably due to the parenchymal changes.

Various degrees of dilatation of the splenic and superior mesenteric veins also occur in portal hypertension (Fig. 2). The upper limit of the normal splenic and superior mesenteric veins ranges from 10 to 12 mm.[3,27,29,30] Weill reports that a calibre of the splenic vein of 20 mm, or greater, should be considered a specific sign of portal hypertension.[34] Gross splenomegaly is usually associated with dilatation of the splenic vein, possibly due to the increased blood flow through the spleen (Fig. 3). Marked splenomegaly always leads to dilatation of the splenic vein and it may be difficult to establish whether this indicates portal hypertension or is simply a consequence of the splenomegaly. The demonstration of other signs of portal hypertension, such as dilatation of the superior mesenteric

Table 1 Maximum diameter of the portal vein in normal subjects

	Calibre of the portal vein (in mm)
Webb et al[5]	10
Weinreb et al[24]	15
Cottone et al[25]	17
Niederau et al[26]	14
Bolondi et al[3,27]	13
Zoli et al[28]	14
Kurol and Forsberg[29]	16
Goyal et al[30]	16

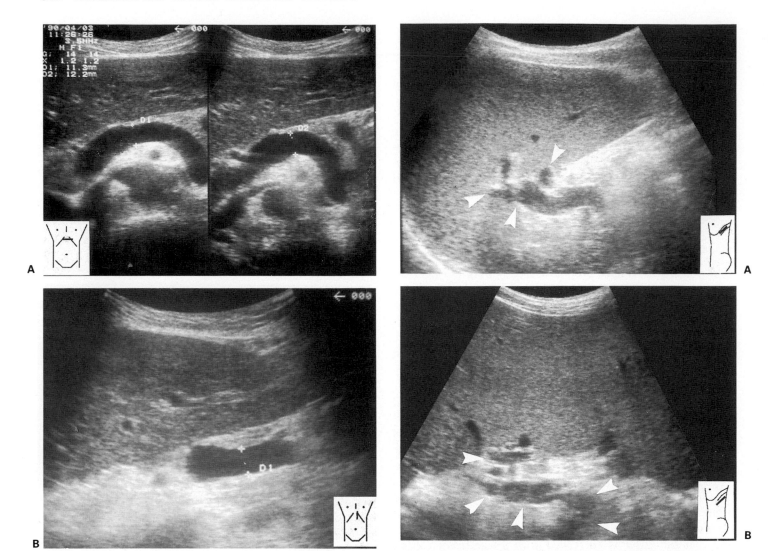

Fig. 2   Dilated splanchnic vessels. A: Dilatation of the splenic vein. During respiration there is only a slight calibre variation of the vessel; expiration (left) 11.3 mm; inspiration (right) 12.2 mm. **B:** Dilatation of the superior mesenteric vein.

Fig. 3   Splenomegaly. A: Mild and **B:** severe splenomegaly with a dilated splenic vein at the splenic hilum (arrowheads).

vein, which does not depend on spleen size, may be helpful.

Another important sign of portal hypertension is the respiratory calibre variation in the splenic (Fig. 2A) and superior mesenteric veins.[3] In normal subjects, during suspended inspiration there may be dilatation of the portal vein, related to the reduced venous outflow from the liver.[35] In patients with portal hypertension the intrahepatic resistance is increased anyway and this prevents further dilatation of the portal vessels during the Valsalva manoeuvre. The sign of the lack of respiratory calibre variation has good sensitivity (80%) and is specific.[3]

Detection of spontaneous portosystemic collaterals

Dilatation of the collateral vessels connecting the high pressure portal venous system with the low pressure systemic circulation usually occurs in patients with portal hypertension. It is a highly specific ultrasonographic sign.

The umbilical vein runs within the ligamentum teres in the left lobe of the liver and is easily visible as a channel greater than 3 mm in diameter when recanalised in portal hypertension (Fig. 4).[6,8,12] Though not always apparent, the demonstration of recanalisation of the umbilical vein is a highly specific sign of portal hypertension. The detection of hepatofugal flow in this vein outside the liver is pathognomonic. Para-umbilical collaterals may sometimes be located within the liver parenchyma close to the falciform ligament, and in some cases two (or, rarely, more) umbilical veins are detectable (Fig. 4B). The umbilical vein may also be visible distally[9] where it can be followed along the abdominal wall superior to the umbilicus. Ultrasonography

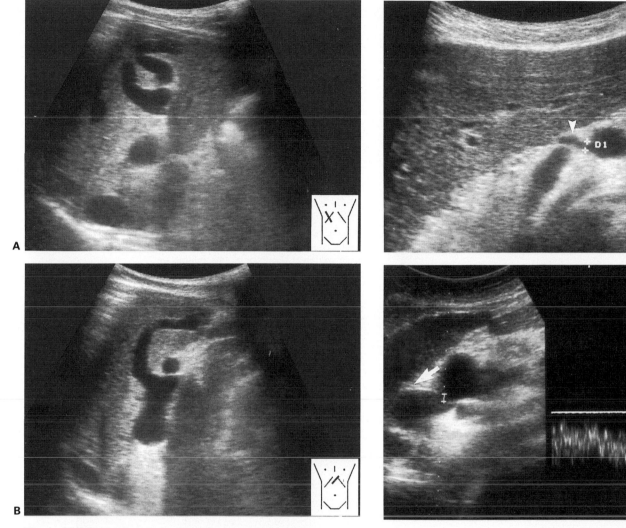

Fig. 4 **Umbilical vein** may be dilated in portal hypertension. In this case the umbilical vein is seen both in **A**: in the ligamentum teres and **B**: also in the surrounding liver parenchyma.

Fig. 5 **Left gastric vein. A:** Normal left gastric vein (arrowhead) joining the splenic vein. **B:** Marked dilatation of the left gastric vein (arrow) suggests the presence of oesophageal varices confirmed by the Doppler trace showing reversed flow.

has been reported to be more sensitive than portography,[16] which may give false negative results related to the lack of opacification of the umbilical vein in case of stagnant or low velocity flow.

Other collaterals, such as the left gastric vein and the retroperitoneal veins around the pancreas may be difficult to visualise owing to intestinal gas. The left gastric vein usually joins the distal portion of the splenic vein or the confluence between the splenic and the superior mesenteric veins, and may appear very enlarged. In most cases it runs with a winding course close to the posterior surface of the left lobe of the liver (Fig. 5). Significant dilatation of the left gastric vein suggests the presence of large oesophageal varices.[6]

Direct ultrasound visualisation of oesophageal varices is often difficult. Their presence may be inferred by the demonstration of:

a) thickening of the oesophageal wall;
b) irregularity of the air-containing lumen;
c) variation of oesophageal wall thickness with respiration.

These features have been reported to detect all endoscopically confirmed moderate or large varices.[36]

Short gastric veins may be detectable between the upper portion of the spleen and the gastric wall; their visualisation suggests the presence of gastric (and oesophageal) varices (Fig. 6). Since good quality coronal views are almost always achievable in these patients, these collateral vessels are the most reliably demonstrated with ultrasound.

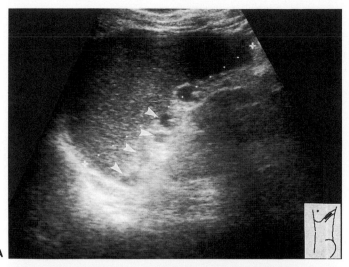

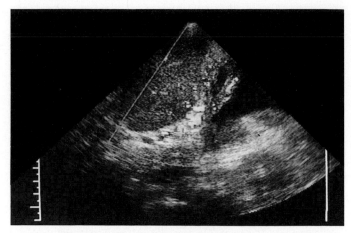

Plate 1 Colour Doppler scan showing portal collaterals in the gallbladder wall. This figure is reproduced in colour in the colour plate section at the front of this volume.

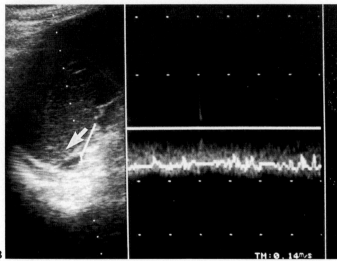

Fig. 6 A: Short gastric veins appear as small winding vessels near the upper pole of the spleen (arrowheads). **B:** The Doppler trace demonstrates flow towards the diaphragm (arrow).

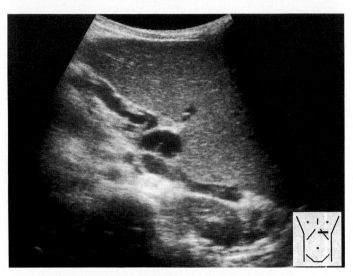

Fig. 7 Splenorenal collaterals originate from the hilum of the spleen and run around the left kidney.

Splenorenal pathways connecting the splenic varices with the left renal vein may have a large calibre, thus relieving the portal hypertension; they may lead to flow reversal in the splenic and even in the portal vein.[37] They appear as tortuous vessels near the lower pole of the spleen (Fig. 7). This type of spontaneous shunt is associated with a low incidence of gastro-oesophageal varices and so carries a good prognosis because haematemesis is much less common.

Infrequently collaterals may be seen within the gallbladder wall (Plate 1),[38] connecting the extrahepatic portal venous system with the intrahepatic portal branches; this also occurs in portal thrombosis.[39]

Other unusual sonographically detected portosystemic collaterals, such as omphalo-ilio-caval, spleno-retroperitoneal and splenoportal anastomoses, have been described by Di Candio et al in patients with uncomplicated portal

hypertension.[40] In these cases the presence of large spontaneous shunts prevents the development of ascites and gastrointestinal bleeding.[41]

Portal vein thrombosis

In adults portal vein thrombosis may be caused by haematological and coagulation disorders, acute inflammatory diseases of the digestive tract (necrotising enteritis, intestinal infarction, acute cholecystitis, pancreatitis, etc.), pancreatic or gastric tumours or surgical complications. Liver cirrhosis is however the most important cause of thrombosis of the portal vein. The incidence of this complication is unknown, since an old autopsy series reports 11%,[42] whereas a more recent angiographic study shows an incidence of about 1%.[43]

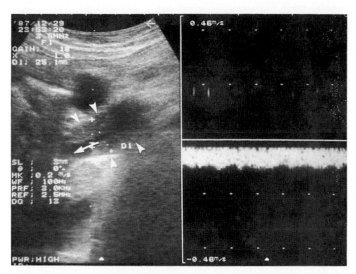

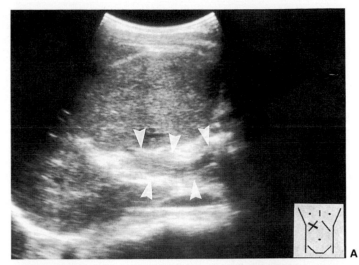

Fig. 8 Portal vein thrombosis. The portal vein is markedly dilated with a thrombus adherent to the anterior and posterior walls (arrowheads). The vessel appears partially patent. The Doppler trace demonstrates hepatopetal flow (arrow) thus confirming the patency of the lumen.

Ultrasonography is routinely utilised in patients with suspected portal thrombosis, being simple, non-invasive and accurate.[18,27] Partial thrombosis appears as an echogenic band on the wall of the vessel (Fig. 8). Recent thrombosis may be undetectable with ultrasound imaging, since early thrombus is echo-poor and indistinguishable from blood. In these cases Doppler ultrasound (especially colour Doppler) is essential in confirming the absence of portal flow. As the thrombosis organises the reflectivity increases and it is visualised as non-mobile echogenic material within the lumen of the vessel (Fig. 9A). In chronic thrombosis, highly reflective fibrous tissue replaces the portal vein (Fig. 10).[27] Complete occlusion may lead to cavernous transformation of the portal vein in which small collateral vessels develop around the thrombosed portal vein.[20,27] This appears as a solid elongated structure at the porta hepatis, surrounded by small, thin winding channels (Fig. 11). In cases of tumour invasion of the portal vein, the thrombus may present an echo pattern similar to that of the surrounding (neoplastic) liver parenchyma and there is often marked dilatation of the vessel probably related to growth of the tumour within the vessel itself (Fig. 9B). Tumour thrombus is seen in up to 25% of patients with hepatocellular carcinoma. It may also be seen in patients with metastases where the incidence is less than 1%.

Doppler ultrasound findings in portal hypertension

Clinical applications of Doppler flowmetry of hepatic vessels include the assessment of a) the presence, b) the direction and c) the characteristics of blood flow. Quantification of the volume of blood flow has also been attempted in some of the major abdominal arteries and

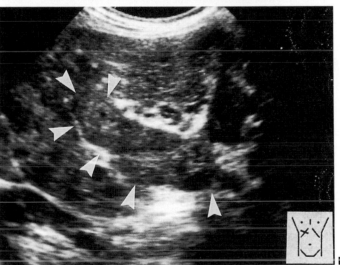

Fig. 9 Complete thrombosis of the portal vein. A: The portal trunk is filled with echogenic material (arrowheads). **B:** Tumour thrombus of the portal vein (arrowheads) in a case of diffuse hepatocellular carcinoma. The vessel is markedly dilated.

veins, but though important clinically, the reliability of these measurements is still questioned. Failing this, the qualitative information about the flow pattern provided by pulsed Doppler is of established value, since it not only clarifies doubtful images on real time ultrasonography, but also provides new insights in many clinical conditions.

Detection of blood flow

Establishing the presence of blood flow within the portal vein is the simplest Doppler finding and it is easily detected (Fig. 12). Colour Doppler further facilitates the evaluation of vascular haemodynamics by directly visualising flow within the vessels (Plate 2).

In cases of chronic portal vein thrombosis, when the portal vein is small and highly reflective, Doppler investigation of the porta hepatis will reveal no evidence of blood

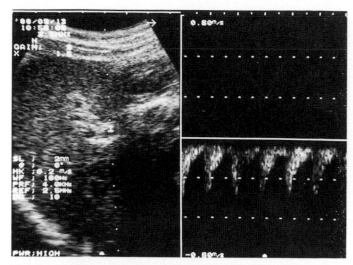

Fig. 10 Chronic thrombosis. The portal vein is replaced by echogenic fibrous tissue. Doppler ultrasound demonstrates only arterial signals.

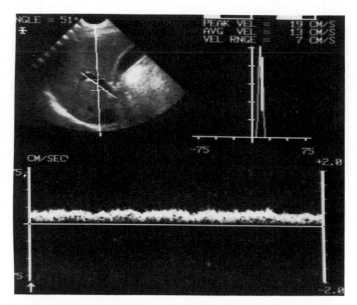

Fig. 12 Doppler of the normal portal vein. The mean velocity in this case was 16 cm/sec.

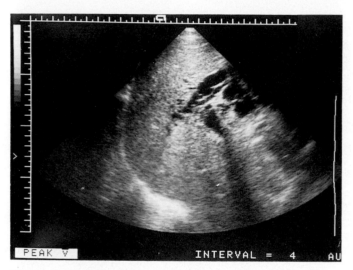

Fig. 11 Cavernous transformation of the portal vein. The portal vein is replaced by a series of tortuous small vessels (see also Plate 3).

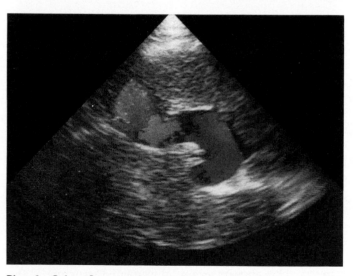

Plate 2 Colour flow mapping of a dilated and tortuous intrahepatic portal branch in a patient with portal hypertension. Flow is represented in red (towards the probe) or blue (away from the probe) depending on the vessel direction with respect to the ultrasound beam. This figure is reproduced in colour in the colour plate section at the front of this volume.

flow. When cavernous transformation has occurred, continuous low velocity flow can be demonstrated within the small tortuous vessels, best depicted with colour Doppler (Plate 3). Because the hepatic artery takes over the entire hepatic blood supply in portal thrombosis, the demonstration of high frequency arterial signals within the liver with no accompanying portal vein signal may be considered an indirect sign of portal thrombosis.

The sensitivity of Doppler ultrasound in diagnosing portal vein thrombosis is similar to that of dynamic computed tomography,[44] but it is less reliable in partial thrombosis and in portal branch thrombosis.[45] In some instances Doppler flowmetry may be even more accurate than arterioportography, which can erroneously suggest portal thrombosis when there is reverse flow in the portal vein.[46]

Doppler ultrasound may therefore be considered extremely sensitive in the diagnosis of portal thrombosis.[47] The extensive application of Doppler ultrasound in non-selected patients affected by liver cirrhosis should clarify the actual prevalence of portal thrombosis.

An important practical point is the value of the detection of blood flow within anechoic abdominal structures whether or not suspected as portosystemic collaterals (Figs 5B, 6 and 13); this may clarify a difficult ultrasound diagnosis, especially in cases of retroperitoneal and

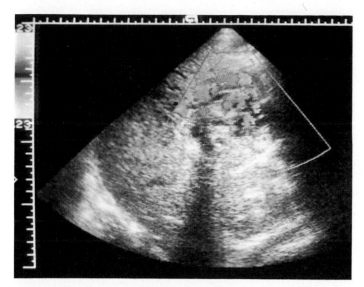

Plate 3 Cavernous transformation of the portal vein. Colour Doppler demonstrates blood flowing in small collaterals. This figure is reproduced in colour in the colour plate section at the front of this volume.

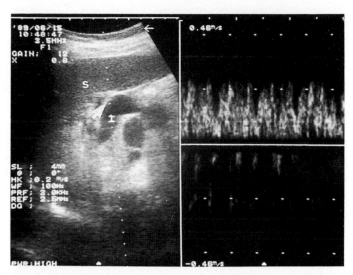

Fig. 13 Splenorenal shunt. Dilated collateral vessels near the lower pole of the spleen (s). Doppler ultrasound demonstrates phasic flow away from the spleen (arrow).

splenorenal collaterals. The latter can be so enlarged as to simulate renal cysts.[48]

Direction of blood flow

Flow direction is another unequivocal qualitative finding provided by Doppler ultrasound (Fig. 14). Its importance in the investigation of hepatic haemodynamics is obvious. The actual prevalence of reversed flow in the portal venous system in an unselected cirrhotic population is not known. L'Herminè et al[49] reported reversed intrahepatic portal flow (demonstrated by arterioportography) in about 5% of their cases, one third of whom had a complete hepatofugal flow. However, the rate of reversed flow detected by arterioportography may not accurately reflect its prevalence in a non-selected population of cirrhotics, because only patients with complicated portal hypertension or who are surgical candidates are subjected to this invasive procedure. Kawasaki et al[50] report a prevalence of spontaneous hepatofugal flow of 6.1% in cirrhotic patients and of 5.3% in patients with hepatocellular carcinoma. In our experience[51] the overall prevalence of hepatofugal flow in liver cirrhosis (without hepatocellular carcinoma) was 8.3% (19 in 228). Reversed portal flow was associated with a significantly reduced calibre of the portal vein. It is not clear if reversed portal vein flow carries a poor prognosis, but hepatofugal flow in the splenic vein has proved to be closely correlated with hepatic encephalopathy,[52] probably due to the drainage of large amounts of blood into large splenorenal collaterals.

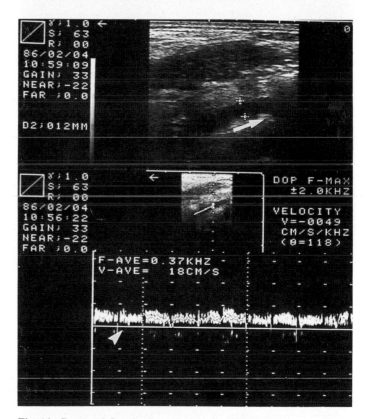

Fig. 14 Reversed flow in the splenic vein. The Doppler trace above the reference line (arrowheads) corresponds to flow directed towards the spleen (arrow).

Characteristics of blood flow and its disturbances

One of the most valuable deductions that can be obtained from the Doppler signals derives from the fact that the features of the waveform and spectral distribution of

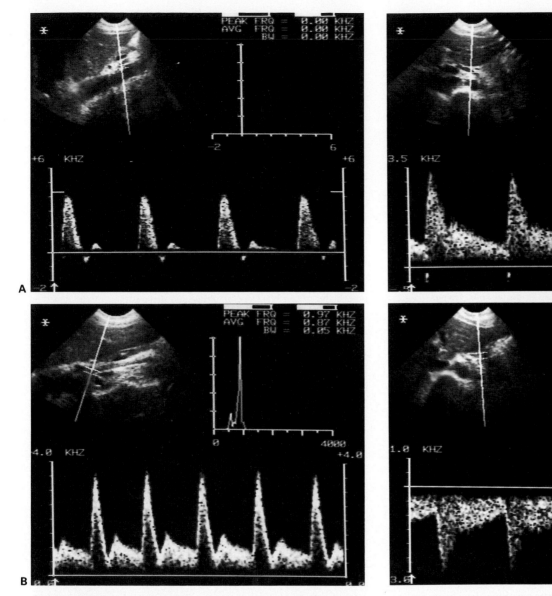

Fig. 15 Superior mesenteric artery. A: Doppler ultrasound study of the superior mesenteric artery in a normal subject shows a low diastolic flow with reversed end systolic phase. **B:** In a patient with portal hypertension there is increased and continuous diastolic flow due to the decreased resistance of the splanchnic vascular bed.

Fig. 16 Normal hepatic and splenic arteries. Doppler ultrasound studies of **A:** the hepatic and **B:** splenic artery show a flow profile with high diastolic phase, due to the low resistances of hepatic and splenic vascular beds.

frequencies are mainly consequences of haemodynamic factors and location of the vessel.

Therefore the pattern of the Doppler signal (whether presented as an audio signal or a spectral tracing) identifies its origin, even when the ultrasound image is equivocal. Vessels tend to have a Doppler 'signature', from which they can be recognised.[53] The assessment of flow disturbances from waveform data includes semiquantitative methods based on the analysis of the velocity profile and the calculation of ratios between maximum, minimum and mean frequencies of the spectrum. Numerous indices have been proposed to describe waveforms of arterial flow. One

of the most commonly used is the pulsatility index (PI) defined as:

$$PI = \frac{A - B}{mean}$$

where A is the maximum value over the cardiac cycle, B the minimum and mean the average value. The resistance index is an alternative.

$$RI = \frac{A - B}{A}$$

Because it is not necessary to know the angle of incidence of the ultrasonic beam when calculating these indices, they can be assessed in vessels that are too small or tortuous to be imaged (e.g. the intrahepatic arteries). Since the pulsatility of an artery is determined by the impedance of the distal vascular bed, this variable could prove useful in the investigation of liver diseases.

An example is provided by the study of the superior mesenteric artery. One of the striking findings in cirrhotic patients is the hyperdynamic circulation associated with a fall in arterial resistance.[54] In a study of this phenomenon utilising Doppler[55] the PI of the superior mesenteric artery was found to be significantly decreased in patients with liver cirrhosis (Fig. 15) and acute hepatitis, but not in cases of portal vein thrombosis unrelated to liver cirrhosis. Changes in the waveform of the hepatic and splenic arteries during the development of portal hypertension has not been adequately investigated. These vessels normally have good diastolic flow due to a low resistance peripheral bed and therefore their waveform differs significantly from that of the superior mesenteric artery (Fig. 16).[53]

Doppler examination of the hepatic veins may also provide useful data. The hepatic veins in healthy humans display a triphasic waveform depending upon the cardiac cycle, particularly the fluctuating right atrial pressure. These phasic variations of flow are completely lost in some 25% of cases of liver cirrhosis with portal hypertension (Fig. 17) and greatly reduced in another 25%.[56] The pathophysiology of this alteration is still unclear but is presumably attributable to increase in liver stiffness.

Quantitative measurement of blood flow

The haemodynamic evaluation of the portal venous system in portal hypertension should include the measurement of three fundamental variables: a) the volume of portal venous flow (Q_{pv}), b) the portal perfusion pressure (pressure gradient between the portal vein and the hepatic veins) ($P_{pv} - P_{hv}$) and c) the portal vascular resistance (P_{vr}), which is calculated by the formula:[57]

$$P_{vr} = \frac{P_{pv} - P_{hv}}{Q_{pv}}$$

from the volume and gradient.

While several invasive methods have been developed recently to measure portal and hepatic venous pressure,[58,59] measurement of flow volume has always proved much more difficult; so non-invasive measurements using Doppler ultrasound have attracted a great deal of attention. The measurement is based on the principle of uniform insonation in which the entire volume of blood in a cross-section of the vessel is exposed to a uniform ultrasonic beam. The instantaneous mean velocity (V), calculated from the mean Doppler shift, is multiplied by the cross-sectional area (A) of the vessel, to give the volume flow (Q): Q = VA.

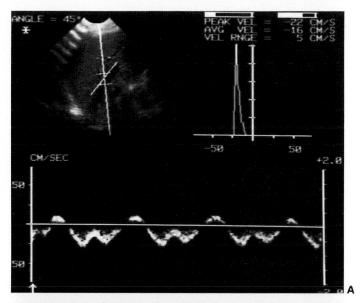

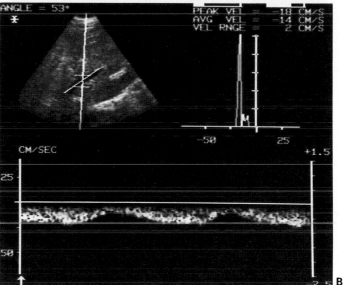

Fig. 17 Hepatic vein Doppler. A: Doppler flow profile in a normal hepatic vein is characterised by a triphasic waveform. **B**: In some patients with liver cirrhosis the flow profile may be continuous. This tracing also shows superimposed velocity changes due to respiration.

Sources of errors, however, are the assessment of the beam vessel angle (necessary to convert the frequency shifts of the Doppler signal into velocity) and measurement of the cross-sectional area of the vessel; the angle errors increase rapidly with increasing obliquities of approach (see Ch. 5).[60] Measurement of the cross-sectional area of the vessel presents even greater problems because most vessels, especially veins, are not circular in section[26] and their calibre varies through the cardiac and respiratory cycles. For these reasons flow velocity and volume calculations taken at angles over 60° or in small and tortuous vessels, show a poor reproducibility and are unacceptable in clinical practice.

One additional critical point is the calculation of the mean velocity. Its determination as a fixed fraction of the maximum velocity[61,62] may be inaccurate because the velocity profile in the portal vein varies from patient to patient. It is therefore necessary to calculate V_{mean} directly from the Doppler spectrum; this can be automated by the software of modern scanners (see Ch. 5).

Although ultrasound cannot directly measure the portal pressure this can be indirectly assessed by use of the 'congestion index'. This combines measurement of the portal vein diameter and the time averaged mean portal blood velocity. An increased diameter gives a high index implying increased portal pressure.[62]

For the portal vein, its 3 to 4 cm straight course, its relatively large calibre and its oblique position with respect to the abdominal wall are all favourable factors for the Doppler investigation. Measurements of V_{mean} should be made on Doppler traces of 4 to 6 seconds in order to average the effects of flow velocity fluctuations. The temptation to make these measurements during suspended respiration should be avoided since this reduces flow. Errors in measuring the cross-sectional area do affect the calculation of flow volume in the portal vein, but repeated measurements of the diameter reduce the error of flow calculation to within 10%.[63]

The accuracy of Doppler flowmetry for measuring flow volume in the portal vein has been validated: it correlates well with the results of lipiodol droplet cine-angiography[61] and electromagnetic flowmetry.[62,64] However, Dauzat and Pomier Layrargues[64] found that the coefficient of variation for Doppler measurements was higher than for electromagnetic measurements (10.9% versus 5.9%).

In a recent study[65] the intra- and interobserver variability of Doppler ultrasound measurements was assessed in normal volunteers. Intra-observer variability was low in repeated examination in the same day, with a tendency to increase in consecutive days (this could be due to physiological changes in the portal flow). The interobserver agreement was always poor. Instrumentation variation[66] is also a factor that can be eliminated if follow up examinations are carried out on the same equipment and transducer.

Based on these findings it is reasonable to affirm that the Doppler spectrum reflects the actual blood flow in the portal vein, even though the absolute values expressed in ml/min may not correspond to the real flow volumes. Changes of V_{mean} and in flow volume assessed by Doppler flowmetry in the same subject under different conditions are more acceptable, since possible sources of errors in measuring the absolute values would be expected to affect different measurements in the same way. The method seems to be suitable for monitoring acute haemodynamic changes in the portal vein in vivo such as those induced by feeding, hormones and drugs.[64,67,68]

Despite these limitations, many papers dealing with

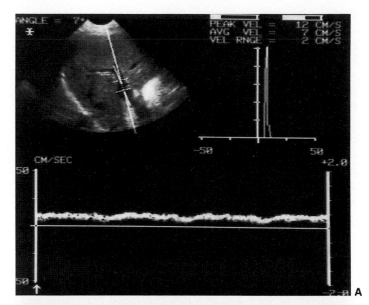

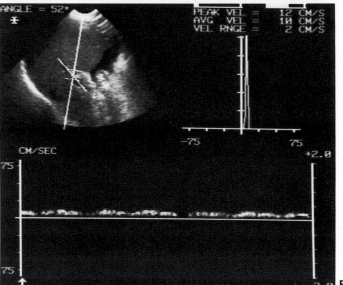

Fig. 18 **Doppler of the portal vein. A:** Slight decrease of flow velocity (9 cm/sec) in a patient with liver cirrhosis. **B:** Marked decrease of flow velocity (4 cm/sec) in a patient with decompensated liver cirrhosis and gross ascites.

quantitative measurements of flow in the portal vein have been published in recent years[33,57,61,67–70] and they agree in that velocity is reduced, to a greater or lesser degree, in cirrhotic patients in comparison with the healthy subjects (Fig. 18) (Tables 2 and 3). The variation of reported values for portal vein flow velocity is partly dependent on the methodology (see Ch. 5) and partly on the variation of the haemodynamic patterns in relation to the stage and aetiology of the cirrhosis. Data about portal flow volumes in liver cirrhosis are even more variable (Table 3) because the development of collateral pathways, whose extent varies from case to case, greatly influences portal flow volume. A patent and dilated umbilical vein (Plate 4) may explain a

Table 2 Portal blood flow in healthy subjects

	Velocity (cm/sec)	Volume (ml/min)
Ohnishi et al[61]	17 ± 3.9	648 ± 186
Moriyasu et al[62]	15.3 ± 4	899 ± 284
Zoli et al[69]	16 ± 0.5*	694 ± 23*
Brown et al[67]	12.3 ± 5.9	864 ± 188
Gaiani et al[33]	16 ± 4.1	832 ± 245

average ± SD; * average ± SE

Editors note.
These values in Tables 2 and 3 may be overestimates as the mean velocities were calculated from the means of the peak velocity envelopes rather than the correct time averaged weighted mean velocities (see Ch. 5).

Table 3 Portal blood flow in liver cirrhosis

	Velocity (cm/sec)	Volume (ml/min)
Ohnishi et al[61]	12 ± 3	690 ± 258
Ohnishi et al*[61]	7.1 ± 2.3	326 ± 145
Moriyasu et al[62]	9.7 ± 2.6	870 ± 289
Zoli et al[69]	10.5 ± 0.6	736 ± 46
Gaiani et al[33]	12.4 ± 2.3	1160 ± 426

average ± SD
* patients with spontaneous splenorenal shunts

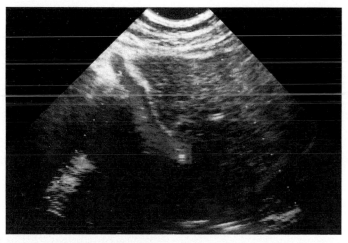

Plate 4 Colour Doppler of the umbilical vein. The red colour indicates flow towards the transducer (hepatofugal). This figure is reproduced in colour in the colour plate section at the front of this volume.

case of high velocity and volume portal flow while large splenorenal collaterals may reduce portal flow and even produce reversal.

In portal hypertensive patients lack of the normal post-prandial increase of portal flow has been demonstrated,[33] probably related to the hypertensive state in the splanchnic venous bed and to the diversion of blood flow by portosystemic collaterals.

Flow volume in the splenic and superior mesenteric veins has been reported in several studies that show the different contribution of these vessels to the post-prandial increase of portal flow[70] and in the attempt to draw new insights in the pathophysiology of portal hypertension.[71,72] However, the course of the superior mesenteric vein, parallel to the abdominal wall, sometimes makes it difficult to orientate the beam at less than 60° to the vessel, while the curved course of the splenic vein makes the measurement of the angle uncertain, greatly diminishing the reliability of quantitative Doppler flowmetry of this vessel. In a recent study, investigating the feasibility of Doppler flow measurements in splanchnic vessels in non-selected patient population and in cirrhotics,[73] the splenic and superior mesenteric veins were adequately visualised in only about 60% of cases.

More severe problems are encountered when attempting to measure flow in the winding and irregular collateral vessels which develop in portal hypertension, with the exception of the recanalised umbilical vein. In this vessel flow volume can be calculated in most cases, due to its long straight course, and this measurement has some clinical importance because it demonstrates how much the effective portal perfusion of the liver is reduced by diversion of blood flow into this hepatofugal pathway.[74] Only the presence and direction of flow can be assessed in the splenorenal collaterals, while flow velocity measurements in the coronary vein (left gastric vein) can sometimes be attempted. Other collateral vessels are even more difficult to visualise and therefore to measure by Doppler ultrasound. Overall a reliable quantitative evaluation of collateral flow is still impossible. This implies that caution has to be maintained in the clinical interpretation of any measurement taken at the level of the portal vein.

Volume flow has also been measured in the splenic and superior mesenteric arteries.[75-78] The reliability of absolute values of flow reported for the splenic artery is doubtful in view of its curved course and the difficulty in visualisation,[73] while flow volume calculations for the superior mesenteric artery seem to be more acceptable and values reported by various authors on normal subjects are in agreement.[75-78]

Diagnosis of Budd-Chiari syndrome

The Budd-Chiari syndrome is a rare disorder in which the hepatic veins are obstructed. The most important sonographic findings are hepatomegaly with enlargement of the caudate lobe (because the inferior hepatic veins are spared), non-visualisation or dilatation and irregularity of the main hepatic veins, non-visualisation of the confluence of the hepatic veins with the inferior vena cava and narrowing or obstruction of the inferior vena cava.[79-81] Since the IVC is often also included in the Budd-Chiari syndrome, confirmation may be obtained by demonstrating

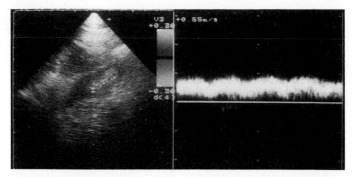

Plate 5 Budd-Chiari syndrome. Colour Doppler ultrasound of the inferior vena cava shows reversed (red) and continuous flow (arrow). This figure is reproduced in colour in the colour plate section at the front of this volume.

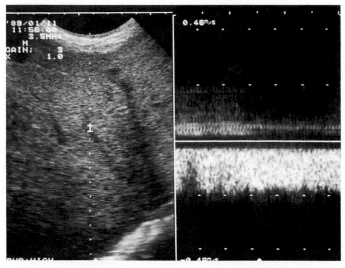

Fig. 19 Budd-Chiari syndrome. Doppler ultrasound of the hepatic vein shows a flat and broad band waveform corresponding to continuous and disturbed flow.

steady reversed flow in the lower portion of the IVC (Plate 5). In other instances flow in the IVC is in the normal direction (towards the heart) but it loses its phasic oscillation; this suggests partial obstruction. Another Doppler finding, which may help in the diagnosis, is the change of the Doppler waveform of the hepatic veins. Absence of phasic variations, resulting in steady flow (Fig. 19) suggests obstruction of the upper portion of the IVC or of the hepatic vein outlet, preventing retrograde transmission of the pressure variations of the right atrium. This has been advocated as a major Doppler sign of Budd-Chiari Syndrome[82] but a similar pattern is found in advanced liver cirrhosis[56] so that its specificity is poor. Reversed flow in the hepatic veins is pathognomonic, though seldom found, while reversed flow in the portal vein is more commonly seen, though non-specific.

Evaluation of portosystemic surgical shunts

Ultrasonography is a useful method in the follow up of patients after portosystemic shunt surgery.[23,27] The patency of the shunt may be assessed in 75% of cases,[27] splenorenal shunts being more easily detected than portocaval shunts (Fig. 20),[34] which may be obscured by abdominal gas. The shunt is patent when a direct confluence between the portal vein and the inferior vena cava, or between the splenic and left renal vein can be demonstrated.

When the shunt itself is not displayed, indirect signs may suggest its patency: in portocaval shunts the decrease in calibre of the portal vein is a useful sign of patency, as is widening of the inferior vena cava above the level of the anastomosis (Fig. 20).[83] In the same way dilatation of the left renal vein is consistent with a patent distal splenorenal shunt. Ultrasonography may also demonstrate atrophy of other collaterals, confirming shunt patency.

Doppler has proved to be extremely useful both in pre-operative evaluation of patients as well as post-operative follow up. Pre-operatively, Doppler can be of great help in guiding the choice of surgery. Thrombosis or flow reversal in the portal vein suggests that shunts may be technically impossible or unhelpful. In the post-operative period Doppler is the investigation of choice to assess shunt patency and the haemodynamic consequences of the procedure. Provided pre-operative baseline studies have been performed, it is possible within certain limits to assess flow through the shunt and to gauge the change in portal perfusion.

With regard to the direct assessment of flow through the anastomosis, the series published in the literature show considerable variations of sensitivity ranging from 55% to

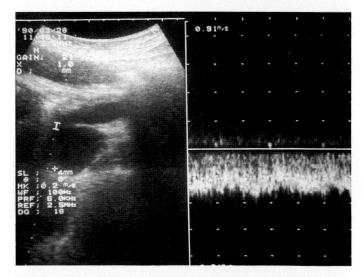

Fig. 20 Side to side portocaval shunt. The anastomosis between the portal vein (above) and the inferior vena cava (below) is easily detectable. Doppler examination demonstrates flow towards the systemic circulation.

87%.[84–88] Turbulent, high speed flow towards the systemic circulation can be detected within the shunt itself (Fig. 20). In some cases this flow may show a phasic profile in response to variations in caval pressure.

Indirect signs of patency can be found in practically all patients on the basis of the direction of flow in the portal vein or characteristics of the flow towards the shunt. When a side to side portocaval shunt cannot be visualised on conventional real time ultrasound, the presence of hepatofugal flow in the intrahepatic portal branches is a reliable indicator of patency of the shunt.[86] However it must be remembered that the haemodynamics change gradually and thus, in the immediate post-operative period, slow hepatopetal portal flow may still be detected despite a patent shunt. Conversely, hepatopetal portal flow detected in a late post-operative study raises the suspicion of thrombosis of the shunt, especially if in a previous examination flow was hepatofugal.

In end to side portocaval shunts portal flow is absent or hepatofugal in the intrahepatic branches despite the literature reports[86] of the appearance of hepatopetal flow in an intrahepatic branch due to anomalous pathways, such as arterioportal fistulae.

Demonstration of reversal of flow in the splenic, and sometimes also the portal veins is proof of patency of the conventional splenorenal shunt.

Visualisation of distal splenorenal shunts is not always feasible on real time ultrasound (53.5% in our group of patients) (Fig. 21).[88] In this case useful information can be obtained from the flow pattern in the splenic vein which displays a typical phasic profile synchronous with caval pulsatility. The goal of this kind of shunt is to decompress gastro-oesophageal varices selectively while maintaining

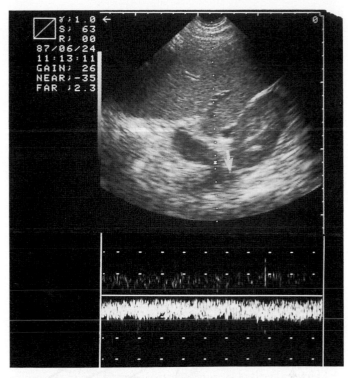

Fig. 21 Distal splenorenal shunt (Warren). Doppler study shows continuous flow directed from the splenic to the left renal vein (arrow).

hepatopetal flow in the mesoportal venous bed in order to reduce the incidence of encephalopathy. Using Doppler low velocity hepatopetal flow was maintained at 12 months after surgery in 77% of cases,[88] with a low incidence of late reversal of flow.[89]

REFERENCES

1 Benoit J N, Womack W A, Hernandez L, Granger D N. 'Forward' and 'backward' flow mechanisms of portal hypertension. Relative contribution in the rat model of portal vein stenosis. Gastroenterology 1985; 89: 1092

2 Sikuler E, Groszmann R J. Interaction of flow and resistance in maintenance of portal hypertension in a rat model. Am J Physiol 1986; 250: 205

3 Bolondi L, Gandolfi L, Arienti V, et al. Ultrasonography in the diagnosis of portal hypertension: diminished response of portal vessels to respiration. Radiology 1982; 142: 167

4 Duvauferrier R, Duvauferrier-Pellenc H C, Bretagne J F, Duval J M, Gastard J. Exploration échographique su sistème porte. J Radiol 1980; 61: 559

5 Webb L J, Berger L A, Sherlock S. Gray-scale ultrasonography of portal vein. Lancet 1977; 2: 675

6 Lafortune M, Marleau D, Breton G, et al. Portal venous measurements in portal hypertension. Radiology 1984; 151: 27

7 Funston M R, Goudie E, Richter I A, Butterworth A M, Allan · J C. Ultrasound diagnosis of the recanalised umbilical vein in portal hypertension. JCU 1980; 8: 244

8 Glazer G M, Laing F C, Brown T W, Gooding G A W. Sonographic demonstration of portal hypertension: the patent umbilical vein. Radiology 1980; 136: 161

9 Weill F S. Ultrasonic visualisation of an umbilical vein. Radiology 1976; 120: 159

10 Fakhry J, Gosing B B, Leopold G R. Recanalised umbilical vein due to portal vein occlusion: documentation by sonography. AJR 1981; 137: 410

11 Aagaard J, Jensen L I, Sorensen T I A, et al. Recanalised umbilical vein in portal hypertension. AJR 1982; 139: 1107

12 Schabel S I, Rittenberg G M, Javid L H, Cunningham J, Ross P. The 'bull's-eye' falciform ligament: a sonographic finding of portal hypertension. Radiology 1980; 136: 157

13 Kane R A, Katz S G. The spectrum of sonographic findings in portal hypertension: a subject review and new observations. Radiology 1982; 142: 453

14 Juttner H U, Jenney J M, Ralls P W, Goldstein L I, Reynolds T B. Ultrasound demonstration of portosystemic collaterals in cirrhosis and portal hypertension. Radiology 1982; 142: 459

15 Dach J L, Hill M C, Pelaez J C, et al. Sonography of hypertensive portal venous system: correlation with arterial portography. AJR 1981; 137: 511

16 Dokmeci A K, Kimura K, Matsutani S, et al. Collateral vein in portal hypertension demonstrated by sonography. AJR 1981; 137: 1173

17 Subramanyan B R, Balthazar E J, Madamba M R, et al.

Sonography of portosystemic venous collaterals in portal hypertension. Radiology 1983; 146: 161

18 Merrit C R. Ultrasonographic demonstration of portal vein thrombosis. Radiology 1979; 133: 425

19 Brunelle F, Alagille D, Pariente D, Chaumont P. Etude echotomographique de l'hypertension portale chez l'enfant. Ann Radiol 1981; 24: 121

20 Sassoon C, Douillet P, Cronfalt A M, Odievre M, Chaumont P, Doyon D. Ultrasonographic diagnosis of portal cavernoma in children: a study of twelve cases. Br J Radiol 1980; 53: 1047

21 Miller E L, Thomas R H. Portal vein invasion demonstrated by ultrasound. JCU 1979; 7: 57

22 Berger L A, Sagor G, George P. The ultrasonic demonstration of portocaval shunts. Br J Surg 1979; 66: 166

23 Goldberg B B, Patel J. Ultrasonic evaluation of portocaval shunt. JCU 1977; 5: 304

24 Weinreb J, Kumari S, Phillip G, et al. Portal vein measurements by real time sonography. AJR 1982; 139: 497

25 Cottone M, Sciarrino E, Marceno M P, et al. Ultrasound in the screening of patients with cirrhosis with large varices. BMJ 1983; 533: 287

26 Niederau C, Sonnen A, Muller J E, et al. Sonographic measurements of the normal liver, spleen, pancreas and portal vein. Radiology 1983; 149: 537

27 Bolondi L, Mazziotti A, Arienti V, et al. Ultrasonographic study of portal venous system in portal hypertension and other portosystemic shunt operation. Surgery 1984; 95: 261

28 Zoli M, Dondi C, Marchesini G, et al. Splanchnic vein measurements in patients with liver cirrhosis: a case-control study. J Ultrasound Med 1985; 4: 641

29 Kurol M, Forsberg L. Ultrasonographic investigation of respiratory influence on diameters of portal vessels in normal subjects. Acta Radiol Diagn 1986; 27: 675

30 Goyal A K, Pokharna D S, Sharma S K. Ultrasonic measurements of portal vasculature in diagnosis of portal hypertension. J Ultrasound Med 1990; 9: 45

31 Rahim N, Adam E J. Ultrasound demonstration of variation in normal portal vein diameter with posture. Br J Radiol 1985; 58: 313

32 Bellamy E A, Bossi M C, Cosgrove D O. Ultrasound demonstration of changes in the normal portal venous system following a meal. Br J Radiol 1984; 57: 147

33 Gaiani S, Bolondi L, Li Bassi S, Santi V, Zironi G, Barbara L. Effect of meal on portal hemodynamics in healthy humans and in patients with chronic liver disease. Hepatology 1989; 9: 815

34 Weill F S. Cirrhosis and portal hypertension. In: Weill F S. ed. Ultrasound diagnosis of digestive diseases. Berlin: Springer Verlag. 1990

35 Moreno A H, Burchell A R, Van der Woude R, Burke J H. Respiratory regulation of splanchnic and systemic venous return. Am J Physiol 1967; 213: 455

36 Saverymuttu S H, Wright J, Maxwell J D, Joseph A E A. Ultrasound detection of oesophageal varices – comparison with endoscopy. Clin Radiol 1988; 39: 513–515

37 Takayasu K, Moriyama N, Shima J, et al. Sonographic detection of large spontaneous splenorenal shunt, and its clinical significance. Br J Radiol 1984; 57: 565

38 Marchal G F J, Van Holsbeeck M, Tshibwabwa-Ntumba E, et al. Dilatation of cystic veins in portal hypertension: sonographic demonstration. Radiology 1985; 154: 187

39 Gaiani S, Bolondi L, Barbara L. Duplex Doppler evaluation of cystic veins in prehepatic portal hypertension. Ital J Gastroenterol 1988; 20: 19

40 Di Candio G, Campatelli A, Mosca F, Santi V, Casanova P, Bolondi L. Ultrasound detection of unusual spontaneous portosystemic shunts associated with uncomplicated portal hypertension. J Ultrasound Med 1985; 4: 297

41 Wexler M J, MacLean L D. Massive spontaneous portal-systemic shunting without varices. Arch Surg 1975; 110: 995

42 Hunt A H, Whittard B R. Thrombosis of the portal vein in cirrhosis hepatis. Lancet 1954; i: 281–284

43 Okuda K, Ohnishi K, Kimura K, et al. Incidence of portal vein thrombosis in liver cirrhosis. An angiographic study in 708 patients. Gastroenterology 1985; 89: 279

44 Miller V E, Berland L L. Pulsed Doppler duplex sonography and CT of portal vein thrombosis. AJR 1985; 145: 73

45 Alpern M B, Rubin J M, Williams D M, Cape K P. Porta hepatic: duplex Doppler ultrasound with angiographic correlation. Radiology 1987; 162: 53

46 Raby N, Meire H B. Duplex Doppler ultrasound in the diagnosis of cavernous transformation of the portal vein. Br J Radiol 1988; 61: 586–588

47 Scoutt L M, Zawin M L, Taylor K J W. Doppler ultrasound. Part II. Clinical applications. Radiology 1990; 174: 309

48 Bolondi L, Zironi G, Gaiani S, Testa S, Li Bassi S, Barbara L. Cyst of the kidney or spontaneous splenorenal shunt? Differentiation by pulsed Doppler sonography. AJR in press

49 L'Herminè C. Radiology of liver circulation. Dordrecht: Martinus Nijhoff. 1985

50 Kawasaki T, Moriyasu F, Nishida O, et al. Analysis of hepatofugal flow in portal venous system using ultrasonic Doppler duplex system. Am J Gastroenterol 1989; 84: 937

51 Gaiani S, Bolondi L, Li Bassi S, Zironi G, Barbara L. Prevalence of spontaneous hepatofugal portal flow in liver cirrhosis. Clinical and endoscopic correlation in 228 patients. Submitted to Gastroenterology.

52 Ohnishi K, Saito M, Sato S, et al. Direction of splenic venous flow assessed by pulsed Doppler flowmetry in patients with a large splenorenal shunt. Relation to spontaneous hepatic encephalopathy. Gastroenterology 1985; 89: 180

53 Taylor K J W, Burns P N, Woodcock J P, et al. Blood flow in deep abdominal and pelvic vessels: ultrasonic pulsed Doppler analysis. Radiology 1985; 154: 487

54 Benoit J N, Granger N. Splanchnic hemodynamics in chronic portal venous hypertension. Semin Liver Dis 1986; 6: 287

55 Darnault P, Bretagne J F, Raoul J, et al. Assessment of the role of portal hypertension and liver failure in lowering splanchnic vascular resistance. Gastroenterology 1989; 96: A590

56 Bolondi L, Gaiani S, Li Bassi S, et al. Changes in the hepatic vein waveform detected by Doppler ultrasound in liver cirrhosis. J Hepatol 1989; 9: S117

57 Moriyasu F, Nishida O, Ban N, et al. Measurement of portal vascular resistance in patients with portal hypertension. Gastroenterology 1986; 90: 710

58 Paton A, Reynolds T B, Sherlock S. Assessment of portal venous hypertension by catheterisation of hepatic vein. Lancet 1953; 1: 918

59 Groszmann R J, Glickmann M, Blei A, et al. Wedged and free hepatic venous pressure measured with a balloon catheter. Gastroenterology 1978; 76: 253

60 Burns P N. Interpretation and analysis of Doppler signals. In: Taylor K J W, Burns P N, Wells P N T. eds. Clinical applications of Doppler ultrasound. New York: Raven. 1988

61 Ohnishi K, Saito M, Nakayama T, et al. Portal venous hemodynamic in chronic liver disease: effects of posture change and exercise. Radiology 1985; 155: 757

62 Moriyasu F, Ban N, Nishida O, et al. 'Congestion index' of the portal vein. AJR 1985; 146: 735

63 Eik-Nes S H, Marsal K, Kristoffersen K. Methodology and basic problems related to blood flow studies in the human fetus. Ultrasound Med Biol 1984; 10: 329–337

64 Dauzat M, Pomier Layrargues G. Portal vein blood flow measurements using pulsed Doppler and electromagnetic flowmetry in dogs: a comparative study. Gastroenterology 1989; 96: 913

65 Sabbà C, Nakamura T, Weltin G, et al. Intra- and inter-observer variability of echo-Doppler measurements of portal flow in normal volunteers. 39th Annual Meeting of the American Association for the Study of Liver Disease. Chicago: Nov 5–8, 1988; Abstracts Book. p 54

66 Kimme-Smith C, Hussain R, Duerinckx A, Tessler F, Grant E. Reproducibility of Doppler abdominal flow rates: instrumentation variability. J Ultrasound Med 1988; 7 (supplement): 90; abstract 1242

67 Brown H S, Halliwell M, Qamar M, Read A E, Evans J M, Wells PNT. Measurement of normal portal venous blood flow by Doppler ultrasound. Gut 1989; 30: 503

68 The value of Doppler ultrasound in the study of hepatic hemodynamics. Consensus conference. Bologna, Italy: 12

September, 1989. Chairman: L.Barbara. J Hepatol 1990; in press

69 Zoli M, Marchesini G, Cordiani M R, et al. Echo-Doppler measurement of splanchnic blood flow in control and in cirrhotic subjects. JCU 1986; 14: 429

70 Pugliese D, Ohnishi K, Tsunoda T, Sabba C, Albano O. Portal hemodynamics after meal in normal subjects and in patients with chronic liver disease studied by echo-Doppler flowmeter. Am J Gastroenterol 1987; 10: 1052

71 Ohnishi K, Saito M, Sato S, et al. Portal hemodynamics in idiopathic portal hypertension (Banti's syndrome). Gastroenterology 1987; 92: 751–758

72 Darnault P, Bretagne J F, Fournier V, Raoul J. Splanchnic hemodynamics assessment in patients with liver cirrhosis and hypersplenism. Gastroenterology 1989; 96: A589

73 Sabba C, Ferraioli G, Sarin S K, Groszmann R J, Taylor K J W. Feasibility for Doppler flow measurements in splanchnic vessels in non-selected patient population and in cirrhotics. Gastroenterology 1989; 96: A432

74 Mostbeck G H, Wittich G R, Herold C, et al. Hemodynamic significance of the paraumbilical vein in portal hypertension: assessment with duplex ultrasound. Radiology 1989; 170: 339

75 Jaeger K, Bollinger A, Valli C, Ammann R. Measurement of mesenteric blood flow by duplex scanning. J Vasc Surg 1986; 3: 462

76 Qamar M I, Read A E, Skidmore R, Evans J M, Wells P N T. Transcutaneous Doppler ultrasound measurement of superior mesenteric artery blood flow in man. Gut 1986; 27: 100

77 Sato S, Ohnishi K, Sugita S, Okuda K. Splenic artery and superior mesenteric artery blood flow: non-surgical Doppler ultrasound measurement in healthy subjects and patients with chronic liver disease. Radiology 1987; 164: 347

78 Moneta G L, Taylor D C, Helton W S, Mulholland M W, Strandness D E. Duplex ultrasound measurement of postprandial intestinal blood flow. Effect of meal composition. Gastroenterology 1988; 95: 1294

79 Weill F S, Le Mouel A, Bihr E, Rohmer P, Zeltner F, Perrisney G. Ultrasonic patterns of acquired Budd-Chiari's syndromes. Eur J Radiol 1981; 1: 236

80 Baert A L, Fevery J, Marchal G, et al. Early diagnosis of Budd-Chiari syndrome by computed tomography and ultrasonography: report of five cases. Gastroenterology 1893; 84: 587

81 Makuuchi M, Hasegawa H, Yamazaki S, et al. Primary Budd-Chiari syndrome: ultrasonic demonstration. Radiology 1984; 152: 775

82 Hosoki T, Kuroda C, Tokunaga K, et al. Hepatic venous outflow obstruction: evaluation with pulsed Doppler sonography. Radiology 1989; 170: 733

83 Holmin T, Alwmark A, Forsberg L. The ultrasonic demonstration of portacaval and interposition mesocaval shunt. Br J Surg 1982; 69: 673

84 Forsberg L, Holmin R. Pulsed Doppler and B-mode ultrasound features of interposition meso-caval and porta-caval shunts. Acta Radiol (Diagn) 1983; 24: 353

85 Ackroyd N, Gill R, Griffiths K, Kossoff G, Reeve T. Duplex scanning of the portal vein and portosystemic shunts. Surgery 1986; 99: 591

86 Lafortune M, Patriquin H, Pomier G, et al. Hemodynamic changes in portal circulation after portosystemic shunts: use of Duplex sonography in 43 patients. AJR 1987; 149: 701

87 Moryiasu F, Nishida O, Ban N, et al. Ultrasonic Doppler duplex study of hemodynamic changes from portosystemic shunt operation. Ann Surg 1987; 205: 151

88 Bolondi L, Gaiani S, Mazziotti A, et al. Morphological and hemodynamic changes in the portal venous system after distal spleno-renal shunt: an ultrasound and pulsed Doppler study. Hepatology 1988; 8: 652

89 Tylen U, Simert G, Vang J. Hemodynamic changes after distal spleno-renal shunt studied by sequential angiography. Radiology 1986; 121: 585

Liver transplants

Hylton B. Meire and Pat Farrant

INTRODUCTION

Liver transplantation is now an acceptable option for patients with end-stage chronic liver disease[1] and fulminant hepatic failure[2] and may also offer prolonged survival for certain patients with hepatic malignancies. The progressive improvement in patient survival from liver transplantation over the past few years has been due to a combination of factors including better patient selection, improved organ preservation, developments in surgical technique, modern immunosuppressive agents and improved post-operative management. Medical imaging, especially ultrasound, plays an important role in patient selection and management. Ultrasound is used in the pre-operative, operative and post-operative periods[3,4] depending upon factors such as the surgical technique and the patient's original diagnosis.

Pre-operative assessment

The initial role for ultrasound in the pre-operative assessment of patients considered for liver transplantation is in confirming the diagnosis. For patients with fulminant hepatic failure or end-stage liver disease, the changes associated with the disease can be identified though the cause of the disease cannot, of course, be determined by ultrasound. An exception to this rule is the Budd-Chiari syndrome where ultrasound imaging and Doppler studies can confirm occlusion of the hepatic veins and usually also shows enlargement of the caudate lobe, together with any other lobe or segment in which the major vein has been spared.

If transplantation is being considered as a treatment for hepatic tumours it is essential that the malignant nature of the lesion is confirmed histologically. Patients referred for liver transplantation with liver tumours have, on occasion, proved to have complex hydatid cysts, amoebic abscesses or haemangiomas. In addition true tumours may be difficult to identify, particularly for pathologists not used to evaluating the rarer types. Both focal nodular hyperplasia and hepatic adenoma can be indistinguishable from hepatocellular carcinoma on ultrasound imaging and these diagnoses should therefore always be borne in mind and, if necessary, ultrasound guided biopsy, angiography and dynamic CT should be undertaken.

In addition to confirming the diagnosis, ultrasound imaging should be directed towards assessing the complications of the disease. In patients with chronic liver disease this includes confirmation of portal vein patency and assessment of paraportal collaterals. If the liver failure is secondary to biliary atresia, associated anatomical abnormalities should be sought and for those patients with malignant disease the size and extent of the tumour and the presence of extrahepatic spread should be assessed. The exact role of ultrasound in the pre-transplant patient therefore varies somewhat according to the patient's diagnosis and each of the main diagnoses is considered separately below. However, perhaps the most important role for ultrasound is that of confirming portal vein patency as portal vein occlusion may be a contra-indication to surgery.

Portal vein patency

Successful liver transplantation depends upon several factors but amongst the most important are successful vascular anastomoses. Portal vein occlusion is a recognised sequela of long-standing liver disease and causes rapid hepatic decompensation; it is therefore important for the status of the portal vein to be assessed pre-operatively. Until recently patency of the portal vein was an essential prerequisite for liver transplantation. Some transplant surgeons now attempt portal thrombectomy or construct portal conduits[5] but, if either of these procedures is to be undertaken, it is important that accurate pre-operative information is available. In the majority of patients this can all be obtained from an ultrasound examination.

The extrahepatic components of the portal venous system can normally be assessed via subcostal scans and the combination of imaging and colour flow Doppler usually rapidly confirm their patency (Fig. 1). In patients with gaseous distension and very small livers, imaging of the extrahepatic portal vein may be difficult or impossible and angiography remains necessary in a minority of patients.

Both imaging and Doppler studies of the intrahepatic portal venous system are best achieved via right lateral intercostal scans which allow visualisation of the main and right portal veins even in the smallest of livers (Fig. 2). It is important to be aware that flow within the intrahepatic portal vein does not necessarily imply patency of the extrahepatic venous system; low velocity forward intrahepatic flow can occur in patients in whom splenic and superior mesenteric venous occlusion have been proven. Both components of the portal system must be examined.

If duplex and colour flow studies fail to detect flow within the portal vein the equipment control settings must be optimised to detect low velocity flow. In particular the high pass filter (wall thump filter), often invaluable for arterial studies, should be set at the lowest possible value consistent with excluding artefactual noise from the spectrum analysis tracing. In addition the Doppler shift frequency must be optimised by minimising the beam/vessel angle, particularly by use of lateral intercostal scans. Even if all these measures fail to detect portal flow, portal occlusion cannot be considered proven as flow velocities below 2 or 3 cm per second are below the threshold of some scanners. If no flow is found, the examination should be repeated after an interval or after a meal, particularly if the patient's clinical condition improves. If doubt exists after a second or subsequent examination, angiography is essential.

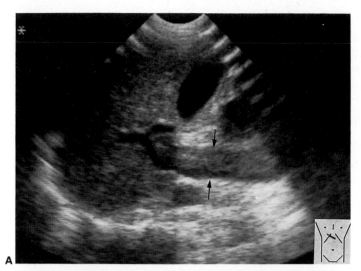

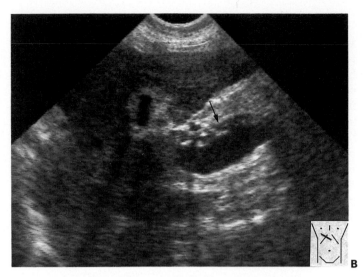

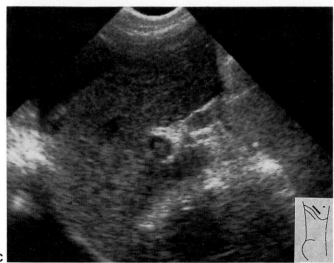

Fig. 1   Assessment of portal vein patency. A: Oblique subcostal scan of extrahepatic portal vein. The main portal vein (arrows) is dilated and there is thrombus adherent to its anterior wall. **B:** There is old partially calcified thrombus adherent to the anterior portal vein wall (arrow). **C:** Same patient as B. There is fresh thrombus within the intrahepatic portal vein.

vein thrombosis and this is particularly likely if the flow velocity is low (see Plate 1).

A further source of error in the diagnosis of portal vein occlusion is cavernous transformation of the portal vein which develops as a long-term sequel to portal vein thrombosis. Imaging alone may suggest the diagnosis by detecting numerous serpiginous channels replacing the portal vein at the porta hepatis. However, in a minority of patients with this condition, a single large collateral channel may be present and may be mistaken for the main portal vein (Fig. 5). In the majority of patients with cavernous transformation the intrahepatic portal vein branches

The direction and absolute velocity of portal flow are unimportant in this context (Fig. 3) and, in patients with severe decompensated liver disease, rapid changes in both velocity and direction of flow may be observed as the patient's condition varies.

If little or no flow is detected in the intrahepatic portal veins and if there is imaging evidence of either fresh or old thrombus in the intrahepatic portal system, the superior mesenteric vein must be assessed. If the superior mesenteric vein remains patent at the level of the splenic vein confluence, the surgeon may be able to use this as a source of portal supply to the grafted liver.

In those patients in whom low velocity flow is detected within the portal vein, the examination should be repeated if transplantation is not undertaken within 1 to 2 weeks (Fig. 4). Similarly, even if flow is normal or high, the examination should be repeated if transplantation is not undertaken within 4 to 6 weeks. All patients with chronic liver disease are at increased risk for spontaneous portal

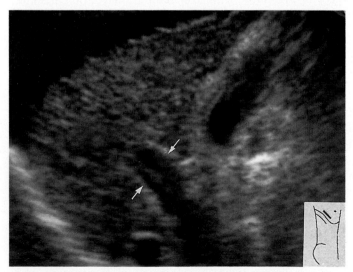

Fig. 2   Lateral intercostal scan of portal vein. In this patient with a small cirrhotic liver and ascites, this approach shows partial thrombosis of the intrahepatic portal vein. Arrows – portal vein walls.

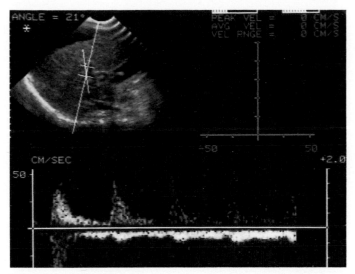

Fig. 3 Portal vein Doppler. There is low velocity reversed flow in the portal vein. The simultaneous acquisition of an arterial signal confirms that the venous signal is portal in origin.

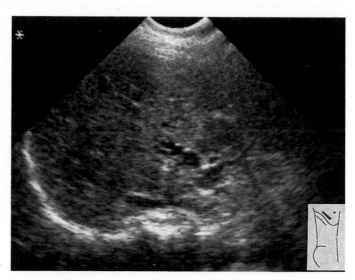

Fig. 5 Cavernous transformation of the portal vein. In this patient with long-standing portal vein thrombosis there has been cavernous transformation with the production of a dominant collateral anteriorly within the porta; this can easily be mistaken for the main portal vein.

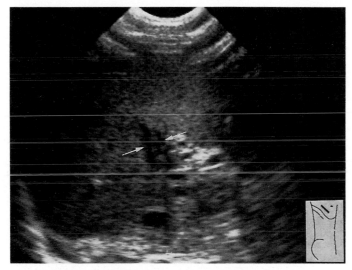

Fig. 4 Acute portal thrombosis. The portal vein (arrows) contains fresh thrombus 4 weeks after an initial pre-transplant study confirmed portal vein patency.

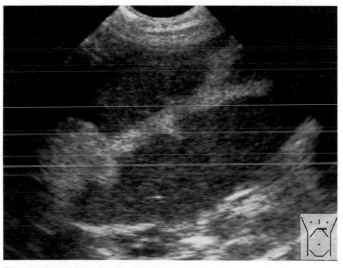

Fig. 6 Portal invasion by hepatocellular carcinoma. Transverse scan of the left lobe of the liver showing a highly reflective primary hepatocellular carcinoma which has extended into the left intrahepatic portal system.

are either abnormally small or absent and, therefore, the assessment should include both the intra- and extrahepatic components of the portal vein.

In patients in whom transplantation is being considered for malignant liver disease it is important to determine whether or not there is vascular invasion by the tumour, particularly in primary hepatocellular carcinoma (Fig. 6). Up to 25% have been reported to invade the intrahepatic portal venous system and tumour thrombus may occupy the whole of the intrahepatic system and extend into the extrahepatic portal vein (Fig. 7).

The final component of portal assessment is the detection of paraportal collaterals, particularly those in the right side of the abdomen which may give rise to surgical problems during hepatectomy. Foreknowledge of the presence of major subhepatic collaterals helps the surgeon to plan the operative approach.

It is customary to measure the maximum diameter of the spleen when assessing patients with liver disease and this should always be recorded prior to liver transplantation. Though the presence and degree of splenomegaly are of no importance at this stage in the patient's management,

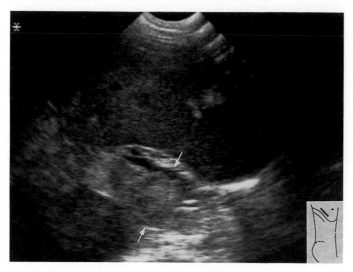

Fig. 7 Tumour thrombus in main portal vein. In this patient with hepatocellular carcinoma the main portal vein (arrows) is greatly expanded and is filled with tumour thrombus.

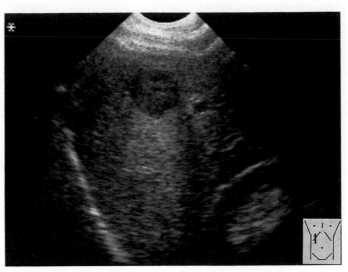

Fig. 8 Hepatocellular carcinoma in chronic liver disease. In this routine pre-transplant examination a 2.5 cm diameter poorly reflective and poorly attenuating mass has developed and was proved to be a hepatocellular carcinoma.

progressive splenic enlargement in the post-operative period may be the first indication of portal vein stenosis or occlusion. A pre-operative baseline measurement is therefore important and, in a minority of patients with successful transplantation, the spleen may be found to decrease in size post-operatively as successful transplantation immediately reduces the portal pressure to normal.

Hepatocellular carcinoma

Patients with chronic liver disease, especially that due to the hepatitis B virus, have a greatly increased incidence of hepatocellular carcinoma (HCC) (Fig. 8). Liver transplantation as a treatment for primary HCC is now used less frequently as the large majority of patients transplanted for HCC during the past decade have died from recurrent tumour. The most important factor in selection of patients for liver transplantation is the total tumour volume, while the number of tumours is also important. Survival beyond 1 year is uncommon in patients with multiple tumours or those with a single lesion greater than 3 cm in diameter.

Pre-operative assessment of the HCC patient for transplantation is therefore aimed at confirmation of the number and size of tumours (Fig. 9). If the total tumour bulk is greater than 15 ml, the chances of 1 year survival are less than 5% and liver transplantation is therefore contra-indicated.

HCC is particularly prone to invade the portal vein and may also extend into the hepatic veins. The ultrasound examination should be directed towards exclusion of vascular invasion.

In those patients with HCC superimposed on a relatively normal or only moderately compromised liver, the question of resectability should always be considered. The patient is likely to have a longer survival with a curative resection. If the tumour is relatively small and can be shown to be confined to a single segment or lobe of the liver with no vascular invasion, a partial hepatectomy may be the most appropriate course of treatment.

HCC most often metastasises to the lungs and bones which are best investigated by CT and nuclear medicine studies. Occasionally lymphatic spread gives rise to adenopathy in the porta hepatis or upper abdomen and ultrasound examination can confirm the presence of lymph node enlargement.

Other tumours

Liver transplantation may occasionally be offered to patients with other forms of hepatic malignancy which are not amenable to resection. Tumours in this group include cholangiocarcinoma, other very rare primary hepatic tumours, and metastases from carcinoid (Fig. 10), provided the tumour is confined to the liver. Liver transplantation is seldom curative in this group of patients but may extend the period of good quality survival and palliate the severe endocrine manifestations of the neuro-endocrine tumours.

In this group of patients ultrasound is aimed at confirmation of the original diagnosis, assessment of the resectability and possible spread of the disease process and confirmation of portal vein patency.

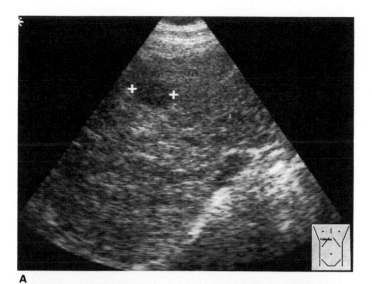

A

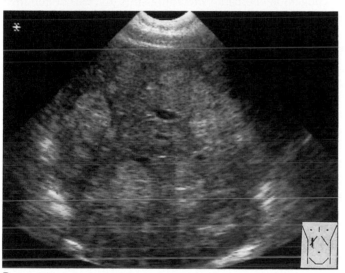

B

Fig. 9 Assessment of hepatocellular carcinoma. A: In this child with tyrosinaemia, a solitary 15 mm diameter nodule has arisen; its presence expedited transplantation. **B:** In this adult patient, multifocal hepatoma has developed and excludes the possibility of curative transplantation.

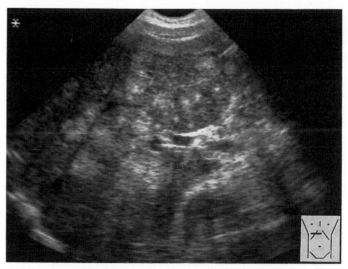

Fig. 10 Metastatic carcinoid of the liver. The symptoms associated with carcinoid are related to the tumour volume within the liver. Carcinoid deposits are almost always clearly defined and highly reflective.

Budd-Chiari syndrome

Budd-Chiari syndrome (BCS) may present as acute hepatic venous congestion, fulminant hepatic failure (FHF) or established cirrhosis. Patients in the first category may achieve almost complete recovery if an early porto-systemic shunt is created, those with FHF or late decompensated cirrhosis may require transplantation.

The role of ultrasound in BCS is firstly in confirmation of the original diagnosis.[6] Imaging and Doppler studies, especially colour flow imaging, should be directed towards confirming occlusion of all the major hepatic veins. In patients with long-standing BCS, numerous serpiginous in-

trahepatic collaterals are usually detected and retrograde flow may occasionally be seen in patent central segments of the major hepatic veins (see Ch. 18). Rarely the hepatic vein occlusion may be secondary to an inferior vena caval abnormality, particularly a web, and attempts should be made to assess the IVC. However, this is often difficult in the presence of a swollen liver and biplane contrast vena cavography is more accurate than ultrasound in assessment of the IVC.

Many patients with BCS also suffer thrombotic occlusion of the portal venous system, either in the acute phase or later in the disease process. In acute complete BCS, flow within the portal vein is almost always reversed but, as hepatic venous collaterals develop, flow within the portal vein may reduce thus increasing the risk of spontaneous thrombosis, particularly if the original vascular occlusions were secondary to an underlying abnormality of thrombogenesis.

Fulminant hepatic failure

The clinical management of fulminant hepatic failure has changed rapidly in recent years with a marked improvement in survival. However, there remains a group of patients in whom liver recovery can be predicted to be very unlikely and these patients may be offered emergency liver transplantation. Their clinical diagnoses vary widely and include paracetamol and other drug overdoses, Wilson's disease and acute viral hepatitis (Fig. 11) and are often uncertain until after transplantation. The role of preoperative ultrasound in these patients is to exclude exten-

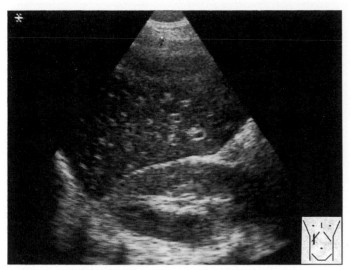

Fig. 11 Acute viral hepatitis. This child presented with fulminant hepatic failure. The ultrasound reveals uniform decrease in parenchymal reflectivity, the portal vein branches standing out against the poorly reflective parenchymal background.

sive hepatic malignancy as the cause of the failure and to confirm portal vein patency.

Chronic liver disease

Patients with a variety of chronic liver disorders comprise the largest group considered for liver transplantation. Pre-operative ultrasound imaging is directed to confirming the presence of severe liver disease, if necessary with the use of ultrasound guided liver biopsy in those patients with very small livers.

These patients are at increased risk for development of primary HCC and it is therefore essential that the whole volume of the liver is examined carefully to detect any focal lesion. If focal lesions or suspicious areas are detected on ultrasound imaging, further investigations are indicated, including ultrasound guided biopsy, angiography and CT scanning after lipiodol injection into the hepatic artery. If imaging procedures confirm the presence of a small HCC, this finding will generally expedite transplantation but, if larger volumes of tumour are present, transplantation is unlikely to be appropriate.

Confirmation of the patency of the intra- and extra-hepatic portal vein is important and any patient with low velocity flow or in whom there is a significant delay before transplantation, should be re-examined in the pre-operative period to exclude subsequent thrombosis of the portal vein.

Biliary atresia

Patients with severe progressive liver failure secondary to a failed Kasai procedure or undiagnosed biliary atresia con-

stitute an important group in whom liver transplantation offers the only hope of prolonged survival. These patients are almost always children varying in age from a few months to a few years. In this group ultrasound assessment is technically difficult as a result of several factors including previous surgery, associated congenital anomalies, ascites, heterogeneous and highly reflective livers (Fig. 12) and a lack of patient co-operation.

Previous surgical intervention, particularly the Kasai procedure, usually gives rise to adhesions in the upper abdomen with gas-filled bowel in the subhepatic space extending up to the porta hepatis. This may make visualisation of the extrahepatic portal venous system difficult or impossible and may necessitate recourse to angiography if doubt about their patency persists.

Patients with biliary atresia have an increased incidence of congenital anomalies including situs inversus abdominis, malrotation of the gut, abnormalities of the hepatic artery, portal vein and inferior vena cava and polysplenia or asplenia. It is important that as many of these as possible are identified or excluded on the pre-operative investigations so that the surgeon can be warned of their existence.[7] In particular the hepatic artery anatomy is frequently abnormal, with multiple arteries and/or an anomalous extrahepatic course. Very rarely the portal vein may drain directly into the vena cava or may lie in a preduodenal position. The IVC may be absent, left sided or subject to a number of other anomalies, the commonest of which is caval interruption with azygos continuation.

The heterogeneous and highly reflective liver in end-stage secondary biliary cirrhosis may render imaging of the intrahepatic portal venous system difficult and indeed the portal vein radicals may be compressed by the abnormal

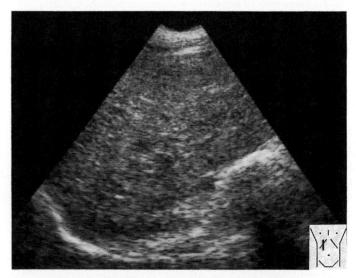

Fig. 12 Heterogeneous liver of secondary biliary cirrhosis. In this child with a failed Kasai procedure, the liver has become extremely heterogeneous and the main portal vein and portal tracts can no longer be identified by ultrasound imaging.

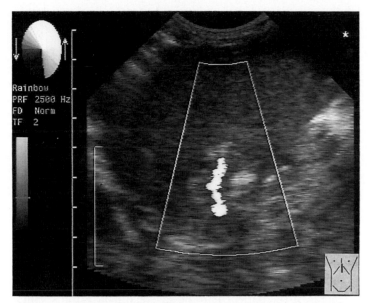

Plate 1 Arterial signal in portal vein occlusion. There is a strong forward flow signal in the region of the porta hepatis. This is due to continuous high velocity flow in the hepatic artery in the absence of portal vein flow. This figure is reproduced in colour in the colour plate section at the front of this volume.

liver. In this situation colour flow imaging usually permits confirmation of portal vein patency. However, care should be exercised when interpreting colour flow images as these patients often have a particularly rapid flow in relatively large hepatic arteries (Plate 1). Any high velocity forward flowing colour signal within the liver must also be subjected to spectrum analysis to determine whether it is arterial or venous in origin.

Per-operative scanning

Intra-operative ultrasound is now an accepted technique (see Ch. 15) and may fulfil a number of roles in the transplant patient.

Pre-hepatectomy intra-operative ultrasound may be helpful to confirm the number and extent of neoplasms and to assess vascular invasion. Absence of the intervening abdominal wall permits better quality images to be obtained on intra-operative scans than is possible pre-operatively and thus makes the technique worthwhile even when pre-operative imaging has been reassuring.

If the donor liver is too large for the recipient it may be necessary to reduce its size, usually using segments II, III and IV.[8,9] Scanning of the donor liver to identify the major intrahepatic vessels may be helpful in speeding reduction operations.

After successful transplantation, intra-operative Doppler studies are invaluable in confirming good flow through the vascular anastomoses, especially if conduits have been used or if the anatomy is abnormal, for example if a donor liver reduction procedure has been performed.

Post-operative

The role of ultrasound in the post-operative period varies according to the time elapsed since the operation. There are cogent arguments in favour of performing routine imaging and Doppler examinations during the early post-operative period,[10] though the need for and the frequency of these examinations remains subject to controversy. If circumstances permit, it is probably ideal to perform routine examinations on days 1, 3, 5 and 7 and weekly thereafter, unless otherwise indicated by clinical or biochemical findings.

Before undertaking post-operative examinations it is important for the equipment operator to be fully conversant with the surgical details. In particular it is important to

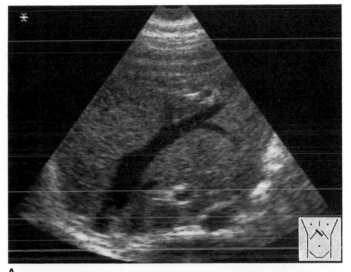

A

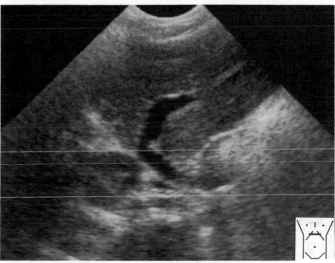

B

Fig. 13 Cutdown liver. A: Oblique subcostal scan and **B:** transverse subcostal scan. The unusual hepatic vein anatomy (A) and portal vein anatomy (B) result from transplantation of segments II, III and IV only from the donor liver.

know whether or not a cutdown procedure has been employed (Fig. 13) and to have detailed information concerning the hepatic artery, portal vein, IVC and biliary anastomoses. Many different variants of these anastomoses may be used, according to the preference of the surgeon, the nature of the underlying disease process or the anatomy of the donor and recipient vessels. For example, patients with biliary atresia, sclerosing cholangitis and other bile duct abnormalities are likely to have a Roux loop for the biliary conduit. Patients with abnormal arterial anatomy or who are being retransplanted for arterial occlusions may have an arterial conduit, often arising anteriorly from the distal abdominal aorta.

The operator should follow a predetermined protocol to ensure that all aspects of the transplant anatomy are carefully assessed and that all possible sites for fluid collections are evaluated.

Hepatic artery

Problems related to the hepatic artery anastomosis are the most common vascular complications after liver transplantation.[11] Most patients suffer a minor degree of post-operative haemorrhage giving rise to haematomas of 3 to 5 cm diameter at the porta hepatis (Fig. 14). In adults early arterial occlusion occurs in 1% to 3% of patients but is much more common in the paediatric age group, rising to 25% in patients below 1 year of age. Early arterial occlusion is almost always a catastrophic event with rapid and irreversible liver cell death. The resultant hepatic necrosis can usually be diagnosed on ultrasound scanning by the detection of areas of liquefaction (Fig. 15). Rarely surgical revascularisation procedures may be successful[12] but, in general, if the patient is to be saved, urgent retransplantation is necessary.

Post-operative occlusion of the hepatic artery most commonly occurs at the site of the vascular anastomosis but may occur elsewhere in the main vessel (possibly as a result of clamp injury) and intrahepatic obstructions of individual major branches have also been documented.

Impending or complete occlusion of the hepatic artery is often indicated by generalised non-specific deterioration of the liver function tests with a characteristic rise in the AST, or with a bile leak.

Ideally all segments of the arterial system should be studied including the extrahepatic and intrahepatic main hepatic artery and the right and left intrahepatic branches. In practice, the extrahepatic artery is often difficult to identify owing to upper abdominal bowel gas. The intrahepatic

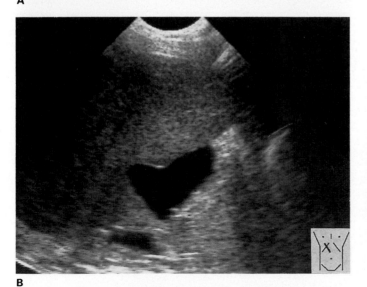

A

B

Fig. 14 Porta hepatis fluid collections. These small periportal fluid collections are almost invariable in the early post-transplant phase and are usually of no clinical significance.

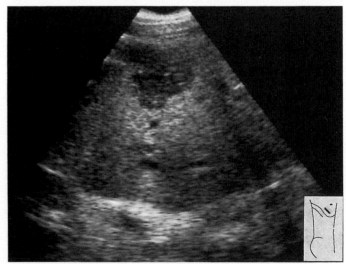

Fig. 15 Hepatic infarction. Segmental infarction due to occlusion of a branch artery gives rise to an irregular area of reduced reflectivity which may be the first indicator of arterial occlusion.

portion of the main hepatic artery and the right hepatic arterial branch can normally be identified via the right lateral intercostal approach and the left branch can be visualised on transverse subcostal scans using the left portal vein branch as a landmark. The anatomical location of the artery and its branches is somewhat variable and colour flow imaging (CFI) may be helpful in its detection (Plates 2 and 3). However, difficulties may arise with CFI owing to the inability of the majority of current scanners to resolve the portal vein and hepatic artery separately. Both vessels have flow in the same direction and the high velocity and disturbed flow within the portal vein may partially or completely mask the small adjacent hepatic artery. A spectral Doppler trace should therefore be obtained from the hepatic artery before its patency can be confirmed with certainty (Fig. 16).[13] The velocity of flow within the artery is very variable in the early post-operative phase and both colour flow and spectral scans may show the artery to have flow either higher or lower in velocity than that in the adjacent accompanying portal vein (Plate 3). Where the flow velocity is low and CFI is not available, duplex scanning alone may fail to detect the artery.[14,15]

The flow velocity waveform obtained from the hepatic artery in the acute post-transplant phase is variable and, as with velocity values, the significance of the various waveforms is uncertain. However, if the velocity is found to be extremely low or the waveform very damped (Fig. 17) this strongly raises the suspicion of a significant anastomotic stenosis. Similar appearances may result from hepatocellular problems due either to poor preservation of the donor organ or early acute rejection. Occasionally

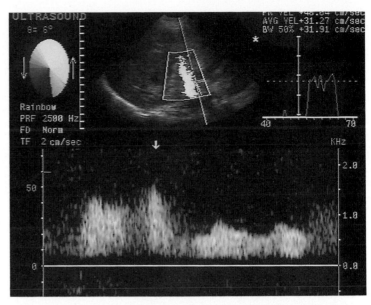

Plate 3 Low velocity arterial flow. The high velocity flow within the portal vein prevented identification of the artery on the colour flow image. Spectral Doppler studies reveal the presence of a low velocity arterial signal adjacent to the high velocity venous signal. This figure is reproduced in colour in the colour plate section at the front of this volume.

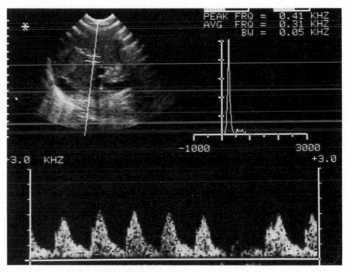

Fig. 16 Hepatic artery Doppler. Patency of the main and right hepatic artery are confirmed by this lateral intercostal duplex Doppler study.

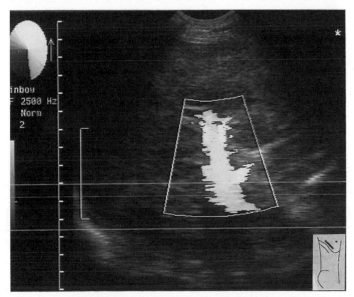

Plate 2 Colour Doppler detection of the hepatic artery. The colour map velocity coding has been adjusted to highlight the higher systolic velocities in the artery as orange against the slower red portal vein flow. This figure is reproduced in colour in the colour plate section at the front of this volume.

waveforms are found in which there is no evidence of diastolic flow (Fig. 18). Although this was initially thought to indicate the presence of acute rejection, this waveform is now known to be non-specific[16] and may indicate liver parenchymal problems, kinking of the hepatic artery or merely the existence of a long and compliant arterial conduit. Usually the arterial waveform is unremarkable and therefore any patient in whom the waveform is felt to be abnormal should receive frequent follow up examinations

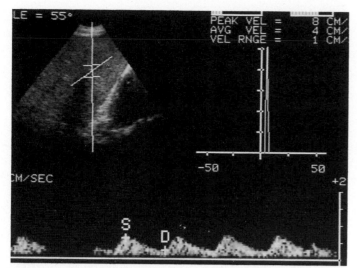

Fig. 17 Damped arterial flow. This low amplitude intrahepatic arterial signal raises the suspicion of significant anastomotic stenosis.

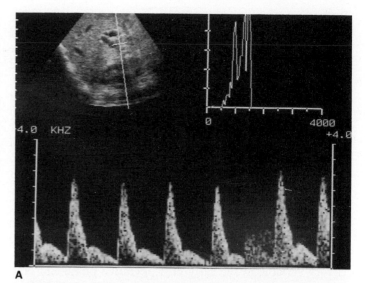

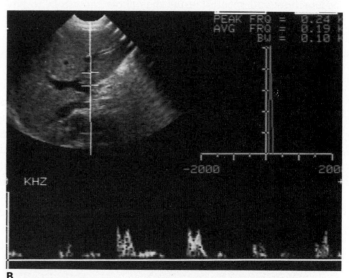

Fig. 18 Absence of hepatic artery diastolic flow. A: There is good systolic and early diastolic perfusion with very little end diastolic flow. This was a transient finding of uncertain origin. **B:** There is a low velocity biphasic systolic pulse and no diastolic flow. This trace indicates poor arterial perfusion, possibly as a result of severe parenchymal damage.

to confirm continuing vascular patency. If the Doppler studies show a progressive reduction in arterial velocity or a fall-off in diastolic flow in the absence of obvious parenchymal abnormality, the possibility of a progressive arterial obstructive lesion should be considered and angiography must be advised. Operative relief of a stenosis or inadequate anastomosis is much more satisfactory than an urgent retransplantation.[17] Percutaneous hepatic artery angioplasty probably has no role in the acute post-transplant phase, a period of at least 2 weeks being necessary for the anastomosis to heal to a point where it can withstand balloon dilatation.

When the liver is transplanted all possible collateral arterial routes are interrupted. After transplantation potential collaterals readily develop, particularly in children, and may be capable of maintaining adequate arterial perfusion by the third post-operative week.[18] In adults they develop more slowly, though are probably both quicker and more efficient if a Roux loop has been used in place of the recipient's common duct.

Doppler studies of the intrahepatic arterial tree become more difficult to interpret with increasing time after the operation. If good collateral supply has been established an entirely normal intrahepatic arterial waveform may be detected, even in the presence of total occlusion of the main hepatic artery. More commonly, however, there is some damping of the intrahepatic systolic arterial wave with maintenance of the diastolic flow (Fig. 19).[15] Conversely, the technical limitations of colour and duplex Doppler systems may prevent the operator from obtaining a Doppler signal even in the presence of a patent hepatic artery. Doppler studies of the hepatic artery are important but, in any patient in whom the Doppler findings do not concur with the clinical context, angiography must be per-

formed, particularly if there is likely to be a therapeutic implication.

If the hepatic artery remains patent but the portal vein becomes occluded, there is almost always a marked increase in arterial flow with increase in systolic velocity and a reduction in the resistance index (Fig. 20).

Very rarely liver biopsy may lead to an arterio-portal shunt and this may also give rise to high arterial flows but the true nature of the lesion can generally be established by detecting alteration in the portal flow, usually manifested by flow reversal in the portal vein branch draining the affected segment. Such arterio-portal shunts are of

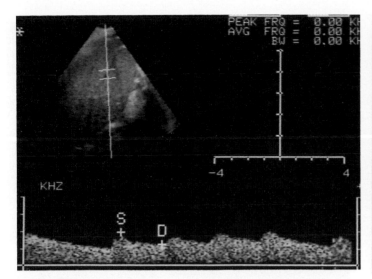

Fig. 19 Hepatic artery perfusion via collaterals. There was total occlusion of the hepatic artery developing several weeks after transplantation. The intrahepatic branches remain perfused via collaterals with a very damped waveform.

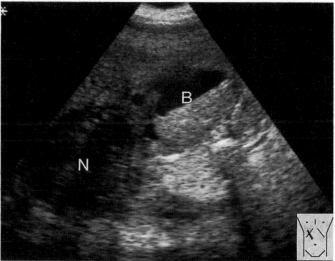

Fig. 21 Consequences of arterial occlusion. This patient with complete arterial occlusion has developed an area of necrosis in the right lobe (N) and a biliary leak with subhepatic biloma (B) in which the bile is sedimenting out.

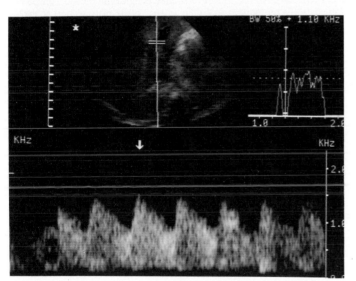

Fig. 20 Hepatic arterial waveform in portal occlusion. In this patient late portal occlusion had occurred but liver perfusion was maintained by a compensatory increase in arterial flow.

little clinical significance and almost always resolve spontaneously.

Although some patients with late onset arterial obstruction may show little clinical evidence of this, the majority suffer one or more complications. In the first few weeks after transplantation the most likely consequence is breakdown of the biliary anastomosis. Bile leaks should therefore be searched for in any patient thought to have a compromised artery and the artery should be studied in any patient thought to have a biliary leak (Fig. 21). If the biliary anastomosis survives the arterial deprivation, a biliary stricture may develop, either at the site of anastomosis or, more commonly, at the junction of the left and right hepatic ducts.[19,20] A consequence of this may be segmental or asymmetrical intrahepatic duct dilatation and, once again, it is important to study both ducts and artery.

A further complication of hepatic artery occlusion is the increased risk of intrahepatic abscess formation. Even if Doppler studies reveal an adequate collateral supply, the risk remains and is further enhanced if there is associated biliary stenosis, with intrahepatic bile duct dilatation and stasis increasing the chance of cholangitis. Therefore the whole volume of the liver must be scanned in any patient with known or suspected arterial occlusion or biliary stenosis, with a view to detecting abscess formation as early as possible (Fig. 22). If a suspected abscess is identified, this should be confirmed by CT scan and its communication with the biliary tree can be demonstrated by ascending cholangiography. Ultrasound may be helpful for both diagnostic and therapeutic drainage of liver abscesses and, with aggressive treatment, these may resolve despite continuing arterial occlusion.

If the arterial stenosis is treated by trans-luminal angioplasty serial Doppler studies are invaluable for confirming improvement in the arterial flow and for monitoring the patient's subsequent progress. It is not yet clear what percentage of arterial stenoses can be treated by angioplasty alone and how many ultimately require re-operation.

The intrahepatic arterial flow velocity waveform is very variable and can be affected by a large number of different factors. Loss of diastolic flow has been reported in rejection but this association seems to be very rare and there would

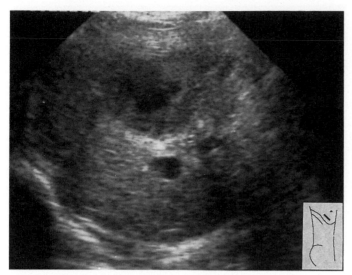

Fig. 22   Hepatic abscess secondary to ischaemia. The area of necrosis shown in Figure 15 has progressed to frank abscess formation.

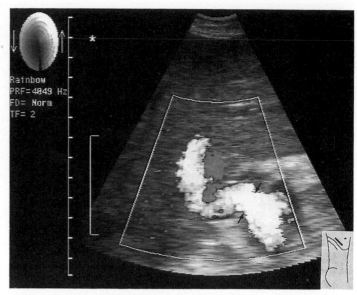

Plate 4   Post-transplant portal vein study. There is a mild narrowing at the anastomosis (arrows) with a moderately high velocity jet through the anastomosis (coded yellow). Within the intrahepatic portal vein there is a coarse vortex, the reverse flow component is coded purple. This figure is reproduced in colour in the colour plate section at the front of this volume.

not appear to be any reliable correlation between rejection and the arterial waveform.

Portal vein

Early post-operative occlusion of the portal vein is rare in adults and uncommon in paediatric patients. However early occlusion may have catastrophic consequences with early graft dysfunction or variceal bleeding; confirmation of portal patency is therefore very important. Colour flow imaging alone is almost always sufficient for confirmation of patency (Plate 4), problems being experienced only when the anatomy is abnormal after liver reduction procedures. Patients with BCS, abnormal portal vein anatomy, including those with a cutdown liver, a portal vein conduit or who have had an operative thrombectomy are all at increased risk of portal vein thrombosis and deserve special attention.

The flow characteristics within the transplanted portal vein are almost always abnormal due to a degree of infolding at the portal anastomosis (Fig. 23). There is severe flow disturbance beyond the anastomosis (Fig. 24) and a relatively high velocity jet is found at the anastomosis. For this reason, velocity measurements distal to the anastomosis are difficult or impossible. However, spectral Doppler studies should be attempted using colour flow imaging to detect the high velocity and a peak velocity estimate should be performed. If this is greater than 100 cm/sec the anastomosis is likely to be unacceptably tight (Fig. 25) and the patient must be carefully monitored for the development of portal stenosis and evidence of extrahepatic portal hypertension. Kinked vessels are also at increased risk of thrombosis. In those patients with significant subhepatic fluid collections, the portal vein can be compressed or displaced and this may give rise to stenosis or kinking.

Aspiration of the collection may prevent subsequent portal vein thrombosis.

Transient highly reflective foci within the portal vein lumen indicate gas bubbles. These may be an incidental finding[21] but can also indicate grave intra-abdominal pathology such as bowel infarction. We have seen only one example of intraportal gas bubbles in many thousands of examinations (Fig. 26); the patient died within 48 hours because of overwhelming gas gangrene.

As with pre-operative investigations, assessment of the portal system includes measurement of spleen size. Many post-transplant patients show a small reduction in spleen size; a significant enlargement suggests unresolved portal hypertension.

Late stenosis of the portal vein is uncommon and can usually be predicted by detection of a narrow anastomosis on the early post-operative scans (Fig. 27). In these patients serial measurements of the jet velocity permits detection of a progressive stenosis and the spleen is seen to enlarge if the lesion becomes haemodynamically significant.

Portal vein stenosis may rarely occur as a very late complication, even several years after successful transplantation. The diagnosis may be made incidentally by detection of intrahepatic post-stenotic dilatation of the portal vein (Fig. 28) with an associated high velocity jet and increasing splenomegaly. These patients may also present with ascites or haematemesis.

Late and sudden portal vein occlusion is rare and usually presents with sudden deterioration in liver function tests,

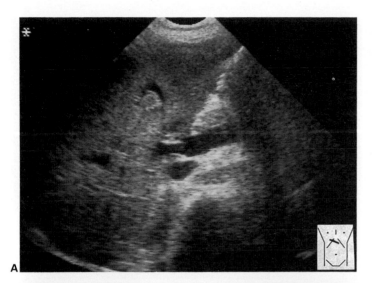

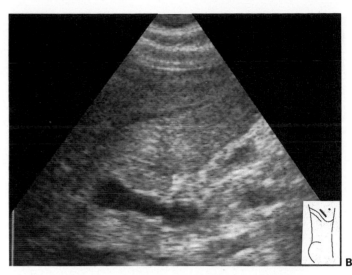

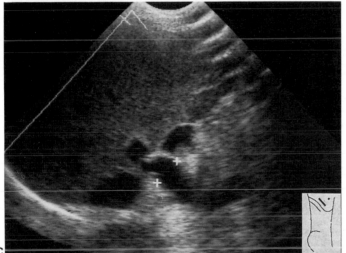

Fig. 23 Portal vein anastomoses. The portal vein anastomosis is frequently visible and may appear **A:** as a sudden change in calibre, **B:** a circumferential flap or **C:** an eccentric flap.

the onset of resistant ascites and rapidly increasing splenomegaly. Occasionally the only symptom is acute gastrointestinal haemorrhage indicating the recurrence of portal hypertension. Any patient with one or more of these signs or symptoms should receive immediate and thorough ultrasound examination of the liver and spleen with full Doppler assessment.

Hepatic veins and IVC

In the majority of liver transplant patients examination of the hepatic veins need be only fairly cursory. Hepatic vein

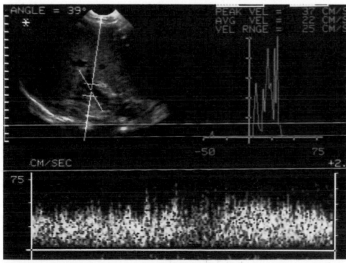

Fig. 24 Normal post-transplant portal vein Doppler. The irregularity at the portal anastomosis almost invariably gives rise to disturbed flow distal to the anastomosis.

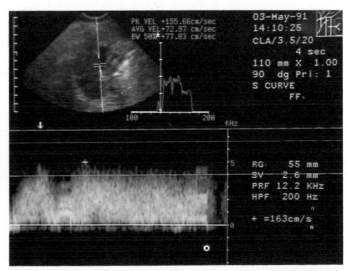

Fig. 25 Portal vein stenosis. In this early post-transplant patient the lumen at the portal vein anastomosis is very small and the peak velocity through the anastomosis is 163 cm/sec.

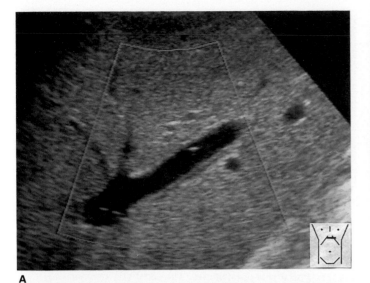

A

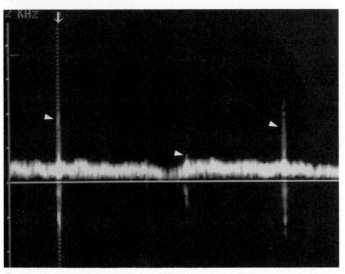

B

Fig. 26 Intraportal gas. A: Rapidly moving highly reflective foci were seen within the lumen of the portal vein; three are captured in this still frame. **B:** Passage of gas bubbles through the Doppler range gate gives rise to high amplitude transient signals (arrowheads) superimposed on the portal venous signal.

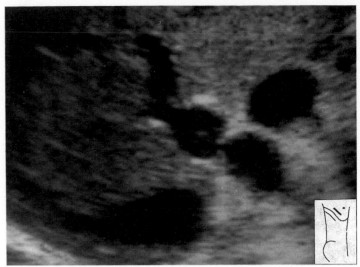

Fig. 27 Late onset portal vein stenosis. There is a very tight stenosis with a residual lumen of only 2 mm and both pre- and post-stenotic dilatation.

waveform and the presence of liver abnormality and duration of patient survival. More encouraging shorter term results have recently been reported in which deterioration of pulsatility of the hepatic waveforms was 100% correlated with deterioration in the patient's liver status (Fig. 29).[22] Our own experience suggests that there is a large number of extraneous factors affecting the hepatic vein pulsatility including the presence and severity of ascites, pleural effusions and other collections, patient obesity and the degree to which the transplanted liver matches the size of the recipient abdomen. For the moment it seems prudent to study the hepatic vein waveform and to be aware that significant progressive reductions in pulsatility may be a non-specific indicator of the presence of one of many clinical complications.

Stenosis of the IVC is extremely rare and generally presents with ascites and increasing lower limb oedema. The diagnosis can be established with ultrasound by demonstration of a dilated and pulseless cava below the level of the stenosis (Fig. 30) but contrast cavography is the definitive diagnostic test.

Fluid collections

Upper abdominal fluid collections are common in the early post-operative period and are seldom of any clinical significance.[3] The commonest causes are unresolved ascites, small periportal haematoma (Fig. 31) and subcapsular intrahepatic haematomas (Fig. 32), which usually occur on the superior aspect of the left lobe or inferior lateral aspect of the right lobe. Of these the periportal haematomas are the only collections likely to become of significance since they may compress or displace the portal vein or bile duct.

dilatation due to upper IVC anastomotic stenosis is rare and early hepatic vein thrombosis is almost unheard of, except in those patients who have been transplanted for BCS. In these patients the major hepatic veins and IVC must be scanned carefully to confirm flow and to exclude the presence of thrombi.

A non-specific correlation has been shown between the pulsatility of the hepatic vein waveform and the presence and severity of a range of hepatic parenchymal abnormalities. The clinical relevance of hepatic vein Doppler studies in liver transplantation remains uncertain. After some initial enthusiasm, our own results have been disappointing, showing no correlation between hepatic vein

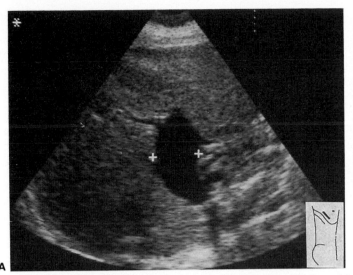
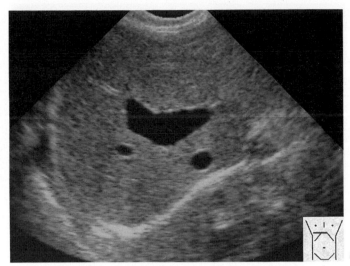

Fig. 28   Portal vein stenosis with post-stenotic dilatation. A: Lateral intercostal scan and **B:** transverse scan. There is marked dilatation of the intrahepatic portal vein associated with a high velocity vortex secondary to anastomotic stenosis.

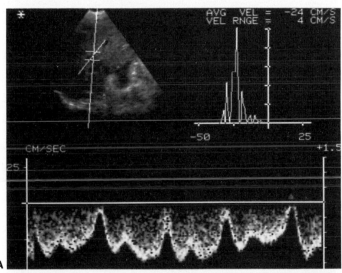
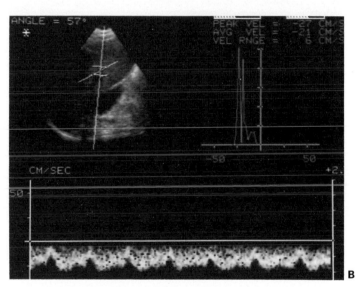

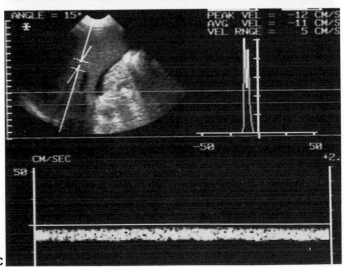

Fig. 29   Doppler studies of the hepatic veins. A: Normal hepatic vein tracing. **B:** The tracing is moderately damped and **C:** severely damped indicating increased liver stiffness.

Fine linear echoes are frequently detected within haematomas, thus differentiating them from bile collections, which may contain amorphous and unstructured reflective material which may precipitate with time (Fig. 33). During the first week or two of post-operative management the majority of haematomas are comprised of clotted blood (Fig. 34) and aspiration is seldom either necessary or possible.

An early post-operative scan to identify and measure fluid collections is an important component of post-operative care, the majority of collections stabilising in size in the first few days. Any collections which arise de novo

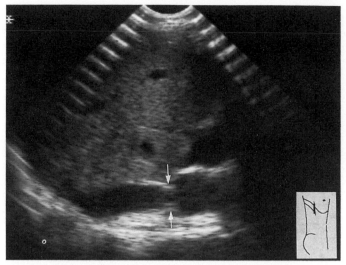

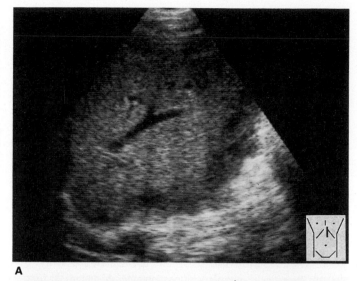

Fig. 30 Stenosis of the IVC. The inferior IVC anastomosis (arrows) is rather tight with dilatation of the IVC inferior to the anastomosis.

A

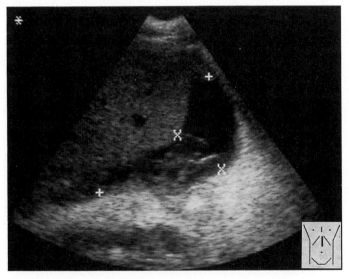

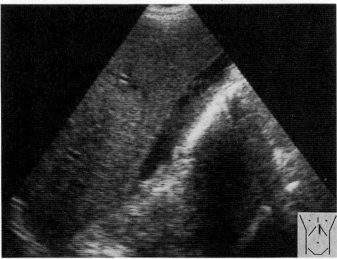

B

Fig. 32 Subcapsular haematoma. A: In the early post-transplant phase the inferior subcapsular haematoma is only just detectable as an irregular area of reduced reflectivity. **B:** As the haematoma matures it acquires the more typical 'lens' shape with indentation of the liver margin.

Fig. 31 Periportal haematoma. This subhepatic periportal haematoma shows retraction of the blood clot inferiorly with clear serous fluid superiorly.

several days after a transplant, or any which progressively increase in size, may compress adjacent structures and warrant further investigation.

In our experience infection of fluid collections during the early post-operative phase is rare. However, if the patient's clinical condition suggests the presence of infection the fluid collections should be examined in detail to determine whether the nature of the fluid within any of them has altered, especially with the development of gas bubbles (Fig. 35). Any collection with features suspicious of infection warrants ultrasound guided diagnostic aspiration.

Large right sided (Fig. 36) and small left sided pleural effusions are very common and are almost never of any clinical consequence.

The fluid collections occurring in the early post-operative period may be slow to clear, haematomas frequently persisting for 6 to 12 weeks or more. However, the development of new collections in the late post-operative period is of serious significance and raises the possibility of a bile leak, (possibly indicating hepatic artery occlusion) or ascites, raising questions about the patency of the portal vein and IVC.

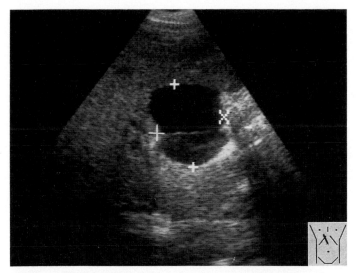

Fig. 33 Subhepatic bile collection. Bile salts have precipitated out to give a fluid/fluid level. This is suggestive but not definitely diagnostic of a biloma.

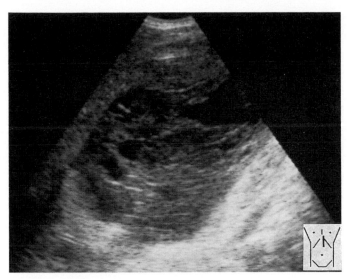

Fig. 34 Subhepatic haematoma. In this fresh haematoma the true fluid nature is indicated by the marked distal accentuation and the linear echoes of freshly clotted blood are well-seen within the haematoma.

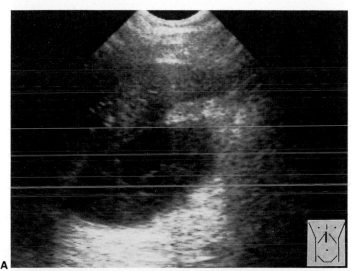

A

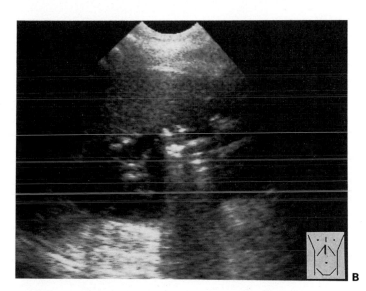

B

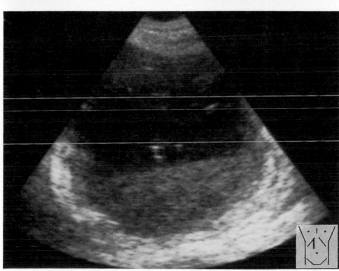

C

Fig. 35 Infected haematoma. A: In the early post-operative phase an uncomplicated haematoma is noted. **B:** Several days later the patient developed a pyrexia and gas bubbles have arisen within the haematoma, indicating a pyogenic infection. **C:** This subhepatic bile collection had been known to be present for several days. Repeat examination when the patient developed a pyrexia revealed small gas bubbles rising slowly to the surface within the fluid collection.

Fluid collections which have been confidently demonstrated to be persistent and unchanged in size can usually be successfully drained by ultrasound guided catheter placement in the late post-operative phase.[3] By this stage the majority of collections consist of only thin fluid, usually liquefied blood or bile-stained ascites. In those patients with proven bile leaks catheter placement and subsequent continuous drainage of the collection may promote healing of the biliary leak and prevent the need for more radical reconstructive surgery.

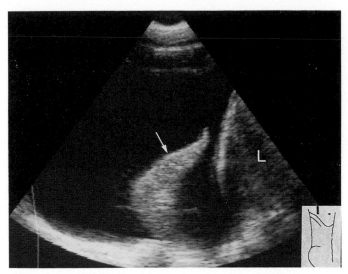

Fig. 36   Large right pleural effusion. There is a large right pleural effusion with a compressed and airless right lower lobe of the lung (arrow) above the diaphragm. L – liver.

The bile ducts

Many surgical variations of the bile duct anastomosis have been used but current practice almost always employs an end-to-end anastomosis.

Bile duct dilatation in the early post-operative period is unusual, the biliary system normally being drained by an indwelling T-tube (Fig. 37). Rarely inspissated bile may occlude the T-tube and common duct with consequent obstruction (Fig. 38). It is however important to identify and measure the common, left and right hepatic ducts to confirm their normality and to establish baseline values for comparison with subsequent examinations (Fig. 39).

A biliary stent is sometimes used instead of a T-tube. Obstruction of the anastomosis in these cases does not seem to be particularly common but, because a T-tube cholangiogram cannot be performed, ultrasonography is heavily relied on for monitoring change.

Patients who have received a cutdown liver may be at increased risk of biliary anastomotic complications, and the altered anatomy makes imaging of these livers more taxing. This group of patients deserves particularly careful monitoring of the intrahepatic duct diameters.

The bile ducts within transplanted livers seem less compliant than normal and may fail to return to a normal calibre after early and successfully treated bile duct dilata-

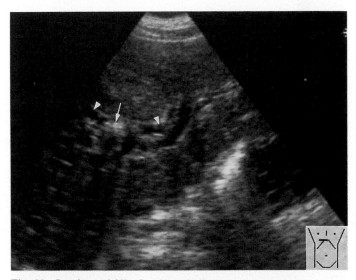

Fig. 38   Inspissated bile. Inspissated bile (arrow) has become adherent to the upper limb of the T-tube with subsequent obstruction and intrahepatic duct dilatation (arrowheads).

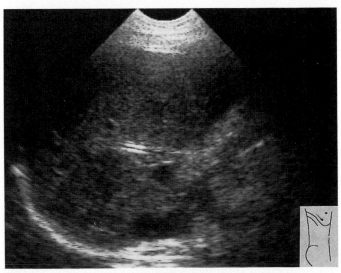

Fig. 37   Biliary T-tube. The intrahepatic limb of the T-tube is frequently identified as parallel highly reflective linear echoes within the non-dilated common hepatic duct.

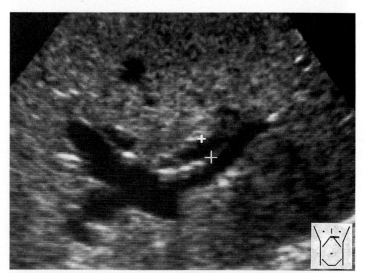

Fig. 39   Measurement of bile duct diameter. The proximal left hepatic duct diameter has been measured for monitoring in this patient receiving balloon dilatation of a late biliary stricture.

tion (Fig. 40). This persistent bile duct dilatation is generally of little clinical significance, though it is important to monitor the patient's serum bilirubin carefully. Ascending cholangitis and biliary sludge formation with concretions are more likely to develop in these patients (Fig. 41).[3]

The late onset of biliary strictures is not uncommon after liver transplantation and may occur either at the anastomotic site or higher within the biliary tree (Fig. 42), possibly at a vascular watershed. The former are probably complications of surgical technique and generally respond satisfactorily to percutaneous trans-hepatic dilatation. Non-anastomotic stenoses are likely to be ischaemic in origin and the hepatic arterial tree must be studied in these patients.

Late onset biliary leaks are extremely uncommon.

Gas within the intrahepatic bile ducts may be noted on routine examination (Fig. 43). If the patient is afebrile and asymptomatic this is of no significance and is almost certainly a consequence of a previous sphincterotomy or the use of a Roux loop as a biliary conduit. There may be an increased incidence of ascending cholangitis in these patients and careful monitoring for early hepatic abscesses is therefore indicated though large quantities of intrahepatic gas may prevent a complete evaluation with ultrasound.

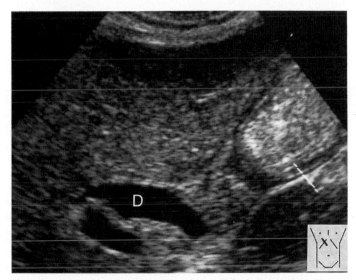

Fig. 40   Persistent duct dilatation after relief of obstruction. This patient received surgical correction for a biliary stenosis but the dilatation of the common hepatic duct (D) never resolved despite good bile drainage.

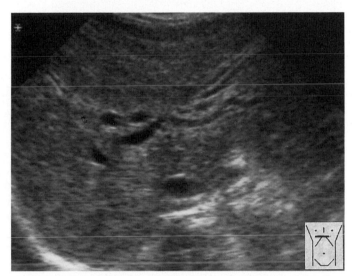

Fig. 42   Ischaemic biliary stricture. This patient became jaundiced several weeks post-transplant. There is mild dilatation of the left and right duct systems but the common hepatic duct was collapsed. This pattern of bile duct dilatation suggests an ischaemic cause.

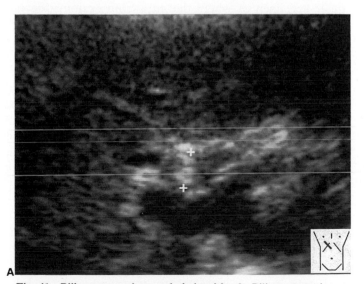

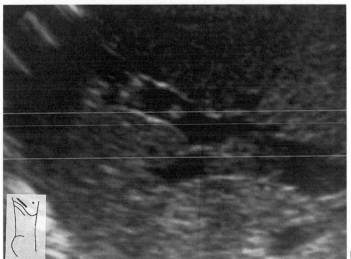

Fig. 41   Biliary concretions and cholangitis. A: Biliary concretions are seen within a non-dilated common duct (between calipers) and **B:** within a dilated system. Cholangitis cannot be diagnosed by ultrasound unless frank abscess formation is detected.

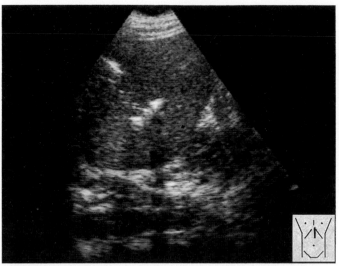

Fig. 43 Gas within the biliary tree. The highly reflective foci with shadowing are due to gas within the left duct system. The diameters cannot be assessed.

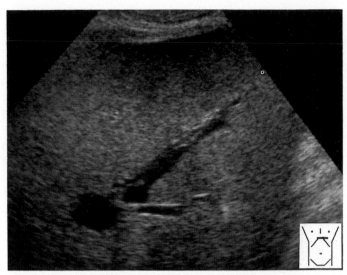

Fig. 44 Post-transplant fatty change. The uniform increase in parenchymal reflectivity in this transplanted liver was associated with normal liver function and is probably due to moderate fatty change. Note the non-dilated left hepatic duct is outlined anterior to the left portal vein branch.

Parenchymal changes

Subjective assessment of the parenchymal echo pattern and reflectivity seldom reveals any significant change in the majority of liver transplant patients. A minority show a variable degree of progressive increase in reflectivity (Fig. 44), possibly indicating fat deposition, which is of no clinical significance.

In patients who are acutely unwell a generalised reduction in reflectivity may occasionally be detected and should raise the possibility of viral hepatitis, particularly in the first few months after transplantation.

There are no identifiable parenchymal changes in patients with either acute or progressive chronic rejection.

If the original transplantation was undertaken for malignancy, both the liver and the upper abdominal cavity must be checked for any evidence of tumour recurrence. Once the acute post-operative phase has been successfully overcome, the commonest cause of death in these patients is recurrent tumour, usually in the transplanted liver.

There is also a significantly increased risk in all liver transplant patients from new primary malignancies, especially lymphoma, as a consequence of prolonged immunosuppression.[23]

Ultrasound guided procedures

Although the majority of post-operative fluid collections do not require diagnostic or therapeutic aspiration, ultrasound remains a useful technique for guiding needle or catheter placement where collections of bile, blood or ascites are slow to resolve or are thought to have become infected. Similarly, intrahepatic abscesses can be diagnosed and treated by ultrasound guided catheter placement and chronic drainage of bile collections may permit spontaneous healing of bile duct leaks.

Ultrasound guided biopsy may be helpful in those patients where blind biopsy has failed to produce an adequate specimen or where the ultrasound examination has shown suspicion of a focal lesion in patients at risk for malignant disease.

In patients with biliary or portal stenoses in whom percutaneous trans-hepatic balloon dilatation is considered, ultrasound imaging may be invaluable in guiding the initial needle and catheter into the appropriate vessel. Once the dilatation has been successfully accomplished imaging, and where relevant, Doppler studies, are important for monitoring subsequent progress and assessing the need for further intervention.

REFERENCES

1 Bismuth H, Castaing D, Ericzon B G, et al. Hepatic transplantation in Europe. First report of the European liver transplant registry. Lancet 1987; 2: 674–676

2 Bismuth H, Samuel D, Gugenheim J. Emergency liver transplantation for fulminant hepatitis. Ann Intern Med 1987; 10: 337–341

3 Raby N, Meire H B, Forbes A, Williams R. The role of ultrasound screening in management after liver transplantation. Clin Radiol 1988; 39: 507–510

4 Lengley D G, Skolnick M L, Zajko A B, Bron K M. Duplex Doppler sonography in the evaluation of adult patients before and after liver transplantation. AJR 1988; 151: 687–696

5 Tzakis A G, Todo S, Steiber A, Starzl T E. Venous jump grafts for liver transplantation in patients with portal vein thrombosis. Transplantation 1989; 48: 530–531

6 Powell-Jackson P R, Karani J, Ede R J, et al. Ultrasound and ^{99m}Tc sulphur colloid scintigraphy in diagnosis of Budd-Chiari syndrome. Gut 1986; 27: 1502–1506

7 Bisset III G S, Strife J, Balistrevi W F. Evaluation of children for liver transplantation: value of MR imaging and sonography. AJR 1990; 155: 351–356

8 De Hamptinne B, de Goyet J de V, Kestens P J, Otte J B. Volume reduction of the liver graft before orthotopic transplantation. Transplantation Proceedings 1987; 19: 3317–3322

9 Broelsch C E, Emond J C, Whitington P F, Thistlethwaite J R, Baker A L, Lichtor J L. Application of reduced-size liver transplants as split grafts, auxillary orthotopic grafts and living related segmental transplants. Ann Surg 1990; 212: 368–377

10 Kubota K, Billing H, Ericzon B G, Kelter U, Groth C G. Duplex Doppler ultrasonography for monitoring liver transplants. Acta Radiol 1990; 31: 279–283

11 Wozeney P, Zajko A B, Bron K M. Vascular complications after liver transplantation: a five year experience. AJR 1986; 147: 657–663

12 Klintmalm B G, Olson L M, Nery J R, Husberg B S, Paulsen A W. Treatment of hepatic artery thrombosis after liver transplantation with immediate vascular reconstruction: a report of three cases. Transplant Proceedings 1988; 20 (Suppl. 1): 610–612

13 Flint E W, Sumkin J H, Zajko A B. Duplex sonography of hepatic artery thrombosis after liver transplantation. AJR 1988; 151: 481–483

14 McDiarmid S V, Hall T R, Grant E G, et al. Failure of duplex sonography to diagnose hepatic artery thrombosis in a high risk group of pediatric liver transplant recipients. J Pediatr Surg 1991; 26: 710–713

15 Hall T R, McDiarmid S V, Grant E G, Boechat M I, Busultil R W. False negative duplex Doppler studies in children with hepatic artery thrombosis after liver transplantation. AJR 1990; 154: 573–575

16 Longley D G, Skolnick M L, Sheahan D G. Acute allograft rejection in liver transplant recipients: lack of correlation with loss of hepatic artery diastolic flow. Radiology 1988; 169: 417–420

17 Marujo W C, Langnas A N, Wood R P, Stratta R J, Li S, Shaw B W Jnr. Vascular complications following orthotopic liver transplantation: outcome and the role of urgent revascularisation. Transplant Proceedings 1991; 23: 1484–1486

18 Pariente D, Riou J Y, Schmit P, Verlhac S, Bernard O, Devictor D. Variability of clinical presentation of hepatic artery thrombosis in paediatric liver transplantation: role of imaging modalities. Pediatr Radiol 1990; 20: 253–257

19 Zajko A B, Campbell W L, Logsdon G A, et al. Cholangiographic findings in hepatic artery occlusion after liver transplantation. AJR 1987; 149: 485–489

20 Evans R A, Raby N D, O'Grady J G, et al. Biliary complications following orthotopic liver transplantation. Clin Radiol 1990; 41: 190–194

21 Chezmar J L, Nelson R C, Bernardino M E. Portal venous gas after hepatic transplantation: sonographic detection and clinical significance. AJR 1989; 153: 1203–1205

22 Coulden R A, Britton P D, Farman P, Noble-Jamieson G, Wight D G D. Preliminary report: hepatic vein Doppler in the early diagnosis of acute liver transplant rejection. Lancet 1990; 336: 273–274

23 Nalesnik M A, Makowka L, Starzl T E. The diagnosis and treatment of post-transplant lymphoproliferative disorders. Current Problems in Surgery 1988; 25: 367–472

The spleen

A. N. Dardenne

Anatomy and ultrasound appearances

Technique, shape, position

Visualisation of the normal sized spleen is improved with the patient in the right lateral decubitus position, scanning through the respiratory cycle. Occasionally standing the patient upright may give more satisfactory images of the spleen. A posterior and rarely an anterior approach can be useful (Fig. 1).[1,2]

The borders of the spleen are normally well-defined, smooth and convex along its superior and lateral borders, concave medially. The inferior medial aspects of the spleen are often lobulated because of focal impressions made on its surface by surrounding viscera. The hilar region is normally umbilicated or lobulated where the vascular pedicle attaches.[1,2]

Normal splenic parenchyma displays a homogeneous pattern which consists in the main of low level echoes.[1,2]

The splenic hilum, unlike the splenic substance, returns high level echoes.[3] The normal splenic tissue is generally of slightly lower reflectivity than hepatic tissue.[4,5] In some normal subjects, however, the spleen appears to be slightly more reflective than the liver[1] but its internal vasculature cannot ordinarily be identified,[2] assisting in the distinction.

Anomalies

The incidence of accessory spleens in autopsy series has been reported to range from 10% to 31%.[6,7] Characteristically, they are smooth with a round or oval shape and are 1.0 to 1.5 cm in diameter[8] and are rarely larger than 4 cm in diameter, though one example of an accessory spleen weighing 750 g and receiving blood supply from the splenic hilum has been described.[9] The majority lie at or near the splenic hilum, but a location in the left lower quadrant of the abdomen is not unusual.[3,6,7,10,11]

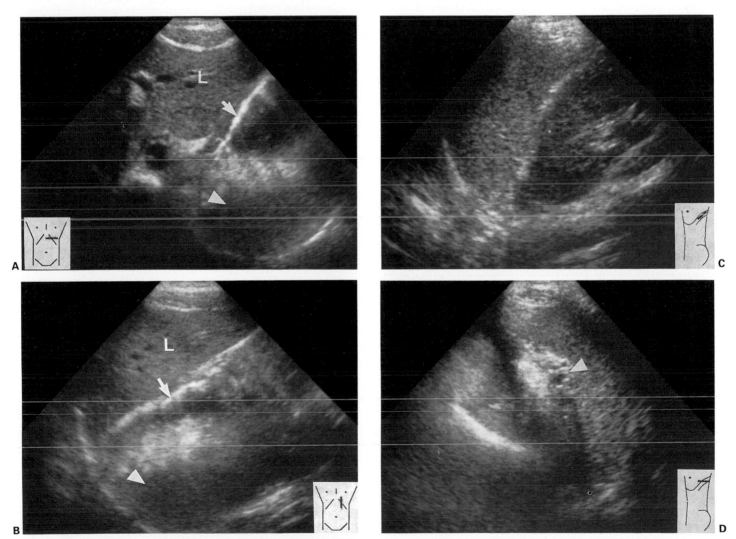

Fig. 1 Normal spleen. A: Transverse epigastric, **B:** longitudinal epigastric scans. The spleen (arrowheads) is poorly visualised because of gas in the overlying stomach (arrow). **C:** Oblique left intercostal scan shows the length of the spleen and its relationship with the kidney. **D:** Transverse left intercostal scan through the hilum (arrowhead). L – liver.

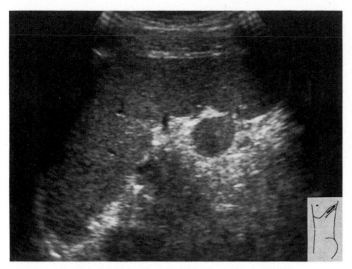

Fig. 2 **Accessory spleen.** Oblique intercostal scan. The echo texture of the accessory spleen is the same as the main spleen.

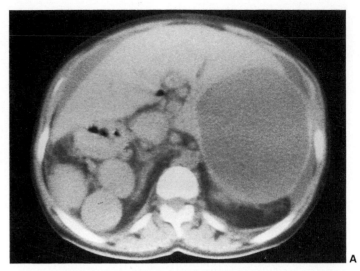

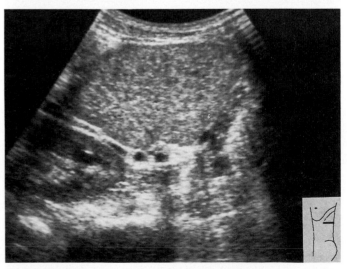

Fig. 3 **Polysplenia and situs inversus. A:** Computed tomography. Right-sided polysplenia and cyst in the left-sided right hepatic lobe. **B:** Ultrasound of the spleens.

Ultrasound identification depends on its shape, location at or near the splenic hilum and echo texture identical to that of the main spleen (Fig. 2).[9] Hypertrophy of an accessory spleen in post-splenectomy patients with haematological or rheumatoid disease is well-known.[12]

Polysplenia is a syndrome characterised by multiple individual splenules and a tendency for normally asymmetrical organs to occur symmetrically (e.g. double liver, situs ambiguous).[11,13,14] Cardiac defects are frequently associated. The aetiology of polysplenia is uncertain, but some familial cases have been described.[15] One hypothesis is that failure of fusion of the splenic precursors at an early stage in development results in polysplenia.[11] 10% of children with biliary atresia have an associated complex of anomalies, including polysplenia, continuation of the inferior vena cava into the azygos vein, preduodenal portal vein, hepatic arterial anomalies, bilaterally bilobed lungs and situs inversus abdominis (see Ch. 26).[16] The abnormal arrangement of the viscera and associated vascular anomalies such as interruption of the inferior vena cava may be identified by ultrasound[13,17] though in general CT is more informative (Fig. 3).[14]

Asplenia is a rare isolated anomaly and may be associated with congenital immune deficiency.

Ectopic or wandering spleen is also rare.[18] It refers to the condition in which a long pedicle allows the spleen to migrate from its normal position in the left upper quadrant.[19] It primarily affects women of childbearing age and usually remains asymptomatic unless torsion occurs.[19,20] Torsion of a wandering spleen can occasionally produce chronic disabling symptoms that are mistaken for a variety of digestive disturbances. Ultrasound not only delineates the typical comma shape of the spleen, but also shows that the spleen is enlarged, ectopic and malrotated,

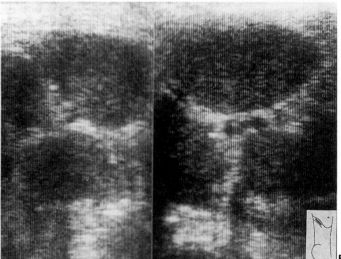

Fig. 4 **Wandering spleen.** Transverse scan showing the spleen at the level of the left kidney.

with a coarse, echo-poor texture due to infarction and splenic congestion. The demonstration of an abdominal or pelvic mass with seeming asplenia should suggest splenic torsion.[21] Ultrasound, CT, and radionuclide scanning may all be helpful, and occasionally angiography may also be required (Fig. 4).[11,20]

Another relatively common congenital anomaly is a pronounced posterior location of the spleen which may even lie posterior to the left kidney.[8]

Special techniques

Size measurement

Ultrasound offers accurate three-dimensional information on splenic morphology.[22] Although exact volume measurements may be difficult to obtain, ultrasound can readily demonstrate splenomegaly and can be used to determine changes in the spleen's size with serial examinations.[2] The long axis of the spleen is normally less than 12 cm.[3,21] More sophisticated methods for determining the spleen's volume have been employed, using serial transverse sections and computed analysis for determining the area of individual slices.[23] However computed tomography, unlike ultrasonography, provides cross-sectional contours of organs methodically without interruption and thus is probably more precise for volume measurement.[22]

Contrast media

Fluosol-DA 20%, an emulsion of perfluorodecalin and perfluorotripropylamine, has been used to produce echo enhancement of the liver and spleen. Many lesions are seen only after administration of contrast material, with an increase in ultrasound sensitivity.[24]

Pathology

Diffuse diseases

Diffuse diseases can change the echo pattern or the size of the spleen or both. Increased reflectivity of the spleen can be due to malignant involvement but, generally, analysis of the splenic echo texture is not particularly helpful as it is dependent on so many other factors, such as the vascularity of the organ or reactive changes.[25,26]

Splenic enlargement occurs in a wide range of systemic or focal diseases: acute and chronic infections (malaria, tuberculosis), blood dyscrasias, tumours, hereditary storage diseases (Gaucher's), chronic liver disease (portal hypertension), portal and splenic vein thrombosis, amyloid, sarcoid etc. As splenomegaly becomes increasingly pronounced, the spleen becomes easier to visualise by ultrasound and enlarged splenic vessels can frequently be identified, particularly in the region of the splenic hilum. In the great majority of patients with splenomegaly the shape and contour of the spleen remain normal despite its large size.[2] Splenomegaly due to lymphoma is usually more pronounced than splenomegaly due to portal hypertension.[1] However ultrasound may not detect very small deposits.[27]

Lymphoma, leukaemia, Castelman's disease Lymphoma is the most common malignant tumour affecting the spleen.[27] Different ultrasound patterns are produced, depending on the particular pathological changes: involvement may be diffuse or focal.[3] Homogeneous spleen enlargement is frequently found during staging[28] and the spleen may be echo-poor or have increased reflectivity.[2] More frequently however, splenic reflectivity is quite normal.[3] Detection of splenomegaly is not reliable evidence of splenic involvement,[29] moreover, a normal sized spleen does not exclude the possibility of splenic involvement.[28,30] A large spleen has a sensitivity of 36% and specificity of 61% in the diagnosis of splenic lymphoma; if splenic hilar adenopathy is also present the likelihood of splenic involvement by lymphoma is increased.[27]

In chronic myeloid leukaemia the spleen is often very enlarged with a normal homogeneous structure.[3]

Castelman's disease, or angiofollicular hyperplasia, is a rare disorder characterised by the development of tumour-like masses of lymphoid tissue. The spleen may be moderately enlarged.[31]

Tuberculosis Tuberculosis of the spleen is usually miliary.[32] The texture is uniform, with increased reflectivity. Focal tuberculosis of the spleen is rare: echo-poor or reflective areas are seen.[33]

Focal diseases

Focal splenic masses are rarer than focal liver masses.[34] Although ultrasound is sensitive in detecting focal splenic lesions, as with other non-invasive imaging modalities, it often lacks specificity. Furthermore, the ultrasound appearances in a particular pathological process can vary greatly. The spleen may lose its normal contour if there is a space occupying lesion within it.[2]

Lymphoma In addition to diffuse splenic infiltration, lymphoma can also involve the spleen as multiple nodules or a single large lesion.[27] These focal forms of involvement are often detectable by imaging techniques but are rare.[27,29,35] In most patients with focal lymphoma the spleen is not enlarged. The echo patterns of splenic nodules are similar to those of hepatic lymphomatous foci. Most are echo-poor with poorly defined margins (Fig. 5).[29] Rarely, lymphoma may be more reflective than the surrounding spleen.[27] When large they are generally heterogeneous, although any pattern such as target lesions (Fig. 6) may be found.[35] Bulging of the organ contours is frequent.[29] The ultrasound appearance of splenic lymphoma is non-specific so that differentiation from other benign or malignant splenic foci such as cysts,

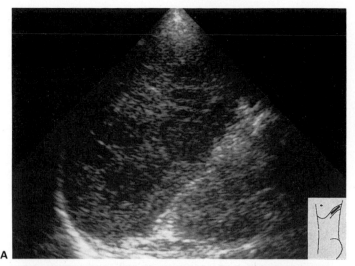

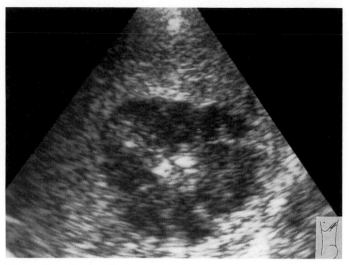

Fig. 6 Lymphoma. Single target lesion.

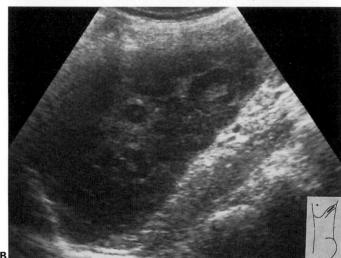

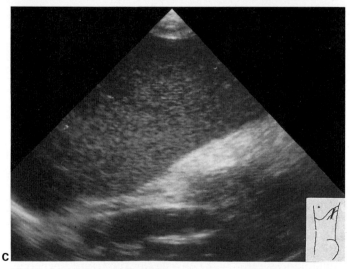

Fig. 5 Lymphoma. A: Typical echo-poor masses. **B:** Complex masses are typical of higher grade lymphoma. **C:** Small foci of lymphoma may be difficult to discern and microscopic involvement usually does not alter the appearance of the spleen.

haematomas, abscesses, metastases or accessory spleens may be difficult. However, the overall incidence of focal lesions of the spleen is so low (0.1%) that nodule formation in a patient with lymphoma almost always represents lymphomatous involvement.[29] Overall the accuracy of ultrasound in the diagnosis of splenic involvement in lymphoma is approximately 75%.[27]

Abscess, inflammatory pseudotumour Splenic abscesses are uncommon; they are usually caused by haematogenous spread of infection but may develop after trauma or infarction. The usual bacteria are *Streptococci*, *Staphylococci* and *Salmonella* but, except for *Gonococcus*, every conceivable pyogenic organism has been incriminated. Amoebic splenic abscess is very rare.[36] Similar to abscesses elsewhere in the body, the ultrasound appearances vary greatly with respect to number, size, echo texture, wall definition and attenuation.[2] Typically they appear as focal echo-free defects or as lesions with solid and cystic components.[36] They may also appear like cysts, but the abscess wall is often thick and irregular and they may contain echoes due to debris, septation, or gas bubbles (Fig. 7).[36,37] It is impossible to distinguish between gas within splenic abscess and non-suppurative gas formation due to a splenic infarct.[38] In some cases, abscesses appear more highly reflective with irregular margins.[36]

In fungal abscesses of the spleen (splenic candidiasis) four patterns have been described: 'wheel within a wheel' lesions seen early in the course of the disease, 'bull's-eye' lesions, uniformly echo-poor lesions (Fig. 8) and, finally, reflective foci with variable degrees of acoustic shadowing.[39]

The splenic lesions of cat scratch disease are usually multiple, and consist of granulomata with abscess formation. Multiple small echo-poor lesions develop into multiple abscesses that later heal and form calcified granulomas.[37]

Inflammatory pseudotumours are benign well-circumscribed masses that are usually solitary and composed of foci of inflammatory cells and lymphocytes in a fibroblastic stroma. It is considered by most pathologists to represent repair of an inflammatory lesion.[40] Splenic involvement is extremely rare. Ultrasound shows a large, partially calcified, well-defined reflective mass.[40,41] The differential diagnosis of calcified splenic foci is extensive and includes granuloma, venous congestion (Fig. 9),[42] splenic cysts, hamartoma, haemangioma and lymphangioma.

Metastases Intrasplenic metastases are uncommon except from lymphoma.[43,44] They vary in appearance, as in the liver (Fig. 10); those from a melanoma for example may be either reflective or echo-poor.[45]

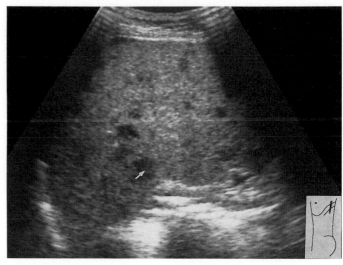

Fig. 8 Fungal abscesses. Small echo-poor foci with irregular walls scattered through the spleen. Note the reflective central focus (arrow) in one lesion; this typical appearance is probably due to a blood vessel.

Trauma and splenosis The spleen often increases in volume after blunt abdominal trauma; this enlargement is not an indicator of a clinical deterioration but most likely due to marked adrenergic stimulation and changing blood volume.[46]

Sub-capsular haematomas are seen as echo-free areas outside the main body of the spleen and separated from it (Fig. 11).[3] A normal anatomical structure can cause confusion with subcapsular haematoma: the left lobe of the liver in some individuals extends between the spleen and left hemidiaphragm and, when echo-poor, can resemble a perisplenic (subcapsular) fluid collection.[2]

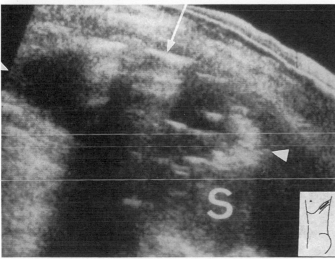

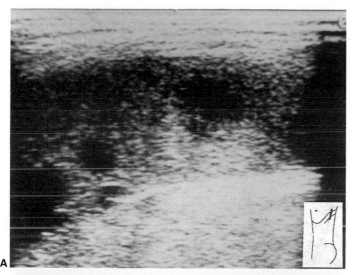

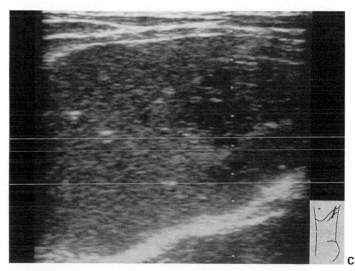

Fig. 7 Abscesses. A: Multiple abscesses. Echo-poor cavities were seen in this patient with a fever. (Figure courtesy of Dr C Bossi, Milan.)
B: Gas-containing abscess. Highly reflective band (arrow) in a cavity (arrowheads). Splenic tissue (S) is obscured by reverberation artefacts.
C: Brucellosis. Typical abscess cavity found in this patient with brucellosis. More commonly the spleen is enlarged with a non-specific appearance.

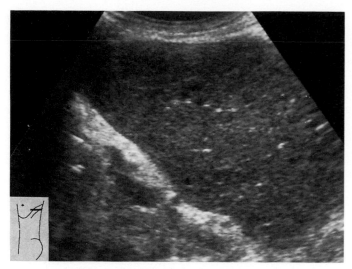

Fig. 9 Calcified foci. Multiple small highly reflective foci are seen in this patient with portal hypertension. This is thought to represent multiple small phleboliths.

Splenic rupture produces an irregular region of reduced reflectivity due to haemorrhage. The focal pattern is rarer and causes localised areas of decreased reflectivity or fluid spaces (Figs 11 and 12).[3] Splenic lacerations may not be detectable on ultrasound making it difficult to identify risk factors for delayed rupture.[47] In one series, in three cases with apparently minimal parenchymal lesions, surgery showed frank parenchymal tears. The discrepancy can be attributed to the fact that haematomas may have the same echo intensity as the surrounding spleen.[48]

An acute haematoma is a highly reflective lesion that may be well or poorly defined and is characteristically crescentic in shape. Initially the haematoma may enlarge and later become echo-poor (Fig. 13), so much so that they may on occasion mimic a cyst.[2,3] Demonstration of bleeding within both peritoneal compartments (lesser and greater sac) suggests extensive splenic damage.[48]

In the evaluation of splenic trauma, computed tomography and magnetic resonance imaging seem to be more sensitive than ultrasonography or radionuclide examination (Figs 12 and 14).[49] However, the sensitivity of ultrasound to free peritoneal fluid makes it important in these cases; the pelvis should be examined carefully – fluid here may be the only sign of splenic rupture.

Splenic clefts, notches, or lobulations that persist from fetal lobulations should not be mistaken for splenic fractures due to trauma. Clefts usually occur on the diaphragmatic surface of the spleen, whereas lobulations occur along the medial part of the spleen.[8]

Traumatic disruption of the spleen may result in seeding of splenic tissue (splenosis), usually restricted to the peritoneal cavity but occasionally also in other sites such as the pleura, pericardium, subcutaneous tissue, stomach, liver, and left renal space.[50–53] This uncommon

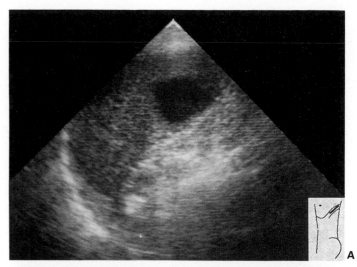

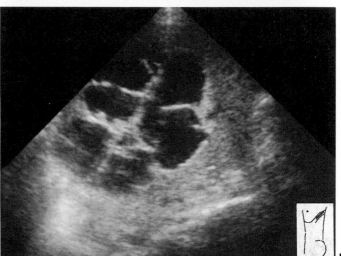

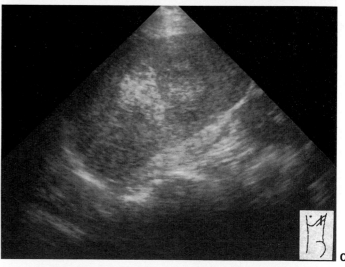

Fig. 10 Metastases. A: Solitary lesion. **B:** Multiloculated lesion. Both these cases arose from carcinoma of the ovary. **C:** Reflective metastasis. As with liver metastases, splenic metastases may have any appearance. A pair of reflective deposits is seen in this patient with carcinoma of the ovary.

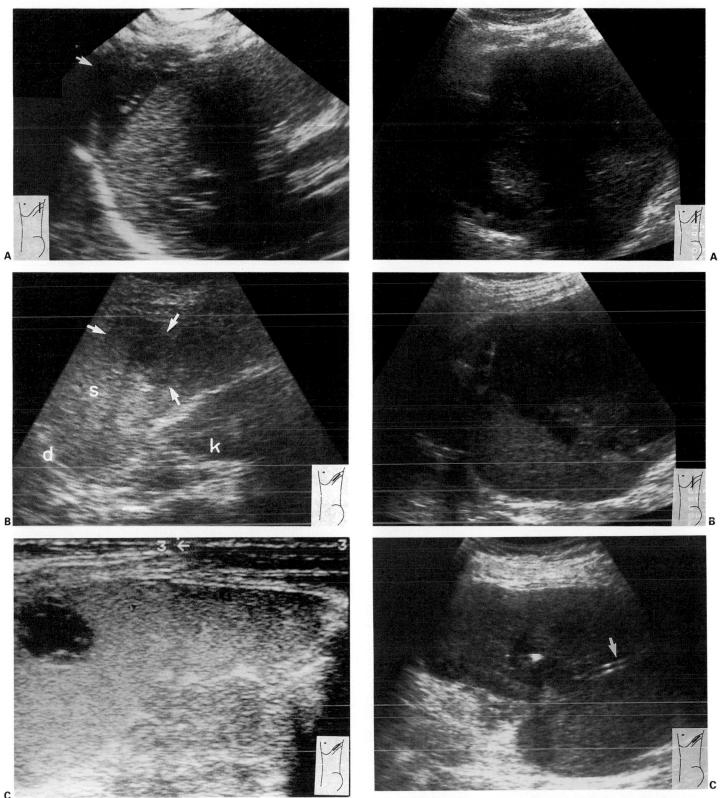

Fig. 11   Splenic trauma. A: Subcapsular haematoma (arrow).
B: Intrasplenic haematoma (arrows). s – spleen, k – kidney,
d – diaphragm. **C:** Well-defined resolving intrasplenic haematoma.

Fig. 12   Ruptured spleen. A and **B:** Longitudinal scans showing
disruption of the spleen with a large haematoma. **C:** Conservative
management by ultrasound guided catheter (arrow) placement.

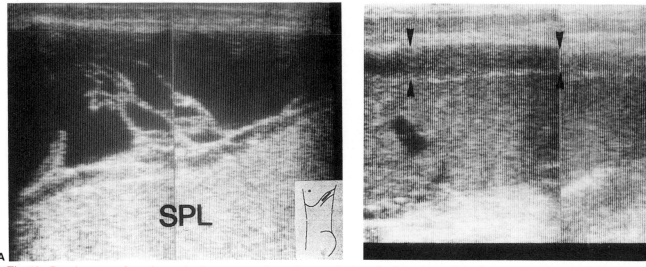

Fig. 13 Development of a subcapsular haematoma. Coronal scans. **A:** 1 week after trauma. Echo-free spaces with septa. SPL – normal splenic tissue. **B:** 4 weeks after trauma. Residual collection (arrowheads).

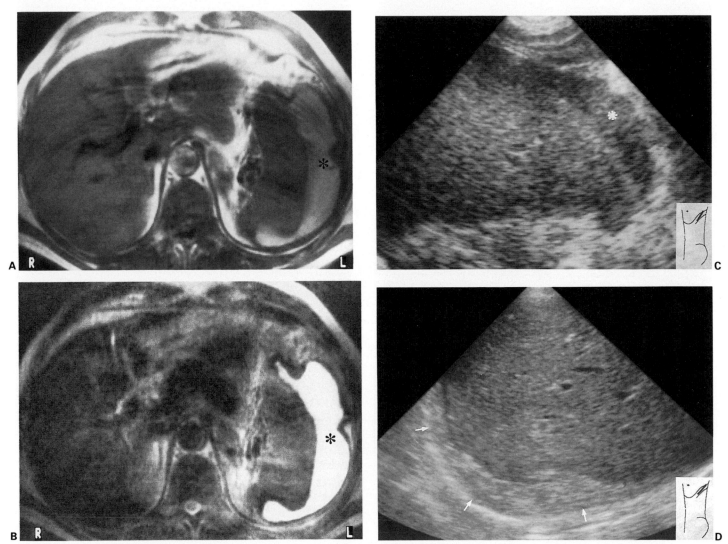

Fig. 14 Perisplenic lesions. Magnetic resonance imaging. **A:** T1 and **B:** T2 weighed images demonstrate the haematoma (*). **C:** Echo-poor crescentic space partly covering the spleen represents a perisplenic haematoma (*) in another case. **D:** Peritoneal tumour producing reflective plaque (arrows) aroundhe spleen (carcinoma of the ovary).

complication usually appears as an incidental finding long after the injury. The small nodules in the peritoneum are difficult to detect by ultrasound so that computed tomography and radionuclide scans are more suitable.[50,51]

Cysts, tumours Non-parasitic cysts of the spleen are classified as primary or epithelial cysts if their inner surface has a cellular lining which may be mesothelial or epidermoid.[54,55] Both have usual echo-free appearances with posterior enhancement. They may calcify (Fig. 15). On ultrasound they are indistinguishable from the more common post-traumatic cysts.

Splenic cysts sometimes contain cholesterol crystals which can make the lesion seem solid (Fig. 16).[2,56] In haemorrhagic cysts, the two types of fluid produce a gravitational layering effect.[3]

Haemangiomas are rare in the spleen (Fig. 17) (autopsy incidence of 0.1% to 14%). Hamartoma is a term used interchangeably by some authors although others make a distinction based on the histological appearance.[57] Three ultrasound patterns of splenic haemangiomas have been described:

a) well-defined echo-poor lesions displaying acoustical enhancement;
b) homogeneous reflective lesions;
c) a mixed pattern of reflective and echo-poor lesions.[58]

A complex pattern of multiple cystic areas (some anechoic and others containing reflective debris) may occur. High level echoes with acoustic shadowing can be seen and correspond to areas of calcification.[59]

Lymphangiomas are benign congenital malformations of the lymphatic system. Splenic involvement is quite rare. Ultrasound shows splenomegaly due to multiple echo-poor lesions of the spleen.[60]

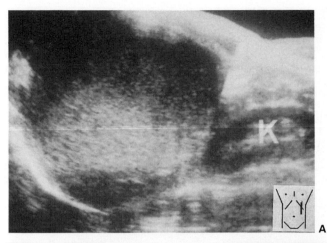

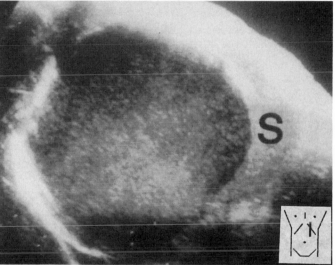

Fig. 16   Splenic post-traumatic cyst. A and **B:** Sagittal scans. The fluid is reflective owing to the presence of cholesterol crystals. K – kidney, S – splenic tissue.

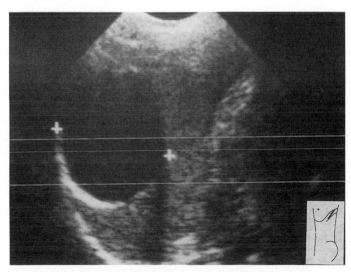

Fig. 15   Splenic cyst. Note the thickened wall superiorly; this probably represents calcification in the wall. (Figure courtesy of Dr C Bossi, Milan.)

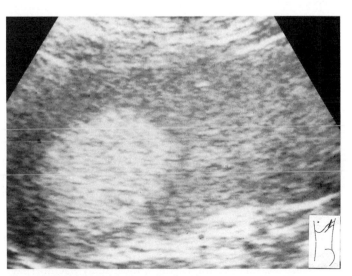

Fig. 17   Haemangioma. Rounded, highly reflective mass. The appearance is identical to that in the liver.

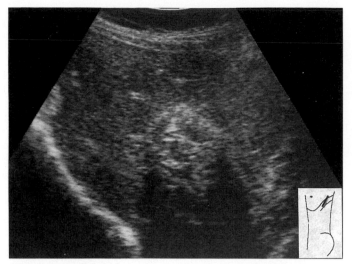

Fig. 18 Complicated hydatid. The hydatid membrane is infolded and this, together with hydatid sand, gives rise to a complex reflective lesion with acoustic shadowing.

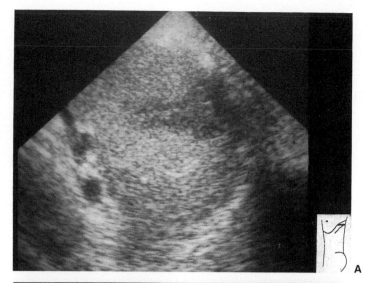

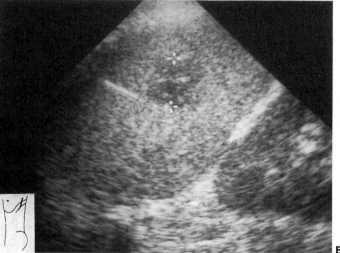

Fig. 19 Infarct. A: Transverse scan shows the wedge shape. **B:** Seen as a circular shape in a coronal scan.

Primary malignant tumours of the spleen are very rare and consist mainly in different types of sarcoma. Their ultrasonic patterns are non-specific.[1] A splenic plasmacytoma is described.[61]

Parasites Splenic hydatid cysts are uncommon, being found in about 2% of all patients with echinococcosis.[62] Hydatid cysts may present a typical appearance when multiple daughter cysts are present.[3] However, the ultrasound findings of splenic hydatid cysts are frequently not specific,[62] an echo-free cyst being the commonest finding;[27] its true nature can be suspected if the wall is thick and highly reflective.[3] The mixture of infolded membranes, scolices, and hydatid sand may produce a highly reflective lesion (Fig. 18).[62]

Most tropical parasitic diseases can produce non-specific splenomegaly. The commonest is chronic malaria.

Infarcts Splenic infarction is usually embolic and due to intravenous drug abuse or atrial fibrillation but it may occur spontaneously in splenomegaly and is a feature of sickle cell disease.

Acute splenic infarction typically appears as a well-demarcated wedge-shaped echo-poor area with its apex at the splenic hilum and its base directed toward the periphery of the spleen (Fig. 19).[2,63] Not infrequently however, splenic infarcts are atypical in shape: round irregular or smooth, echo-poor and anechoic lesions can also be found.[2,34]

Scarring following infarction may appear as hetero-geneity of the splenic texture and is not usually detectable until months later (Fig. 20).[63] Findings that require surgical referral are: increasing subcapsular haemorrhage, extravasation of blood into the peritoneal cavity and flow in the area of infarction demonstrated by Doppler.[63] When

caused by septic emboli, infarcts may progress to form focal abscesses.

In sickle cell anaemia vaso-occlusion due to sickling results in recurrent splenic infarctions leading to fibrosis and autosplenectomy (Figs 21 and 22). Splenomegaly occurs initially, usually after the first 6 months of life and generally persists throughout childhood. Micro-infarctions lead to gradual shrinkage and ultimately fibrosis and calcification which may be amorphous, punctate, or rarely curvilinear.[64]

Miscellaneous

Gaucher's disease is a familial disorder of lipid metabolism resulting in the accumulation of glucocerebrosides in the reticuloendothelial cells. It produces splenomegaly and focal echo-poor lesions in the spleen.[1,44] The nodules are

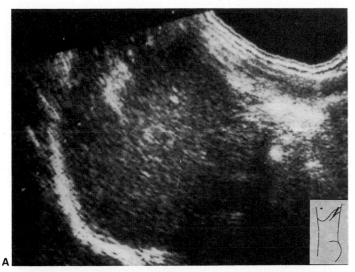

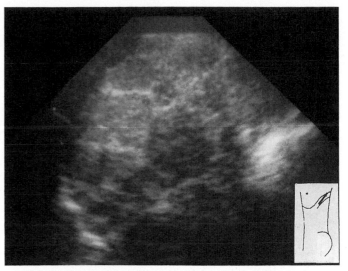

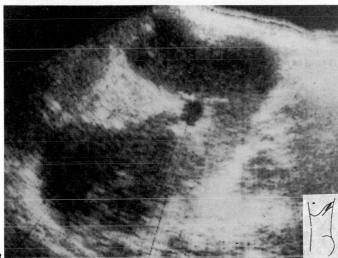

Fig. 21 Sickle cell anaemia. Multiple intrasplenic reflective lines corresponding to fibrous septa.

Fig. 20 Healed infarct. As the infarct organises it becomes replaced by wedge-shaped or linear highly reflective tissue. (Figure courtesy of Dr C Bossi, Milan.)

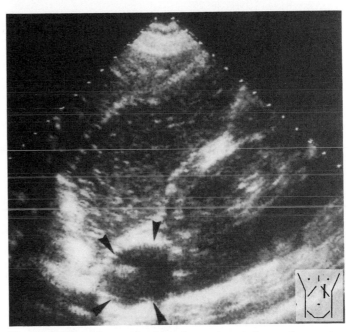

Fig. 22 Sickle cell anaemia. Sagittal scan through liver and stomach. Very small residual spleen (arrowheads).

circumscribed areas of fibrosis with entrapped Gaucher cells.[55]

Glycogen storage diseases may be associated with splenomegaly as a result of portal hypertension secondary to hepatic fibrosis or cirrhosis.

Hepatosplenomegaly occurs in systemic amyloidosis.[65]

Diagnostic puncture of the spleen is not widely used though ultrasound guided biopsy of focal lesions with 22-gauge needles, or biopsies with use of 21-gauge Surecut needles in patients with lymphoma have been recommended.[55,66,67]

REFERENCES

1 Weill F S. L'ultrasonographie en pathologie digestive. 4th edition. Paris: Editions Vigot. 1989

2 Laing F C, Filly R A, Gooding G A W. Ultrasonography in alimentary tract radiology. In: Margulis AR, Burhenne H. eds. St Loius: CV Mosby. 1989: volume 2(58): p 1421

3 Bolondi L, Labo G, Gandolfi L. Diagnostic ultrasound in gastroenterology. Piccin/Butterworths. 1984

4 Arenson A M, McKee J D. Left upper quadrant pseudolesion secondary to normal variants in liver and spleen. JCU 1986; 14: 588

5 Li D K B, Cooperberg P L, Graham M F, Callen P. Pseudo perisplenic 'fluid collections' a clue to normal liver and spleen echogenic texture. J Ultrasound Med 1986; 5: 397

6 Halpert B, Gyoerkey F. Lesions observed in accessory spleens of 311 patients. Am J Clin Pathol 1959; 32: 81

7 Curtis G M, Mevitz D. The surgical significance of the accessory spleen. Ann Surg 1946; 123: 276

8 Dodds W J, Taylor A J, Erickson S J, Stewart E T, Lawson T L. Radiologic imaging of splenic anomalies. AJR 1990; 155: 805

9 Subramanyam B R, Balthazar E J, Horii S C. Sonography of the accessory spleen. AJR 1984; 143: 47

10 Mostbeck G, Sommer G, Haller J, et al. Accessory spleen: presentation as a large abdominal mass in an asymptomatic young woman. Gastrointest Radiol 1987; 12: 337

11 Hine A L, Wilson S R. Ultrasonography of splenic variants. Can Assoc Radiol J 1989; 40: 25

12 Beahrs J R, Stephens D H. Enlarged accessory spleens: CT appearance in postsplenectomy patients. AJR 1980; 135: 483

13 Curran J G, Ryan M J. Hodgkin's disease in a patient with polysplenia. Br J Radiol 1987; 60: 929

14 Vossen P G, Van Hedent E F, Degryse H R, De Schepper A M. Computed tomography of the polysplenia syndrome in the adult. Gastrointest Radiol 1987; 12: 209

15 Arnold G L, Bixler D, Girod D. Probable autosomal recessive inheritance of polysplenia, situs inversus and cardiac defects in an Amish family. Am J Med Genet 1983; 16: 35

16 Abramson S J, Berdon W E, Altman R P, Amodio J B, Levy J. Biliary atresia and noncardiac polysplenic syndrome: US and surgical considerations. Radiology 1987; 163: 377

17 Garris J B, Kangaloo H, Sample W F. Ultrasonic diagnosis of infrahepatic interruption of the inferior vena cava with azygos (hemiazygos) continuation. Radiology 1980; 134: 179

18 Phillips G W L, Hemingway A P. Wandering spleen. Br J Radiol 1987; 60: 188

19 Bollinger B, Lorentzen T. Torsion of a wandering spleen: ultrasonographic findings. JCU 1990; 18: 510

20 Franic S, Pirani M, Stevenson G W. Torsion of a wandering spleen. Can Assoc Radiol J 1988; 39: 232

21 Shiels W E, Johnson J F, Stephenson S R, Huang Y C. Chronic torsion of the wandering spleen. Pediatr Radiol 1989; 19: 465

22 Kashiwagi T, Mitsutani N, Koizumi T, Kimura K. Three-dimensional demonstration of liver and spleen by a computer graphics technique. Acta Radiol 1988; 29: 27

23 Koga T. Correlation between sectional area of the spleen by ultrasonic tomography and actual volume of the removed spleen. JCU 1979; 7: 119

24 Mattrey R F, Strich G, Shelton R E, et al. Perfluorochemicals as US contrast agents for tumor imaging and hepatosplenography: preliminary clinical results. Radiology 1987; 163: 339

25 Siler J, Hunter T B, Weiss J, Haber K. Increased echogenicity of the spleen in benign and malignant disease. AJR 1980; 134: 1011

26 Carroll B A, Ta H N. The ultrasonic appearance of extranodal abdominal lymphoma. Radiology 1980; 136: 149

27 Shirkhoda A, Ros P R, Farah J, Staab E V. Lymphoma of the solid abdominal viscera. Radiol Clin North Am 1990; 28: 785

28 Goerg C, Schwerk W B, Goerg K, Havemann K. Sonographic patterns of the affected spleen in malignant lymphoma. JCU 1990; 18: 569

29 Wernecke K, Peters P E, Krüger K-G. Ultrasonographic patterns of focal hepatic and splenic lesions in Hodgkin's and non-Hodgkin's lymphoma. Br J Radiol 1987; 60: 655

30 Zornoza J, Ginaldi S. Computed tomography in hepatic lymphoma. Radiology 1981; 138: 405

31 Libson E, Fields S, Strauss S, et al. Widespread Castelman disease; CT and US findings. Radiology 1988; 166: 753

32 Choi B I, Im J-G, Han M C, Lee H S. Hepatosplenic tuberculosis with hypersplenism: CT evaluation. Gastrointest Radiol 1989; 14: 265

33 Dafiri R, Zakari S, Iraqui G, Bouzekri M, Imani F. Apport de l'échographie dans la tuberculose des viscères pleins de l'abdomen. J Radiol 1990; 71: 73

34 Skolnick M L. Real-time ultrasound imaging in the abdomen. Springer-Verlag. 1981

35 Bonmati L M, Ballesta A, Chirivella M. Unusual presentation of non-Hodgkin lymphoma of the spleen. Can Assoc Radiol J 1989; 40: 49

36 Gupta R K, Pant C S, Ganguly S K. Ultrasound demonstration of amebic splenic abscess. JCU 1987; 15: 555

37 Cox F, Perlman S, Sathyanarayana. Splenic abscesses in cat scratch disease: sonographic diagnosis and follow-up. JCU 1989; 17: 511

38 Williamson S L, Stevers Golladay E. Gas-containing splenic infarct masquerading as gastric bezoar: ultrasound elucidation. JCU 1988; 16: 678

39 Pastakia B, Shawker T, Thaler M, O'Leary T, Pizzo P A. Hepatosplenic candidiasis: wheels within wheels. Radiology 1988; 166: 417

40 Franquet T, Montes M, Aizcorbe M, Barberena J, Ruiz de Azua Y, Cobo F. Inflammatory pseudotumor of the spleen: ultrasound and computed tomographic findings. Gastrointest Radiol 1989; 14: 181

41 Sheahan K, Wolf B C, Neiman R S. Inflammatory pseudotumor of the spleen: a clinicopathologic study of three cases. Hum Pathol 1988; 19: 1024

42 Logan H, Meire H B. Calcified splenic and portal vein thrombosis: an unusual case of multiple high amplitude echoes in the spleen. Br J Radiol 1991; 64: 366–367

43 Carrington B M, Thomas N B, Johnson R J. Intrasplenic metastases from carcinoma of the ovary. Clin Radiol 1990; 41: 418

44 Stevens P G, Kumari-Subaiya S S, Kahn L B. Splenic involvement in Gaucher's disease: sonographic findings. JCU 1987; 15: 397

45 Murphy J F, Bernardino M E. The sonographic findings of splenic metastases. JCU 1979; 7: 195

46 Goodman L R, Aprahamian C. Changes in splenic size after abdominal trauma. Radiology 1990; 176: 629

47 Sutton C S, Haaga J. CT evaluation of limited splenic trauma. J Comput Assist Tomogr 1987; 11: 167

48 Weill F, Rohmer P, Didier D, Coche G. Ultrasound of the traumatized spleen: left butterfly sign in lesions masked by echogenic blood clots. Gastrointest Radiol 1988; 13: 169

49 Erasmie U, Mortensson W, Persson U, Lännergen K. Scintigraphic evaluation of traumatic splenic lesions in children. Acta Radiol 1988; 29: 121

50 Delamarre J, Capron J P, Drouard F, Joly J P, Deschepper B, Carton S. Splenosis: ultrasound and CT findings in a case complicated by an intraperitoneal implant traumatic hematoma. Gastrointest Radiol 1988; 13: 275

51 Derin H, Yetkin E, Özkilic H, Özekli K, Yaman C. Detection of splenosis by radionuclide scanning. Br J Radiol 1987; 60: 873

52 Fleming C R, Dickson E R, Harrison E G Jnr. Splenosis: autotransplantation of splenic tissue. Am J Med 1960; 61: 414

53 Maillard J C, Menu Y, Scherrer A, Witz M O, Nahum H. Intraperitoneal splenosis: diagnosis by ultrasound and computed tomography. Gastrointest Radiol 1989; 14: 179

54 Bürrig K F. Epithelial (true) splenic cysts: pathogenesis of the mesothelial and so-called epidermoid cyst of the spleen. Am J Surg Pathol 1988; 12: 275

55 Jequier S, Guttman F, Lafortune M. Non-surgical treatment of a congenital splenic cyst. Pediatr Radiol 1987; 17: 248

56 Glancy J J. Fluid filled echogenic epidermoid cyst of the spleen. JCU 1979; 7: 301

57 Pakter R L, Fishman E K, Nussbaum A, Giargiana F K, Zerhouni

E A. CT findings in splenic hemangiomas in the
Klippel-Trenaunay-Weber syndrome. J Comput Assist Tomogr
1987; 11: 88

58 Manor A, Starinsky R, Garfinkel D, Yona E, Modai D.
Ultrasound features of symptomatic splenic hemangioma. JCU
1984; 12: 95

59 Ros P R, Moser R P, Dachman A H, Murari P J, Olmsted W W.
Hemangioma of the spleen: radiologic-pathologic correlation in ten
cases. Radiology 1987; 162: 73

60 Pistoia F, Markowitz S K. Splenic lymphangiomatosis: CT
diagnosis. AJR 1988; 150: 121

61 Adler D D, Silver T M, Abrams G D. The sonographic appearance
of splenic plasmacytoma. J Ultrasound Med 1982; 1: 323

62 Franquet T, Montes M, Lecumberri F J, Esparza J, Bescos J M.
Hydatid disease of the spleen: imaging findings in nine patients.
AJR 1990; 154: 525

63 Goerg C, Schwerk W B. Splenic infarction: sonographic patterns,
diagnosis, follow-up, and complications. Radiology 1990; 174: 803

64 Rao V M, Mapp E M, Wechsler R J. Radiology of the
gastrointestinal tract in sickle cell anemia. Semin Roentgenol 1987;
22: 195

65 Pear B L. Other organs and other amyloids. Semin Roentgenol
1986; 21: 150

66 Solbiati L, Bossi M C, Belloti E, Ravetto C, Montali G. Focal
lesions in the spleen: sonogaphic patterns and guided biopsy. AJR
1983; 140: 59

67 Suzuki T, Shibuya H, Yoshimatsu S. Ultrasonically guided staging
splenic tissue core biopsy in patients with Hodgkin's lymphoma.
Cancer 1987; 60: 879

The retroperitoneum

Anton E. Joseph, Caroline Lewis and David O. Cosgrove

Anatomy

The retroperitoneum is that part of the abdomen which is bounded anteriorly by the posterior parietal peritoneum, posteriorly by the transversalis fascia and laterally by the lateroconal ligaments (Figs 1 and 2). It is largest posteriorly but continues anteriorly as the properitoneal fat compartment. It extends from the pelvic brim inferiorly to the diaphragm superiorly. The retroperitoneum contains the adrenals, kidneys and ureters, the duodenal loop and the pancreas, the great vessels with their branches and the ascending and descending portions of the colon including the caecum. It can be divided into three distinct compartments by the fascial planes it contains.

The anterior pararenal space lies between the posterior parietal peritoneum and the anterior renal fascia with the lateroconal ligament laterally, blending with the parietal peritoneum anteriorly. The space is continuous across the midline and contains the pancreas, duodenum, ascending and descending colon, the caecum and the appendix when it lies in a retrocaecal position.

The perirenal space is confined by the anterior and posterior renal fasciae which fuse laterally to form the lateroconal ligament. The precise site at which the lateroconal ligament blends with the renal fascia varies widely. The posterior renal fascia (Gerota's fascia) is generally thick whereas the anterior renal fascia is generally thin. Gerota's fascia has at least two layers, the anterior of which is continuous with the anterior renal fascia while the posterior layer continues into the lateroconal ligament. Superiorly the renal fascial layers fuse above the adrenals and become attached to the diaphragm. Inferiorly the renal fasciae extend into the pelvis where they thin out so that the anterior and posterior pararenal spaces become continuous in the iliac fossa. The fascia consists of dense connective tissue which blends with the connective tissue enveloping the aorta, the IVC and the roots of the superior mesenteric vessels. The perirenal space contains the kidneys, adrenals, fat and blood vessels.

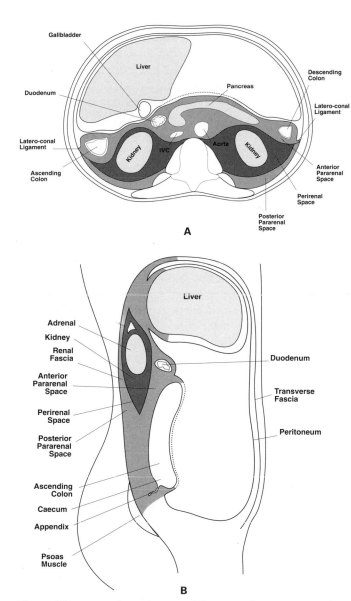

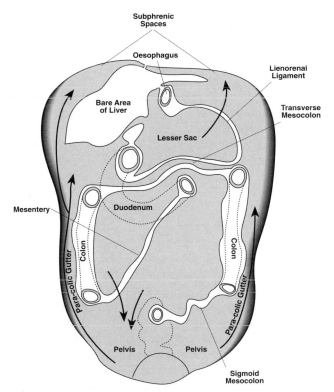

Fig. 1 The retroperitoneal spaces. Diagrammatic transverse section through the kidneys **A**: transverse, **B**: parasagittal, to show the perirenal and pararenal spaces and the lateroconal ligaments. IVC – inferior vena cava.

Fig. 2 The peritoneal cavity. The pathways along which infections tend to track are indicated in this diagram of the peritoneum. The commonest origins for infections are the pelvis and from the lower bowel and appendix. (Redrawn from Meyers M. Fig. 2.65 in: Dynamic radiology of the abdomen. Berlin: Springer Verlag. 1982.)

The posterior pararenal space lies between the posterior renal and lateroconal ligament anteriorly and the transversalis fascia posteriorly. Its medial border is formed by the psoas major and quadratus lumborum muscles. Laterally it communicates with the properitoneal fat compartment (flank stripe). It contains no organs.[1-4]

All the retroperitoneal spaces contain varying amounts of adipose tissue, depending on body habitus, but the right anterior and both posterior pararenal spaces are usually thin compartments.

The diaphragmatic crura extend inferiorly as tendinous fibres that attach to the vertebrae and their transverse processes down to L3 on the right and L1 on the left. The right crus is more prominent and usually more lobular than the left. It is bounded by the IVC antero-laterally with the right adrenal gland and the right lobe of the liver posterolaterally. Its fibres diverge as they ascend – the lateral fibres insert on the central tendon of the diaphragm, whilst the medial fibres ascend on the left side of the oesophageal hiatus, decussating with those of the left crus in front of the abdominal aorta. On parasagittal scans the right crus can be seen as a longitudinal echo-poor structure immediately posterior to the IVC or, on the left of the midline, anterior to the aorta. The intra-abdominal portion of the oesophagus begins at the cephalic end of the right crus. The left crus ascends along the anterior lumbar vertebral bodies and inserts into the central tendon of the diaphragm. It is closely related to the adrenal gland, splenic vessels and oesophago-gastric junction. Occasionally, the medial fibres of the left crus cross the aorta and run toward the IVC.

The right crus is more readily seen on ultrasound than the left. The left crus, rarely seen on a parasagittal scan, is often apparent on transverse scans.[5] The prevertebral spaces at the level of the crura contain the aorta, nerves, portions of the azygos venous system, lymph nodes and the cisterna chyli.

Scanning techniques

Using transverse and longitudinal scans, the superior reaches of the retroperitoneum are well-seen as the liver and spleen can be used as acoustic windows. Little if any patient preparation is required for retroperitoneal ultrasound. Fasting the patient for 12 hours before the scan may reduce gas but is not always necessary. Parenteral fluid or fluid enemas may occasionally be helpful. Barium studies should be performed after rather than immediately before an ultrasound because barium is a strong reflector.

The diaphragmatic crura, pancreas, kidneys, duodenum, psoas muscles and prevertebral vessels should all be detected and, in the lower abdomen, the iliopsoas, quadratus lumborum, and the prevertebral vessels can be visualised when scanning conditions are optimal. The oblique coronal view is a valuable addition to the standard views in visualising the retroperitoneum, particularly for the great vessels.[6-8] This is best performed from the right flank with the patient in a left posterior oblique position so that the right lobe of the liver and the right kidney move antero-inferiorly and act as acoustic windows. At the same time fat and gas filled bowel loops move anteriorly, facilitating acoustic access posterior to them. Similarly, scans can be performed from the left flank in the right posterior oblique position but these are usually less valuable than on the right where the better window provided by the liver is available.

With oblique coronal views the proximal renal arteries can be demonstrated in up to 90% of patients[7] though success is lower in the presence of an aortic aneurysm, presumably because of the anatomical distortion it causes.[6] The proximal portions of the common iliac arteries can be seen in 80% of patients. Enlarged posterior abdominal lymph nodes can be detected with an accuracy, sensitivity and specificity of around 90% and they can easily be differentiated from the para-aortic vessels.[8] Anomalous or duplicated venae cavae can be displayed in sagittal or oblique coronal scans.[6]

Ultrasound is generally held to be less reliable than CT in imaging the retroperitoneum;[1] this is because ultrasound access to the retroperitoneum is often impaired by bowel gas, bone, and thick muscle or fat layers. However, the solid parenchymal organs of the abdomen and pelvis can almost always be visualised by both CT and ultrasound. Ultrasound may be more accurate than CT in a thin patient, is rapidly performed and involves no X-rays or contrast agents; it should, therefore, be the first imaging choice in very thin patients, those who are too ill to move to the CT suite and in children, adolescents and pregnant women where radiation is particularly to be avoided. Most often the diagnostic information obtained from CT and ultrasound is complementary, the weaknesses of one technique being offset by the strengths of the other.

Aorta

The great vessels lie anterior to the spine in the retroperitoneum. The abdominal aorta enters the abdomen at approximately L1 and descends to L4 where it bifurcates into the common iliac arteries (Fig. 3). It is closely related to the anterior surface of the spine: any separation is suspicious, suggesting a space occupying lesion such as a haematoma, lymphadenopathy or fibrosis. At the level of the crura the aortic lumen measures 2.5 cm in diameter, tapering to 1 cm at the bifurcation (Fig. 4).

The coeliac axis, superior mesenteric artery and renal arteries are all usually visualised on ultrasound (Fig. 5). The inferior mesenteric artery is occasionally seen arising from the anterior surface of the aorta, several centimetres above the bifurcation. The common iliac arteries are often visible in the decubitus views.

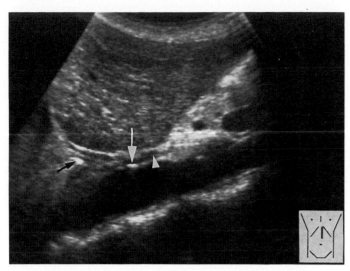

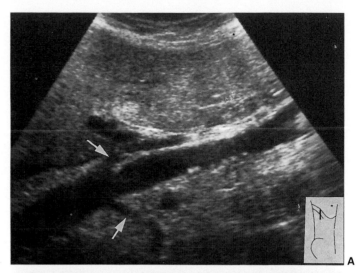

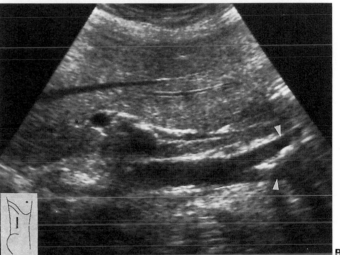

Fig. 3 The aorta and crus. The aorta is shown in longitudinal section as it enters the abdomen under the crus (arrowhead) with the lower thoracic oesophagus above it (black arrow). In this subject there is a small calcific plaque (white arrow) in the anterior wall of the aorta.

Fig. 4 Coronal sections of the aorta. A: The renal artery origins are shown (arrows). **B:** The bifurcation into the common iliac arteries (arrowheads).

Congenital anomalies of the aorta are rare; in situs inversus all the abdominal contents are transposed so that the aorta lies on the right – apart from its position, the appearances are normal.

In atheroma, the normally thin, smooth endothelial lining of the aorta thickens and becomes irregular, often with calcification. The aorta may also dilate slightly so that it looses its normal tapering configuration (Fig. 6). Such ectatic aortas may produce a pulsatile epigastric 'mass' that suggests an aneurysm; ultrasound readily makes the distinction. The ectatic aorta is often very tortuous (Fig. 7).

Ultrasound has long been the diagnostic procedure of choice in evaluating abdominal aortic aneurysms.[9] It is used initially to confirm the diagnosis and to differentiate it from other causes of a pulsatile mass such as a tortuous atheromatous aorta, a hyperdynamic aorta in a thin person (Fig. 8) or a para-aortic mass. These distinctions may often be difficult to establish on clinical examination.[10] About a third of abdominal aortic aneurysms do not contain enough calcification to allow a measurement of their size on a plain film but ultrasound can be used to assess aneurysm size to within ±3 mm[11] and has an advantage over angiography in that it demonstrates both the true lumen and the amount of mural thrombus (Fig. 9). An aneurysm with a true luminal diameter of 5 cm or larger is at slight risk of rupture but half of those larger than 6 cm in diameter rupture within the first year.

Ultrasound is useful for serial measurements of the aneurysm: progressive expansion of more than 1 cm per annum[10,12] is an indication for surgical intervention. The relationship of the aneurysm and the renal arteries affects the surgical treatment as well as the associated morbidity and mortality, so visualisation of the renal arteries is

important. Though the renal arteries are usually seen in normal subjects, they are more difficult to visualise in the presence of an abdominal aortic aneurysm, so that aortography or a dynamic CT scan are required.[7] Extension of the aneurysm into the iliac arteries can usually be demonstrated on ultrasound.

Acute aortic rupture is a surgical emergency with a high mortality so that imaging studies are not useful or appropriate. However, in chronic aortic rupture, a pulsating haematoma or a peri-aortic collection extending into the flanks may be demonstrated. Post-operatively these collections may show transmitted pulsation from the graft rather than intrinsic pulsatility of the vessel walls.

Aortic dissection gives a characteristic ultrasound appearance with a 'flapping' inner (media-intima) wall which has become separated from the outer (media-adventitia) wall and the extent of the dissection, within the abdomen,

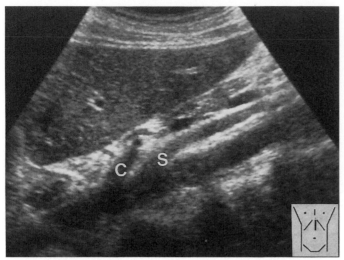

Fig. 5 Midline branches of the aorta. The coeliac axis (C) and the superior mesenteric artery (S) are seen in this sagittal section through the upper abdominal aorta.

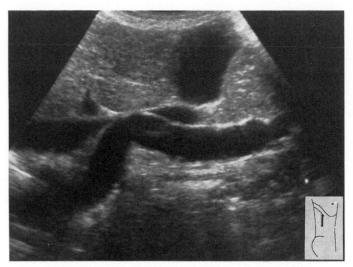

Fig. 7 Tortuous aorta. In this coronal section the extreme tortuosity that the aorta may achieve is well-shown. Here the cava is compressed by the elongated tortuosity.

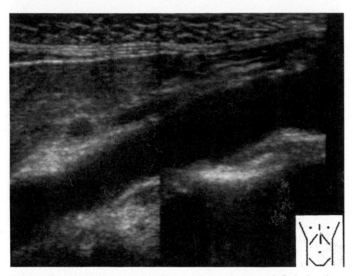

Fig. 6 Ectatic aorta. Instead of narrowing as it passes inferiorly, the ectatic aorta has the same calibre throughout its length or, as in this case, expands progressively. Such an aorta may be easily palpable and is readily confused for an aneurysm on clinical examination.

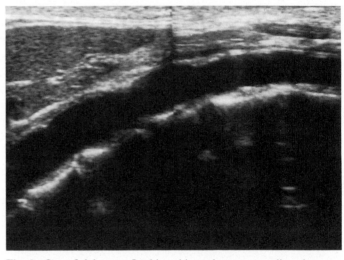

Fig. 8 Superficial aorta. In thin subjects the aorta may lie only a few cm deep because of the normal lumbar lordosis. This patient was referred to confirm an aortic aneurysm but this is excluded by the normal tapering configuration.

can often be defined (Fig. 10).[13–15] Colour Doppler is particularly helpful in demonstrating the separate vascular channels with their different flow velocities shown as distinct colour values.

In aortic occlusion, the aorta typically remains anechoic but there is no pulsation.[16] Doppler studies are essential to confirm the occlusion.

Aortic grafts are identified by their typical sharply-defined parallel, reflective walls (Fig. 11). Abdominal aortic aneurysms are repaired by incising the aneurysm, implanting the graft and then wrapping the aneurysm sac around the graft to stabilise it. Post-operative bleeding

tends to track between the graft and the encircling aneurysm wall to produce a characteristic 'lumen within a lumen' appearance on ultrasound.[17] False aneurysms are the commonest graft complication. They occur at the anastomotic sites and are usually due to breakdown of sutures but also occasionally to graft infection. False aneurysms are less common at the proximal anastomotic site but more serious than those affecting the distal (femoral) anastomosis because they may erode into the overlying duodenum producing an aorto-duodenal fistula with massive gastrointestinal bleeding.

Usually, even recently implanted grafts are not

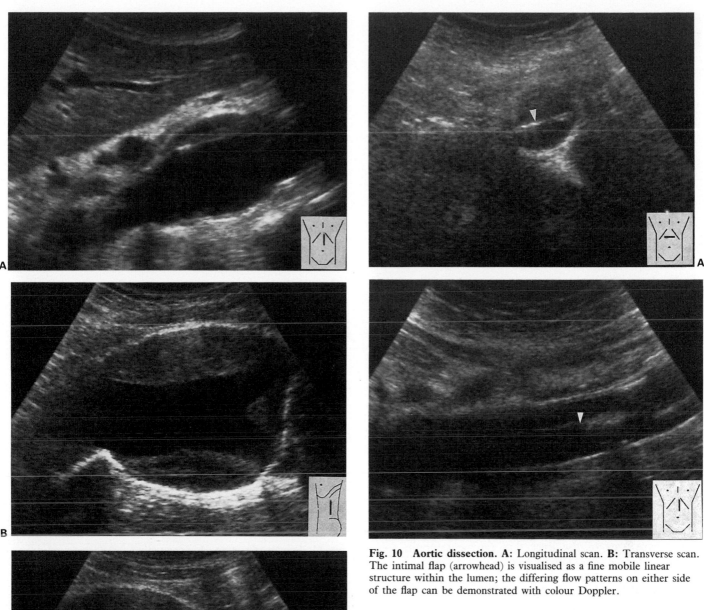

Fig. 9 Aortic aneurysm. All three components of an aneurysm, the wall, the lumen and the thrombus are well-shown by ultrasound. There is calcific atheroma (arrowhead) in the aortic wall in **C**.

Fig. 10 Aortic dissection. A: Longitudinal scan. **B:** Transverse scan. The intimal flap (arrowhead) is visualised as a fine mobile linear structure within the lumen; the differing flow patterns on either side of the flap can be demonstrated with colour Doppler.

associated with significant fluid collections. Perigraft fluid, either proximal, distal, or tracking along the length of the graft is a serious and important finding that suggests an abscess, haematoma or lymphocele. Collections at the distal anastomoses can be aspirated under ultrasound control to exclude early infection. CT is more sensitive for graft abscesses because the characteristic gas pocket is readily detected. Small haematomas tend to occur at the anastomotic sites and resorb within a few weeks of surgery. Persistent or enlarging collections suggest the formation of a false aneurysm, abscess or aorto-duodenal fistula.[17] Ultrasound may be used to distinguish a false aneurysm, which is intrinsically pulsatile, from a simple perigraft fluid collection which only has transmitted pulsations (and then only where the fluid lies adjacent to a pulsatile vessel).

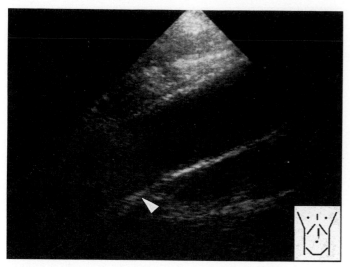

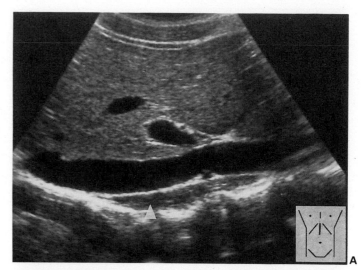

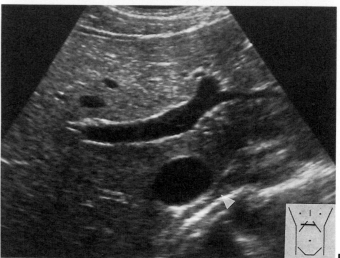

Fig. 11 Aortic graft. The graft's strong echoes and parallel walls are characteristic. In this case the texture of the weave of the Dacron® (arrowhead) can be discerned in the graft wall.

Fig. 12 Inferior vena cava. A: Longitudinal and **B:** transverse sections showing the normal cava in the distended state (held inspiration) closely applied to the posterior surface of the liver and lying over the right crus of diaphragm (arrowheads).

However, in practice, this distinction is often difficult to make.

In graft occlusion, as with aortic occlusion, the only ultrasound signs may be lack of pulsatility so Doppler is required for a definitive diagnosis.[10,17]

Inferior vena cava

The inferior vena cava originates at the junction of the two common iliac veins to the right of L5 and continues cephalad on the right side of the spine, widening after receiving the renal veins (Fig. 12). It lies within a groove in the bare area of the liver that can occasionally completely enclose it. Just before penetrating the diaphragm at the level of T8 to T9, it turns anteriorly towards the right atrium and receives the hepatic veins.

In the supine position, the upper portion of the inferior vena cava is usually accessible but it is often obscured distally by overlying bowel gas. The right coronal view often gives better visualisation of the entire length of the inferior vena cava.

The calibre of the inferior vena cava varies greatly, depending on the phase of respiration; it can normally appear thin and slit-like. A Valsalva manoeuvre can be used to distend a normal inferior vena cava so it becomes more obvious on ultrasound.

Anomalies of the cava are common because of its complex embryological origins from several primitive segments. Left sided cava, with an incidence of 0.2%, occurs in various degrees of completeness, the usual form consisting of a left cava below renal level, draining into a large left renal vein that crosses over the aorta to a normal upper caval segment (Fig. 13).

Pathological distension of the inferior vena cava not related to respiration is seen in congestive cardiac failure, cardiac tamponade and proximal inferior vena cava obstruction. If the lesion is above the hepatic veins, these are also distended.[18]

The inferior vena cava is invaded in approximately 10% of renal cell carcinomas when reflective material is visualised within its lumen. The connection with the tumour in the appropriate renal vein can usually be demonstrated (see Vol. 2, Ch. 30).

The inferior vena cava may be displaced anteriorly by posterior lesions such as lymphadenopathy, right adrenal and renal masses. It is displaced posteriorly by anteriorly sited masses such as lymph nodes, masses in the pancreatic head and by caudate lobe enlargement due to liver tumours (see Ch. 17) or the Budd Chiari syndrome (see Ch. 18).

A large mass can severely compress or even obstruct the

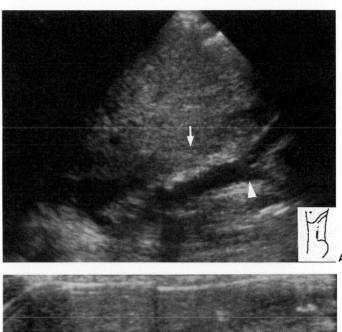

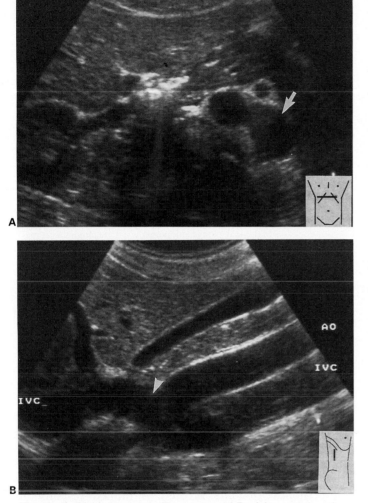

Fig. 13 Left-sided cava. A: Transverse and **B:** right coronal sections showing a left-sided cava (arrow) discharging into the left renal vein (arrowhead). AO – aorta, IVC – inferior vena cava.

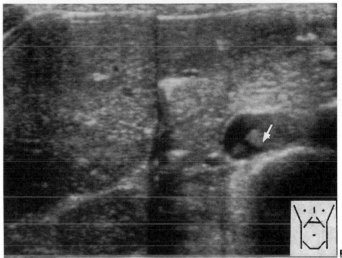

Fig. 14 Caval thrombus. A: Left coronal section at the pelvic brim. **B:** Transverse section in the epigastrium. The caval thrombus is seen as reflective material within the caval lumen (arrows). **A** shows the aortic bifurcation (arrowhead).

inferior vena cava. Caval obstruction at a site of narrowing can be difficult to evaluate on ultrasound since the inferior vena cava may normally be slit-like; lack of distension on Valsalva, with dilatation below the apparent site of compression, are suggestive features.[18] Confirmation is best made by a Doppler examination.

Thrombus within the cava has the same general appearances as thrombus elsewhere, typically being seen as reflective material in the lumen (Fig. 14). However, it is important to note that fresh thrombus may be poorly reflective and so difficult to distinguish from blood. In this situation Doppler is invaluable; either spectral (pulsed) or colour Doppler may be used, the anatomical display of the latter revealing the position of the thrombus better as well as demonstrating blood flowing through recanalisation channels. Ultrasound cannot reliably distinguish between blood and tumour thrombus.

Filters, made of metallic or plastic wire, placed under angiographic control, are used to prevent pulmonary emboli from deep venous or pelvic or caval thrombosis. The filter material is strongly reflective and appears as a complex of linear echoes in the caval lumen (Fig. 15).

Retroperitoneal tumours

Most retroperitoneal tumours arise in the kidneys (see Vol. 2, Ch. 30) or adrenals (see Ch. 23). Of the remainder, primary retroperitoneal tumours other than lymphomas are uncommon.[18,19] Approximately 80% are malignant.[20,21] Most retroperitoneal tumours in the adult are mesenchymal in origin (Table 1), the three commonest being liposarcoma, leiomyosarcoma and malignant fibrohistiocytoma.[22] Metastatic disease in the retroperitoneum

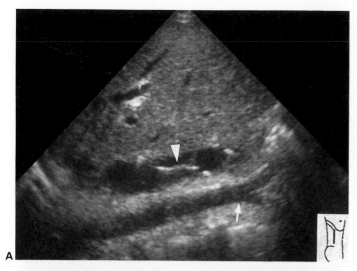

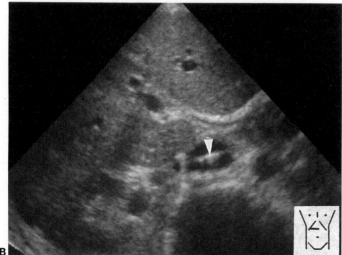

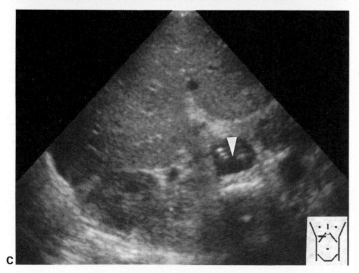

Fig. 15   Caval filter. A: Right coronal, **B** and **C:** low and high transverse sections showing the strong intracaval echoes (arrowheads) from a Greenberg filter. The aortic bifurcation is well-seen (arrow in **A**).

Table 1   Classification of retroperitoneal tumours (Hsu-Chong Yeh[20])

	Malignant	Benign
Mesenchymal		
	Liposarcoma	Lipoma
	Leiomyosarcoma	Leiomyoma
	Rhabdomyosarcoma	Rhabdomyoma
	Fibrosarcoma	Fibroma, fibromatosis
	Malignant fibrous histiocytoma	
Vascular		
	Haemangiopericytoma	
	Angiosarcoma	(haemangioma)
	Lymphangiosarcoma	(lymphangioma)
Neurogenic		
	Malignant Schwannoma	Neurilemmoma
		Neurofibroma
Tumours of sympathetic nerve origin		
	Neuroblastoma	
	Ganglioneuroblastoma	Ganglioneuroma
	Malignant paraganglioma	Paraganglioneuroma
	Extra-adrenal phaeochromocytoma	
Germ cell tumours		
	Malignant teratoma	Benign teratoma
	Embryonal carcinoma	
	Seminoma*	

* occasionally arises in the retroperitoneal space as a primary tumour.

is usually recurrence of a urological or gynaecological malignancy.

Clinically, retroperitoneal tumours are insidious in onset with few early manifestations, so that they reach a large size by the time of diagnosis (Table 2). Abdominal pain is the commonest presentation, probably attributable to bowel and renal obstruction and 80% of the tumours are palpable. Surgery offers the best hope of cure for malignant retroperitoneal tumours as there is limited response to radiotherapy and chemotherapy. However, most are invasive and cannot be resected completely, so the prognosis is poor.[23–25]

Table 2   Presenting features of retroperitoneal tumours (S. Jacobsen et al[21])

Abdominal pain	88%
Fatigue	44%
Weight loss	32%
Anorexia	24%
Fever	20%
Radiating nerve root pain	16%
Back pain	12%

Although it may not always be possible to confirm the retroperitoneal origin of the tumour with ultrasound, some characteristic features may be helpful in locating their origin. Anterior displacement of the pancreas, kidneys, great vessels, or of the ascending or descending colon are highly suggestive of a retroperitoneal lesion (Fig. 16). Encasement of retroperitoneal structures such as the aorta,

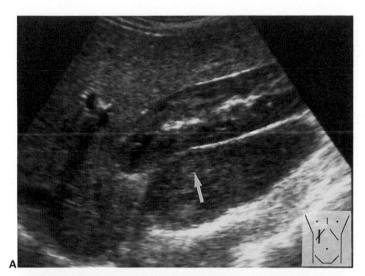

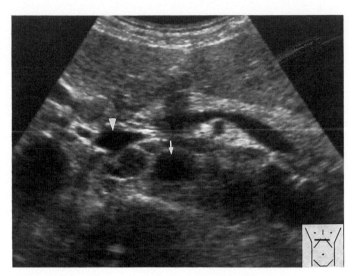

Fig. 17 Retroperitoneal tumour encasing the aorta. Numerous retroperitoneal masses are seen surrounding the aorta (arrow) and elevating the inferior vena cava (arrowhead).

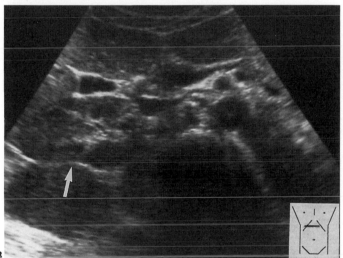

Fig. 16 Retroperitoneal sarcoma. A: Longitudinal right parasagittal and **B:** transverse sections of a retroperitoneal mass elevating the right kidney (arrow). The uniform echo texture is typical of a sarcoma.

IVC, renal vessels, kidney and pancreas or compression of the iliopsoas or quadratus lumborum muscles are also typical features (Fig. 17).

It is usually impossible to determine the histology of the tumour from the ultrasound appearances but features suggestive of a specific diagnosis have been described. Many retroperitoneal tumours are large (particularly haemangiopericytomas) but functioning tumours (e.g. extra-adrenal phaeochromocytoma) and tumours associated with disease elsewhere (e.g. a Schwannoma in a patient with neurofibromatosis) may be small at diagnosis. Neurogenic tumours are generally parvertebral and tumours of sympathetic nerve origin tend to be para-aortic in position but extra-adrenal phaeochromocytomas or paraganglionomas often arise in the organ of Zuckerkandl which is usually found below the renal hilum, or at the origin of the inferior mesenteric artery. Teratomas often involve the

sacrococcygeal area whereas a malignant fibrohistiocytoma typically lies very close to the kidney (necessitating nephrectomy in 50% of cases).[26] The patient's age may also provide a clue to the tumour type, rhabdomyosarcoma, neuroblastoma, ganglioneuroblastoma and teratomas all tending to occur in children, whereas malignant fibrohistiocytoma is the commonest soft tissue sarcoma of late adult life.

The ultrasound appearances are very variable with strongly and poorly reflective or mixed tumours all occurring, both with and without central anechoic zones due to necrosis.[27] Tumours with a uniform cell type and a paucity of connective tissue and fat have fewer internal echoes so that they produce lesions that are echo-poor or nearly anechoic as is typical of a malignant Schwannoma or fibrohistiocytoma. A highly reflective tumour suggests a liposarcoma, although these are not always reflective when poorly differentiated. The reflectivity of a lipoma varies from highly intense to weak, depending on the content and distribution of fat and fibrous tissue (Fig. 18). Vascular tumours such as haemangiopericytomas are also reflective, presumably because of the abundant interfaces produced by the vessel walls.

A solid mass typically of mixed reflectivity with an echo-poor centre suggests a sarcoma as these rapidly progressive tumours tend to outgrow their blood supply causing central necrosis with haemorrhage. This is particularly true of leiomyosarcomas.

A teratoma has a characteristically heterogeneous mixed echo pattern with solid areas, calcification (50%) and cystic spaces (76%) (similar to ovarian teratomas). They occur in female infants under 6 months of age with a second peak in incidence in young adult males. However, a retro-

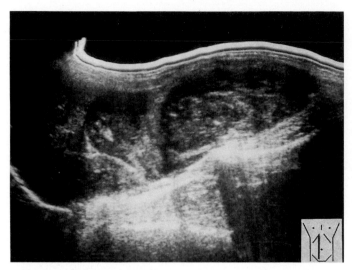

Fig. 18 Liposarcoma. The strong echoes that are typical of a liposarcoma are attributable to the admixture of fatty and watery soft tissue elements; for this reason, only well-differentiated tumours (i.e. those that retain the ability to form fat) have this appearance.

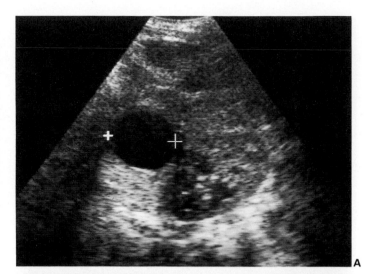

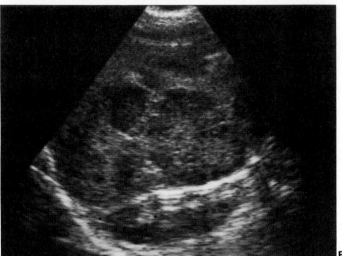

Fig. 19 Retroperitoneal cyst. A: Transverse scan through a left intercostal space in a 4-month-old with a congenital retroperitoneal cyst. The distinction from a pancreatic cyst cannot be made on imaging grounds but, at laparotomy, the clear fluid that was aspirated had a very low amylase level. **B:** Scan through the liver showing multiple echo-poor lesions which were haemangioendotheliomas; the purpose of the laparotomy was to tie off the hepatic artery. The discovery of one developmental anomaly should prompt a careful search for others.

peritoneal teratoma discovered in a young adult male is more likely to represent a metastasis from a testicular primary, hence the testes should also be scanned. Contrary to early reports, it is not possible to distinguish benign from malignant teratomas on the basis of whether they are predominantly cystic or solid.[28]

The benign or malignant nature of any retroperitoneal tumour cannot be reliably determined on ultrasound. A smooth, round, well-demarcated cystic mass may be benign or malignant. However, an irregular lesion is more likely to be malignant, benign fibromatosis being an exception since it may be very irregular and show features of muscle invasion.

Retroperitoneal cysts

Primary retroperitoneal cysts are rare. They include simple inclusion cysts (teratomatous cysts) and cysts arising from embryonic gastrointestinal and genitourinary tract rests (e.g. Wolffian or Müllerian duct remnants in the male). They may be lymphatic, parasitic, traumatic or inflammatory and are usually asymptomatic, being discovered incidentally on routine physical examinations as a soft, non-tender abdominal mass.

Retroperitoneal cysts meet the usual ultrasound criteria for simple cysts: they are smooth walled and echo-free with increased through transmission of sound (Fig. 19). The absence of internal echoes helps distinguish them from abscesses, haematomas and complex cysts such as dermoids or hydatids, although lymphangioma may consist of multi-septated cysts.[29] The history helps distinguish cysts from urinomas or lymphocele which are usually post-operative or follow urinary obstruction.

The recommended treatment for retroperitoneal cysts is surgical removal as they tend to recur after simple aspiration.[30]

Retroperitoneal fluid collections

Retroperitoneal fluid collections tend to spread by gravity along the path of least resistance, namely between the fascial planes. Although occasionally more than one compartment is involved or the fascia is destroyed by the disease process (e.g. in trauma), it is generally possible to localise the fluid to a specific compartment and thereby

Table 3 Features of retroperitoneal collections

Compartment	Direction of fluid movement within the compartment	Renal displacement	Likely source of fluid
Perirenal space	Fluid localises in fat postero-laterally and drains posteriorly (i.e. collects dorso-laterally to lower renal pole)	Antero-medially and superiorly	Intrarenal infection
Posterior pararenal space	Infero-laterally parallel to psoas	Anteriorly and superiorly	Spontaneous retroperitoneal haemorrhage (e.g. bleeding diathesis, anticoagulant therapy)
Anterior pararenal space	Bulges anteriorly into peritoneal cavity, displacing small bowel loops	Superiorly ± laterally (anterior or descending antero-laterally)	Exudates from lesions of colon, pancreas, duodenum, bile ducts, retroperitoneal appendix. Haemorrhage from trauma or rupture of splenic or hepatic artery aneurysm

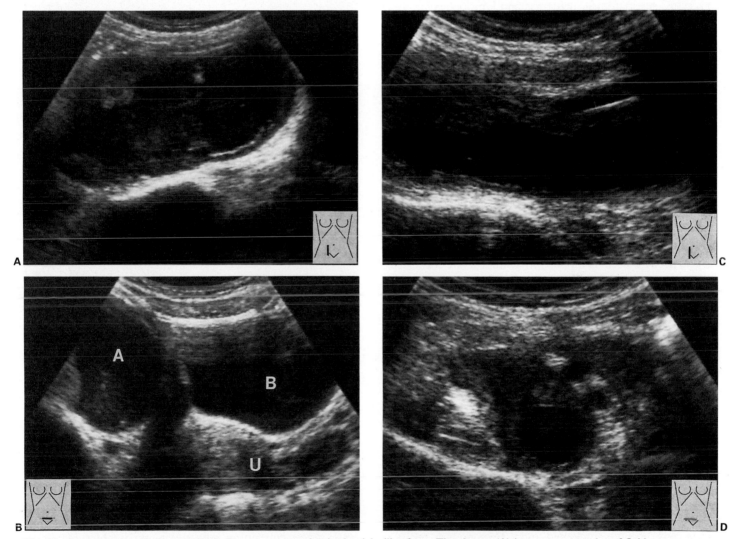

Fig. 20 Psoas abscess. A: Longitudinal, **B:** transverse section in the right iliac fossa. The abscess (A) is seen as a complex of fluid spaces, many with internal echoes, extending into the false pelvis. Tubercle bacilli were cultured and antituberculous drugs started. B – bladder, U – uterus. **C:** Longitudinal and **D:** transverse sections in similar positions 1 month later. The changes of organisation are seen with an increase in the solid elements.

deduce the likely source of the fluid, from anatomical considerations (Fig. 1 and Table 3).[2]

Although ultrasound is very accurate in detecting retroperitoneal collections, it is often unhelpful in distinguishing between the types of collection so that needle aspiration should be considered an integral part of the examination. Subsequently ultrasound may be used to establish therapeutic drainage and to follow the progress of the lesion. Scans performed with the patient supine allow a comparison between the two sides. However, gas often obscures the views in this position and coronal decubitus and prone views (both transverse and longitudinal) are often more helpful.

Retroperitoneal fluid collections can be divided into abscesses, haematomas, urinomas and lymphoceles.

Retroperitoneal abscesses are most commonly encountered as a post-operative complication or following extension from renal, spinal or paraspinal infection (Fig. 20). Less often they are due to haematogenous spread, trauma or infection following perforation of an abdominal viscus such as colon, appendix or duodenum. They often involve the psoas muscles (psoas abscess) and the perirenal spaces.[18]

As elsewhere, abscesses may have thick irregular walls, septa, layering of internal debris and, occasionally, gas bubbles (Fig. 21). Large pockets of gas, although uncommon, may completely obscure views of the abscess so, where there is a strong clinical suspicion of a retroperitoneal abscess but a negative ultrasound, a CT scan should be performed.

The psoas muscle is a relatively common site for abscess formation, formerly mostly due to TB but now more often following appendicitis, perirenal pathology and nontuberculous bacterial spondylitis. Clinically there is often unilateral flank, hip or back pain aggravated by hip extension. There may be a palpable tender abdominal mass (particularly in children) or occasionally a lump in the upper thigh. Typically there is fever, leucocytosis and a raised ESR. The plain X-ray may show bone destruction but this is a late finding and not always present. Ultrasound reveals the psoas outline to be enlarged and rounded. The size and extent of the abscess can be assessed as well as its relationship to adjacent structures, particularly the kidneys and blood vessels. The muscle may be generally echo-poor if the infection has spread diffusely, or may contain a localised fluid collection.

The right anterior pararenal space and anterior perirenal fascia may become thickened and reflective as a result of extension of inflammation from retroperitoneal organs into the pararenal space. While this is typical of acute pancreatitis, it has also been reported in association with acute cholecystitis and acute appendicitis.[18,31]

Retroperitoneal haematomas are not uncommon, especially in anticoagulated patients, those with bleeding diatheses (such as haemophilia) and in association with a

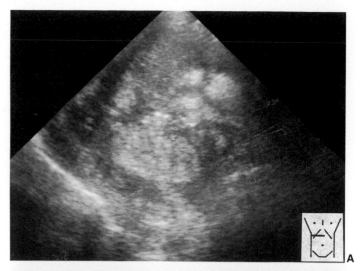

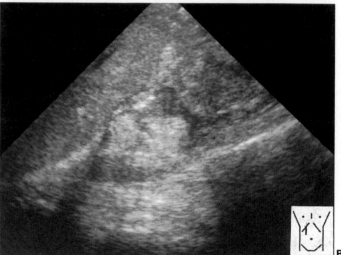

Fig. 21 Retroperitoneal abscess. A: Transverse and **B:** longitudinal sections in the right upper quadrant showing an abscess that followed a nephrectomy. The intense echoes are due to multiple minute gas bubbles in the purulent fluid.

leaking abdominal aortic aneurysm (Fig. 22). Haematomas in the perirenal space most often follow renal trauma whereas those in the posterior pararenal space or psoas muscle are more likely to occur spontaneously.

There is a spectrum of ultrasound appearances: very fresh haematomas may be anechoic and thus difficult to differentiate from other retroperitoneal fluid. A more chronic haematoma often develops complex multiseptate cystic spaces containing reflective material which may layer and move with changes in the patient's position (Fig. 23). Diffusely infiltrating haematomas may be very poorly defined in shape and size. A chronic haematoma may become so well-organised that it cannot be distinguished from a solid mass; it may also calcify.

The psoas muscle is a site for spontaneous retroperitoneal haemorrhage particularly in haemophiliacs. Pain

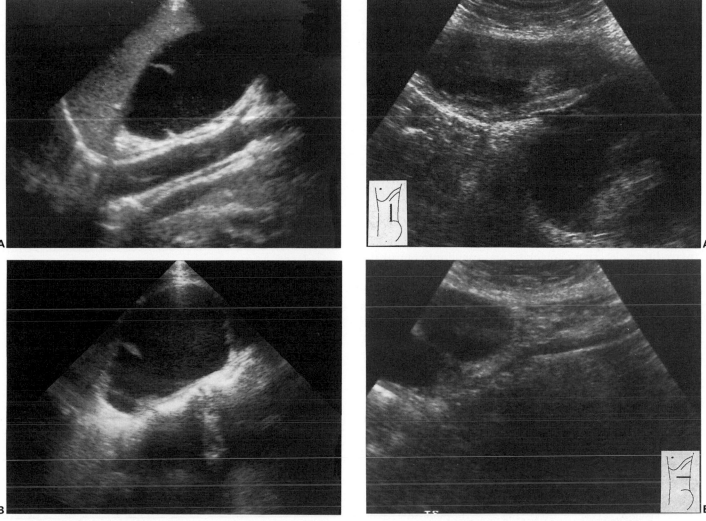

Fig. 22 Retroperitoneal haematoma. A and **B:** Left coronal sections showing two views of a well-demarcated collection in the left para-aortic position. Note the low level internal echoes and the septa. The bleed in this patient was from retroperitoneal metastases from a malignant melanoma.

Fig. 23 Retroperitoneal haematoma. A: Left longitudinal and **B:** transverse sections through an old retroperitoneal haematoma. The increased echo intensity indicates organisation (compare Fig. 22).

and stiffness in the flank, hip or groin are typical presenting symptoms and flexion deformities of the hip may develop secondary to iliopsoas spasm. Large psoas haematomas may cause anorexia, constipation, fever, leucocytosis, urinary frequency and dysuria (due to pressure on the bladder) and may even mimic acute appendicitis or ureteric colic.[32] Femoral nerve encroachment at the level of the inguinal canal can cause loss of sensation on the anterior surface of the thigh and, more seriously, paralysis of the quadriceps. Early diagnosis of a psoas haematoma is particularly important in haemophiliacs as prompt treatment with Factor VIII is very effective in preventing femoral nerve entrapment and any resultant neurological deficit.

In addition to infection and haematoma, the differential diagnosis of psoas muscle enlargement includes invasion by retroperitoneal tumour and hemihypertrophy (occasionally also seen as a normal variant in young West Indian adults when it is typically bilaterally symmetrical). It must also be differentiated from adjacent lymphadenopathy.

Both urinomas and lymphoceles are mainly postoperative complications, although a urinoma may also result from urinary extravasation following renal obstruction (see Vol. 2, Ch. 29). Both appear as anechoic fluid spaces on ultrasound. Urinomas tend to remain within the perirenal space whereas lymphoceles are more typically seen in the pelvis following renal transplantation (see Vol. 2, Ch. 34) or pelvic lymphadenectomy.

Retroperitoneal fibrosis

Retroperitoneal fibrosis was first described by Albarron in

1905.[33] It is a proliferation of fibrous tissue generally confined to the central and paravertebral regions of the retroperitoneum in the perirenal space between the renal hila and the dome of the bladder.[34] It is typically thickest immediately anterior to the sacrum and lower lumbar spine.[35] Rarely, extension into the mediastinum, porta hepatis and mesentery have been reported.[36] Infiltration of the small bowel, uterus, vagina, bladder and rectum are also recognised.[37,38] The tissue is sharply delineated but is not encapsulated. It tends to envelop rather than displace adjacent structures such as ureters, blood and lymphatic vessels and, rarely, bowel loops. Approximately 70% of cases are idiopathic.[34] Other cases are associated with drugs (notably methysergide), inflammation, infection, trauma, retroperitoneal haemorrhage and with both primary and metastatic tumours. The rare association with Riedel's thyroiditis, sclerosing cholangitis and pseudotumour of the orbit suggests an autoimmune basis in some cases.

The insidious onset and progressive nature of the fibrosis make this a serious clinical problem. Presentation tends to be delayed until symptoms of ureteral or vascular obstruction appear. There is a peak incidence in the fifth or sixth decade and a preponderance of males to females (2:1). Symptoms are often minimal and the clinical features, in general, are non-specific: patients present with abdominal or flank pain and tenderness, weight loss, anorexia, malaise, hypertension and renal failure. There may be scrotal or leg oedema due to lymphatic obstruction. A palpable abdominal or rectal mass is found in approximately 30%.[39] Laboratory investigations are also non-specific, with anaemia, a raised ESR and hypoalbuminaemia.

Ultrasound reveals a mass that is echo-poor due to its homogeneous consistency (Fig. 24). It may be bulky, with an ill-defined irregular margin, or flat and plaque-like with a smooth margin. Adjacent solid organs such as the kidney may be displaced. Typically the plaque extends below the aortic bifurcation into the upper pelvis.

The classic diagnostic triad of urographic findings in retroperitoneal fibrosis (hydronephrosis with compressed and medially deviated ureters) is not entirely reliable: occasionally, there is no hydronephrosis and medial deviation of the ureters may be a normal finding[34] so that further imaging is required when retroperitoneal fibrosis is suspected. CT is better able to delineate the extent of retroperitoneal fibrosis and to detect minimal or localised

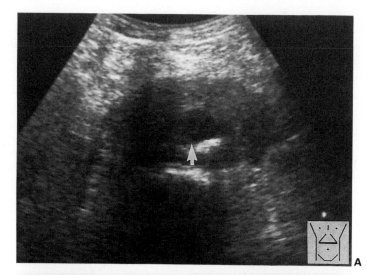

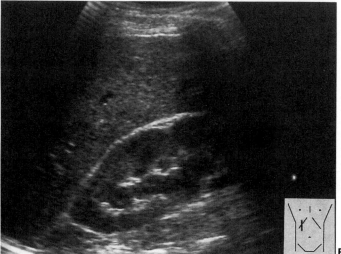

Fig. 24 Retroperitoneal fibrosis. A: Transverse section across the aorta (arrow) showing the echo-poor cuff of fibrous tissue which is thicker anteriorly. **B:** Right longitudinal section through the kidney showing the hydronephrosis.

areas of fibrosis; it is the investigation of choice.[40] However, there is a role for ultrasound in follow up, particularly in assessing the associated hydronephrosis. It may not always be possible to distinguish retroperitoneal fibrosis from other retroperitoneal masses such as lymphoma, sarcoma or haematoma. A needle biopsy, which can be performed under ultrasound guidance, is often needed.

REFERENCES

1 Raskin M. Combination of CT and ultrasound in the examination of the retroperitoneum and pelvis. Crit Rev Diag Imaging 1980; 13: 173–228
2 Meyers M A, Whalen J P, Peele K. Radiological features of extraperitoneal effusions. Radiology 1972; 104: 249–257
3 Raptopoulos V, Kleinman P K, Marks S, Snyder M, Silverman

P M. Renal fascial pathway: posterior extension of pancreatic effusions within the anterior pararenal space. Radiology 1986; 158: 367–374
4 Belli A M, Joseph A E. The renal rind sign: a new ultrasound indication of inflammatory disease in the abdomen. Br J Radiol 1988; 61: 806–810

5 Callen P W, Filly R A, Sarti D A, Sample W F. Ultrasonography of the diaphragmatic crura. Radiology 1979; 130: 721–724

6 Pardes J G, Auh Y H, Kneeland J B, et al. The oblique coronal view in sonography of the retroperitoneum. AJR 1985; 144: 1241–1247

7 Creagh-Barry M, Adam E J, Joseph A E. The value of oblique scans in the ultrasonic examination of the abdominal aorta. Clin Radiol 1986; 37: 239–241

8 Grunebaum M, Ziv N, Kornreich L. The sonographic evaluation of the great vessels' interspace in the pediatric retroperitoneum. Pediatr Radiol 1986; 16: 384–387

9 LaRoy L L, Cormier P J, Matalon T A, Patel S K, Turner D A, Silver B. Imaging of abdominal aortic aneurysms. AJR 1989; 152: 785–792

10 Gomes M N. Clinical and surgical aspects of abdominal aortic aneurysms. Semin Ultrasound 1982; 3: 156–169

11 Leopold G R, Goldberger L E, Bernstein E F. Ultrasonic detection and evaluation of abdominal aortic aneurysms. Surgery 1980; 72: 939–945

12 Mittlestaed C A. Vascular Ultrasound. Abdominal ultrasound. Chapter 6. New York: Churchill Livingstone. 1987: p 441–580

13 King P S, Cooperberg P L, Madigan S M. The anechoic crescent in abdominal aortic aneurysms: not a sign of dissection. AJR 1986; 146: 345–458

14 Bondestam S, Hekali P, Landtman M. Sonographic diagnosis of dissection of the descending thoracic aorta. Ann Chir Gynaecol 1981; 70: 210–212

15 Schopp D, Wimmer B. Current diagnosis of dissecting aortic aneurysm. Radiology 1989; 29: 237–244

16 Harter L P, Gross B H, Callen P W, Barth R A. Ultrasonic evaluation of abdominal aortic thrombus. J Ultrasound Med 1982; 1: 315–318

17 Gooding G A, Effeney D J, Goldstone J. The aortofemoral graft: detection and identification of healing complications by ultrasonography. Surgery 1981; 89: 94–101

18 Koenigsberg M, et al. Sonographic evaluation of the retroperitoneum. Semin Ultrasound 1982; 3: 79–95

19 Yeh H C. Adrenal gland and non-renal retroperitoneum. Urol Radiol 1987; 9: 127–140

20 Jacobsen S, Juul-Jørgensen P. Primary retroperitoneal tumours. Act Chir Scand 1974; 140: 498–500

21 Felix E L, et al. Tumours of the retroperitoneum. Current Problems in Cancer 1981; 6: 3–47

22 Davidson A J, Hartman D S. Imaging strategies for tumors of the kidney, adrenal gland, and retroperitoneum. CA 1987; 37: 151–164

23 Goldman S M, Davidson A J, Neal J. Retroperitoneal and pelvic haemangiopericytomas: clinical, radiologic and pathologic correlation. Radiology 1988; 168: 13–17

24 Kryger-Baggesen N, Kjaergaard J, Sehested M. Nonchromaffin paraganglionoma of the retroperitoneum. J Urol 1985; 134: 536–537

25 Skaane P. The right iliac fossa features of a large retroperitoneal liposarcoma. Fortschr Rontgenstr 1986; 145: 351–353

26 Goldman S M, Hartman D S, Weiss S W. The varied radiographic manifestations of retroperitoneal malignant fibrous histiocytoma revealed through 27 cases. J Urol 1986; 135: 33–38

27 Rubenstein W A, Gray G, Auh Y H, et al. CT of fibrous tissues and tumors with sonographic correlation. AJR 198; 14: 1067–1074

28 Davidson A J, Hartman D S, Goldman S M. Mature teratoma of the retroperitoneum. Radiologic, pathologic and clinical correlation. Radiology 1989; 172: 421–425

29 Davidson A J, Hartman D S. Lymphangioma of the retroperitoneum: CT and sonographic characteristic. Radiology 1990; 175: 507–510

30 Derchi L E, Rizzatto G, Banderali A, Sala P, Larghero G C, Solbiati L. Sonographic appearance of primary retroperitoneal cysts. J Ultrasound Med 1989; 8: 381–384

31 Hoddick W, Jeffrey R B, Goldberg H I, Federle M P, Laing F C. CT and sonography of severe renal and perirenal infections. AJR 1983; 140: 517–520

32 Kumari S, Pillari G, Phillips G, Pochachaczevsky R. Fluid collections of the psoas in children. Semin Ultrasound 1982; 3: 139–155

33 Albarran J. Retention renale par periureterite: libération externe de l'uretere. Assoc Fran d'Urole 1905; Proc-verb 511

34 Fagan C J, Amparo E G, Davis M. Retroperitoneal fibrosis. Semin Ultrasound 1982; 3: 123–138

35 Sanders R C, Duffy T, McLoughlin M G, Walsh P C. Sonography in the diagnosis of retroperitoneal fibrosis. J Urol 1977; 118: 944–946

36 Arger P H, Stolz J L, Miller W T. Retroperitoneal fibrosis: an analysis of the clinical spectrum and roentgenographic signs. AJR 1973; 119: 812–821

37 Coleman P K. Radiologic/pathologic correlation conference. Case 15: abdominal mass in a 73 year old man. Applied Radiology 1980; 12: 121–126

38 Kittredge R D, Nash A D. The many facets of sclerosing fibrosis. AJR 1974; 122: 288

39 Fagan C J, Larrieu A J, Amparo E G. Retroperitoneal fibrosis: ultrasound and CT features. AJR 1979; 133: 239–243

40 Brooks A P. Computed tomography of idiopathic retroperitoneal fibrosis ('periaortitis'): variants, variations, patterns and pitfalls. Clin Radiol 1990; 42: 75–79

The adrenals

Keith C. Dewbury

INTRODUCTION

Demonstration of the normal adrenal glands and small adrenal lesions remains a challenge for abdominal ultrasound. These small organs are high in location, deep within the rib cage and adjacent to the vertebrae. They are, therefore, easily obscured by the ribs, transverse processes and by stomach and bowel gas. A clear understanding of the anatomy and careful technique are essential to show them. Successful demonstration of the normal glands was reported by Sample in 1977[1] and by Yeh in 1980.[2] Both authors used static grey scale equipment and achieved high success rates of about 80% for the right adrenal gland and rather less for the left gland. These results were not universally achieved and computed tomography became pre-eminent for the routine examination of the adrenals.[3-6] The routine availability of real time ultrasound equipment with its ease and flexibility of use, particularly for intercostal scanning, has rekindled interest in adrenal ultrasound imaging. The progressive technical improvements in transducers, and particularly beam focusing capabilities, have led to a further reappraisal of the situation. There can be no doubt that routine visualisation of the adrenal glands during abdominal ultrasound is now commonplace and worthwhile.[7]

The normal adrenal gland

The normal adrenal glands are a pair of rather small flat organs lying anteromedial to the upper pole of the kidneys, extending partly over the kidneys.

Each gland consists of three parts, an anteromedial ridge from which two thin wings extend posteriorly. These are the lateral and medial wings which straddle the anteromedial aspect of the upper pole of the kidney. The general shape of the glands is illustrated diagrammatically in Figure 1.

The right adrenal gland is triangular or pyramidal in shape. The medial wing is largest superiorly and may be absent inferiorly; the opposite is true of the lateral wing.

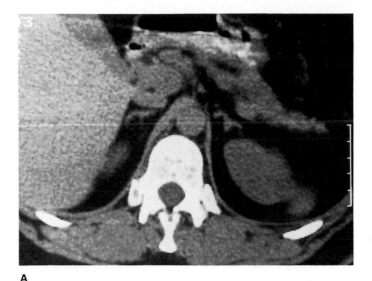

A

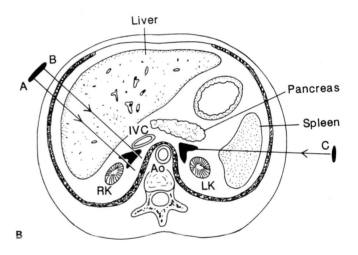

B

Fig. 2 **Anatomy of the adrenals. A**: CT scan showing the position of the normal adrenal glands. **B**: Diagrammatic section taken at the same level as the CT scan to show the ideal scanning approach to the two sides. Scan lines A and B will show the wings and anteromedial ridge of the right gland respectively. Scan line C through the spleen will show the left adrenal gland.

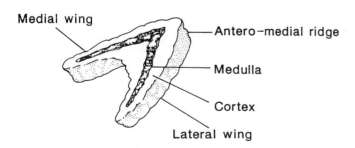

Fig. 1 **Anatomy of the adrenals.** Diagrammatic representation of the general shape and make up of the adrenal gland.

The anteromedial ridge of the gland is located immediately posterior to the IVC. It lies between the crus of the diaphragm and the posteromedial margin of the right lobe of the liver.

The left adrenal gland is more crescentic in shape and more cranial than the right. The anteromedial ridge of the gland may be slightly convex in outline and the lateral and medial wings are shorter than on the right. The gland lies lateral or slightly posterior to the aorta and lateral to the left crus of the diaphragm. It is posterior to the lesser sac superiorly and posterior to the pancreas inferiorly. As on the right, the adrenal is anteromedial to the upper pole of the kidney. The bulk of the adrenal gland is composed of

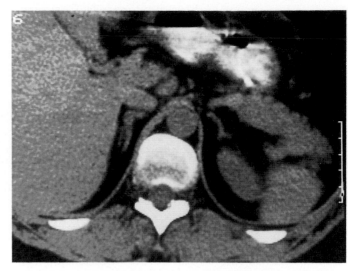

Fig. 3 Right adrenal – transverse sections. A: A slightly oblique transverse view through a right intercostal space showing both wings of the adrenal gland (arrows) lying parallel to the diaphragmatic crus (arrowhead). **B:** CT scan at the corresponding level.

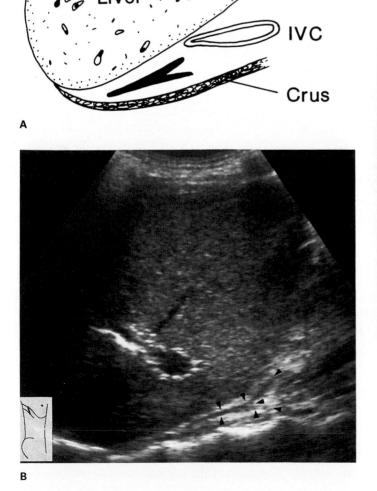

Fig. 4 Right adrenal – coronal sections. A: Diagrammatic representation of the shape and appearance of the right adrenal gland shown on a coronal section. **B:** Corresponding ultrasound section where both wings of the gland are displayed as a long inverted 'Y' shaped structure lying above the diaphragmatic crus. **C:** Similar section in another patient shows the gland to be more 'V' shaped and with rather bulkier limbs.

the adrenal cortex with a thin central medulla. The glands are 3 to 6 cm in overall length, 2 to 3 cm in width but only 2 to 6 mm in thickness.

Scanning technique and normal appearances

The position of the adrenals as described (Fig. 2A) dictates an intercostal approach using the acoustic window of the liver on the right and the spleen on the left. Figure 2B diagrammatically illustrates the preferred scanning approach with the patient lying supine. For the right side the transducer is placed in the ninth or tenth intercostal space in the mid or anterior axillary line. Scanning transversely the transducer is gently rotated to move the field of view

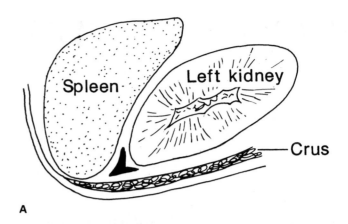

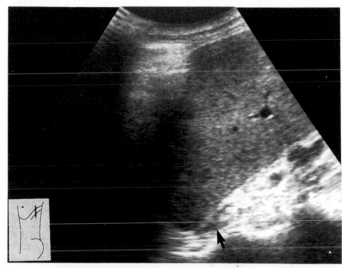

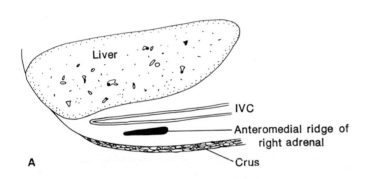

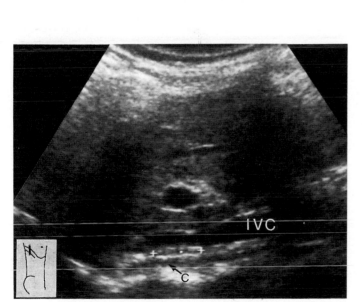

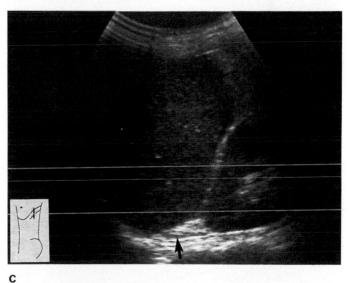

Fig. 5 Right adrenal – coronal sections. A: Diagrammatic representation of the position and appearance of the anteromedial ridge of the right adrenal gland lying sandwiched between the inferior vena cava and the diaphragmatic crus. **B:** Corresponding ultrasound section (c – crus, IVC – inferior vena cava). Small crosses mark the position of the anteromedial ridge.

Fig. 6 Left adrenal – coronal section. A: Diagrammatic representation of a coronal view of the left adrenal gland. **B and C:** Corresponding ultrasound sections in different patients mirroring this appearance (arrows).

from the renal hilum upwards to a few centimetres above the kidney, concentrating on the region behind the IVC and lateral to the right diaphragmatic crus. The adrenal area will be completely covered in such a sequence. In the upper transverse section on the right a vertical linear or curvilinear structure corresponding to the anteromedial ridge and medial wing is seen. In the middle section both wings are seen as an inverted 'V' or 'Y' (Fig. 3). Through the inferior portion of the gland only the lateral wing may be seen as a horizontal band. Coronal or longitudinal sec-

tions are obtained by rotating the transducer through 90°. The upper pole of the right kidney is located and the transducer angled medially. Both wings of the gland may be simultaneously displayed as a thin, long inverted 'V' or 'Y' shaped structure up to 6 cm in length (Fig. 4). A further small medial angulation is necessary to visualise the anteromedial ridge of the gland in this plane where it lies posterior to the IVC (Fig. 5).

The left adrenal gland is more difficult to image because of the smaller acoustic window available through the

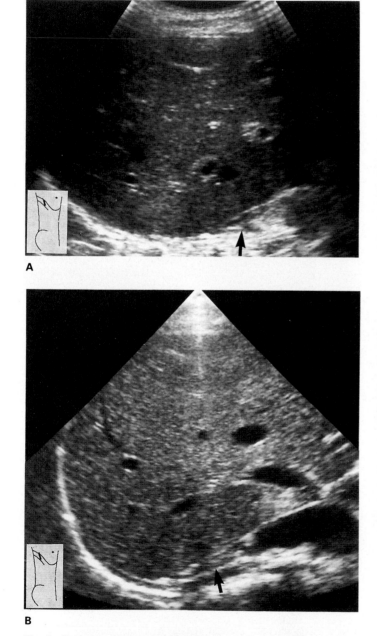

A

B

Fig. 7 Structure of the adrenal gland. A and **B:** Views of the right adrenal gland (arrow) in two adults clearly showing the distinction between cortex and medulla.

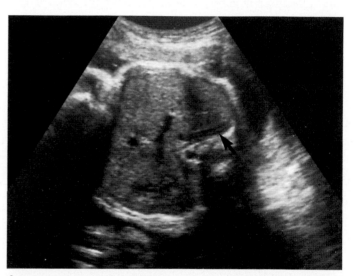

A

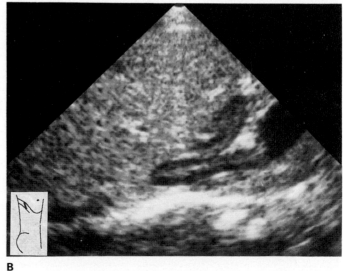

B

Fig. 8 Fetal and neonatal adrenal. A: Transverse scan through the fetal abdomen at 32 weeks of gestation. The right adrenal gland is well-visualised (arrow) with clear distinction between cortex and medulla. **B:** Coronal view of the right adrenal gland in a neonate which shows the relatively large size of the gland at this age and the marked contrast between cortex which has a low reflectivity and the central medulla having a high reflectivity.

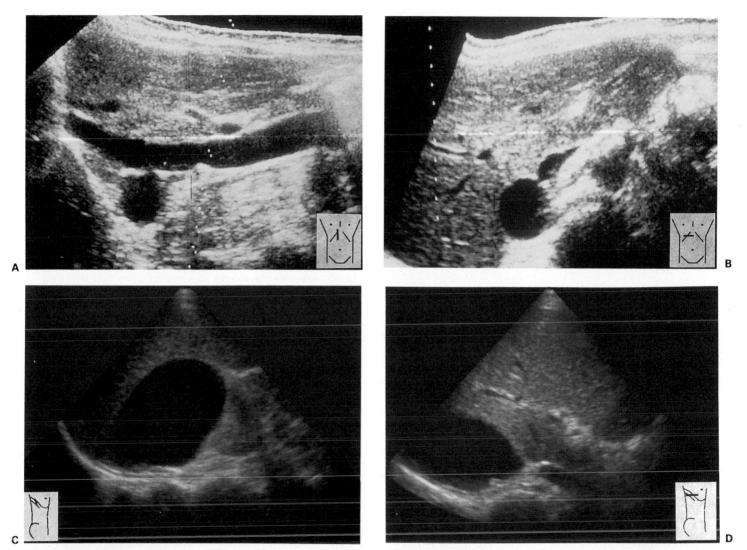

Fig. 9 Adrenal cysts. A: Longitudinal and **B:** transverse scans showing a 2.5 cm right adrenal cyst. **C** and **D:** Intercostal views of the right adrenal gland showing a larger adrenal cyst. Note the clear plane between the cyst and the upper pole of the kidney.

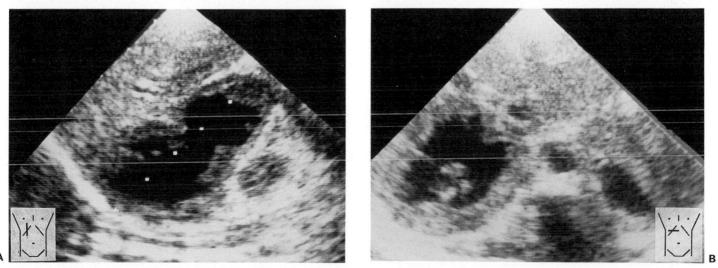

Fig. 10 Adrenal haemorrhage. A: Longitudinal and **B:** transverse scans in a neonate showing a large lobular right adrenal haemorrhage. This has a low reflectivity overall with a slightly irregular wall and a few centrally placed high level echoes.

spleen. The transducer is placed on the eighth or ninth intercostal space in the posterior axillary line, avoiding stomach or bowel gas, to give a coronal scan. The upper pole of the kidney should first be located through the spleen. A small angulation of the transducer towards the anterior aspect of the kidney will demonstrate the left adrenal gland in the perirenal space between spleen, kidney and left diaphragmatic crus. This is best recognised when both wings are shown, displaying the characteristic 'V' shape (Fig. 6). A transverse section is obtained by rotating the transducer through 90°. Because of the relative difficulty in demonstrating the left adrenal gland, additional views in right lateral decubitus and erect positions may be helpful. With high resolution real time scanning the right adrenal gland is demonstrated in 92% of patients and the left gland in 71%.[7]

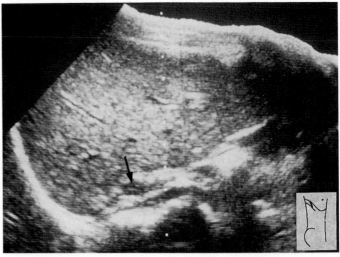

Fig. 12 Adenoma. An oblique scan showing a tiny echo-poor mass arising within one limb of the right adrenal gland. This measures < 1 cm in diameter. It proved to be a small Conn's tumour.

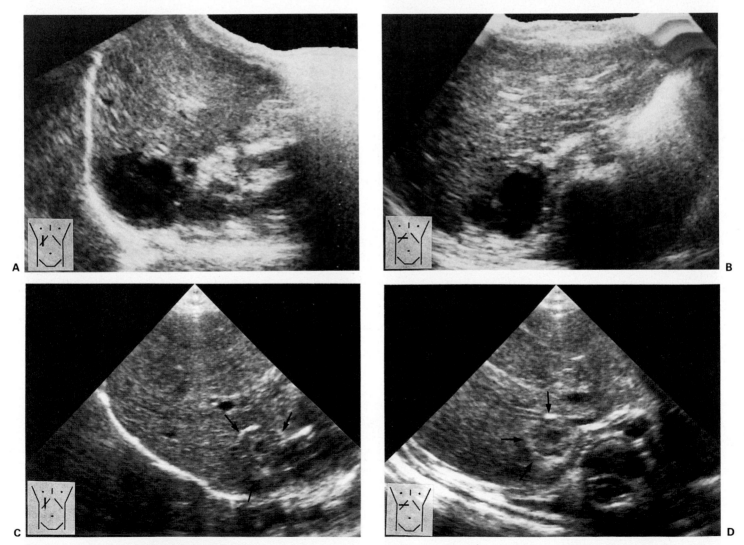

Fig. 11 Adrenal haemorrhage. A: Longitudinal and **B:** transverse scans showing a typical right adrenal haemorrhage in a 6-week-old. **C** and **D:** Longitudinal and transverse scans taken 2 months later showing almost complete resolution of the haemorrhage which is now replaced by an area of higher reflectivity with the suggestion of a peripheral calcific rim (arrows).

The adrenal cortex appears echo-poor on ultrasound. The medulla is regularly seen as a thin reflective structure in the centre of the cortex in up to 13% of adults (Fig. 7).[7] This is a particularly prominent feature in the neonatal or fetal adrenal gland (Fig. 8). At birth the neonatal adrenal cortex is relatively thick and is composed of two layers: the thick fetal zone occupying 80% of the gland and the thin peripheral zone that becomes the adult cortex.[8] The fetal cortex synthesises most of the precursors for maternal oestrogens and is one of the main consumers of placental progesterone. It involutes after birth. The neonatal adrenal gland is readily visualised for several reasons:

a) the infant gland is proportionally larger. At birth it is a third of the size of the kidney as compared to only a thirteenth the size of the kidney in the adult;

b) the small amount of perirenal fat in neonates allows for better resolution;

c) the small size of the subject means that higher frequency transducers are routinely used, further optimising overall resolution.[8]

The contours of the normal adrenal glands are straight or concave and convexity should be regarded with suspicion. It is important to examine the whole of each gland

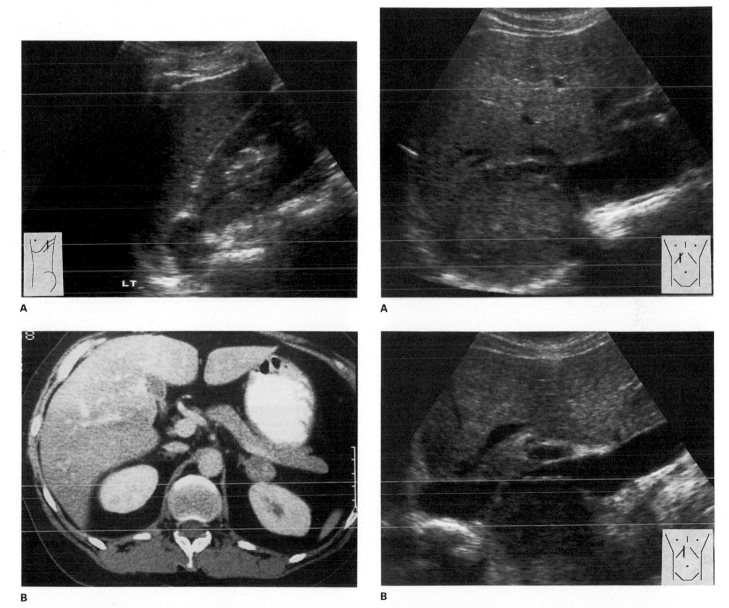

A

B

Fig. 13 Adrenal mass. A: Coronal ultrasound view of the left adrenal gland and kidney. There is a very well-defined 2 cm mass in the left adrenal gland. Clear separation from the left kidney is shown. **B:** Corresponding CT scan.

A

B

Fig. 14 Adrenal tumour. A: Longitudinal and **B:** oblique views showing a 5 cm mass in the right adrenal gland causing marked anterior bowing of the posterior wall of the inferior vena cava. The inferior vena cava has been compressed by the tumour.

since small masses may affect only part of the gland leaving the remainder with a normal appearance.

Pathology

Adrenal cystic lesions

The most common adrenal cyst is an endothelial cyst, accounting for nearly half of all reported cases.[9] They are mostly lymphangiomatous in origin but some are angiomatous. Some adrenal cysts are sequelae of haemorrhage or epithelial glandular cysts. Occasionally, the cyst wall may calcify. Adrenal cysts are rarely symptomatic, mostly being encountered as incidental findings (Fig. 9) which do not require active intervention.[10]

Adrenal haemorrhage The large adrenal gland of the neonate undergoes a marked reduction in size following birth. The vessels in the primitive adrenal cortex become distended and are prone to haemorrhage. The exact cause of haemorrhage in neonates is unknown but stress and birth trauma, anoxia and systemic disease are all implicated. Infants usually present within 2 to 7 days of birth (Fig. 10). Haemorrhage is more commonly seen on the right side although up to 10% are bilateral.[11-13]

In adults the hypertrophic adrenal gland due to ACTH therapy or severe stress may also be more prone to haemorrhage. Sepsis secondary to meningococcal infection and anticoagulant therapy may also predispose to haemorrhage. The resulting adrenal haematoma is usually echo-free, but may be more reflective due to fibrin strand formation as resolution occurs (Fig. 11). The haematoma may resolve, calcify or remain as a residual adrenal cyst.[11]

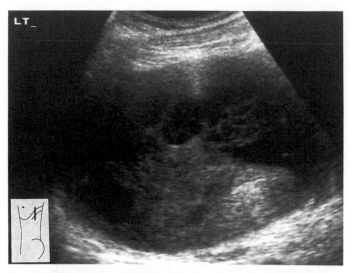

Fig. 16 Adrenal metastasis. Coronal view of a large left adrenal metastasis. The tumour mass is heterogeneous. This is a typical pattern often seen as tumours increase in size.

Adrenal tumours

It is most common for adrenal tumours to enlarge the adrenal gland focally, although diffuse enlargement may occur. A focal mass is usually oval or round and may vary in size from 0.5 to 20 cm. A small adrenal mass is easier to delineate than the normal adrenal gland because its diameter usually exceeds that of the adrenal. Its overall reflectivity is low, in contrast to the high reflectivity of the surrounding fat (Fig. 12). Ultrasound has been reported to have an

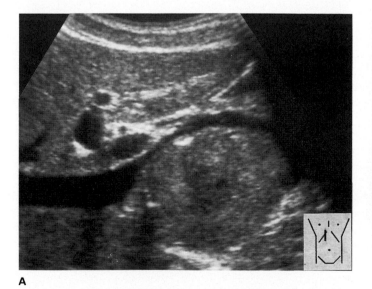

A

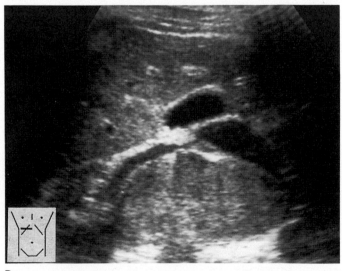

B

Fig. 15 Adrenal tumour. A: Longitudinal and **B:** transverse scans showing a relatively homogeneous right adrenal tumour which is causing anterior displacement and bowing of the inferior vena cava. The tumour has extended downwards anterior to the kidney producing very little renal displacement. In the transverse section the bowing of the renal vessels is well shown.

overall accuracy of 95% in the evaluation of adrenal masses.[14] Even when a normal adrenal gland is not visualised, if the adrenal area is thoroughly scanned and no mass can be identified, tumour can be fairly confidently excluded.[15] To differentiate an adrenal from a renal mass a separating interface must be demonstrated (Fig. 13). A right adrenal tumour typically compresses or displaces the inferior vena cava forwards (Fig. 14).[16] A large adrenal tumour usually displaces the upper pole of the kidney laterally or the whole kidney inferiorly. Occasionally, the tumour may extend downwards anterior to the kidney without much displacement (Fig. 15). Larger masses may indent liver or kidney. While smaller tumours are usually fairly homogeneous, focal areas of necrosis or haemorrhage are more likely to occur in larger masses. This produces heterogeneity (Fig. 16).[16]

Cortical adenoma These tumours are common incidental findings being reported in up to 2% of adult autopsies. Whilst most are non-steroid producing, they may be part of an endocrine neoplastic syndrome (MEN type 2). They are usually small, 1 to 2 cm in diameter (Fig. 17).[17]

Carcinoma Adrenal carcinomas in children usually produce steroids and are associated with one of the hyperadrenal syndromes (see Vol. 2, Ch. 55). In adults adrenal carcinomas are only rarely endocrinologically active

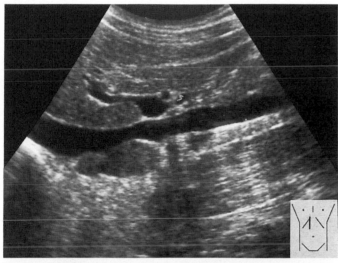

A

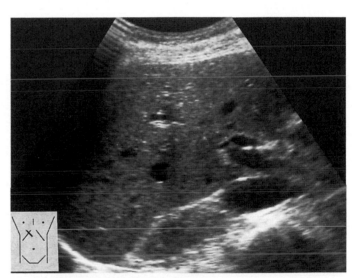

Fig. 18 **Adrenal carcinoma**. Oblique scan showing a moderate sized right adrenal carcinoma. This has a relatively uniform reflectivity and its typical position tucked posterior to the IVC is clearly shown.

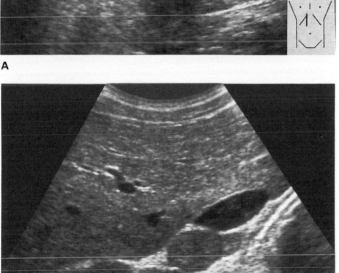

B

Fig. 17 **Adrenal adenoma**. A: Longitudinal and B: transverse scans showing two small rounded masses in the right adrenal gland. The upper and more medial mass measures under 1 cm in diameter and the inferior and more laterally placed mass about 2 cm in diameter. Note the characteristic position behind the inferior vena cava which is slightly bowed by the small cortical adenoma.

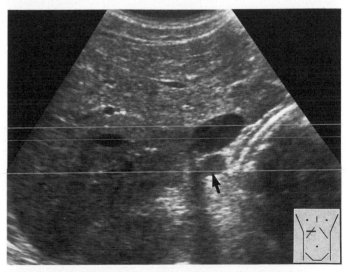

Fig. 19 **Phaeochromocytoma**. Transverse scan showing a tiny phaeochromocytoma only 1 cm in diameter lying posterior to the IVC and on the diaphragmatic crus.

and are therefore large and commonly have invaded the adrenal vein and IVC by the time they present (Fig. 18). Nodal and blood-borne metastases are common.[17]

Myelolipoma Adrenal myelolipoma is a rare cortical tumour composed of varying proportion of fat and bone marrow elements.[18] There is no malignant potential and the lesions are endocrinologically non-functioning. On ultrasound these rare tumours are characteristically highly reflective which may confirm the fatty nature of the lesion.[19]

Phaeochromocytoma Phaeochromocytomas are uncommon tumours occurring in up to 1% of patients with hypertension. The majority arise within the chromaffin cells of the adrenal medulla but up to 10% arise in the autonomic nervous tissue, particularly in the organs of Zuckerkandl.[20,21] The majority of phaeochromocytomas are benign but 5% to 10% are malignant and up to 5% are multiple. Multiple lesions are frequently associated with various hereditary syndromes, e.g. Sipple's syndrome and von Hippel-Lindau syndrome. The clinical presentation is typically with paroxysmal hypertension. The diagnosis may be confirmed by biochemical assay for catecholamines in the urine.[21] Phaeochromocytomas may present when small (Fig. 19) (< 2 cm in diameter) or when larger. Typically, when small they are well-defined round or oval masses with a uniform reflectivity. Larger

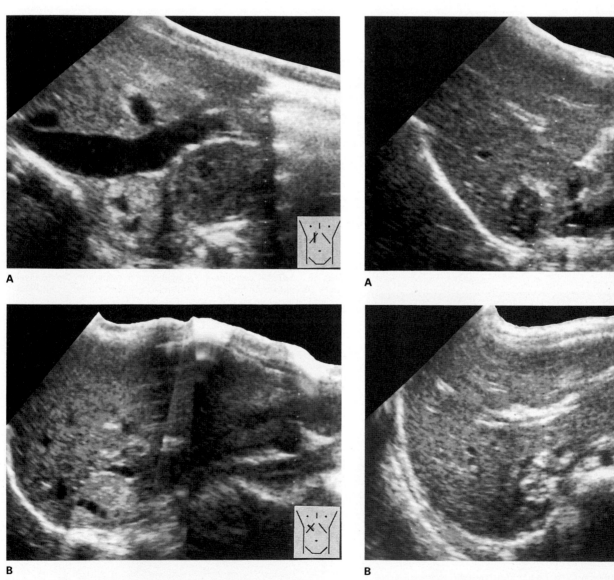

A

B

Fig. 20 Phaeochromocytoma. A: Longitudinal and **B:** oblique scans showing a 3 cm phaeochromocytoma of the right adrenal gland. Note the slightly high reflectivity of the main tumour mass with small central echo-poor necrotic areas. This is a typical pattern of phaeochromocytomas.

Fig. 21 Neuroblastoma. A: Longitudinal and **B:** transverse scans of a right neuroblastoma. This shows the typical appearances of marked heterogeneity and areas of high reflectivity within and on the periphery of the tumour, which lies above the right kidney as shown on the longitudinal scan.

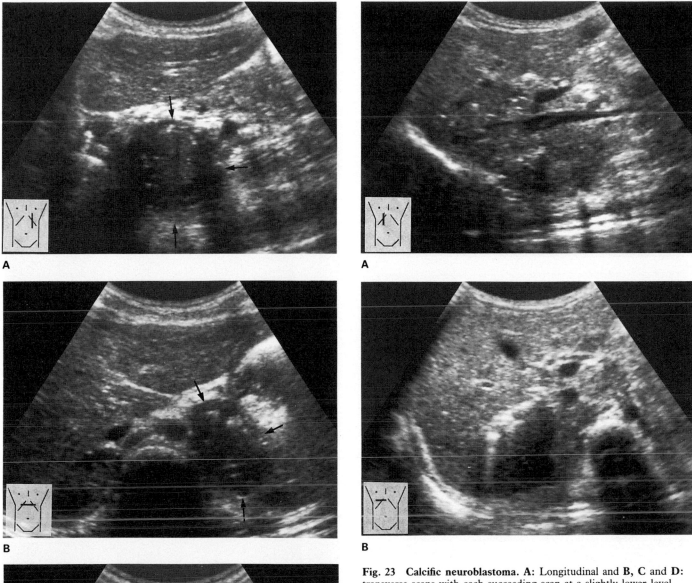

Fig. 23 Calcific neuroblastoma. A: Longitudinal and **B, C** and **D:** transverse scans with each succeeding scan at a slightly lower level. There is a large right neuroblastoma which contains calcification with distal acoustic shadowing. The tumour has infiltrated diffusely across the midline, around the coeliac axis and up towards the hilum of the liver. The tumour margins are extremely poorly defined. This pattern of extension of neuroblastoma around the IVC and aorta is typical and a more precise delineation may often be made with CT.

Fig. 22 Neuroblastoma. A: Longitudinal and **B** and **C:** transverse scans through the upper abdomen of a 3-year-old showing a left neuroblastoma (arrows). Note the marked heterogeneity of the tumour with areas of very high reflectivity within the tumour mass.

tumours frequently undergo necrosis or haemorrhage with loss of the homogeneity (Fig. 20).

Neuroblastoma   The neuroblastoma is one of the most common tumours of childhood with 80% occurring in children of less than 5 years of age and a third under 2 years of age. Under 1 year of age the tumour may spontaneously regress or differentiate into a ganglioneuroma.[21] The great majority of neuroblastomas arise in the adrenal medullary tissue, but the posterior mediastinum is the second most

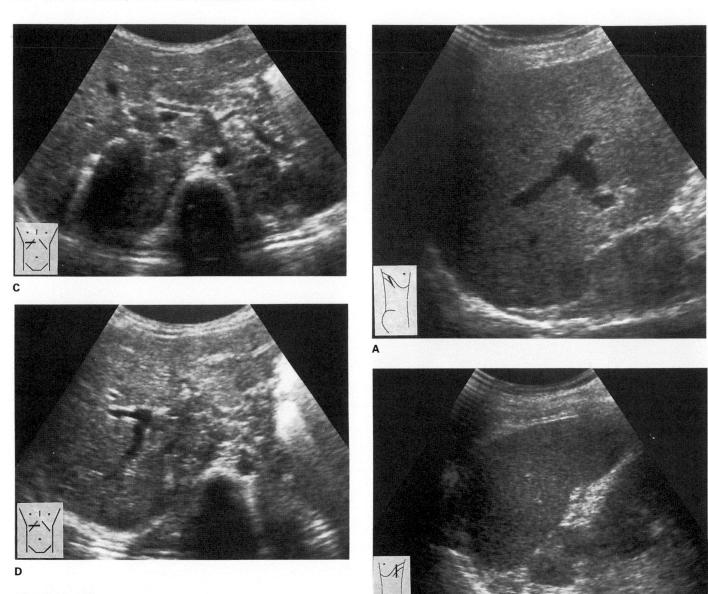

C

D

Fig. 23 (cont'd)

Fig. 24 Adrenal metastases. A: Coronal scan through the right and **B**: left adrenal glands. These sections are taken from a patient with a known bronchial carcinoma and the appearances are typical of metastases. No focal lesions were demonstrated in either liver or spleen.

common site. The clinical presentation of neuroblastoma is related to its rapid growth and its secretions. There may be generalised debility with weight loss and fever. An abdominal mass may be palpable. Most tumours produce catecholamines. Up to three quarters of patients have metastases at the time of presentation.[21] Neuroblastoma is often well-demonstrated by ultrasound and must be distinguished from the other common childhood abdominal tumour, the Wilms' tumour (see Vol. 2, Ch. 50). Neuro-

blastomas are typically heterogeneous with areas of high reflectivity which may represent calcification and areas of lower reflectivity (Figs 21 and 22). The margins of the tumour are ill-defined. Neuroblastoma will often cross the midline (Fig. 23).[22] It is important to delineate the relationship of the mass to the IVC and aorta before surgery is planned. Ultrasound is particularly valuable in the follow up of those children who undergo chemotherapy to monitor the response of the tumour.

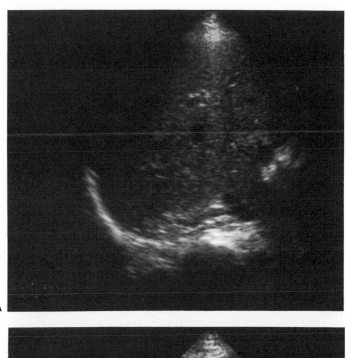

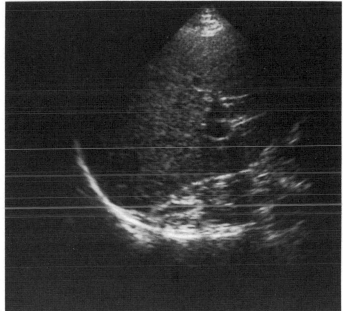

Fig. 25 **Adrenal hyperplasia. A** and **B:** Minor enlargement of the right adrenal gland affecting the echo-poor peripheral cortex resulting in exaggeration of the trilaminar appearance.

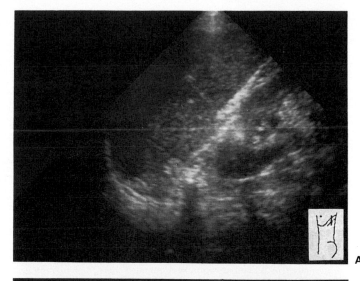

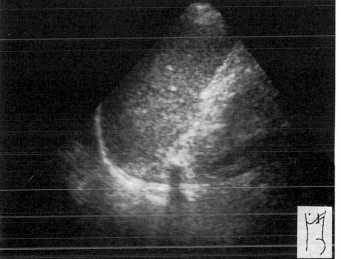

Fig. 26 **Adrenal calcification. A** and **B:** Coronal views of the left kidney showing a small area of calcification in the region of the left adrenal gland beyond which there is clear acoustic shadowing. A small amount of calcification was visible on the plain abdominal X-ray in this patient who was asymptomatic.

Adrenal metastases The adrenal glands are the fourth most common site in the body for metastases after the lungs, liver and bones. Common primaries to metastasise to the adrenals include bronchial and breast carcinomas. The adrenals are also commonly involved with non-Hodgkin's lymphoma. Metastases are usually rounded or oval and poorly reflective.[23-25] Visualisation of both adrenal areas should be part of the routine assessment of any patient with primary malignancy (Fig. 24). Imaging alone will

not differentiate between a metastasis and a benign adenoma – serial scans may be needed.

Diffuse adrenal enlargement

Diffuse adrenal enlargement may occur in diffuse bilateral hyperplasia. In most patients the enlargement will be slight and this is extremely difficult to detect with confidence using ultrasound. When the glands are significantly enlarged demonstration of the medulla allows differentiation of hyperplasia from a diffuse infiltrative process such as lymphoma, when the medulla will not be identified (Fig. 25).[26,27]

Adrenal calcification

Adrenal calcification is not uncommonly noted as an inci-

dental finding on plain abdominal X-rays or on standard examination of the upper abdomen (Fig. 26). It is a recognised sequel of adrenal haemorrhage and, perhaps more commonly in the past, of adrenal tuberculous infection. A less commonly seen pattern of curvilinear calcification may be seen in the wall of an adrenal cyst.

REFERENCES

1 Sample W F. A new technique for the evaluation of the adrenal gland with grey scale ultrasonography. Radiology 1977; 124: 463

2 Yeh H C H. Sonography of the adrenal glands: normal glands and small masses. AJR 1980; 135: 1167

3 Hattery R R, Sheedy P F 2nd, Stevens D H. Computed tomography of the adrenal glands. Semin Roentgenol 1980; 16: 4

4 El-Sherief M A, Hemmingson A. Computed tomography of the normal adrenal gland. Acta Radiol 1982; 23: 433

5 Wilms G, Baert A L, Marchal G. Computed tomography of the normal adrenal glands: correlative study with autopsy specimens. J Comput Assist Tomogr 1979; 3: 467

6 Abrahams H L, Siegelman S S, Adams D F. Computed tomography verses ultrasound of the adrenal glands: a prospective study. Radiology 1982; 143: 121

7 Marchal G, Gelin J, Verbeken E, Baert A, Lauwerijns J. High resolution real time sonography of the adrenal glands: a routine examination? J Ultrasound Med 1986; 5: 65–68

8 Oppenheimer D A, Carroll B A, Yousem S. Sonography of the normal neonatal adrenal glands. Radiology 1983; 146: 157

9 Foster D G. Adrenal cysts: review of literature and report of case. Arch Surg 1986; 92: 131–143

10 Scheible W, Coel M, Siemers P T, Siegel H. Percutaneous aspiration of adrenal cysts. AJR 1977; 128: 1013

11 Pery M, Kaftori J K, Bar-Maor J A. Sonography for diagnosis and follow up of adrenal haemorrhage. JCU 1981; 9: 397

12 Mittelstaedt C A, Volberg F M, Merten D F, Brill P W. The sonographic diagnosis of neonatal haemorrhage. Radiology 1979; 131: 453

13 Mineau D E, Koehler P R. Ultrasound diagnosis of neonatal adrenal haemorrhage. AJR 1979; 132: 443

14 Sample W F. Adrenal ultrasonography. Radiology 1978: 127: 461

15 Yeh H C. Ultrasonography of normal adrenal gland and small adrenal masses. AJR 135: 1980; 1167–1177

16 Yeh H C, Mitty H A, Rose J, et al. Ultrasonography of adrenal masses: unusual manifestations. Radiology 1978; 127: 475

17 Robbins S L, Cotran R S. The endocrine system – adrenal cortex. In: Pathologic basis of disease. Philadelphia: W B Saunders. 1979: p 1387

18 Behan M, Martin E C, Meucke E C, Kazam E. Myelolipoma of the adrenal: two cases with ultrasound and CT findings. AJR 1977; 129: 993

19 Vick C W, Zeman R K, Mannes E, et al. Adrenal myelolipoma: CT and ultrasound findings. Urol Radiol 1984; 6: 7

20 Bowerman R A, Silver T M, Jaffee M H. Sonography of adrenal phaeochromocytoma. AJR 1981; 137: 1227

21 Robbins S L, Cotran R S. The endocrine system – adrenal medulla. In: Pathologic basis of disease. Philadelphia: W B Saunders. 1979: p 1402

22 White S J, Stuck K J, Blane C E, Silver T M. Sonography of neuroblastoma. AJR 1983; 141: 465

23 Cunningham J J. Ultrasonic findings in 'primary ' lymphoma of the adrenal area. J Ultrasound Med 1983; 2: 467

24 Antoniou A, Spetseropoulos J, Vlahos L, Pontifex G. The sonographic appearance of adrenal involvement in non-Hodgkins lymphoma. J Ultrasound Med 1983; 2: 235

25 Forsythe J R, Gosink B B, Leopold G R. Ultrasound in the evaluation of adrenal metastases. JCU 1977; 5: 31

26 Paling M R, Williamson B R J. Adrenal involvement in non-Hodgkins lymphoma. AJR 1983; 141: 303–305

27 Yeh H C. Ultrasonography of the adrenals. Semin Roentgenol 1988; 23: 250–258

24

The lymph nodes

The normal para-aortic nodes
Lymphadenopathy
Differential diagnosis

Keith C. Dewbury

The normal para-aortic nodes

Lymphatic glands surround the major vessels such as the abdominal aorta and its branches, the inferior vena cava and the splanchnic system. Para-aortic nodes may lie directly anterior to the spine while some of the splanchnic nodes lie in the gut mesentery and are difficult to image with ultrasound. The special drainage of the gonads should be borne in mind: as a consequence of their descent from the mid-abdomen, the first nodes from the testis lie at renal level. For the ovaries the arrangement is the same except that they also drain to the uterus along the uterine tubes.

Lymphadenopathy

Since normal lymph nodes are rarely identified on ultrasound, to search for lymphadenopathy it is necessary to identify the associated vessels and trace their abdominal course looking for paravascular masses (Fig. 1).[1] Enlarged nodes may be found at the porta hepatis, renal hila, splenic hilum and in the mesentery as well as around the coeliac axis and along the pancreas.

Enlarged nodes typically have low and uniform reflectivity on ultrasound; indeed they may be almost anechoic, especially when very large. This is presumably because of their relatively homogeneous structure so that there are few interfaces to produce echoes. When there is calcification or, rarely, lipid deposition (e.g. Whipple's,[2]) they may have the same reflectivity as fat or even be more strongly reflective (Fig. 2). Abnormal nodes as small as 1.5 to 2 cm may be visualised with ultrasound, particularly if they distort the normal anatomy, for example, in the retrocrural or retrocaval spaces (Fig. 3). Apart from the intense echoes

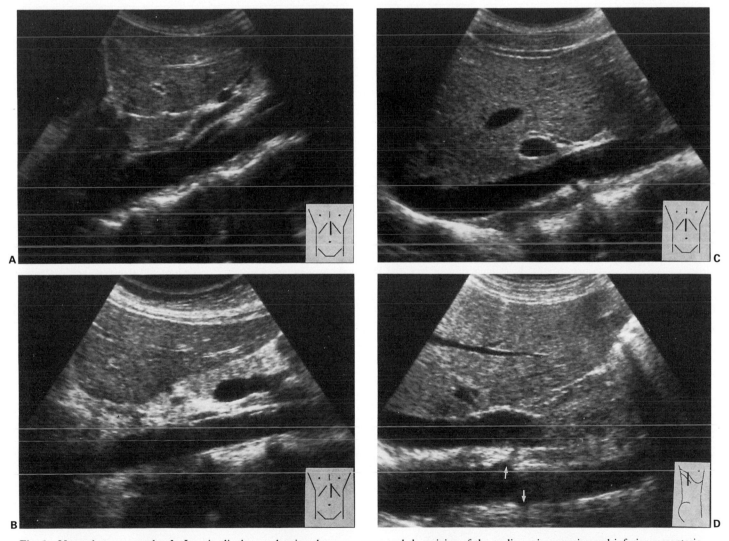

Fig. 1 Normal great vessels. A: Longitudinal scan showing the upper aorta and the origins of the coeliac axis, superior and inferior mesenteric arteries. Note the anomalous hepatic artery. **B:** Longitudinal scan of the abdominal aorta. **C:** Longitudinal scan through the IVC. Note the normal common bile duct and the prominent right diaphragmatic crus lying behind the IVC. With clear crural visualisation, retrocrural nodes may be easily detected. **D:** A coronal section taken from the right side showing a portion of the IVC proximal to the aorta. Note the origin of the renal arteries (arrows).

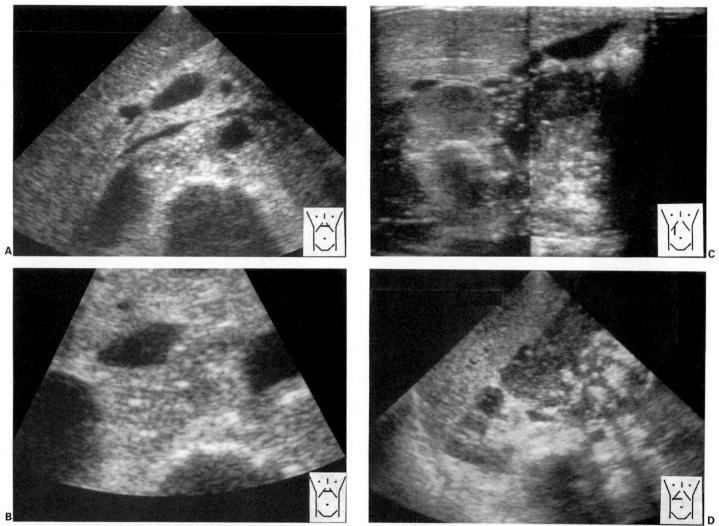

Fig. 2 Calcific nodes. A: Reflective masses surround the aorta and IVC; these were calcific nodes in a patient with carcinoma of the prostate following successful endocrine therapy. **B:** Magnification of A. **C** and **D:** Calcific mass in neuroblastoma (longitudinal and transverse sections); these are either retroperitoneal nodes or infiltration from the primary tumour – the distinction is impossible and not clinically important.

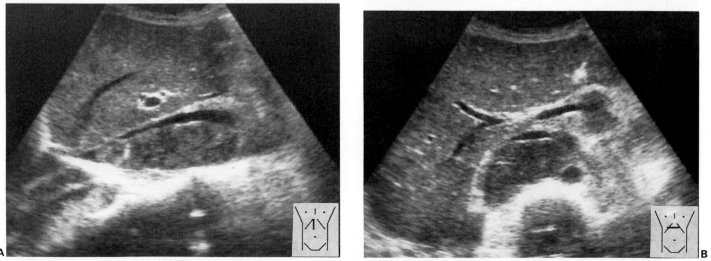

Fig. 3 Enlarged retrocaval nodes. A: A longitudinal scan showing a retrocrural and retrocaval nodal mass. There is anterior bowing of the inferior vena cava. **B:** A transverse scan showing the same nodal mass. There is some extension anteriorly across the front of the aorta.

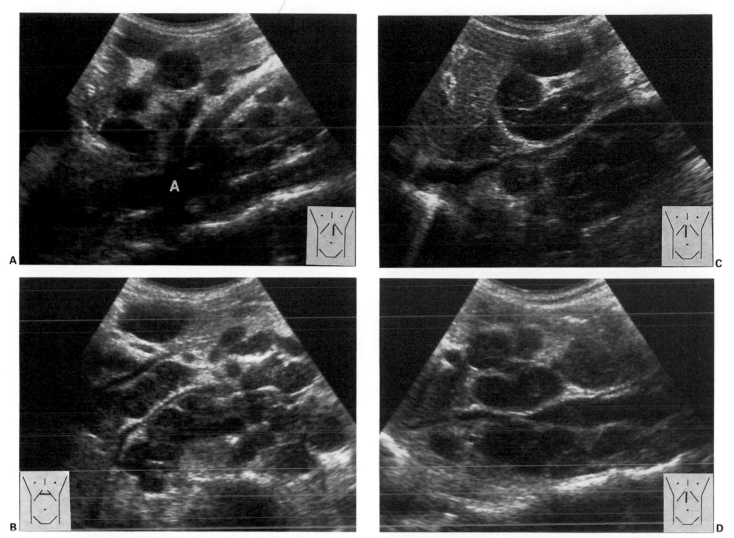

Fig. 4   Non-Hodgkin's lymphoma. A: A longitudinal section through the abdominal aorta. Note the origins of the coeliac axis and superior mesenteric artery which is elevated by enlarged nodes posterior to it. There is a sheet of nodes lying behind the aorta (A) and large nodal masses are seen above the coeliac axis. **B:** A transverse section taken at about the level of the coeliac axis showing lobular nodal enlargement extending around the para-aortic area and laterally towards the flanks. There is anterior extension up towards the liver. **C:** A longitudinal scan through the IVC showing nodes in the region of the porta hepatis. There is also a large mass of nodes behind the inferior vena cava causing elevation and compression. **D:** A similar longitudinal section showing greater detail of the retrocaval nodal mass.

due to calcification and lipids, there is no correlation between the ultrasound appearances of the lymph nodes and the histology. Lymphadenopathy in lymphoma, metastatic disease or in inflammatory reactions, such as retroperitoneal fibrosis, are all indistinguishable from each other. The most florid nodal involvement is characteristically seen in non-Hodgkin's lymphoma (Fig. 4).[3]

Lymphomatous involvement of para-aortic nodes occurs in approximately 25% of patients with Hodgkin's disease and in 40% with non-Hodgkin's lymphoma.[4] Effective therapeutic management in these patients requires accurate histological classification and reliable definition of the anatomical regions involved in the disease process.[4–6]

Classically lymphadenopathy was used, but CT scanning has now become the gold standard. Ultrasound, however, has been shown to detect retroperitoneal nodal lymphoma with an 80% to 90% accuracy.[7] It is also capable of demonstrating lymphadenopathy in the coeliac, perisplenic, mesenteric and perihepatic areas with an accuracy similar to that of CT, although the reliability is not as good due to intervening gas. The ease and cost effectiveness of ultrasound suggest a continuing role in the assessment of nodal disease and its follow up in selected cases.

A variety of patterns of nodal enlargement may be seen in the retroperitoneum:

a) discrete enlargement of individually identifiable nodes

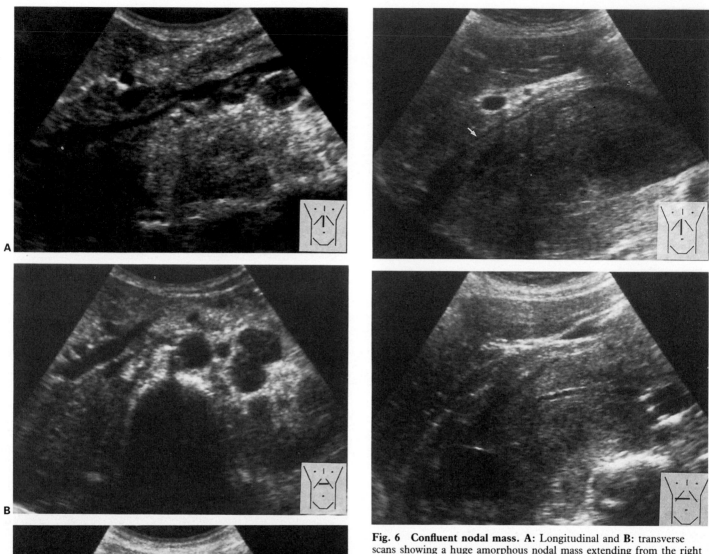

Fig. 5   Discrete nodal enlargement. A: Longitudinal, **B** and **C:** transverse scans. These sections all show discrete nodal enlargement of a relatively small number of individual nodes that can be separately identified. The pattern in each case is similar with a uniform low reflectivity.

Fig. 6   Confluent nodal mass. A: Longitudinal and **B:** transverse scans showing a huge amorphous nodal mass extending from the right kidney to cross the midline and elevate and envelop the inferior vena cava (arrow). No single discrete node can be identified, in contrast to Figure 5.

occurs when a small number of individual nodes is enlarged, retaining the overall morphology (Fig. 5);

b) a homogeneous confluent mass extending anteriorly from the prevertebral space, enveloping and often elevating the great vessels (Fig. 6). The normal outline of the aorta may be lost; this is sometimes misleadingly called the 'silhouette sign' (Fig. 7);

c) compression or displacement of adjacent organs by a nodal mass. Extensive pelvic nodal enlargement characteristically distorts and elevates the bladder (Fig. 8), or other contiguous structures especially those that are less well supported such as the ureters and veins (both portal and systemic);

d) very rarely vascular invasion from malignant lymphadenopathy may accur (Fig. 9).

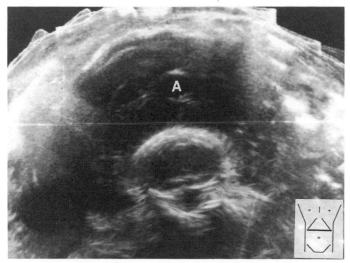

Fig. 7 Lost aortic outline. A compounded transverse section through the mid-abdomen showing partial loss of the outline of the normal aorta (A) and IVC which are elevated and enveloped by a lobular echo-poor nodal mass. This is misleadingly known as the 'silhouette sign'.

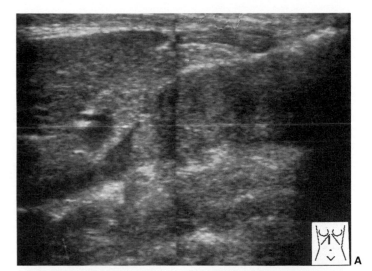

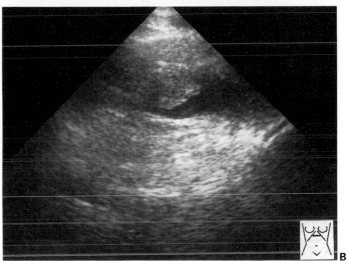

Fig. 9 Nodal invasion of the IVC. A: Longitudinal and **B:** transverse sections. Solid tissue in the upper cava is due to tumour extension from retroperitoneal lymphadenopathy in this patient with carcinoma of the ovary. This is an uncommon occurrence.

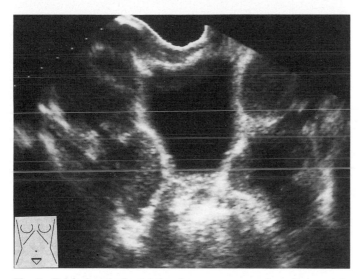

Fig. 8 Pelvic lymphadenopathy. A transverse scan through the pelvis showing the filled bladder which is elevated and distorted by large echo-poor lobular nodal enlargement on the pelvic side walls.

Associated nodal enlargement at other sites in the abdomen is commonly seen in lymphoma. Mesenteric lymphomatous involvement characteristically produces a lobulated confluent anechoic mass surrounding a central more reflective region. This appearance is the result of the nodal mass infiltrating the mesenteric layers and encasing the mesenteric vessels to produce the so-called 'sandwich sign' (Fig. 10).[8] Mesenteric nodal involvement is rare in Hodgkin's disease but occurs commonly in non-Hodgkin's lymphoma (Fig. 11). Generally, mesenteric lymphadenopathy is associated with retroperitoneal or para-aortic adenopathy which should be evaluated systematically.

Peripancreatic, perihepatic and coeliac axis nodes, as well as nodes at the splenic and renal hilum, manifest a spectrum of appearances similar to retroperitoneal lymphadenopathy. Portal nodes may cause biliary obstruction and are characteristic of hepatic lymphomatous involvement (Fig. 12). Nodes that are demonstrated by ultrasound may be accessible to percutaneous biopsy. The enlarged node in the porta (the 'cholecystitis node') is typically observed in patients with viral hepatitis; though not clinically significant, its demonstration is helpful in differential diagnosis.

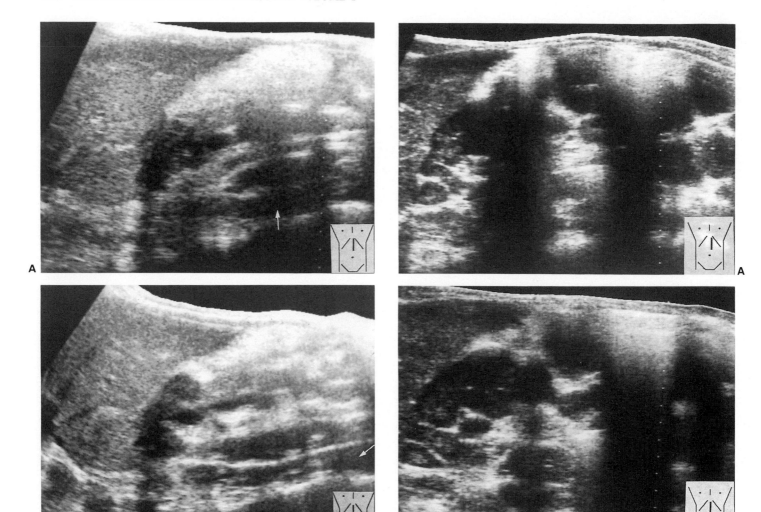

Fig. 10 Mesenteric lymphadenopathy. A and **B:** Longitudinal scans showing confluent echo-poor nodal masses extending into the mesentery. Both the mesenteric artery and vein can be identified producing a relatively reflective central core which is sometimes described as the 'sandwich sign'. Prespinal nodes (arrow) are also identified.

Fig. 11 Mesenteric lymphadenopathy. A and **B:** Longitudinal scans showing large discrete nodal enlargement involving the mesentery in a patient with non-Hodgkin's lymphoma.

Differential diagnosis

Generally the appearances of lymphadenopathy are distinctive, an isolated echo-poor nodule or the multilobulated appearance of multiple enlarged nodes being diagnostic. However, occasionally masses in the same spaces produce confusing appearances. For example small neurofibromata may be identical (Fig. 13). Retroperitoneal fibrosis also produces an echo-poor mass related to the aorta; the differentiation from nodal enlargement may be impossible but the lack of lobulation and the typical thickening of retroperitoneal fibrosis below the sacral promontory are suggestive (Figs 14 and 15). An abdominal aortic aneurysm may also be confusing, the echo-poor thrombus easily being mistaken for para-aortic lymphadenopathy.

The internal echo texture of the solid region may be distinctive if the whorled pattern of the thrombus in an aneurysm can be demonstrated, but otherwise the pattern in a transverse section showing the conformity of the 'mass' to the circular shape of the aorta by comparison with the lateral extension of lymphadenopathy can be helpful.

Masses in organs adjacent to the expected position of nodes can also be very confusing. An example is the way an adrenal mass, especially on the right, simulates high retrocaval lymphadenopathy. The differential diagnosis may be impossible unless the adrenal gland itself can be demonstrated. Similarly, lymphadenopathy in or close to the pancreas can be difficult to distinguish from a pancreatic mass. The uniform echo-poor texture of enlarged nodes can be helpful while demonstration of multiple masses is very suggestive of lymphadenopathy,

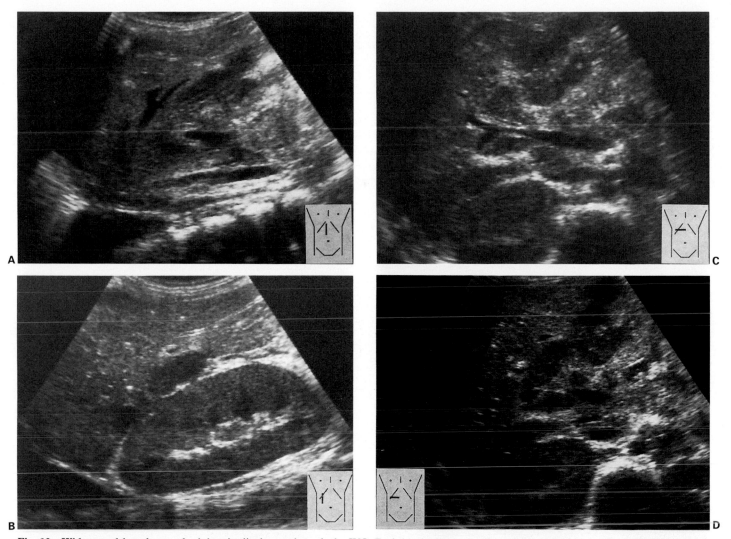

Fig. 12 Widespread lymphoma. A: A longitudinal scan through the IVC. **B:** A longitudinal scan through the right kidney. **C:** A transverse scan through the right branch of the portal vein. **D:** A similar slightly lower transverse section. Widespread abnormalities are demonstrated on these scans with diffuse lymphomatous involvement of the kidney, deposits in the liver and more discrete nodal enlargement particularly around the porta hepatis and in the para-aortic region. A right pleural effusion is also demonstrated in A and B images.

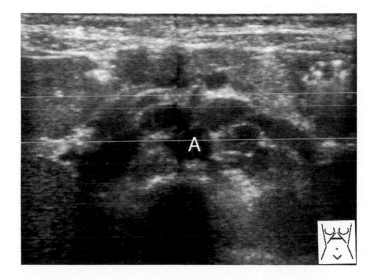

since multicentric pancreatic masses are rare. A splenunculus (accessory spleen) can be very confusing; usually they are solitary and have exactly the same reflectivity and texture as the spleen itself but lymphadenopathy is difficult to exclude (Fig. 16).

Nodes often compress adjacent ducts such as the bile and pancreatic ducts and the ureter. Where anatomically appropriate, features of these should be searched for both because of their diagnostic importance amd because they may be important in management.

Fig. 13 Neurofibroma. Echo-poor retroperitoneal masses with a pattern indistinguishable from lymphadenopathy were seen in this patient with Von Recklinghausen's disease. A – aorta.

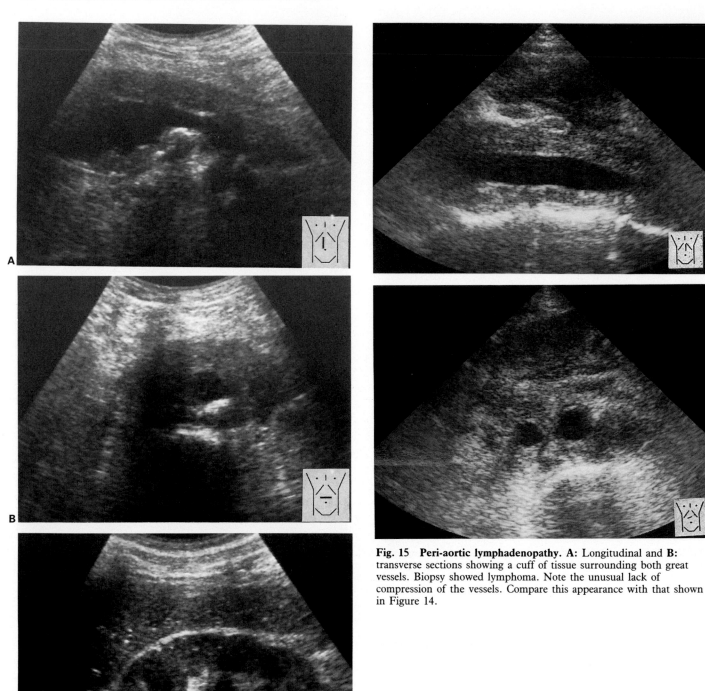

Fig. 15 Peri-aortic lymphadenopathy. A: Longitudinal and **B:** transverse sections showing a cuff of tissue surrounding both great vessels. Biopsy showed lymphoma. Note the unusual lack of compression of the vessels. Compare this appearance with that shown in Figure 14.

Fig. 14 Retroperitoneal fibrosis. A: Longitudinal and **B:** transverse scans. An echo-poor mass surrounding the lower abdominal aorta is typical of retroperitoneal fibrosis (the aorta was atheromatous). **C:** Associated hydronephrosis is shown.

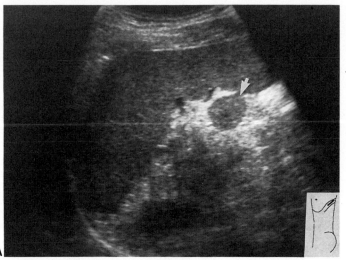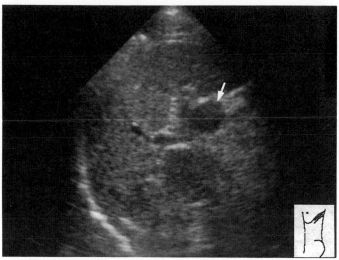

Fig. 16   Splenunculus. A: A rounded mass (arrow) near the hilum with an echo pattern identical to the spleen is typical of a splenunculus. **B:** An echo-poor mass (arrow) in a similar position, but due to lymphadenopathy.

REFERENCES

1 Ritchie W G N. The sonographic demonstration of abdominal visceral lymph node enlargement. AJR 1982; 138: 517

2 Davis S J, Patel A. Distinctive echogenic lymphadenopathy in Whipples disease. Clin Radiol 1990; 42: 60–62

3 Kaude J V, Joyce P H. Evaluation of abdominal lymphoma by ultrasound. Gastrointest Radiol 1980; 5: 249

4 Carroll B A. Ultrasound in lymphoma. In: Raymond H W, Zwiebel W J, eds. Seminars in ultrasound, volume 3. New York: Grunne and Stratton. 1982: p 114

5 Carroll B A, Ta H N. The ultrasound appearance of extranodal abdominal lymphoma. Radiology 1980; 136: 419

6 Carroll B A. Lymphoma. In: Goldberg B B. ed. Clinics in diagnosic ultrasound: ultrasound in cancer. New York: Churchill Livingstone. 1981: p 52

7 Beyer D, Peter P E. Real time ultrasonography: an efficient screening method for abdominal and pelvic lymphadenopathy. Lymphology 1980; 13: 142–149

8 Mueller P R, Ferrucci J T Jr, Harbin W P, et al. Appearances of lymphomatous involvement of the mesentery by ultrasonography and body computed tomography: the 'sandwich sign'. Radiology 1980; 134: 467

25

The paediatric pancreas

Normal appearances and congenital abnormalities
Pancreatitis
Acute pancreatitis
Chronic pancreatitis
Pancreatic masses

Claire Dicks-Mireaux

Normal appearances and congenital abnormalities

The pancreas is more easily visualised in relatively thin children than in adult patients. Fasting is not usually required prior to scanning but, if overlying stomach gas obscures the pancreas, a drink of water and scanning with the child sitting upright may improve visualisation.

The body and tail of the normal pancreas are usually clearly seen and measurements may be taken. Compared to the adult, the pancreas in a child may appear poorly reflective and relatively bulky with a prominent tail. Standard measurements of the pancreas at different ages are available (Table 1).[1]

Table 1 Normal dimensions of the pancreas as a function of age[1]

Age	Maximum antero-posterior dimensions (cm)		
	Head	Body	Tail
< 1 month	1.0 – 1.4	0.6 – 0.8	1.0 – 1.4
1 month to 1 year	1.5 – 2.0	0.8 – 1.1	1.2 – 1.6
1 to 10 years	1.7 – 2.0	1.0 – 1.3	1.8 – 2.2
10 to 19 years	2.0 – 2.5	1.1 – 1.4	2.0 – 2.4

At any age the diagnosis of pancreatic enlargement is made if the width of the body of the pancreas is greater than 1.5 cm. The normal pancreatic duct may be identified as two highly reflective parallel lines in the central portion of the gland. It is usually too narrow for measurements of it to be practicable; a diameter greater than 1.5 mm is considered abnormal. The texture of the normal pancreas is homogeneous with a moderately coarse pattern and it is usually slightly less reflective than normal liver. However, the normal pancreas in children may be markedly echo-poor, particularly in neonates. Unless one is aware of this variation, an erroneous diagnosis of acute pancreatitis may be made.

An annular pancreas is a congenital abnormality which is usually associated with duodenal atresia or a web. Patients usually present in the neonatal period with high intestinal obstruction. However, in some patients the abnormality may not be discovered until later in life. With careful scanning and an awareness of the condition, this abnormality may be detected with ultrasound. The pancreatic head appears more round than normal and the proximal duodenum is seen to run through the head rather than around it.

The difficulty in visualising the normal pancreatic duct with ultrasound means that congenital abnormalities of the pancreatic ducts and pancreas divisum are not reliably detected with ultrasound.

Pancreatitis

Acute pancreatitis

Acute pancreatitis is rare in children and has a number of different aetiologies. In a significant number no cause is found.[2]

Non-specific, poorly localised abdominal pain is the usual presentation and an elevated serum amylase confirms the diagnosis. Ultrasound is usually the first examination and may be useful in confirming the diagnosis and sometimes demonstrating the underlying cause. Ultrasound examination may be difficult because of an associated ileus and abdominal pain. The development of the complications of acute pancreatitis can also be followed with serial ultrasound examinations. The features of acute pancreatitis include generalised or focal enlargement and reduced reflectivity of the pancreas (Fig. 1) – these changes may be difficult to assess because the normal child's pancreas may be echo-poor and seem bulky. A normal ultrasound examination does not exclude the diagnosis of acute pancreatitis. Dilatation of the pancreatic duct, when it can be demonstrated, is the most useful and specific feature of acute pancreatitis. Increased reflectivity of the pararenal space, due to lipolysis of the pararenal fat following release of pancreatic enzymes, is another sign of pancreatitis.[3] Ascites and pleural effusions are often present.

Trauma is the most common cause of acute pancreatitis in childhood and may be due to the classical bicycle handlebar injury, lap seat belts or non-accidental injury. Dilatation of the common bile duct and gallbladder due to

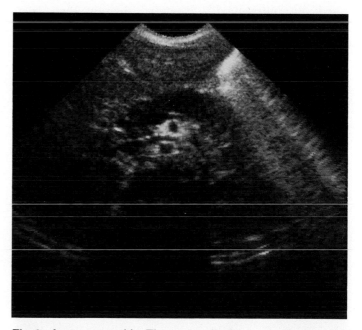

Fig. 1 Acute pancreatitis. The pancreas is of reduced reflectivity and there is enlargement of the body. This episode was secondary to biliary surgery.

oedema and swelling of the head of the pancreas may occur. Fracture of the pancreas with disruption of the duct is suggested by free fluid in the abdomen or collections in the lesser sac or Morrison's pouch. A fractured pancreas is more easily identified on CT scans than with ultrasound.[4] In general CT scanning is more reliable in the evaluation of severe abdominal trauma.

Pseudocyst formation is a common late complication of traumatic pancreatitis[5] and should always be looked for before the patient is discharged from hospital. The pseudocyst commonly arises anterior to the body and tail of the pancreas and extends into the lesser sac (Fig. 2). Initially, focal areas of necrosis with reduced reflectivity are seen within the pancreas; they mature over a few weeks to a well-defined, thick walled, echo-free cyst closely applied to the underlying pancreatic tissue. Haemorrhage into or infection of the cyst produces reflective debris. If the main pancreatic duct is disrupted, there is a high risk of pseudocyst formation which may reach a considerable size. Many pseudocysts resolve spontaneously with a period of conservative management. Percutaneous drainage is a useful method of treatment for those which have not resolved. An ERCP is required prior to percutaneous drainage to demonstrate the pancreatic duct system. If this has been disrupted, surgical resection is the treatment of choice.

In all cases of pancreatitis a careful examination of the gallbladder and biliary tree should be undertaken to exclude choledochal cysts (which may present with acute pancreatitis) and the rare case of gallstones in the paediatric age group (see Ch. 26). Anomalous pancreatic and biliary ducts also predispose to pancreatitis but cannot be diagnosed on ultrasound.[6] Pancreas divisum has been considered a normal variant with an incidence of 3% to 6% but there is an association with 'idiopathic pancreatitis'

– 4 out of 29 cases of childhood pancreatitis in one series. It is suggested that the larger bulk of functioning pancreatic tissue must discharge its secretions through the smaller orifice of the duct of Santorini, thus resulting in a partial obstruction and an increased incidence of acute pancreatitis.

Other congenital abnormalities which may result in pancreatitis include duodenal and gastric duplication cysts. In developing countries pancreatitis may be due to schistosoma or ascaris.

Recurrent episodes of acute pancreatitis occur in a number of conditions. Hereditary pancreatitis is inherited as an autosomal dominant trait. It demonstrates complete penetrance and variable expressivity. Familial hyperlipidaemia, cystic fibrosis and idiopathic pancreatitis may also be associated with repeated episodes of pancreatitis.

Chronic pancreatitis

The ultrasound appearances of chronic and recurrent pancreatitis are of shrinkage and increased reflectivity due to fibrosis or fatty replacement of the gland (Fig. 3). Pancreatic duct dilatation and calcification may be seen (Fig. 4). Associated abnormalities such as increased reflectivity of the liver with effacement of the portal vein walls and irregular rounding of the inferior liver border may identify cirrhosis in children with chronic pancreatitis and cystic fibrosis.[7] Pseudocyst formation, splenic and portal vein thrombosis and biliary obstruction may complicate chronic pancreatitis and can be demonstrated with ultrasound.

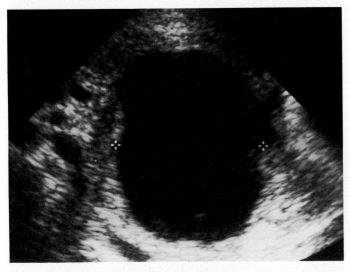

Fig. 2 Pancreatic pseudocyst. An echo-free space in the lesser sac is seen in this 13-year-old child who developed acute pancreatitis after falling off a bicycle.

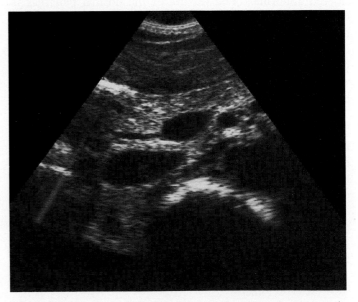

Fig. 3 Chronic pancreatitis. The gland shows increased reflectivity with several foci of high reflectivity in the head. It remains normal in size. The condition was secondary to a congenital anomaly of the duct; an abnormal duct can be seen in the head.

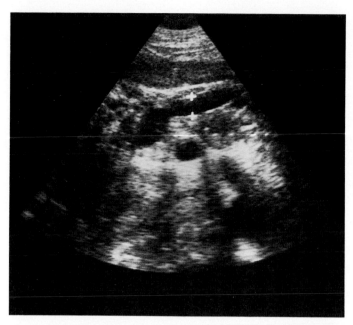

Fig. 4 Pancreatic duct dilatation secondary to chronic pancreatitis. There is marked atrophy of the gland and the duct (calliper markers) is dilated throughout its length.

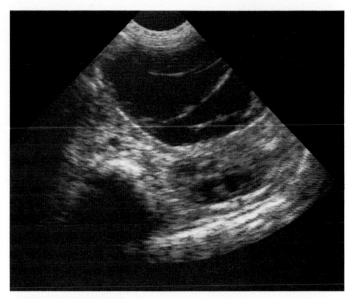

Fig. 5 Pancreaticoblastoma. There is a large septated cyst in the tail of the pancreas in this patient with Beckwith–Wiedemann syndrome.

Increased reflectivity of the pancreas is found in patients with haemosiderosis and Schwachmann's syndrome (pancreatic insufficiency, neutropenia and chest wall deformity). It is seen following the administration of steroids and has been described in sick neonates with severe diffuse oedema of the abdominal wall and abdominal contents including the pancreas.

Pancreatic masses

Pancreatic masses may be cystic or solid. Pseudocysts are the most common cystic masses and are usually associated with a history and clinical evidence of pancreatitis. The rare congenital cysts of the pancreas are usually solitary. They are echo-free and when large, they can be difficult to distinguish from omental or mesenteric cysts. Multiple cysts in the pancreas occur in 5% to 10% of patients with autosomal dominant polycystic kidney disease; they usually develop after adolescence. Multiple cysts may also be seen in patients with von Hippel–Lindau syndrome. Hydatid cysts also occur in and around the pancreas.

Large solitary cysts have rarely been described in patients with cystic fibrosis. A duplication cyst of the foregut may be enveloped in pancreatic tissue and may communicate with the ductal system. Bleeding into the cyst results in a poorly reflective echogenic pancreatic mass. Trauma or surgery to the cyst may result in acute pancreatitis. Pancreaticoblastoma, which is a very uncommon benign neoplasm of the pancreas associated with Beckwith–Wiedemann syndrome, may also present as a cyst in the pancreas (Fig. 5).

Reflective masses in the pancreas are uncommon in children. Fibrosing pancreatitis rarely appears as a solid parenchymal mass, as can a pancreatic abscess or a focal area of pancreatitis. Neoplastic lesions of the pancreas are also rare in children. Cases of adenocarcinoma, mucinous cystadenocarcinomas and islet cell carcinomas have been reported. Similarly, rare cases of hamartoma and lymphangioma of the pancreas have been described. Secondary involvement of the pancreas by other malignancies is more common. This may be seen in lymphoma (with both pancreatic deposits and associated lymphadenopathy) and in neuroblastoma (with displacement or direct infiltration) as well as in lymphoma associated with AIDS (acquired immunodeficiency syndrome).

Functioning lesions of the pancreas may present with severe hypoglycaemia in infancy and childhood. This is due to hyperinsulinaemia secondary to a pancreatic insulinoma or nesidioblastosis. Patients with multiple endocrine neoplasia (MEN) type 1 may have multiple insulinomas. Insulinomas are small, echo-poor lesions and are difficult to identify with conventional ultrasound, though intra-operative scanning is sometimes of great help in directing resection. Evaluation with thin slice CT scans should always be considered when the lesion is not seen on ultrasound.

Nesidioblastosis is characterised by hyperplasia of the insulin-producing b-cells in or around acinar elements but outside the islets of Langerhans. It is a diffuse condition, affecting all or much of the pancreas and is treated surgically with subtotal resection of the pancreas. Although increased reflectivity of the pancreas has been described, this is difficult to evaluate in the neonate and infant and, as there are no specific features, ultrasound is of little value in the diagnosis of this condition.

REFERENCES

1 Siegel M J, Martin K W, Worthington J L. Normal and abnormal pancreas in children: US studies. Radiology 1987; 165: 15–18
2 Boothroyd A E, Dicks Mireaux C, Haughton T. Radiological appearances of acute pancreatitis in children. Journal of Medical Imaging 1989; 3: 180–184
3 Swischuk L E, Hayden C K Jnr. Pararenal space hyperechogenicity in childhood pancreatitis. AJR 1985; 145: 1085–1086
4 Jeffrey R B Jnr, Laing F C, Wing V W. Ultrasound in acute pancreatic trauma. Gastrointest Radiol 1986; 11: 44–46
5 Bass J, Di Lorenzo M, Desjardins J G, et al. Blunt pancreatic injuries in children. The role of percutaneous drainage in the treatment of pancreatic pseudocysts. J Pediatr Surg 1988; 23: 721–724
6 Suarez F, Bernard O, Gauthier F, et al. Bilio-pancreatic common channel in children: clinical, biological and radiological findings in 12 children. Pediatr Radiol 1987; 17: 206–211
7 McHugo J M, McKeown C, Brown M T, et al. Ultrasound findings in children with cystic fibrosis. Br J Radiol 1987; 60: 137–141

The paediatric biliary system

Hylton B. Meire and Pat Farrant

INTRODUCTION

Abnormalities of the biliary tract in children are uncommon but, when they occur, ultrasound now plays a very important role in the diagnosis and management.

In order to obtain the maximum possible diagnostic information it is particularly important for the ultrasonographer to have access to appropriate high frequency, short focus probes, especially for neonates.

In order to improve imaging of the gallbladder, children older than about 5 years of age should be fasted but this is usually counter-productive in younger children as it increases the risk of them being irritable and uncooperative. If imaging of the gallbladder in infants has been unsuccessful in the unfasted state it may be helpful to examine the child during a bottle feed after a 4 hour fast.

NORMAL APPEARANCES

The normal gallbladder should be identifiable, with an appropriate transducer, in all children. If the child is fasted the gallbladder should be well-distended (Fig. 1) but after a feed there may be almost complete obliteration of the gallbladder lumen with apparent thickening of the gallbladder wall (Fig. 2). The size of the gallbladder varies with the patient's age and degree of fasting and no useful measurements for gallbladder size are possible. However, the body of the normal full gallbladder should appear approximately triangular in cross-section whereas the abnormally distended gallbladder tends to have a more circular shape in this view (Fig. 3).

The normal common hepatic duct is identifiable in many neonates and should have a diameter of less than 1 mm (Fig. 4). The normal diameter increases with age up to

6 mm early in the second decade. The parallelism of the normal common duct walls is perhaps more important than the absolute diameter.

Ultrasound assessment for possible biliary disease should always include examination of the pancreas, this is discussed in greater detail in Chapter 25.

NEONATAL JAUNDICE

Mild physiological jaundice occurs in up to 90% of newborn infants, usually between the second and eighth days of life. If the jaundice is noted within the first 24 hours or

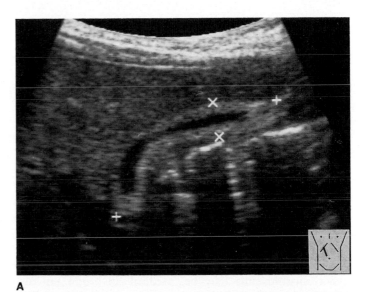

A

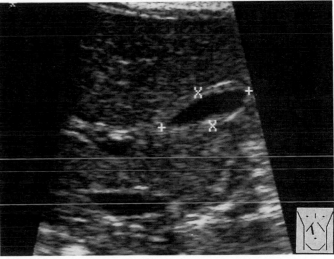

B

Fig. 2 Normal contracted neonatal gallbladder. A: The residual lumen measures only 1 to 2 mm in diameter and the wall is noticeably thickened with an increase in reflectivity. **B:** A further example with a larger residual lumen.

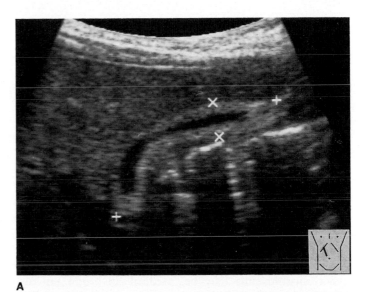

Fig. 1 Normal distended neonatal gallbladder. This degree of distension is unlikely to be seen unless the child has been fasted for more than 4 hours.

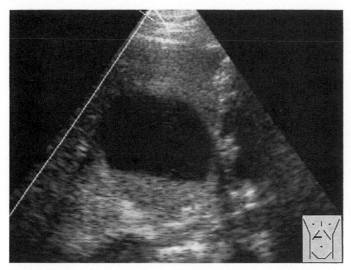

Fig. 3 Distended gallbladder. When the gallbladder is pathologically distended it has a circular cross-section, as seen in this transverse scan. Crystals are precipitating in the hyperconcentrated bile.

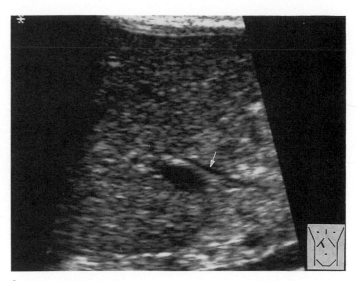

A

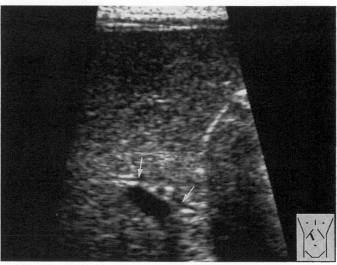

B

Fig. 4 Normal neonatal common duct. A: The duct (arrow) can be seen anterior to the portal vein. **B:** The duct (arrows) is seen anterior to the portal vein and hepatic artery. The lumen should be less than 1 mm in diameter.

the bilirubin exceeds 200 μmol/l or if the jaundice persists or continues to rise after the eighth day there is a high chance that the jaundice is caused by underlying pathology.[1] This group of patients warrants immediate investigation including ultrasound of the liver and biliary system. However, before ultrasound is undertaken it is necessary to determine whether the jaundice is due to to conjugated or unconjugated bilirubin. The latter are due to disorders of the hepatocytes and ultrasound imaging does not contribute in this group of patients. Conjugated hyperbilirubinaemia may be 'medical' in origin but also raises the possibility of a structural defect of the biliary system including:

    extrahepatic biliary atresia
    choledochal cyst
    biliary hypoplasia
    inspissated bile syndrome
    choledocholithiasis
    bile duct stenosis
    spontaneous perforation of the bile duct.

These 'surgical' causes of conjugated hyperbilirubinaemia in infancy frequently present in a manner indistinguishable from infective, metabolic and other medical causes of severe cholestasis and early ultrasound imaging can be very helpful in planning the sequence of investigations. For example, if a confident diagnosis of choledochal cyst or choledocholithiasis is established, no further investigations may be necessary.

JAUNDICE IN CHILDHOOD

Obstructive jaundice in childhood is ideally investigated with ultrasound; a complete and specific diagnosis is often possible. The obstruction is most likely to be associated with a choledochal abnormality, including choledochal cyst and biliary calculi. Rarely bile duct tumours, pancreatic masses, lymphadenopathy and subhepatic benign masses of pancreatic or bowel origin may obstruct the common duct.

BILIARY ATRESIA

Congenital extrahepatic biliary atresia occurs with a frequency of approximately 1 per 10 000 live births and, if undiagnosed or untreated, gives rise to secondary biliary cirrhosis and death within the first 2 years of life.[2,3] The aetiology remains obscure but it is now almost certain that it is not a true atresia, the bile ducts probably being present and normal through much of fetal life. It seems probable that an aggressive inflammatory process damages and destroys segments of the biliary tree, the resultant scarring giving rise to the apparent atresia. The inflammatory process is often still active in the neonatal period and can often be seen in the liver biopsy. It usually destroys part or all of the extrahepatic biliary apparatus and may leave isolated segments of duct which can fill with fluid and give an appearance indistinguishable from a choledochal cyst.

In 25% of babies with biliary atresia there is an associated congenital anomaly which may include intestinal malrotation, situs inversus abdominis, polysplenia, a preduodenal portal vein and a wide range of abnormalities of the inferior vena cava and hepatic artery.[4] There is also an increased incidence in trisomy 17, 18[5] and 21. Early reports of the ultrasound appearances in biliary atresia suggested that the gallbladder was usually absent but, with modern high frequency variable focus transducers, it can be identified in most patients, though it is often abnormal in morphology. Less than 30% of patients with biliary atresia have an apparently normal gallbladder; in the remaining 70% the gallbladder is usually small, often with a thickened wall and an irregular shape (Fig. 5). It may also be entirely intrahepatic and any fluid seen within it may be mucus rather than bile.

Failure to detect the common hepatic duct on ultrasound raises the possibility of biliary atresia (Fig. 6) but does not permit a specific diagnosis as the normal common duct may sometimes be undetectable. Conversely many biliary atresia patients have a large hepatic artery (Fig. 7) which may mimic the common duct but can usually be differentiated from a duct by noting the intrinsic pulsations and using colour flow imaging. If multiple atretic areas are present the isolated segments of duct may dilate and give rise to 'cysts' which may be either intra- or extrahepatic in site (Fig. 8). It may not be possible to differentiate these from primary choledochal cysts but if the latter present with jaundice there is usually dilatation of the intrahepatic biliary system. In biliary atresia no intrahepatic bile ducts can normally be detected.

The ultrasound finding of an anomaly known to be associated with biliary atresia may be the strongest evidence for the diagnosis. Those most likely to be diagnosed by ultrasound include situs inversus (Fig. 9) and polysplenia (Fig. 10). The situs inversus associated with biliary atresia is often an incomplete inversion, the liver may form two approximately equal lobes that lie on either side of the midline. The term 'situs ambiguus' may be more appropriate in this case.

The confident diagnosis of biliary atresia depends upon a combination of tests but especially isotope biliary excretion studies[6] and liver biopsy.

The only potential for cure for biliary atresia is porto-enterostomy (Kasai procedure[7]). Without this operation

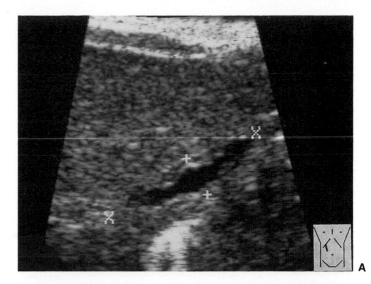

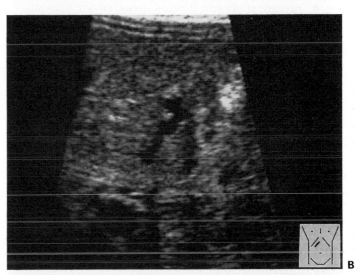

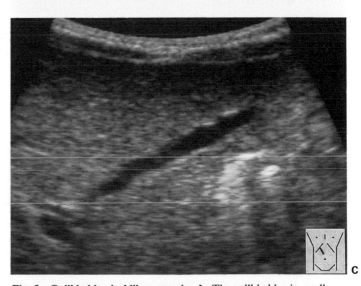

Fig. 5 Gallbladder in biliary atresia. A: The gallbladder is small with a thick irregular wall of low reflectivity (compare with Figure 2A). **B:** The gallbladder is very irregular in shape. **C:** A normal length gallbladder but with a markedly irregular wall.

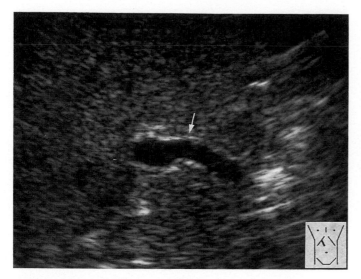

Fig. 6 Absence of bile duct in biliary atresia. Despite good image quality no bile duct can be identified anterior to the portal vein. Arrow – hepatic artery.

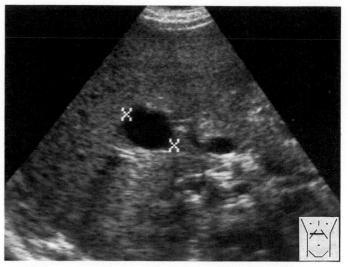

A

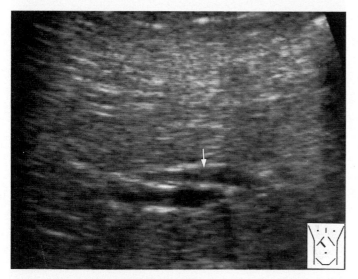

Fig. 7 Abnormal hepatic artery in biliary atresia. No bile duct can be identified and there is a large artery (arrow) passing in an abnormal direction anterior to the portal vein.

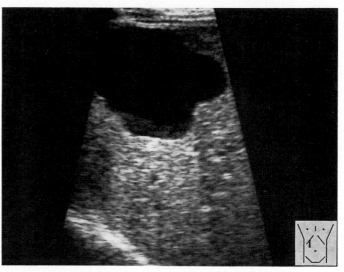

B

Fig. 8 Biliary cysts in biliary atresia. A: 15 mm cyst anterior to the porta hepatis. **B:** Large lobulated intrahepatic cyst.

patients' life expectancy is less than 2 years; if partial biliary drainage is achieved life expectancy may be extended to 10 years or more and rarely the procedure is completely curative. Liver transplantation offers the only alternative form of therapy (see Ch. 20).

The success rate of the Kasai procedure depends upon several factors but one of the most important is the age of the patient at the time of operation.[8] Prior to 8 weeks of age the procedure is successful in more than 50% of patients but after the age of 12 weeks it is unlikely to offer significantly prolonged survival or cure. It is therefore essential that all infants with persistent neonatal jaundice

are investigated early and the diagnosis made with all possible haste.

Ultrasound is employed on a routine basis for the follow up of post-operative biliary atresia patients. If the Kasai procedure has been successful the parenchymal echo pattern should remain normal, the portal vein patent with normal velocity flow and there should be no splenomegaly. Conversely if the procedure has been partially or totally unsuccessful, progressive secondary biliary cirrhosis occurs with increasing heterogeneity of the liver (Fig. 11) and the development of portal hypertension. Ultrasound imaging shows an abnormal rate of increase in spleen size and may show reduction or reversal in portal vein flow (Fig. 12). This form of secondary biliary cirrhosis is one of the few

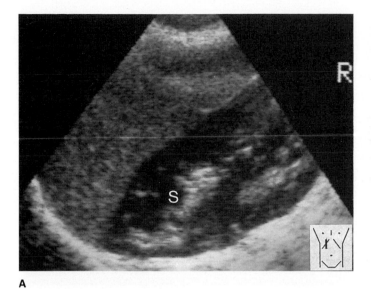

A

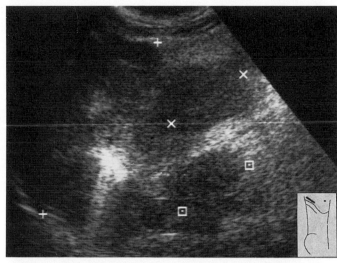

Fig. 10 Polysplenia. Same case as Figure 9. Oblique intercostal scan on the right reveals the presence of three irregular shaped spleens (between caliper markers).

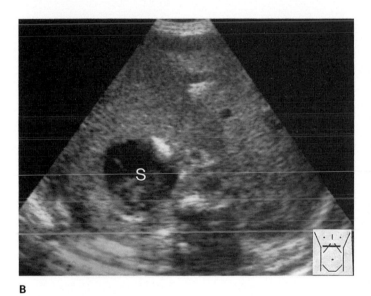

B

Fig. 9 Situs inversus abdominis. A: Longitudinal scan to the right of the midline shows a liver lobe with a left lobe configuration and the stomach (S) posterior to this. **B:** Transverse scan showing a right shaped lobe on the left and the stomach (S) on the right.

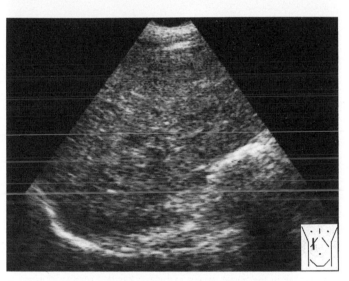

Fig. 11 Secondary biliary cirrhosis after failed Kasai procedure. The liver shows an overall increase in reflectivity and heterogeneous echo pattern. The porta hepatis and portal tracts are difficult to identify.

diseases which gives rise to progressive reduction in hepatic arterial diastolic flow and in severe cases there may be diastolic flow reversal (Fig. 13). The role of Doppler studies in the management of these cases remains to be proven but it is clear that diastolic flow reversal is a late consequence and the majority of these patients require transplantation within a short period of time.

A small number of patients with a failed Kasai procedure develop intrahepatic cysts in association with their secondary biliary cirrhosis (Fig. 14). The exact origin of these cysts is uncertain but they may be isolated bile duct segments and they usually slowly increase in diameter with

time and the fluid within them may become turbid or contain gravity dependent debris.

BILIARY HYPOPLASIA

Hypoplasia of the intrahepatic biliary ducts or ductules may occur as an isolated disorder or as part of Alagille's syndrome.[9] It is rare with an incidence of less than 1 per 100 000 live births. The clinical presentation is with chronic cholestasis and may be indistinguishable from other causes of cholestasis including extrahepatic biliary atresia. The main lesion in this disease is within the biliary

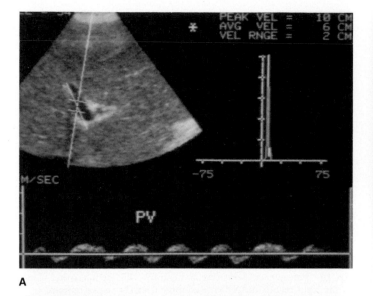

A

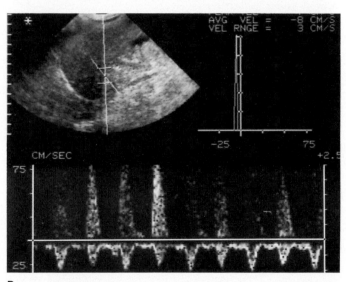

B

Fig. 12 Abnormal portal flow in secondary biliary cirrhosis. A: The flow velocity in the portal vein is extremely low and reverses during arterial systole. **B:** There is established reversal of portal vein flow with a maximum velocity during arterial systole.

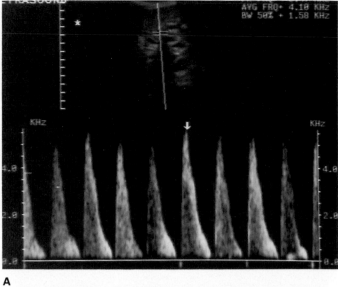

A

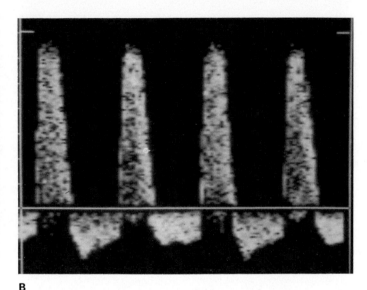

B

Fig. 13 Arterial waveforms in secondary biliary cirrhosis. A: There is high resistance to flow with obliteration of diastolic perfusion. **B:** Very high flow resistance with hepatofugal flow during diastole.

ductules and imaging procedures have no role in the diagnosis of the hepatic abnormality.

CHOLEDOCHAL CYST

Choledochal cysts are congenital cystic dilatations of the common bile duct and the large majority present in childhood, usually with recurrent jaundice. The age at presentation is, however, extremely variable and the diagnosis should always considered whenever a jaundiced child is investigated or when a subhepatic cyst is identified.

There have been several attempts to classify choledochal cysts and most surgeons now use the classification in which they are divided into five types[10] (Fig. 15):

type I – spherical or fusiform dilatation of the extra-hepatic common duct;

type II – diverticulum of the common duct;

type III – choledochocele (cystic dilatation of the intra-duodenal portion of the common duct);

type IV – the combination of extra- and intrahepatic cysts;

type V – intrahepatic biliary cysts with a normal extra-hepatic common duct.

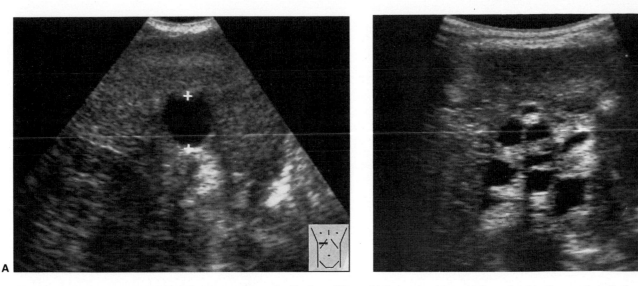

Fig. 14 Hepatic cysts after failed Kasai procedure. A: Single and **B:** multiple intrahepatic cysts have developed approximately 1 year after unsuccessful Kasai procedures.

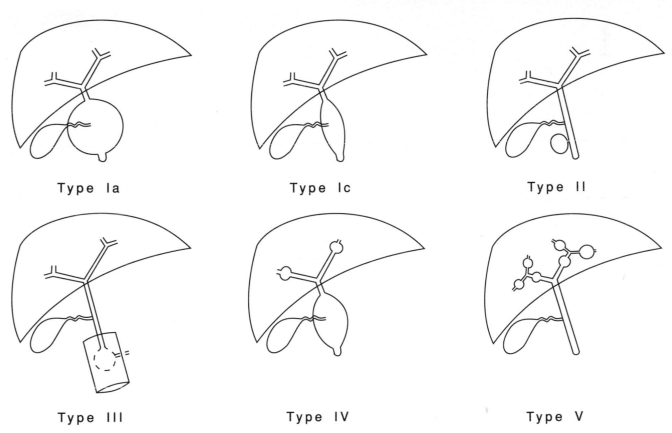

Type Ia   Type Ic   Type II

Type III   Type IV   Type V

Fig. 15 Types of choledochal cyst.

The percentages of these different types vary in the different published series but, in general, the spherical type I is the most common and the type II the least common. Numerous subdivisions of these different types have been suggested; these are primarily of surgical relevance and do not materially affect the ultrasound diagnosis. Many patients with choledochal cyst give a history of recurrent episodes of jaundice of uncertain cause. Although clinically and biochemically it appears to be obstructive, contrast studies seldom show any actual obstruction to bile flow.

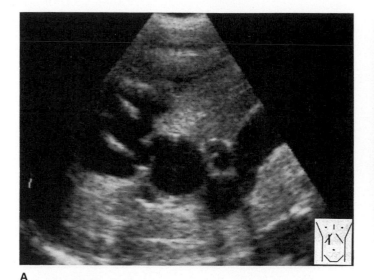

A

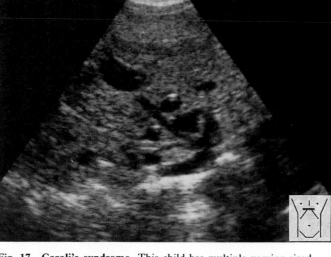

Fig. 17 Caroli's syndrome. This child has multiple varying sized intrahepatic cysts which communicate with the biliary tree.

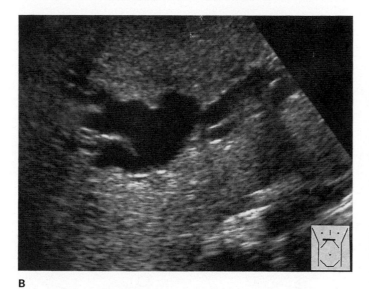

B

Fig. 16 Intrahepatic duct dilatation associated with choledochal cyst. In both these patients there is severe dilatation of the intrahepatic ducts. These returned completely to normal after choledochojejunostomy.

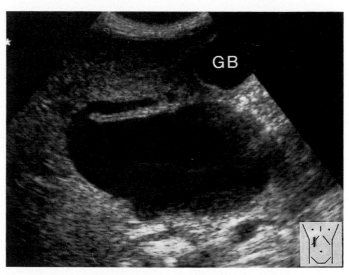

Fig. 18 Type I choledochal cyst. There is a large subhepatic cyst replacing the common bile duct. GB – gallbladder.

The degree of dilatation of the intrahepatic ducts is also variable: often there is little or no dilatation but occasionally gross dilatation may be seen (Fig. 16). This appearance may be indistinguishable from, and can be easily confused with, Caroli's syndrome (Fig. 17) in which there are multiple cystic dilatations of the intrahepatic biliary tree.[11,12] The aetiology may well be similar in the two conditions and choledochal cysts may genuinely coexist with Caroli's syndrome. If the intrahepatic dilatation is secondary to a choledochal cyst, surgical correction leads to complete resolution of the duct dilatation whereas no treatment is effective in Caroli's syndrome. Caroli's syndrome is very rare and is associated with congenital hepatic fibrosis and

medullary sponge kidneys. The diagnosis can only be made with confidence after liver biopsy and renal imaging confirm these components of the syndrome.

The 'classic' and commonest form of choledochal cyst is a large spherical subhepatic cyst (type I) (Fig. 18). Patients with this type of cyst may present at any age from the neonatal period to the eighth decade and several have recently been identified in utero (see the Ultrasound in Obstetrics and Gynaecology volume, Ch. 18). The fluid within the cyst is usually echo-free but occasionally precipitated bile salts may be detected (Fig. 19). Rarely ascites may be associated with the cyst and, in this situation, the differential diagnosis of spontaneous perforation

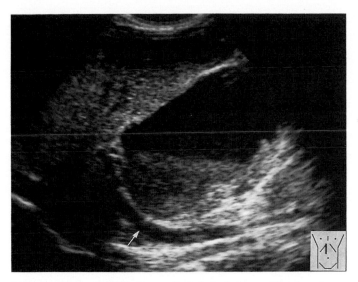

Fig. 19 Inspissated bile in type I choledochal cyst. The chronic stasis in the cyst has predisposed to precipitation of bile salts. The cyst is displacing the portal vein (arrow).

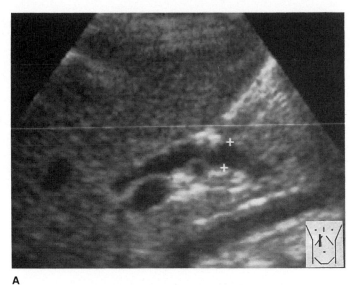

A

of the bile duct must be considered. An additional but very rare differential diagnosis is duplication cyst of the small bowel. These may appear as echo-containing cysts in the right upper abdomen and very rarely give rise to biliary obstruction.

10% to 25% of all choledochal cysts are of the type Ic fusiform variety[13] and, although the clinical presentation with jaundice is identical to patients with larger cysts, many fusiform cysts give rise to only minor degrees of duct dilatation (Fig. 20) that may easily be overlooked or misdiagnosed. In the neonate an identical appearance can be produced by the inspissated bile plug syndrome and this should always be considered as a differential diagnosis.

Type V choledochal cyst comprises between 2% and 4% of most series. These cysts are seldom associated with biliary symptoms and are often an incidental finding (Fig. 21A). Ultrasound alone cannot distinguish these from simple developmental hepatic cysts although, in this variant the cysts typically have a lobulated margin and are often far from spherical in shape. Biliary contrast studies usually establish the correct diagnosis (Fig. 21B).

There is a strong association between choledochal cysts and pancreatic disease. In some patients this is due to an associated congenital anomaly of the insertions of the pancreatic and biliary ducts into the ampulla, possibly with a short common channel.[14] Indeed it is possible that reflux of pancreatic juice into the biliary system may be the cause of some choledochal cysts, a hypothesis supported by the finding that the amylase within the cyst fluid is almost always elevated. At the time of presentation, many choledochal cyst patients also have a raised serum amylase even in the absence of overt pancreatitis. Thus the pancreas should be examined in every patient found to have a choledochal cyst; abnormalities of the pancreatic duct

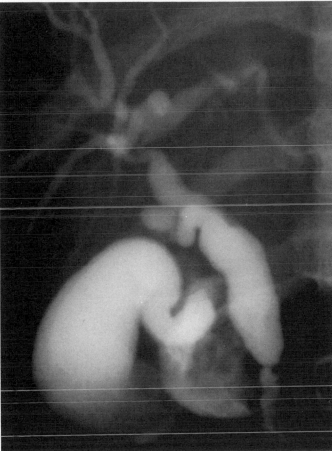

B

Fig. 20 Type Ic choledochal cyst. This child presented with recurrent pancreatitis and was not jaundiced at the time of examination. **A:** There is mild fusiform dilatation of the whole length of the common duct (between caliper markers). In the absence of jaundice this is strongly suggestive of choledochal cyst. **B:** ERCP. There is mild dilatation of almost the whole length of the common duct.

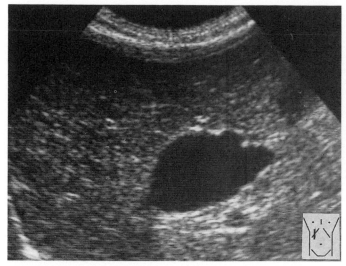

A

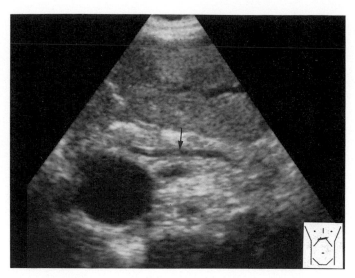

Fig. 22   Dilated pancreatic duct associated with choledochal cyst. There is a type III choledochal cyst with associated dilatation of the pancreatic duct (arrow). The pancreatic parenchymal reflectivity is increased indicating recurrent pancreatitis.

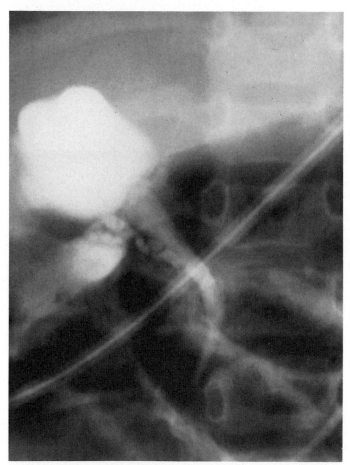

B

Fig. 21   Type V choledochal cyst. A: This lobulated intrahepatic cyst was an incidental finding. **B:** ERCP confirms the communication with the biliary tree.

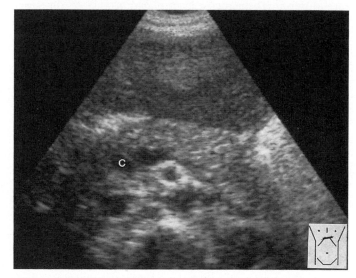

Fig. 23   Pancreatitis secondary to undiagnosed choledochal cyst (C). The pancreas is normal in size but shows a heterogeneous echo pattern with overall increase in reflectivity. (Same case as Figure 20A).

(Fig. 22) indicate a greatly increased risk of pancreatitis and should expedite surgical correction of the cyst, even in the absence of jaundice or other symptoms. Occasionally evidence of previously undiagnosed chronic pancreatitis is seen (Fig. 23). Surgical correction of a choledochal cyst usually produces a prompt post-operative fall in serum amylase but occasionally acute pancreatitis may be precipitated and may progress to pseudocyst formation (Fig. 24).

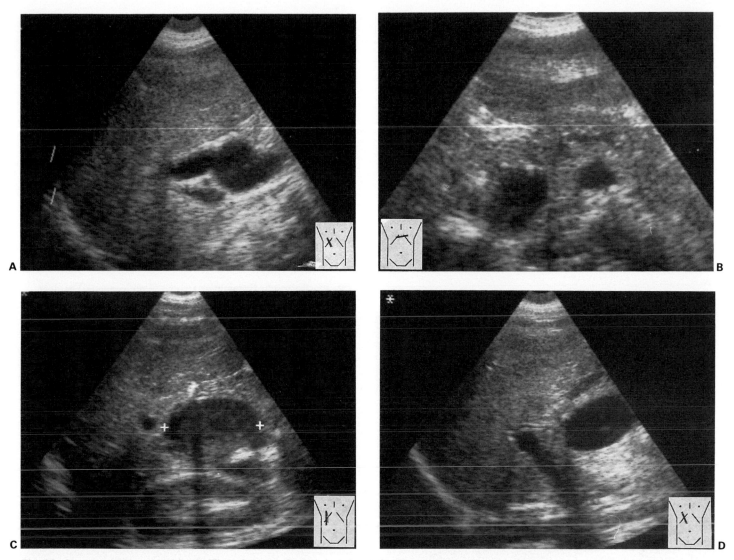

Fig. 24 Post-surgical pancreatitis. A: There is a type Ic choledochal cyst. **B:** The pancreatic duct is irregularly dilated. **C:** An acute pseudocyst (between caliper markers) formed in the pancreatic head post-operatively. **D:** 2 months later the cyst contains clear fluid and has reduced slightly in size.

RHABDOMYOSARCOMA

A further rare differential diagnosis of choledochal cyst is rhabdomyosarcoma of the common bile duct. The clinical presentation is often similar and, on imaging, the common duct is found to be dilated though filled with structured echoes (Fig. 25).[15] Ultrasound does not permit a specific pre-operative diagnosis but, if the echoes within the dilated duct appear structured and the duct is not truly fusiform, this diagnosis may be considered. Rhabdomyosarcoma of the common bile duct comprises less than 1% of all rhabdomyosarcomas. Aggressive treatment with radical surgery and chemotherapy has, as yet, failed to improve the dismal prognosis from this tumour (Fig. 26).[16]

INSPISSATED BILE PLUG SYNDROME

This syndrome has only been recognised relatively recently and is responsible for a minority of cases of neonatal obstructive jaundice.[17] Its incidence is uncertain but is possibly around 1 per 500 000 live births. The extrahepatic biliary obstruction is caused by thick bile plugs within the common duct and may be associated with conditions causing excessive haemolysis, with prolonged total parenteral nutrition or with cystic fibrosis. The common bile duct is usually dilated (Fig. 27), (eight out of nine in the King's College Hospital series over the last 15 years). The obstruction is usually at the lower end of the common duct and may be associated with dilatation of the gallbladder which

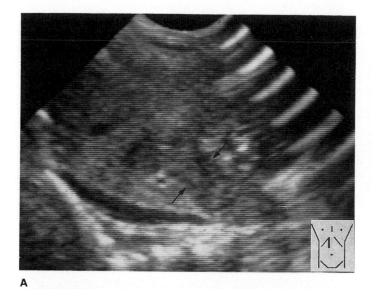

A

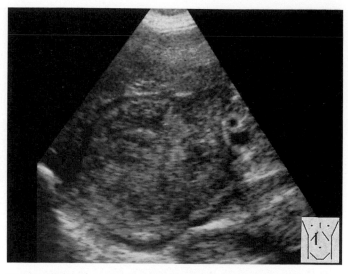

Fig. 26 Recurrent rhabdomyosarcoma of the common bile duct. Same case as Figure 25A. Despite radical surgery and chemotherapy there is a large recurrent tumour 4 years after the initial operation.

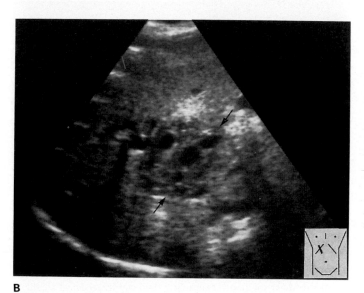

B

Fig. 25 Rhabdomyosarcoma of the common bile duct. A: The bile duct (arrows) is dilated and filled with structured echoes. **B:** There is gross distension of the common duct (arrows) by a partly cystic tumour. The child died of recurrent tumour several weeks after radical surgery.

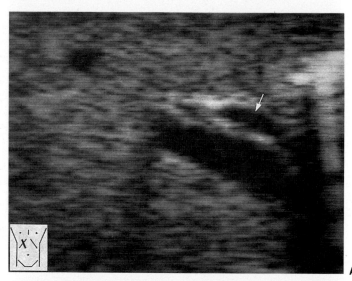

A

itself may also contain inspissated bile or frank calculi. The diagnosis is confirmed by percutaneous cholangiography or ERCP and the latter may permit definitive treatment with removal of the bile plug after sphincterotomy or with a mucolytic agent.[18] Many cases resolve spontaneously (Fig. 28) and the prognosis is generally excellent.

Fig. 27 Inspissated bile plug syndrome. A: This 1-month-old baby presented with conjugated hyperbilirubinaemia of unknown origin. The bile duct (arrow) is dilated to 1.7 mm in diameter. **B:** The bile plug (arrows) in this neonate caused severe duct dilatation and almost filled the extrahepatic duct. This necessitated surgical removal.

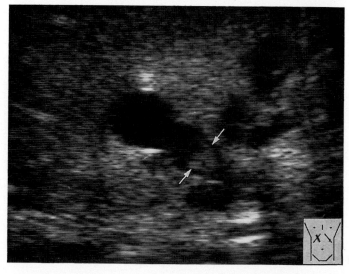

B

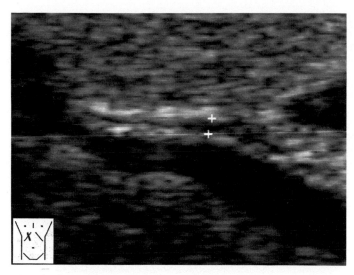

Fig. 28   Spontaneous resolution of inspissated bile plug syndrome.
(Same case as Figure 27A). After 1 month of conservative treatment
the bile duct has reduced to 1.2 mm in diameter (between caliper
markers) and the patient's jaundice had resolved.

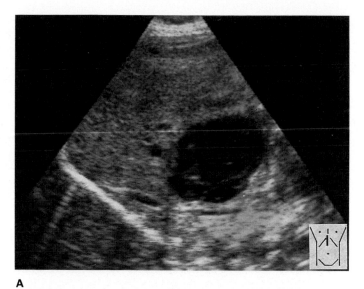

A

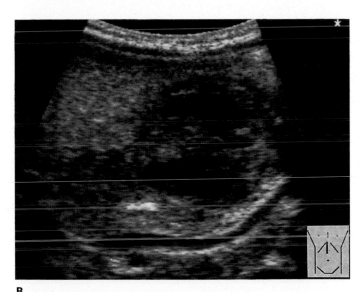

B

SPONTANEOUS PERFORATION OF THE BILE DUCT

Spontaneous perforation of the bile duct is a rare but important condition, there being approximately 70 cases in the world literature.[19] Its importance lies in the high mortality of untreated cases and the excellent results of surgical repair.[20] The spontaneous perforation almost invariably occurs at the junction of the cystic duct and common hepatic duct; its cause is obscure but it may rarely be associated with distal duct obstruction due to inspissated bile plug or calculi (Fig. 29).

Patients present between the ages of 2 and 8 weeks with the onset of jaundice and ascites.

Ultrasound reveals a subhepatic fluid collection and ascites.[21] The subhepatic fluid collection usually contains structured echoes (Fig. 29), particularly if the condition has been present for some weeks prior to diagnosis. In the reported cases there has not been dilatation of the biliary tree or gallbladder and no positive diagnostic features are present on ultrasound. The differential diagnosis is usually between choledochal cyst and duplication cyst of the small bowel.

Fig. 29   Spontaneous perforation of the bile duct. A: The irregular
subhepatic fluid filled space with some contained echoes proved at
operation to be a biloma secondary to spontaneous bile duct
perforation. **B:** There is a large spherical subhepatic mass with some
contained echoes but little attenuation of the ultrasound beam. **C:**
(same case as B). This child was also noted to have calculi within the
gallbladder though none were detected within the common bile duct.

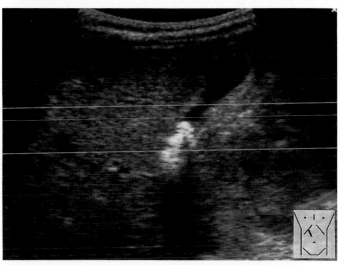

C

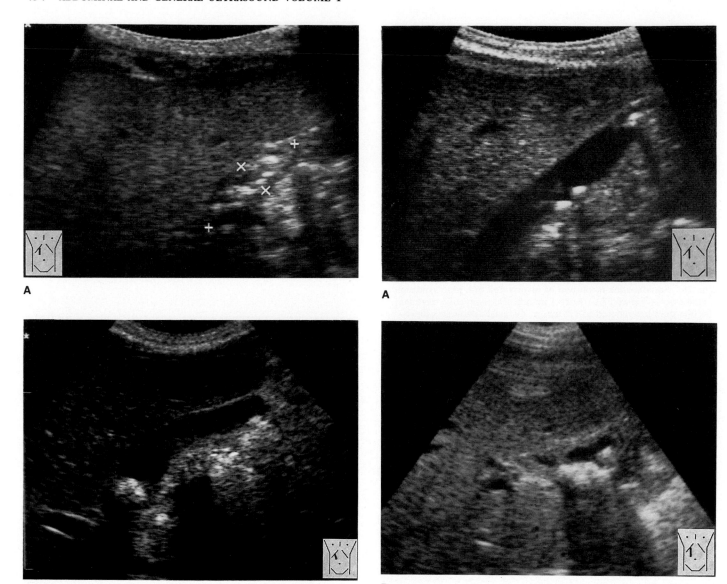

A

B

A

B

Fig. 30   Neonatal gallbladder calculi. A: The gallbladder (between caliper markers) is filled with calculi in this neonate with idiopathic hepatitis. **B:** 2 years later the calculi are still present and several have increased markedly in size.

Fig. 31   Gallbladder calculi associated with liver disease. A: These gallbladder calculi were an incidental finding in this 1-year-old child with persistent hepatitis. **B:** This 5-year-old child with cryptogenic cirrhosis has a small thick walled gallbladder which contained multiple calculi.

GALLBLADDER

The normal gallbladder can always be identified (see Figs 1 and 2) and patency of the cystic duct can be confirmed by pre- and post-prandial scans.

Primary disease of the gallbladder in childhood is uncommon but calculi may be detected in children with metabolic disorders, haemoglobinopathies[22] and after prolonged parenteral nutrition.[23,24] A high proportion (about 60%) of children with sickle cell disease show gallbladder calculi by the age of 12 years. Gallbladder calculi may also be diagnosed in utero and as an incidental

finding in early neonatal scans (Fig. 30A). The cause of and significance of these calculi is uncertain and many of the idiopathic calculi resolve spontaneously in the first few weeks of life[25] whilst others may persist and increase in size (Fig. 30B). They are more common in patients with underlying liver disease (Fig. 31). Biliary colic and obstruction due to calculi migrating into the common duct is extremely rare in childhood (Fig. 32).

Acute cholecystitis is rare in paediatric patients and may be associated with calculi or be acalculous.[26] In the latter group the possibility of cystic duct obstruction by parasitic agents such as giardia, ascaris and clonorchis should be

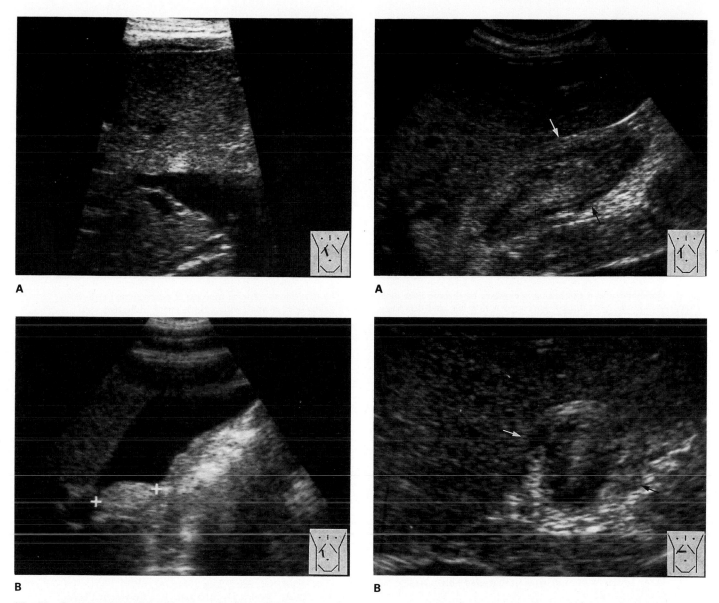

Fig. 32   Common duct obstruction by calculi. A: This 3-month-old child presented with conjugated hyperbilirubinaemia. The dilatation of the common duct is indistinguishable from a type Ic choledochal cyst but was found to be due to duct obstruction by pigment calculi. There was no evidence of a haemoglobinopathy. **B:** This 8-year-old presented with biliary colic and jaundice. Non-shadowing calculi were present in both the gallbladder and common bile duct.

Fig. 33   Gallbladder wall thickening in acute hepatitis. A: The gallbladder lumen appears obliterated in this child with acute viral hepatitis. Arrows – gallbladder. **B:** Transverse scan shows the lumen to be obliterated by gross wall thickening. Arrows – gallbladder.

considered. The ultrasound findings are similar to those in adult cholecystitis (see Ch. 12). Occasionally the gallbladder may be found to be distended in children with acute right upper quadrant pain who are apyrexial and with no leucocytosis. Ultrasound imaging reveals a tense gallbladder with no evidence of calculi and the remainder of the biliary system is normal; the serum bilirubin is normal. This condition has been termed 'acute hydrops of the gallbladder'[27] and, apart from the relatively mild clinical presentation, it cannot be differentiated from genuine cholecystitis. Although the condition is benign and self-limiting, cholecystectomy is usually undertaken and the diagnosis is made when no inflammation is detected in the excised specimen.

Gallbladder wall thickness

The wall of the normal distended gallbladder is seen on ultrasound imaging as a single thin line (see Fig. 1) whilst the wall of the contracted gallbladder appears thickened (see Fig. 2). Real or apparent gallbladder wall thickening may occur in a number of pathological conditions including cholecystitis and is a common incidental finding in many

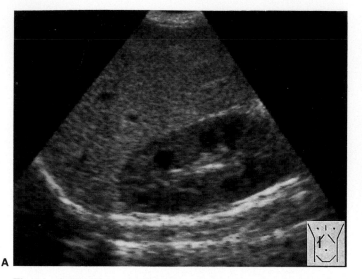

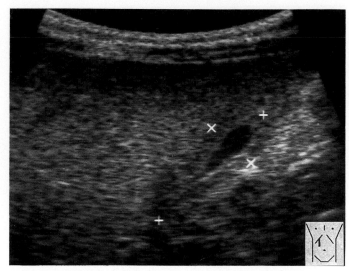

Fig. 34   Gallbladder wall thickening secondary to chronic liver disease. A: The liver shows uniform increase in parenchymal reflectivity secondary to chronic liver disease associated with a bile acid deficiency. **B:** The gallbladder is small with a thick poorly reflective wall.

children with both acute and chronic liver disease (Figs 33 and 34). The aetiology of the gallbladder wall thickening in these patients is uncertain and various hypotheses have been proposed including oedema, venous congestion in portal hypertension and tissue swelling secondary to

hypoalbuminaemia. When gallbladder wall thickening is identified on ultrasound the cause is usually evident from the clinical history and changes in the apparent wall thickness may mirror changes in the patient's clinical condition, especially in those patients with acute liver disease.

REFERENCES

1 Mowat A P. Pathological neonatal unconugated hyperbilirubinaemia. In: Liver disorders in childhood. 2nd edition. London: Butterworths. 1987: p 29

2 Mowat A P. Extrahepatic biliary atresia. In: Liver disorders in childhood. 2nd edition. London: Butterworths. 1987: p 77

3 Hays D M, Snyder W H. Life-span in untreated biliary atresia. Surgery 1963; 64: 373–375

4 Miyamoto M, Kajimoto T. Associated anomalies in biliary atresia patients. In: Kasai M. ed. Biliary atresia and its related disorders. Amsterdam: Excerpta Medica. 1983: p 13–19

5 Alpert L I, Strauss L, Hirschhorn K. Neonatal hepatitis and biliary atresia associated with trisomy 17–18 syndrome. N Engl J Med 1969; 280: 16–20

6 Dick M, Mowat A P. Biliary scintigraphy with DISIDA. A simpler way of showing bile duct patency in suspected biliary atresia. Arch Dis Child 1986; 61: 191

7 Kasai M, Suzuki S. A new operation for 'non-correctable' biliary atresia: hepatic portoenterostomy. Shujitsu 1959; 13: 733

8 Mieli-Vergani G, Howard E R, Portmann B, Mowat A P. Late referral for biliary atresia – missed opportunities for effective surgery. Lancet 1989; i: 421–423

9 Alagille D. Management of paucity of interlobular bile ducts. J Hepatol 1985; 1: 561

10 Alonso-Lej F, Rever W B, Pessagno D J. Congenital choledochal cyst with a report of two, and an analysis of 94 cases. International Abstracts of Surgery 1959; 108: 1–30

11 Caroli J. Diseases of intrahepatic bile ducts. Isr J Med Sci 1968; 4: 21–35

12 Marchal G J, Desmet V J, Proesmans W C, et al. Caroli disease: high frequency US and pathologic findings. Radiology 1986; 158: 507

13 Howard E R. Choledochal cysts. In: Howard E R. ed. Surgery of liver disease in children. Oxford: Butterworth- Heinemann. 1991: p 80

14 Todani K, Yatanabe Y, Fujii T, Uemura S. Anomalous arrangement of the pancreato-biliary duct system in patients with a choledochal cyst. Am J Surg 1984; 147: 672

15 Geoffrey A, Couanet D, Montagne J P, Lectere J, Flamant F. Ultrasonography and computer tomography for diagnosis and follow-up of biliary duct rhabdomyosarcoma. Pediatr Radiol 1987; 17: 127–131

16 Ruymann F B, Raney R B, Crist W M, Lawrence W, Lindberg R D, Soule E H. Rhabdomyosarcoma of the biliary tree in childhood. A report from the intergroup rhabdomyosarcoma study. Cancer 1985; 56: 575–581

17 Bernstein J, Braylan R, Brough A J. Bile-plug syndrome: a correctable cause of obstructive jaundice in infants. Pediatrics 1969; 43: 273

18 Brown D M. Bile plug syndrome: successful management with a mucolytic agent. J Pediatr Surg 1990; 25: 351–352

19 Howard E R, Johnston D I, Mowat A P. Spontaneous perforation of common bile duct in infants. Arch Dis Child 1976; 51: 883–886

20 Davenport M, Howard E R. Spontaneous perforation of the bile ducts in infancy. In: Howard ER. ed. Surgery of liver disease in children. Oxford: Butterworth-Heinemann. 1991: p 92

21 Bahia J O, Boal D K B, Karl S R, Gross G W. Ultrasonic detection of spontaneous perforation of the extrahepatic bile duct in infancy. Pediatr Radiol 1986; 16: 157

22 Bond L R, Hatty S R, Horn M E C, Dick M, Meire H B, Bellingham A J. Gall stones in sickle cell disease in the United Kingdom. BMJ 1987; 295: 234–236

23 Akierman A, Elliott P D, Gall D G. Association of cholelithiasis

with total parenteral nutrition and fasting in the preterm infant. Can Med Soc J 1984; 131: 272

24 Enzenauer R W, Montrey J S, Barcia P J, Woods J. Total parenteral nutrition cholestasis: a cause of mechanical biliary obstruction. Pediatrics 1985; 76: 905

25 Jacir N N, Anderson K D, Eichelberger M, Guzzetta P C.

Cholelithiasis in infancy: resolution of gall stones in three of four infants. J Pediatr Surg 1986; 21: 567–569

26 Bloom R A, Swain V A J. Non-calculous distension of the gallbladder in childhood. Arch Dis Child 1966; 41: 503

27 Appleby G A J, Forestier E, Starck C J. Hydrops of the gallbladder in the neonatal period. Acta Pediatr Scand 1981; 70: 117

The paediatric liver

Claire Dicks-Mireaux

As in other parts of the body, real time ultrasound is ideally suited for imaging disease processes in the paediatric liver and spleen. In many cases of suspected liver disease an ultrasound scan is the first investigation and may make the diagnosis or guide the clinician to the next appropriate investigation.

No special patient preparation is required, unless the gallbladder is to be examined, when a 6 hour or overnight fast is recommended. Using a 5 MHz probe or, in larger children, a 3.5 MHz probe, the entire liver can be examined from the anterior approach. Access to the spleen may be more difficult, particularly as the left side is very ticklish in many children. However, with care and scanning through the intercostal spaces, the whole spleen can be imaged.

Normal anatomy

The ultrasound appearances of the normal liver in a child do not differ greatly from those of the adult liver. Normal liver parenchyma has a homogeneous texture with mid-grey reflectivity, which should be slightly more reflective than normal renal parenchyma. An exception is the premature neonate in whom the reflectivity of the renal parenchyma may be equal to, or greater than that of the liver.

The liver is divided into right and left lobes by a plane that passes through the gallbladder fossa to the inferior vena cava. The falciform ligament further divides the left lobe into medial and lateral segments. The ligamentum teres, which is the obliterated remnant of the left umbilical vein, follows the course of the falciform ligament into the left lobe to join the left portal vein. This is sometimes visualised on ultrasound as a reflective 'mass', particularly in children who are obese or on corticosteroids. This appearance should not be mistaken for an abnormality such as a haemangioma. The major hepatic veins and the portal veins together with their branches can be visualised. Portal veins can be differentiated from hepatic veins by their reflective walls, compared with the absence of echoes from the walls of the hepatic veins. The hepatic veins can be traced to their drainage into the inferior vena cava; they subdivide the lobes of the liver into four segments. The normal change in calibre of the inferior vena cava with respiration can be observed. Examination of the portal vein and hepatic veins with Doppler demonstrates characteristic patterns of blood flow which are altered in disease. The main hepatic artery can be detected lying parallel to the proximal portion of the main portal vein. Doppler studies of the hepatic artery allow its distinction from a dilated common bile duct. The normal bile duct is often only seen with difficulty in children and should not measure more than 1 mm in neonates and 6 mm in adolescents.

Longitudinal scans of the normal liver demonstrate a triangular shaped left lobe with a sharp, acute-angled edge

Table 1 Spleen size

Age	Maximum length (cm)
0–3 months	6.0
3–6 months	6.5
6–12 months	7.0
1–2 years	8.0
2–4 years	9.0
4–8 years	10.0
8–12 years	11.5
12–15 years	12.0

and a straight or concave inferior (visceral) surface. This may become convex when the liver is enlarged. Generally the right lobe of the liver does not extend beyond the lower pole of the right kidney but a Riedel's extension of the right lobe, a normal variant, is recognised by its triangular shape. Studies of measurements of the liver have provided normal ranges[1,2] but are complicated to perform and evaluate. The above guidelines are usually sufficient for assessment of liver size.

The echo pattern of the normal spleen in children is homogeneous, with a reflectivity between that of the kidney and liver. Evaluation of splenic size with percussion and palpation is often inaccurate. Measurement of the spleen is possible with ultrasound. Scanning on the left side in the supine or slightly oblique position enables coronal views of the spleen to be obtained. Normal values of the greatest length of the spleen, from the dome to the tip are available (Table 1).[3]

The splenic vessels are easily visualised at the hilum and Doppler ultrasound may be used to identify the artery and vein.

Congenital abnormalities

Cardiac malpositions in children are associated with abnormalities of position of the liver and spleen. The various cardiac malpositions are complex but mirror image dextrocardia is the most common form. In the majority of these cases there is complete inversion of the cardiac chambers and the cardiac apex points to the right. This is associated with situs inversus and the liver, which is otherwise normal, lies on the left side with the stomach and spleen situated on the right (see Ch. 26). The liver is usually right sided in cases of dextroversion with situs solitus. Asplenia and polysplenia syndromes occur with cardiac malpositions and serious congenital heart disease is often present.[4] In both asplenia and polysplenia the liver often lies in the midline. Microgastria may be present.[5]

It is not possible to confirm the complete absence of a spleen with ultrasound; radionuclide studies are definitive. Polysplenia is more easily diagnosed with ultrasound (see Ch. 26) and when diagnosed associated abnormalities of the abdominal vasculature should be sought as there is a higher incidence of absent inferior vena cava or its continuation into the azygos or hemiazygos veins. A preduodenal portal vein has also been described. In 10% of cases of biliary atresia, there is coincident polysplenia.

If no spleen is detected in the left upper quadrant splenic tissue should be looked for in unusual locations in the abdomen. An 'ectopic spleen' in which the splenic ligaments are thought to be deficient or absent may be associated with intermittent abdominal pain. Torsion around the splenic pedicle and partial occlusion of vessels may occur.[6]

An accessory spleen is seen on ultrasound as a rounded 'mass' near the inferior border of the spleen or in the splenic hilum. Following trauma and rupture of the spleen, nodules of splenic tissue may grow within the abdomen and should not be mistaken for masses (see Ch. 21). Persistence post-natally of splenic connections with hepatic, gonadal and renal tissue result in splenohepatic, splenogonadal or splenorenal fusions.

Congenital cysts of the liver are uncommon; they are derived from the biliary tree and occur in any lobe of the liver. They may be large and present as an abdominal mass in the neonate or may be an incidental finding. A careful examination of the biliary tree should be undertaken to ensure that a choledochal cyst has not been mistakenly called an hepatic cyst. Congenital hepatic cysts are associated with renal, pancreatic and lung cysts and therefore the pancreas and kidneys should also be scanned and a chest X-ray obtained. Hepatic cysts are seen in about 30% of patients with autosomal dominant polycystic kidney disease which is occasionally discovered in children.

Congenital or epidermoid cysts occur in the spleen. They are solitary and on ultrasound a thin walled unilocular cyst is seen.[7] Superimposed infection or haemorrhage may cause the cyst contents to appear slightly reflective.

Diffuse parenchymal disease of the liver

Hepatomegaly and a generalised alteration in the normal reflectivity are the features of diffuse parenchymal disease of the liver. Both acute and chronic liver disease may present in this way.

In acute hepatitis, which has a number of causes (viral – hepatitis A and B, Ebstein Barr virus, cytomegalovirus, toxins, drugs, and Reye's syndrome), the ultrasound appearances may be normal or a diffuse echo-poor pattern may be seen with accentuation of the periportal echoes (Fig. 1). Apart from excluding the presence of biliary tract dilatation and obstructive jaundice, ultrasound is of little clinical value in acute hepatitis. In the neonate, it may be difficult to distinguish between neonatal hepatitis and biliary atresia. Ultrasound may be useful in demonstrating a normal gallbladder (see Ch. 26) and isotope scanning with one of the iminodiacetic acid (IDA) agents demonstrates excretion of radionuclide into the gut unless there is biliary atresia.

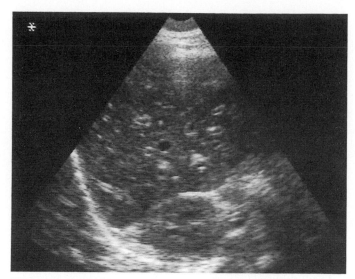

Fig. 1 Acute hepatitis. The liver is of uniformly decreased reflectivity, accentuating the bright echoes from the portal vein walls.

Hepatomegaly with a homogeneous increase in reflectivity and attenuation of the ultrasound beam is seen in numerous conditions:[8]

Reye's syndrome
Malnutrition
Obesity and hyperalimentation
Steroids
Chemotherapeutic agents
Metabolic liver disease
   tyrosinaemia
   fructose intolerance
   glycogen storage disease
   Wilson's disease
   galactosaemia
   Gaucher's disease
   Niemann–Pick disease
Thalassaemia.

In the fatty liver this pattern is thought to be due to the excess intracellular fat itself and is found in obesity and malnutrition, following administration of chemotherapeutic agents and steroids, and in Reye's syndrome. A number of storage disorders produce metabolic disturbances which result in a fatty liver. The glycogen storage disorders, of which there are 12, are autosomally recessive disorders of carbohydrate metabolism with faulty glycogenolysis. Type I glycogen storage disease (von Gierke's disease) is the most frequent and, in addition to a fatty liver, the kidneys may be enlarged. The spleen is not enlarged unless cirrhosis and portal hypertension develop. Types III, IV and VI are also associated with hepatomegaly and fatty liver. Type IV disease is rare and usually progresses to cirrhosis. In hereditary tyrosinaemia, Wilson's disease, Gaucher's disease, Niemann–Pick disease, the mucopolysaccharidoses, galactosaemia and fructose intolerance the liver may become enlarged with increased reflectivity. Several of these conditions eventually progress to cirrhosis and portal hypertension. Hereditary tyrosinaemia is associated with nephromegaly, nephrocalcinosis (Fig. 2) and cirrhosis with a very high incidence of hepatocellular carcinoma. Thalassaemia patients who have repeated blood transfusions may develop haemochromatosis with an enlarged, reflective liver. They also have a higher incidence of gallstones than normal (typically the bilirubin type).

Chronic liver disease with cirrhosis and fibrosis may be due to a number of conditions in children:

Cystic fibrosis
Hepatitis B
Autoimmune chronic active hepatitis
Alpha 1 antitrypsin deficiency
Thalassaemia
Wilson's disease
Caroli's syndrome
Glycogen storage disease
Tyrosinaemia
Langerhans-cell histiocytosis
Conorenal syndrome
Hepatic fibrosis – renal cystic disease
Radiation
Biliary atresia
Sclerosing cholangitis
Schistosomiasis
Meckel syndrome.

Ultrasound scanning of the liver reveals increased parenchymal reflectivity which may be non-uniform with a nodular pattern. The liver may be enlarged or small with an irregular, lobular surface. Fibrosis around the portal triads results in increasing periportal reflectivity. The caudate lobe often appears enlarged relative to the rest of the liver. Although ultrasound may suggest the presence of chronic liver disease and cirrhosis, the changes are often subtle and non-specific and a liver biopsy is required for confirmation. The associated ascites and portal hypertension should be looked for.

Patients with congenital hepatic fibrosis usually present in childhood with hepatosplenomegaly or gastrointestinal bleeding from varices. Congenital hepatic fibrosis most commonly occurs in autosomal recessive infantile polycystic kidney disease. There is usually little clinical evidence of renal disease at presentation – renal failure occurs later. The ultrasound appearances of the liver depend on the degree of fibrosis and cirrhosis. Initially the liver is simply enlarged but later increased reflectivity, nodularity and increased periportal reflectivity are seen. The kidneys are enlarged and appear abnormally reflective due to the numerous small cysts they contain. Congenital hepatic fibrosis is also found in the conorenal syndrome, (nephronophthisis, cone shaped epiphyses, retinitis pigmentosa), Caroli's disease (Fig. 3), asphyxiating thoracic dysplasia and Meckel syndrome (occipital encephaloceles, cleft lip and palate, polycystic kidney, hepatic fibrosis). It may also occur as an isolated lesion.

Hepatic calcification

Calcification in the liver may be seen with congenital infections, toxoplasmosis, rubella, cytomegalovirus and

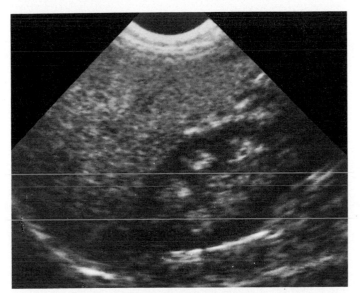

Fig. 2 Nephrocalcinosis in tyrosinaemia. The liver is of increased reflectivity consistent with chronic liver disease. There are areas of increased reflectivity around the margins of the pyramids indicating nephrocalcinosis.

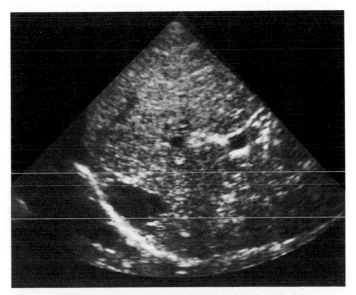

Fig. 3 Congenital hepatic fibrosis. The liver is enlarged with increased reflectivity. There is an irregular cyst posteriorly in the right lobe, possibly indicating a diagnosis of Caroli's syndrome. The patient also had polycystic disease.

herpes simplex. It is also found following tuberculosis and other causes of granuloma formation. Calcification is also found in hepatic masses, such as hepatoblastoma, haemangioma and teratomas. Metastatic neuroblastoma may also calcify in the liver. Strongly reflective nodules or masses are seen, usually accompanied by acoustic shadowing provided the foci are large enough.

Portal hypertension

Portal hypertension follows intrahepatic or extrahepatic obstruction to the portal system. The aetiology, natural history and prognosis of the two types is different although the clinical presentation may be similar. Obstruction to hepatic venous outflow or of the inferior vena cava is an uncommon cause of portal hypertension.

In the examination of a patient suspected of having portal hypertension, the portal vein should be studied with Doppler to ascertain the direction of blood flow, and varices should be specifically sought. In addition enlargement and increased reflectivity of the spleen and ascites may be seen.

Extrahepatic obstruction

This follows obstruction of the portal or splenic veins. Thrombosis of the portal vein may be seen in infants with a history of neonatal sepsis and dehydration or neonatal umbilical venous catheterisation. It may occur as a complication of appendicitis in older children, or following splenectomy, particularly if the operation is carried out to treat hypersplenism. In many cases no cause is found and affected children may be asymptomatic. Clinical presentation is with splenomegaly or haematemesis from bleeding gastro-oesophageal varices. This condition is also known as 'cavernous transformation of the portal vein' (Fig. 4). The cavernous appearance is due to the collaterals that develop around the obstructed portal vein and maintain blood flow to the liver. Ultrasound demonstrates multiple collateral channels in the porta hepatis; they are particularly striking on a colour Doppler study. There is often increased reflectivity in the porta hepatis around the collateral vessels due to previous inflammation and fibrosis.[9]

Dilated collateral veins may be identified around the stomach and spleen, such as the splenorenal gastro-oesophageal and para-umbilical vessels which carry blood away from the liver (hepatofugal flow). Doppler is useful to demonstrate the presence and direction of blood flow within these different channels.

Thickening of the lesser omentum between the left lobe of the liver and the aorta is seen on longitudinal scans in children with portal hypertension.[10] This is presumed to be due to varices too small to be resolved and to dilatation of the left gastric vein within the lesser omentum, or to oedema of the lesser omentum following lymphatic stasis. The thickness of the lesser omentum on longitudinal scans should not exceed 1.7 times the diameter of the aorta at the same level. Lymphadenopathy, obesity or fat deposition secondary to steroid administration may also increase the thickness of the lesser omentum.

Intrahepatic obstruction

Portal hypertension is often due to chronic liver disease with cirrhosis (Fig. 5). Ultrasound demonstrates the fea-

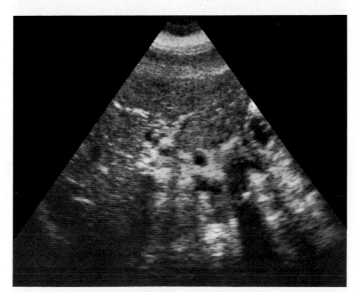

Fig. 4 Cavernous transformation of the portal vein. The portal vein is replaced by multiple irregular vascular channels.

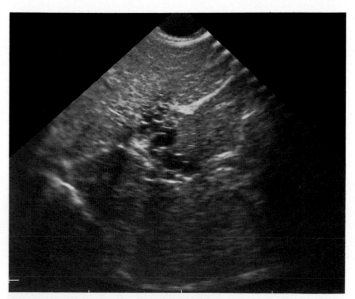

Fig. 5 Varices in hepatic fibrosis. A: There are multiple vascular channels at the porta hepatis consistent with varices secondary to portal hypertension. **B:** Longitudinal scan of the right kidney. There is complete obliteration of the normal architecture with an increase in parenchymal reflectivity.

tures of portal hypertension and also the irregular borders and inhomogeneous reflectivity of the cirrhotic liver.

In developing countries, portal hypertension may be due to infection with schistosoma. Both the ova and worms cause an inflammatory and fibrotic reaction resulting in periportal fibrosis. This is seen on ultrasound as increased reflectivity in the portal triads and around the portal vein.

Hepatic venous obstruction

Obstruction to hepatic venous outflow is also known as the Budd–Chiari syndrome (see Ch. 18). Congenital webs in the hepatic veins or inferior vena cava may result in obstruction to blood flow.[11] Ultrasound scanning can demonstrate the web and any reflective thrombus. Treatment may be surgical or with angioplastic dilatation of the caval web. Other causes of the Budd–Chiari syndrome in children include thrombosis of the hepatic veins, veno-occlusive disease or secondary to cardiac or pericardial disease. The ultrasound appearances are variable and include dilatation or stenosis of the hepatic veins and hypertrophy of the caudate lobe.

Hepatic neoplasms

Primary hepatic neoplasms are the third most common solid abdominal tumour in children. They are derived from the hepatocytes (epithelial tumours) or from the surrounding connective tissues and blood vessels (mesenchymal tumours) or from the biliary system. They may be benign or malignant and primary or metastatic. Metastatic involvement of the liver is much less common in children than in adults.[12]

Malignant hepatic neoplasms

Malignant tumours constitute two thirds of hepatic tumours and approximately 5% of paediatric tumours in general.[13] There are four types, hepatoblastoma, hepatocellular carcinoma, fibrolamellar carcinoma and the mesenchymoma (undifferentiated embryonal sarcoma). Presentation is usually with a mass or hepatomegaly; elevated serum alpha-fetoprotein occurs in both hepatoblastoma and hepatocellular carcinoma.

Hepatoblastoma Hepatoblastoma arises from the primitive epithelial cells of the fetal liver. It is more common than hepatocellular carcinoma in children in Europe and the United States of America. It occurs in children up to 3 years of age and is associated in some cases with hemihypertrophy, Beckwith–Wiedemann syndrome and familial polyposis coli. Lesions may be solitary or multiple and are poorly defined, slightly more reflective than normal liver, occasionally with calcifications (Fig. 6). The tumours are often large and may occupy one, several or even all segments or lobes of the liver; since the extent of involve-

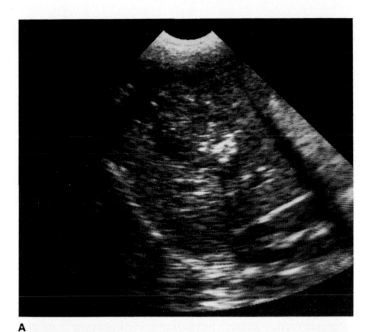

A

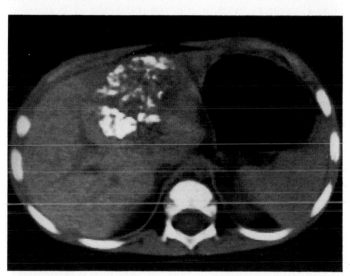

B

Fig. 6 Hepatoblastoma. A: Ultrasound and **B:** CT. There is an irregular heterogeneous mass with numerous foci of calcification.

ment as well as any venous invasion determine resectability these features need careful study. Portal venous amputation or invasion of an adjacent hepatic vein may occur, as may tumour thrombus in the inferior vena cava.[14] Many cases are treated with chemotherapy prior to surgery to shrink the tumour; they often calcify or undergo cystic change.

Hepatocellular carcinoma This tumour arises from mature hepatocytes, and presents throughout childhood with two peaks of incidence at 1 year and 13 years of age. Some cases occur in children with pre-existing cirrhosis and there is a higher incidence in the Far East where cirrhosis is not uncommon in children. There is a very high risk of hepatocellular carcinoma in patients with hereditary tyrosinaemia. The tumour is seen as a poorly defined reflective mass and, in a third of cases, the lesions are multiple. It cannot be distinguished from hepatoblastoma on ultrasound or other imaging techniques. As in hepatoblastoma, invasion of the hepatic and portal veins and the inferior vena cava may occur and should be looked for. If the patient has pre-existing cirrhosis it may be difficult to identify a tumour against the abnormal parenchyma. However, any large irregular mass within the liver should be considered a possible carcinoma. Computerised tomography and magnetic resonance imaging are probably more sensitive techniques for the detection of malignant change.

Fibrolamellar carcinoma This is a rare variant of hepatocellular carcinoma that usually affects older children. It presents as a well-defined reflective mass, and the diagnosis is made after surgical removal and histological examination.

Mesenchymoma The malignant mesenchymoma is more correctly termed 'undifferentiated sarcoma' of the liver. It presents in older children (peak age 11 years) and the appearances on ultrasound are variable. Some resemble the benign mesenchymal hamartoma with a multiseptate, cystic appearance while others are solid and reflective.

Metastatic tumours Tumours that may involve the liver include: Wilms' tumour, neuroblastoma, malignant teratoma, lymphoma and leukaemia. Wilms' tumour may produce solitary or multiple reflective metastases in the liver. Disseminated neuroblastoma (stage 4) may include focal liver metastases. There is a characteristic presentation in infants under 1 year of age with massive hepatomegaly, skin nodules and bone marrow involvement without bony involvement. Ultrasound demonstrates gross hepatomegaly and a diffuse irregular texture with nodules of decreased reflectivity (Fig. 7). The adrenal primary is not always demonstrable because it is often small. This presentation of neuroblastoma is known as stage 4S and has a much better prognosis than disseminated neuroblastoma in older children. Spontaneous regression often occurs and so chemotherapy is withheld unless massive hepatomegaly results in respiratory distress or failure to thrive. Ultrasound is used to monitor shrinkage of the liver though the abnormal reflectivity persists for some time even after the disease has resolved and the baby has recovered.

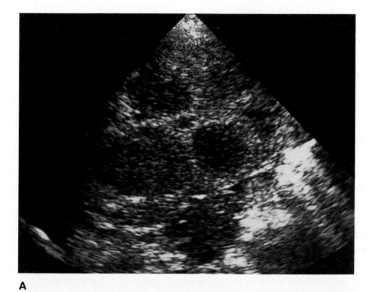

A

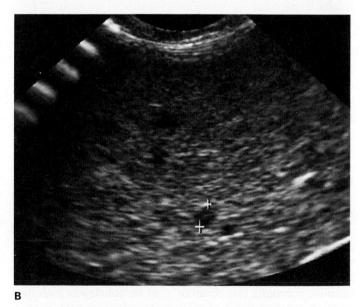

B

Fig. 7 Neuroblastoma stage 4S. This scan in a 3-week-old child with gross hepatomegaly shows diffuse nodularity and a 2 cm mass in the right adrenal region. Neuroblastoma of the unusual 'S' stage was diagnosed.

Fig. 8 Lymphoma. A: Multiple echo-poor lesions are seen in the liver in this child with non-Hodgkin's lymphoma. **B:** Splenic lymphoma. The enlarged spleen contains numerous small echo-poor masses.

Lymphoma and leukaemia both involve the liver and spleen, resulting in marked hepatosplenomegaly. There may be a diffuse, homogeneous increase in reflectivity throughout the liver, focal echo-poor lesions (Fig. 8) or the liver may have a normal echo pattern. Other sites of involvement, such as the para-aortic nodes, kidneys and pancreas can be looked for.

Benign hepatic neoplasms

Benign hepatic tumours comprise about a third of all primary liver tumours in childhood. The majority are mesenchymal in origin and include cavernous haemangioma, haemangioendothelioma and mesenchymal hamartoma. Benign epithelial tumours such as adenomas or focal nodular hyperplasia are rare.[15]

Haemangioma Benign vascular tumours of the liver may be solitary or multiple and may be associated with haemangiomas elsewhere.[16] They can be divided histologically into cavernous and capillary lesions.[17] Cavernous haemangiomas consist of large vascular structures lined by flat endothelial cells, separated by fibrous septa. The commoner capillary haemangiomas and haemangioendotheliomas are more cellular but, when large, necrosis, thrombosis and cystic degeneration may occur in the centre. Cavernous haemangiomas are rare and often an incidental finding in infants. Unlike adults symptomatic benign vascular tumours are not uncommon in children and are usually capillary haemangioendotheliomas. They present with an abdominal mass or congestive cardiac failure or, rarely, thrombocytopenia due to platelet trapping (Kasabach–Meritt syndrome). Unlike older children or adults, neonates may be very sick and require emergency treatment.

The ultrasound appearances of these lesions are variable but they are usually clearly defined with a reflectivity less than that of the surrounding liver (Fig. 9). Very occasionally focal calcifications may occur. Doppler demonstrates high velocity and disturbed blood flow through the mass. The diagnosis is often made by demonstrating changes in the hepatic veins and arteries: the coeliac axis and common hepatic artery are dilated and the calibre of the abdominal aorta reduces below the origin of the coeliac axis while the hepatic veins draining the lesion may be prominent. These vascular abnormalities do not occur with malignant lesions of the liver: they are highly suggestive of a benign vascular tumour.

Alternative methods of imaging such as CT scanning may be helpful, although they have little to add if the characteristic features are seen on ultrasound. Magnetic resonance imaging can be useful and demonstrates high intensity signals on STIR and T2-weighted images. Magnetic resonance imaging is probably superior to other modalities in demonstrating the associated vascular changes, but is more difficult than ultrasound to perform in children.

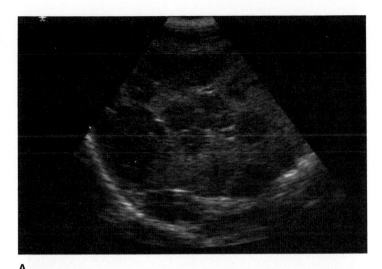

A

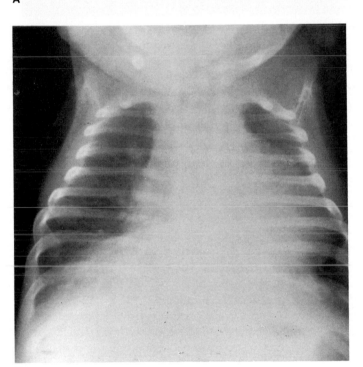

B

Fig. 9 Haemangioendotheliomas. A: Ultrasound scan of the liver showing multiple clearly defined areas of reduced reflectivity in this child who presented with high output heart failure. **B:** Chest radiograph shows the cardiac enlargement.

Rarely, a true arteriovenous malformation occurs within the liver and is seen on ultrasound as numerous echo-poor tubular structures with little or no solid, reflective component. Doppler examination demonstrates blood flow through these channels, with enlarged draining veins.

The management of benign vascular liver tumours depends upon their number, size and on the clinical presentation. If the lesion is small (often an incidental finding), only observation is required as spontaneous regression

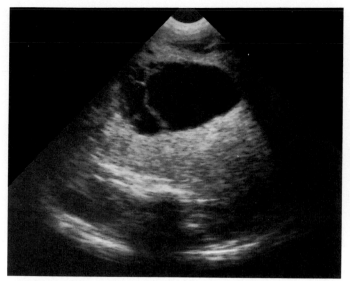

Fig. 10   Mesenchymal hamartoma. Scan of the right lobe of the liver shows a septated cyst.

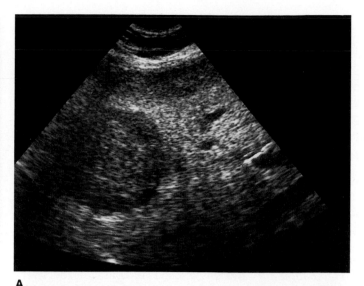

A

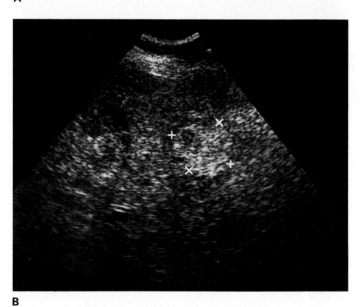

B

Fig. 11   Adenomas in glycogen storage disease type I. A: A 5 cm diameter poorly reflective lesion and **B:** a 3 cm diameter highly reflective lesion in the same patient. Additional lesions of mixed echo patterns were also present.

is usual. Surgical excision may be an option in patients with cardiac failure or thrombocytopenia if the lesion is solitary and confined to one lobe. However, when multiple lesions are present, surgery is not possible. Steroid therapy may be useful and hepatic artery embolisation has been used with some success. Occasionally the diagnosis of a malignant tumour cannot be excluded and surgical excision is required to make a histological diagnosis.

Mesenchymal hamartoma   Mesenchymal hamartoma is a well-defined large liver tumour which usually presents in the first 2 years of life and is slightly more common in males.[18] Ultrasound demonstrates a large, discrete, solitary mass which is predominantly cystic with numerous septa (Fig. 10). Typically the lesion is located in the right lobe of the liver. Patients usually present with a large abdominal mass and most patients are otherwise asymptomatic. Treatment is by surgical excision and the prognosis is good.

Focal nodular hyperplasia   This lesion is rare in childhood and the diagnosis may not be made until surgical excision and histological examination. Ultrasound demonstrates a mass of variable reflectivity supplied by a large hepatic artery best evaluated with Doppler. Radio-isotope imaging is especially useful since the Kupffer cells in the lesion take up colloid and the lesion therefore shows normal or increased uptake. The combination of the ultrasound and isotope features are pathognomonic for focal nodular hyperplasia. CT scanning with intravenous contrast demonstrates uniform, intense enhancement of the lesion, with a central stellate scar.

Hepatic adenoma   Hepatic adenomas are also uncommon in childhood. There is an increased incidence in children with glycogen storage disease (particularly type I) and glucose-6-phosphatase deficiency: in these cases mul-

tiple lesions occur.[19] Hepatic adenomas may also develop in children with aplastic anaemia treated with androgenic steroids: in these patients regular screening with ultrasound should be performed. Well-defined masses which may be more or less reflective than the liver are seen (Fig. 11). If multiple lesions are present, these may vary in reflectivity within the same patient. Lesions are usually followed by serial ultrasound examinations because malignant change has been reported although it is rare, and further investigation or surgery is indicated if the lesion grows rapidly or the serum alpha-fetoprotein rises.

Inflammatory hepatic masses

Hepatic abscesses are uncommon in childhood but are not usually mistaken for tumour because of the typical presentation with fever and signs of infection. They may complicate septicaemia or follow surgery or trauma, when a haematoma becomes infected. In neonates, an umbilical vein catheter or necrotising enterocolitis also predispose to the development of an hepatic abscess. The infective organisms are usually *Staphylococcus* or *E. coli*.

The diagnosis is easily made with ultrasound which, in the early stages, demonstrates a poorly defined echo-poor solid lesion (Fig. 12). Following the formation of pus, the lesion becomes more clearly defined and contains poorly reflective material. Gas in the abscess cavity results in intense echoes. The diagnosis of an hepatic abscess is confirmed by needle aspiration of the pus for bacteriological culture and treatment with percutaneous drainage under ultrasound guidance may be appropriate.

Hepatic abscesses also occur in patients who are immunocompromised or immunodeficient; in this situation they are often multiple. Children with leukaemia treated with chemotherapy are prone to candidiasis and may develop hepatosplenic fungal abscesses. In the early stages, ultrasound is unhelpful and demonstrates only hepatosplenomegaly with a non-specific increase in parenchymal reflectivity. A normal scan does not exclude the possibility of hepatic candida. However, as the lesions progress, multiple small echo-poor foci, typically with reflective centres, are seen (Fig. 13).[20] These lesions can

also be demonstrated with CT and their nature confirmed by biopsy.

Hepatomegaly in children with immune deficiency syndrome is usually due to infective hepatitis or abscess formation. There is also an association with sclerosing cholangitis.[21] Bile duct dilatation and immunodeficiency in children are seen in chronic granulomatous disease. Ultrasound is reliable in the demonstration of hepatic abscesses, hepatomegaly and bile duct dilatation.

Multiple hepatic abscesses may occur in chronic granulomatous disease of childhood (histoplasmosis, tuberculosis); in the chronic phase calcified granulomata form

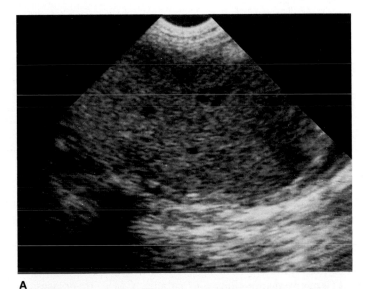

A

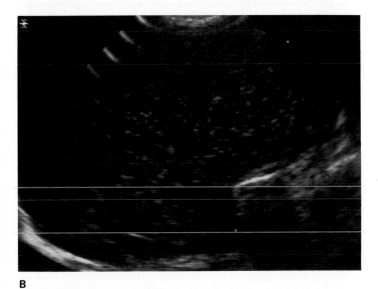

B

Fig. 13   Candida. A: The liver scan in this child on treatment for acute myeloid leukaemia shows a typical echo-poor lesion of disseminated candidiasis. **B:** An additional leukaemic patient with the more typical generalised involvement.

Fig. 12   Abscess. There is a large poorly reflective and heterogeneous mass with good through transmission in this 8-year-old child presenting with a fever and a clinically enlarged liver.

that can be detected with ultrasound as multiple punctate reflective foci.

Hepatomegaly and splenomegaly may be seen in the neonate with congenital infections with rubella, toxoplasmosis, cytomegalovirus, herpes and syphilis. Clotting problems and liver failure with ascites may be present. Calcified foci within the liver may be seen in congenital herpes, toxoplasmosis and cytomegalovirus. Parasitic liver infestations may also occur in children. The ultrasound appearances of infection with amoeba, liver flukes and hydatid cysts have been described.

Splenomegaly

Splenomegaly has a myriad of causes and is often associated with hepatomegaly.

Causes of splenomegaly:

Chronic hepatic diseases
Lymphoma
Leukaemia
Viral infections
Collagen vascular disorders e.g. rheumatoid arthritis
Chronic granulomatous disease
Parasitic infections
Haemolytic anaemias
Gaucher's disease
Glycogen storage disease types III (rarely), IV, and VI (occasionally)
Mucopolysaccharidoses
Mucolipidoses
Congenital infections e.g. rubella, CMV, toxoplasmosis
Felty's syndrome.

The liver must always be scanned and Doppler studies of the splenic vessels made if portal hypertension is suspected. Here the spleen becomes more reflective (because of fibrosis) and the portal blood may flow towards the spleen in extreme cases. Enlargement from infiltration with lymphoma or leukaemia may be quite dramatic with relatively normal parenchymal reflectivity or focal echo-poor areas. Splenic enlargement accompanies viral illnesses and is also seen in immunosuppressed patients with systemic candida infection. As in the liver, when the candida abscesses are large enough to be visualised (about 2 mm), small echo-poor foci are seen throughout the enlarged spleen.

Splenic calcification

Small focal splenic calcifications are often an incidental finding and a cause is not found. Calcified granulomata within the spleen are seen in chronic granulomatous disease of childhood (defective leucocyte function), tuberculosis and histoplasmosis.

Splenic masses

Splenic masses are rare in childhood; they may be cystic or solid; those caused by the parasite *Taenia echinococcus* (hydatid disease) account for over two thirds of cases world-wide. Pseudocysts following trauma, haemorrhage or infarction account for a few cases, and congenital epidermoid cysts occasionally present in children.

Lymphangioma of the spleen may be imaged as a single or multiple 'cysts' when the spaces are large enough to be resolved separately but the multiple minute cysts that may form can simply produce an enlarged reflective spleen.

Splenic abscesses can be of mixed or low reflectivity. Splenic infarcts can have a similar appearance and both are often multifocal so that it may be difficult to differentiate between the two. Patients with splenic abscesses often have a predisposing cause for the infection, such as immunosuppression, polycythaemia with cardiac disease or endocarditis.

Trauma

The liver and spleen may be injured in blunt abdominal trauma, often accompanied by damage to other abdominal organs. Elevation of the serum liver enzymes suggests that the liver has been injured. If trauma has been severe and the patient is unwell, CT scanning is preferred as it is more reliable than ultrasound in demonstrating injury to the liver, spleen, pancreas and kidneys. However, if a CT scanner is not easily available and the child's condition is not critical, abdominal ultrasound is useful.

Examination with ultrasound in a case of suspected hepatic injury should be thorough and include a search for

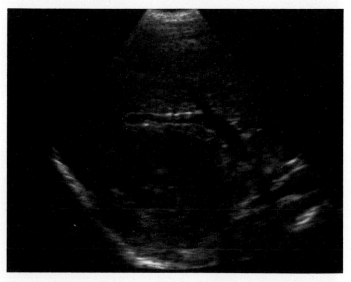

Fig. 14 Trauma. There is an ill-defined haematoma in the right lobe of the liver in this patient who had been subjected to blunt upper abdominal trauma.

free intraperitoneal fluid, examination of the whole liver and a search for injury of other abdominal organs. Free fluid is most common with pancreatic trauma but is also seen in hepatic injury. Lacerations and haematomas in the liver and spleen may be echo-poor (Fig. 14) or of increased reflectivity. Injury to the dome or the lateral segment of the left lobe of the liver is easily missed, particularly if an associated ileus and abdominal pain make the ultrasound scan difficult. Subcapsular collections of blood should be looked for along the borders of the liver and spleen.

Diaphragmatic rupture appears as a discontinuous line on ultrasound scans.

Ultrasound may be particularly useful in the examination of the sick neonate whose clinical condition is too unstable to permit transport to the CT scanner but who may have hepatic haematoma following sepsis, asphyxia, traumatic delivery or resuscitative efforts. The neonate has a falling haematocrit with increasing abdominal distension, and the diagnosis may be confirmed with ultrasound.

REFERENCES

1 Dittrich M, Milde S, Dinkel E, et al. Sonographic biometry of liver and spleen size in childhood. Pediatr Radiol 1983; 13: 206–201

2 Markisz J A, Treves S T, Davis R T. Normal hepatic and splenic size in children: scintigraphic determination. Pediatr Radiol 1987; 17: 273–276

3 Rosenberg H K, Markowitz R I, Kolberg H, et al. Normal splenic size in infants and children: sonographic measurements. AJR 1991; 157: 119–121

4 Hernan Z, Schulman M, Ambrosins M M, et al. Current evaluation of the patient with abnormal visceroatinal situs. AJR 1990; 154: 797–802

5 Mandell G A, Heyman S, Alavi A, et al. A case of microgastria in association with splenic gonadal fusion. Pediatr Radiol 1983; 13: 95–98

6 Setiawan H, Harrell R S, Peiret R S. Ectopic spleen: a sonographic diagnosis. Pediatr Radiol 1982; 12: 152–153

7 Younger K A, Hall C M. Epidermoid cyst of the spleen: a case report and review of the literature. Br J Radiol 1990; 63: 652–653

8 Henschke C I, Goldman H, Teele R L. The hyperechogenic liver in children: cause and sonographic appearance. AJR 1982; 138: 841–846

9 Frider B, Marin A M, Goldberg A. Ultrasonographic diagnosis of portal vein cavernous transformation in children. J Ultrasound Med 1989; 8: 445–449

10 Patriquin H, Tessier G, Grignon A, et al. Lesser omental thickness in normal children. Baseline for detection of portal hypertension. AJR 1985; 145: 693–696

11 Hoffman H D, Stockland B, von der Hayden U. Membranous

obstruction of the inferior vena cava with Budd–Chiari syndrome in children: a report of nine cases. J Pediatr Gastroenterol Nutr 1987; 6: 878–884

12 Boechat M A, Kangarloo H, Gilsanz V. Hepatic masses in children. Semin Roentgenol 1988; 23: 185–193

13 Miller J H, Greenspan B S. Integrated imaging of hepatic tumours in childhood. Part I. Radiology 1985; 154: 83–90

14 Brunelle F, Chaumont P. Hepatic tumors in children: ultrasonic differentiation of malignant from benign lesions. Radiology 1984; 150: 695–699

15 Miller J H, Greenspan B S. Integrated imaging of hepatic tumors in childhood. Part II. Radiology 1985; 154: 91–100

16 Stanley P, Geer G D, Miller J H, et al. Infantile hepatic hemangiomas. Clinical features, radiologic investigations and treatment of 20 patients. Cancer 1989; 64: 936–949

17 Braum P, Ducharme J C, Riopelle J L, et al. Hemangiomatosis of the liver in infants. J Pediatr Surg 1975; 10: 121–126

18 Stanley P, Hall T R, Wooley M M, et al. Mesenchymal hamartomas of the liver in childhood: sonographic and CT findings. AJR 1986; 147: 1035–1039

19 Brunelle F, Tammam S, Odievre M, et al. Liver adenomas in glycogen storage disease in childhood. Ultrasound and angiographic study. Pediatr Radiol 1984; 14: 94–101

20 Pastakia B, Shawker T H, Thaler M, et al. Hepatosplenic candidiasis: wheels within wheels. Radiology 1988; 166: 417–421

21 Garel L A, Pariente D M, Nezelof C, et al. Liver involvement in chronic granulomatous disease: the role of ultrasound in diagnosis and treatment. Radiology 1984; 153: 117–121

Index

Page numbers in **bold type** indicate main discussions; those in *italics* indicate figures. Abbreviations: TRUS: transrectal ultrasound; u.s.: ultrasound